# MODERN TRENDS
## IN
# ENVIRONMENTAL
# BIOLOGY

# MODERN TRENDS
## IN
# ENVIRONMENTAL
# BIOLOGY

*Edited by*

## Dr. G. Tripathi

Ph.D.
Associate Professor, Department of Zoology,
J.N.V. University, Jodhpur

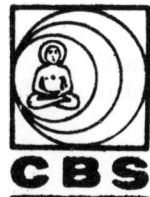

## CBS PUBLISHERS & DISTRIBUTORS
4596/1-A, 11 Darya Ganj, New Delhi - 110 002 (India)

ISBN : 81-239-0798-2

First Edition : 2002

*Published by :*
Satish Kumar Jain for CBS Publishers & Distributors,
4596/1A, 11 Darya Ganj, New Delhi - 110002 (India)

*Production Director :* Vinod Jain

*Printed at :*
Asia Printograph, Shahdara, Delhi - 110 032

# Preface

Life has had an important role in the shaping the environmental evolution of planet earth. The earth has experienced and recovered from many natural disasters in the past. But irresponsible human activities are causing irreparable losses and disturbing the peace of biosphere to a great extent. In fact, living planet is at risk. Now the question is either to stabilize the planet or perish. The current population explosion, the resultant mismanagement of environment and its natural resources may bring grave environmental, economic and human crises in the present millennium. Environmental pollution has become a growing threat to mankind all over the world. Various unplanned activities have altered the man-nature relationship. They have changed not only the economic and sociocultural life of the people but also their values, systems, ideas, beliefs and lifestyle. It is a critical point for scientists facing greater responsibility to highlight the modern emerging trends in the area of environmental biology for future perspective and accomplishment. Therefore, "Modern Trends in Environmental Biology" has been compiled to project the topics of current interest for higher level students, academicians and other professionals.

In the past decade, spectacular advances have been made in various areas of biological and agricultural sciences. However, in contrast, no serious attention has been paid to educate people and save environmental health in order to provide a clean and peaceful biosphere for the coming generations. Each and every person should learn how to live on the living planet and preserve, conserve and promote the global environment for future. Learning environmental biology has become the demand of the day irrespective of subjects offered by students. Educational and research institutions have gradually begun to realize the problem and started incorporating environmental biology courses in various curricula. This book is intended for use by postgraduate and research students, as well as, teachers and research scientists in academic institutions and industries. It is expected to be equally useful to environmental engineers and lawyers. Professionals will find that this book can lead to a better understanding of how various areas of biosciences integrate into harmonious ensemble for human welfare. People in public life, administration, legal system and business will learn much of what they need to know to make wise decisions and take appropriate actions on issues that will effect the environmental stability of the globe. In addition, casual lay readers will learn quite a bit about current environmental problems and their possible remedies. In fact, Modern Trends in Environmental Biology is a multipurpose book in the sense that it can benefit a wide variety of people in different walks of life.

I am grateful to all contributors who could spare their valuable time in writing various important and interesting chapters. I am indebted to Prof. Janardan Singh, Department of Entomology & Agricultural Zoology, BHU, Varanasi for his help bestowed upon me from time to time. I am highly grateful to Dr. Manju Sharma, Secretary, DST, New Delhi and Dr. P.S. Pathak, ADG, ICAR, New Delhi, for their moral support and inspiration. I wish to acknowledge the support extended by Prof. S.C. Tiwari, Department of Zoology, University of Allahabad, Allahabad; Dr. N.S. Shekhawat, Department of Botany, JNV University, Jodhpur; Dr. Y.C. Tripathi, AFRI, Jodhpur; Dr. P. Nath, Department of Entomology, BHU, Varanasi; Dr. G.C. Pandey, Department of Environmental Sciences, Dr. R.M.L. Avadh University, Faizabad; Dr. Y.K. Jaiswal, School of Studies in Biochemistry, Jiwaji University, Gwalior; Dr. P.C. Path,

School of Life Sciences, JNU, New Delhi; Dr. P.R. Yadav, DAV College, Muzaffarnagar and Dr. M. Mishra, MLK College, Balrampur. I would like to thank all my laboratory members Miss P. Verma, Miss P. Bhardwaj and Mr. S.S. Suthar for their valuable assistance. Lastly, I wish to express my grateful thanks to CBS Publishers & Distributors for publishing this important compilation.

G. Tripathi

# List of Contributors

M. Agrawal
*Department of Botany, Banaras Hindu University,
Varanasi - 221005*

S.K. Bahera
*School of Studies in Zoology, Jiwaji University,
Gwalior - 474011*

R. Chandra
*Industrial Toxicity Research Centre, M.G. Marg,
Lucknow - 226001*

N.K. Chaubey
*Law School, Banaras Hindu University,
Varanasi - 221005*

N.J. Chinoy
*Department of Zoology, Gujarat University,
Ahmedabad - 380009*

A.A.K. Dosani
*Konkan Krishi Vidyapeeth, Dapoli,
Ratnagiri - 415712*

S.N. Dube
*Defence Research and Development Establishment,
Jhansi Road, Gwalior - 474002*

S.J.S. Flora
*Defence Research and Development Establishment,
Jhansi Road, Gwalior - 474002*

T.K. Ghosh
*National Environmental Engineering Research
Institute (NEERI), Nagpur - 440020*

P.K. Goel
*Department of Pollution Studies, Y.C. College of
Science, Vidyanagar, Karad - 415124*

B.B. Hosetti
*P.G. Department of Applied Zoology, Kuvempu
University, B.R. Project, Shimoga - 577115*

M. Idris
*Central Arid Zone Research Institute,
Jodhpur - 342003*

F. Kolling
*Mitteilung, Deutsche Gesellschaft fur Technische
Zusammenarbeit (GTZ) GmbH, P3U,
Wachsbleiche 1, 53111 Bonn, Germany*

S. Kumar
*Department of Biosciences, Barkatullah University,
Bhopal - 462026*

S.K. Misra
*Industrial Toxicity Research Centre, M.G. Marg,
Lucknow - 226001*

K.L. Naik
*P.G. Department of Applied Zoology, Kuvempu
University, B.R. Project, Shimoga - 577115*

S.R. Naik
*Department of Gastroenterology, Sanjay Gandhi
Postgraduate Institute of Medical Sciences,
Lucknow - 226014*

T.C. Narendran
*Department of Zoology, University of Calicut,
Calicut - 673635*

A.S. Ninawe
*Department of Biotechnology, Block 2 (7th floor),
CGO Complex, Lodhi Road, New Delhi - 110003*

D.D. Ozha
*Chief Engineer Office, Ground Water Department,
New Power House Road, Jodhpur - 342003*

J. Pandey
*Department of Environmental Sciences,
M.L. Sukhadia University, Udaipur - 313001*

R.K. Pandit
*School of Studies in Zoology, Jiwaji University,
Gwalior - 474011*

M. Parveen
*Department of Biosciences, Barkatullah University,
Bhopal - 462026*

A.G. Powar
*Konkan Krishi Vidyapeeth, Dapoli,*
*Ratnagiri - 415712*

B.D. Rana
*Central Arid Zone Research Institute,*
*Jodhpur - 342003*

R.J. Rao
*School of Studies in Zoology, Jiwaji University,*
*Gwalior - 474011*

B.K. Sahu
*School of Studies in Zoology, Jiwaji University,*
*Gwalior - 474011*

B.M. Sharma
*Department of Zoology, J.N.V. University,*
*Jodhpur - 342001*

K.L. Shrivastava
*Department of Geology, J.N.V. University,*
*Jodhpur - 342005*

B. Singh
*Department of Botany, Banaras Hindu University,*
*Varanasi - 221005*

R.S. Singh
*Central Arid Zone Research Institute,*
*Jodhpur - 342003*

S.S. Suthar
*Department of Zoology, J.N.V. University,*
*Jodhpur - 342001*

S.C. Talashilkar
*Konkan Krishi Vidyapeeth, Dapoli,*
*Ratnagiri - 415712*

S.K. Tandon
*Industrial Toxicology Research Centre,*
*Lucknow*

G. Tripathi
*Department of Zoology, J.N.V. University,*
*Jodhpur - 342001*

K.M. Tripathi
*Law School, Banaras Hindu University,*
*Varanasi - 221005*

R.S. Tripathi
*Central Arid Zone Research Institute,*
*Jodhpur - 342003*

V. Tripathi
*Department of Animal Science, M.J.P. Rohilkhand*
*University, Bareilly - 243006*

Y.C. Tripathi
*Arid Forest Research Institute,*
*Jodhpur - 342005*

M. Venkateshwarlu
*P.G. Department of Applied Zoology, Kuvempu*
*University, B.R. Project, Shimoga - 577115*

P. Verma
*Department of Zoology, J.N.V. University,*
*Jodhpur - 342001*

P.R. Yadav
*Department of Zoology, DAV College,*
*Muzaffarnagar - 251001*

R.S. Yadav
*Department of Botany, DAV College,*
*Muzaffarnagar - 251001*

# Contents

# Environmental Contamination and Human Health Risks

*P. K. Goel*

Environment, in a broader sense, is referred to as the totality of the surroundings which can influence the human beings in diverse ways. It includes both the livings and nonlivings like air, water, land, plants, animals and even microorganisms (Fig.1.1). Any change in the composition of the environment

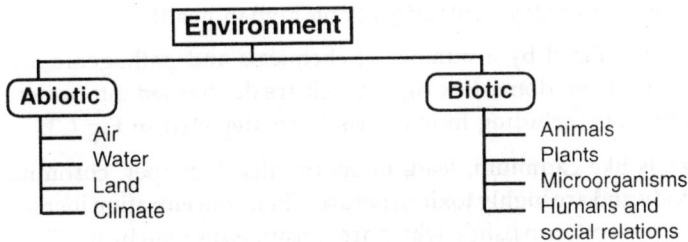

**Fig. 1.1:** Components of environment.

which directly or indirectly affects the Man is considered pollution. For example, addition of various harmful gases like sulphur dioxide, carbon monoxide, hydrocarbons and particulates will cause air pollution; while the contamination of water by organic matter, heavy metals, pesticides and pathogenic microorganisms will cause water pollution. Even the open dumps of solid wastes, noise and radiation can cause pollution of environment. The increasing use of different chemicals in our day to day life has resulted in overall degradation of human life. Sometimes, the accidental release or overdoses of chemicals, which are otherwise safe in usual concentrations, can result in deaths or acute effects on health.

Pollution can be caused by discharge of the pollutants in environment by natural or Man-made activities. Industrialization, agriculture, automobiles, growth of human population and destruction of natural resources are some important factors responsible for increasing pollution in recent days (Fig. 1.2).

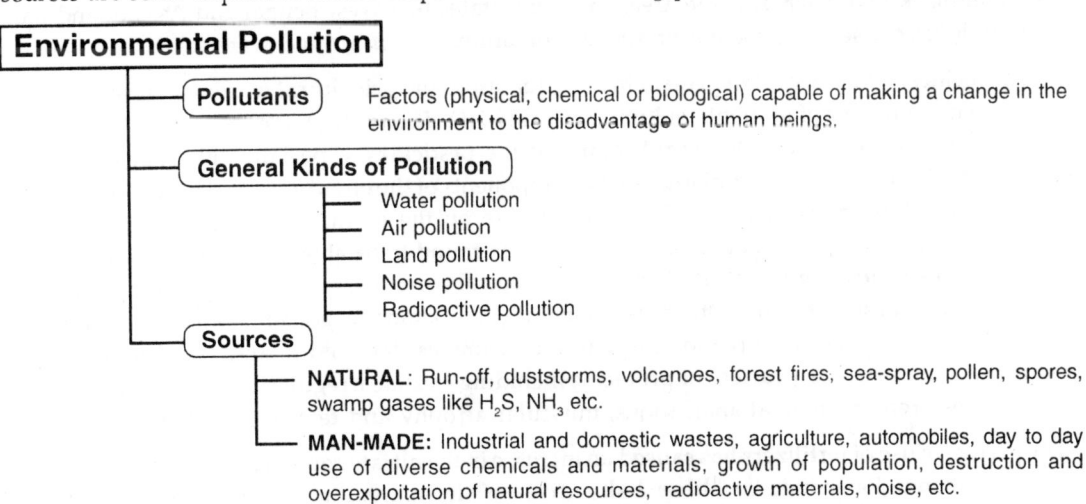

**Fig. 1.2 :** Environmental pollution, its types and sources.

Man, for his existence on the earth, has exploited nature in various ways to his own benefit. He has not only extracted materials from the nature, but also made a variety of synthetic chemicals which were unknown earlier. Many of these chemicals like pesticides and plastics do not degrade in the environment, but go on accumulating and finally contaminating the whole environment. Majority of the synthetic chemicals are highly toxic in nature. The increasing pollution of the environment has made the life of mankind miserable on this planet. The increasing incidents of waterborne diseases, sterility, cancer, heart troubles and many other ailments can be directly related to the environmental pollution.

The following text describes some of the important effects of different kinds of environmental pollutants and common everyday contaminants on human health.

Water pollution is caused by a number of chemicals and pathogenic organisms present in the wastewaters of industrial and domestic origin which are discharged into water resources. The general effects of water pollutants including human health are depicted in Fig.1.3.

The heavy metals like cadmium, lead, mercury, nickel, copper, chromium and arsenic tend to accumulate in the body and are highly toxic in nature. Their concentration increases through food chains in water, reaching highest often in fishes, which are consumed as food by us. The mercury contamination of the Minamata Bay in Japan in 1960s has caused a large number of deaths of the people in that area. The mercury discharged by a factory was accumulated by fish and shellfish from where it reached to Man through food. It caused damage to the central nervous system resulting in death of many. Similarly, cadmium contaminated food and water in Itai Itai village of Japan has caused microfractures of bone of people, ultimately resulting in death. The cadmium has also been reported to cause cancer of prostrate. The mercury and cadmium poisoning are since popularly called Minamata and Itai diseases respectively.

The lead poisoning in humans can result in damage to nervous system and kidney. In mild cases lead can result in insomnia, restlessness, loss of appetite and gastrointestinal troubles. The symptoms of lead poisoning are called plumbism. Chromium may result in skin and respiratory disorders. Chromium is often present in the tannery effluents. Arsenic causes skin cancer, hyper-pigmentation, keratosis and black foot disease. Some areas in Indian states like West Bengal and Assam, and parts of Bangladesh have a severe problem of arsenic contamination of ground waters.

The pesticides, which are often present in high quantities in agricultural wastewaters and sewage, also cause a large number of ailments in humans (Table 1.1). Today, we have more than 10,000 kinds of pesticides produced all over the world. Many of the pesticides, especially chlorinated ones, are nonbiodegradable and go on accumulating in the components of the environment. The use of pesticides has so increased these days, that practically all the life on the earth have some quantity of these accumulated in their flesh. DDT, on an average has been found to be about 12 ppm in an Indian. The DDT group of pesticides more often affect primarily central nervous system. These can cause tremors and incoordination in severe cases. Other effects include liver damage, gonadal and endocrine effects. Other groups of pesticides like, organophosphates, carbamates, rotenoides, and pyrethroids are also quite harmful and can cause a variety of problems including cardiac irregularity, diarrhoea, vomiting, muscle seizures, tremors, mental aberrations, muscular atrophy and teratogenic effects.

The excessive use of fertilizers has caused an increase in the nitrate content of ground waters which can cause methamoglobenemia or "**blue baby disease**" in infants, in which the oxygen-carrying capacity of blood is reduced due to formation of a complex between haemoglobin and nitrate. In India, the disease is quite prevalent in certain parts of Rajasthan and has been found even to occur in adults.

## WATER POLLUTION

**1. Heavy metals**
- *Lead:* Anaemia, disruption of haemoglobin synthesis, damage to nervous system, kidneys and brain, insomnia, restlessness, loss of appetite, lethal dose - 300-700 mg/kg.
- *Mercury:* Brain damage (Minamata disease)
- Cadmium: Disorders of respiratory system, kidneys and lungs; cramps, nausea; vomiting, diarrhoea, micro-fractures of bone (Itai-Itai disease), general decline in health
- *Chromium:* Skin and respiratory disorders, ulceration of skin etc.
- *Arsenic:* Skin cancer, hyper-pigmentation, keratosis, black foot disease

**2. Pesticides**
- Affect central nervous system, Mental aberrations
- Tremors and incoordination in severe cases
- Damage to liver
- Effects on gonads and endocrine system
- Cardiac irregularity and convulsions
- Diarrhoea and vomiting
- Muscle seizure, Muscular atrophy
- Teratogenic effects

**3. Toxic organics**
- Polycyclic aromatic hydrocarbons (PAHs) cause cancers.
- Plastics and plasticizers are extremely toxic
- Dioxins, PCBs, detergents etc. cause disruption of ecosystems; toxic but effects on Man not much known

**4. Toxic inorganics**
- *Cyanide:* Respiratory poison
- *Fluoride:* Bone and dental disorders
- $H_2S$, $NH_3$ in water: Extremely toxic to life

**5. Decomposable organic matter**
- Affects oxygen balance in water
- Determines the biotic structure of water bodies
- Increase in bacterial content of waters

**6. Nutrients (like N & P)**
- Cause eutrophication (Excessive growth of algae)
- Nitrate ($NO_3$) cause methamoglobenemia (Blue baby disease)

**7. Pathogens (Bacteria, viruses, protozoa, worms etc.)**
- Spread of waterborne diseases

**Fig. 1.3 :** Human health and other implications of water pollutants.

### Table 1.1 : Human toxic responses to the major groups of pesticides

| Groups | Effects |
|---|---|
| 1. Naturally occurring organics (Rotenoides, Pyrethroides, Nicotine, Alkaloides | Rotenoids and pyrethroids have usually low toxicity, but kidney and respiratory effects in severe cases. Nicotine compounds highly toxic with convulsions, cardiac irregularity and coma in severe cases. |
| 2. Chlorinated Hydrocarbons | Low to moderate acute toxicity, affect mostly central nervous system (CNS), tremors and incoordination in severe cases, lipid buildup. Heptachlor, aldrin, and dieldrin show CNS disturbance and parasympathetic failures. Other effects include liver damage and gonadal and endocrine effects. |
| 3. Organophosphates | Extremely toxic, absorbed through all routes of entry, symptoms include parasympathetic failures, diarrhoea and vomiting, tremors and muscle seizures, mental aberrations in chronic exposure due to suppression of cholinesterase. Unusually hazardous on direct exposure. Guthion and malathion least toxic of all. |
| 4. Carbamates | Normal dimethyl carbamates are strong inhibitors of cholinesterase. Other actions and symptoms are like organophosphates. |
| 5. Mercurials | Organic mercury, particularly alkyl-Hg is more toxic than inorg.-Hg. Stored in living tissues as methyl-Hg. CNS symptoms appear first (incoordination, parathesias, tremors) followed by muscular atrophy and mental instability. |
| 6. Herbicides | Acute toxicity to Man is low. Chlorophenoxy compounds (2,4-D; 2,4,5-T) produce a mild irritation on exposed areas. Gastro-intestinal effects when taken internally. 2,4,5-T teratogenic on chronic exposure. |
| 7. Rodenticides | Common rodenticides are not chemically related, therefore, have no common symptoms. Sodium fluoroacetate is extremely toxic and disturbs citric acid metabolism with resulting cardiac depression, fibrillation and peripheral nervous system effects. Cyanide (as NaCN in "coyotegetters") is extremely toxic producing respiratory system failure. Strychnine affects all parts of CNS resulting in asphyxia and dyspnea. There are no antidotes for mammal poisons. |

Much of the common water pollution problems occur due to contamination of the water resources by sewage. This often causes the spread of water-borne diseases such as cholera, bacillary dysentery, typhoid and paratyphoid fevers, infantile diarrhoea, leptospirosis, tularaemia, botulism, gastroenteritis, jaundice, colitis and infestation of intestine by various worms. Some common pathogens and diseases caused by them are given in Table 1.2. The jaundice and typhoid are quite prevalent diseases among the populations where the sanitary conditions are poor. India frequently witnesses epidemics of waterborne diseases, however, the most severe were the jaundice epidemics at Delhi and Karad (Maharashtra) where thousands of people have suffered and many died.

### Table 1.2 : Some important water-borne pathogenic organisms/parasites and diseases "caused by them"

| Organisms | Diseases |
|---|---|
| Vibrio cholerae | Cholera |
| Shigella spp. | Bacillary dysentry |
| Salmonella typhi | Typhoid |
| Salmonella paratyphi | Paratyphoid fever |
| Escherichia coli | Infantile diarrhoea |
| Leptospira spp. | Leptospirosis |
| Pasteurella (Brucella or Francisella) tularensis | Tularaemia |
| Clostridium botulinum | Botulism |
| Other Salmonella and Shigella spp., Proteus spp. | Gastroenteritis |
| Hepatitis virus | Jaundice (infective hepatitis) |
| Poliomyelitis virus | Polio |
| Ascaris and other worms | Intestinal infestation |
| Entamoeba histolytica | Intestinal colitis and amoebiasis |

## Air Pollution

The respiratory system (Fig.1.4) and the eye are common targets of air pollution. The eye often gets

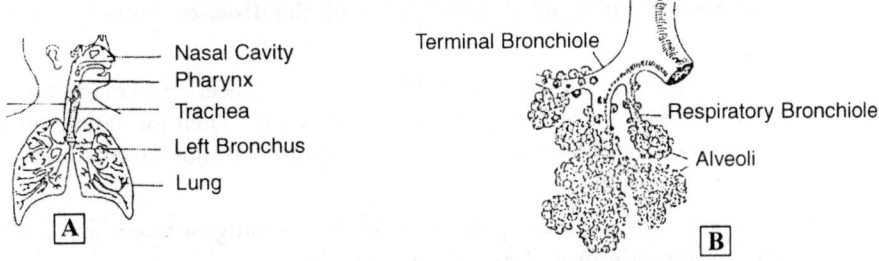

Fig. 1.4 : (A) Respiratory tract of humans. (B) Bronchioles and alveoli of lung.

irritation and tearing in the polluted conditions, especially in high traffic areas. Chronic bronchitis, pulmonary emphysema, lung cancer, bronchial asthma, pulmonary oedema, silicosis and asbestosis are common diseases of the respiratory tract which can be caused by air pollution.The bronchi have a lining of cilia which beat in the opposite direction to push the secreted mucus upwards  into the mouth. The usual function of  the mucus is to entrap the particles which have been inhaled into the bronchi. Air pollutants can cause a progressive degeneration of cilia which reduces the mucus expulsion capacity leading to its excess accumulation in the bronchi from where it can move into the lungs (Fig.1.5).

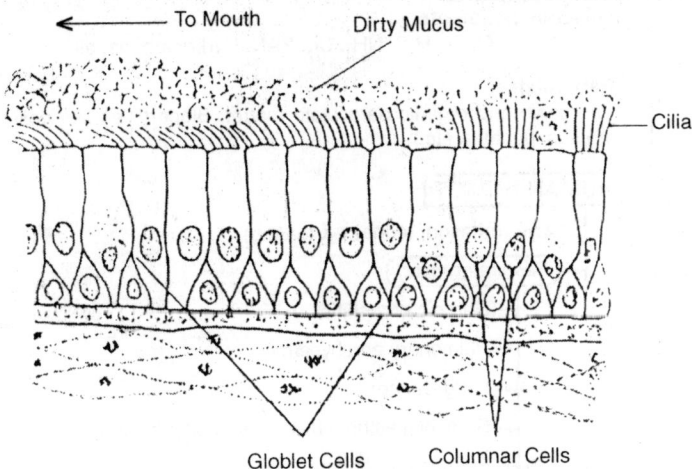

Fig. 1.5 : Expulsion of mucus with impacted particles by the activity of cilia in bronchus.

The chronic bronchitis is characterised by the persistent production of cough. The breathing is hampered by bronchial congestion and fluid, often leading to the production of a bubbling sound as the air passes through this fluid. Over 30,000 people have been killed by chronic bronchitis in 1950 in England and Wales due to particulate and sulphur dioxide pollution. Pulmonary emphysema is the condition of progressive breakdown of alveoli (air sacs) of lungs leading to the joining of many small air sacs into one large volume.

Bronchial asthma is the narrowing of respiratory passage leading to difficulty in breathing. Pulmonary oedema is the condition where excess fluid is accumulated in lungs. Pulmonary fibrosis is toughening of the lung tissues. Pneumoconiosis is inflammation of lung tissues caused by retention of foreign particles. If the foreign particles are silica the disease carries the specific name called silicosis, and if the particles are asbestos, it is called asbestosis. Both the diseases, however, commonly occur as occupational diseases.

Air pollution also promotes certain kinds of skin and lung cancer. However, the lung cancer is by far the most common type of cancers induced by air pollution. When the cancerous tissue breaks after enlargement, it spreads throughout the body, moving rapidly through lymphatic system and blood stream to spread the cancer to other parts of the body.

Benzo(a)pyrene, a common pollutant produced during burning of materials, is a carcinogenic substance encountered commonly in polluted air.

Carbon monoxide is produced in large quantities from automobiles and other combustion activities which affects the oxygen carrying capacity of blood due to its combination with haemoglobin. The effects of carbon monoxide on human body are given in Table 1.3. Pollution checks in automobiles are mainly carried out for the concentration of carbon monoxide in the exhaust. Its concentration should not be more than 3.0 to 4.5% by volume in the exhaust. The components of auto-exhaust react among themselves and oxygen in the air in presence of sunlight to form several oxidants like ozone, peroxy acetyl nitrate (PAN) and free radicals which often lead to the accelerated ageing in humans. Some common ailments caused by air pollutants are given in Fig.1.6.

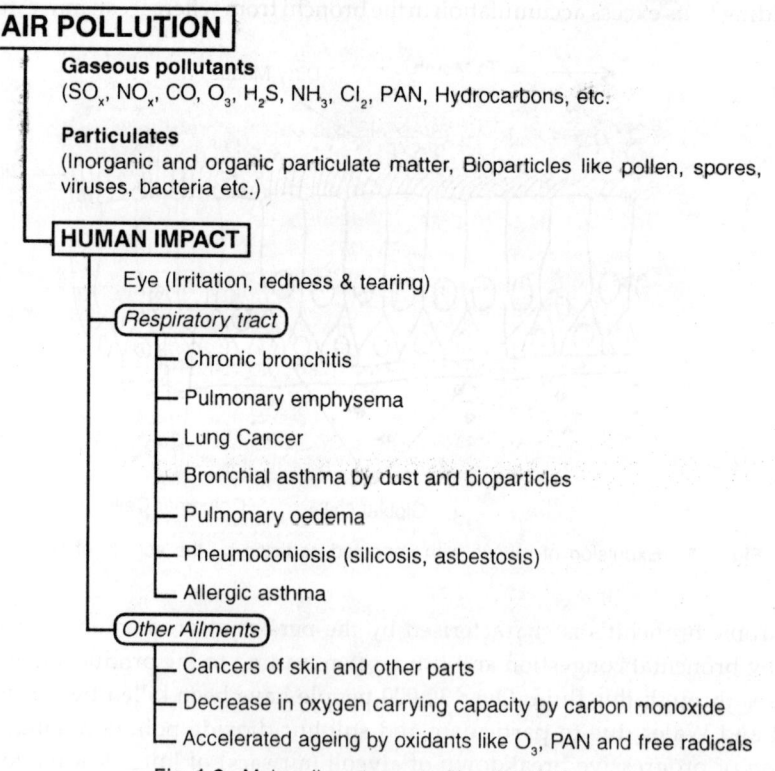

**AIR POLLUTION**

**Gaseous pollutants**
($SO_x$, $NO_x$, CO, $O_3$, $H_2S$, $NH_3$, $Cl_2$, PAN, Hydrocarbons, etc.

**Particulates**
(Inorganic and organic particulate matter, Bioparticles like pollen, spores, viruses, bacteria etc.)

**HUMAN IMPACT**

Eye (Irritation, redness & tearing)

*Respiratory tract*
— Chronic bronchitis
— Pulmonary emphysema
— Lung Cancer
— Bronchial asthma by dust and bioparticles
— Pulmonary oedema
— Pneumoconiosis (silicosis, asbestosis)
— Allergic asthma

*Other Ailments*
— Cancers of skin and other parts
— Decrease in oxygen carrying capacity by carbon monoxide
— Accelerated ageing by oxidants like $O_3$, PAN and free radicals

**Fig. 1.6** : Major ailments caused by air pollution.

**Table 1.3 : Health effect of COHb blood levels (combination of CO + haemoglobin)**

| COHb blood levels % | Demonstrated effect |
| --- | --- |
| Less than 1.0 | No apparent effect. |
| 1.0 to 2.0 | Some evidence of effect on behavioural performance. |
| 2.0 to 5.0 | Central nervous system is affected. Impairment of time interval discrimination and certain other psychomoter functions. |
| Greater than 5.0, 10.0 to 80.00 | Cardiac and pulmonary functional changes headaches, fatigue, drowsiness, coma, respiaratory failure, death. |

## Land Pollution

It is mainly caused by dumping of solid wastes in the open and accumulation of several toxic chemicals in the soil due to atmospheric fall-out or by use in agriculture. The open dumps often become site for habitat of rodents, flies, mosquitoes and other insects. Many of these become vectors of disease carrying germs. The spread of plague in Surat a few years back was the result of the solid wastes accumulation in streets. Certain pathogenic organisms can remain present in the waste which periodically become air-borne due to wind and enter in the body by inhalation of contaminated air. The soluble toxic chemicals, if present in the dumps, can leach and make the groundwater polluted as has been reported quite commonly.

The toxic chemicals, especially heavy metals and radioactive ones, which get deposited over the vegetation due to fall-out can reach Man through foodchains by consuming contaminated milk and meat of the animals those feed upon the vegetation of that area. The general effects of soild wastes including health implications are shown in Fig.1.7.

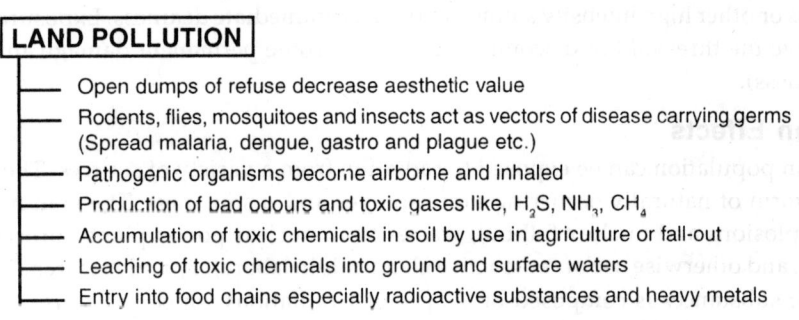

**LAND POLLUTION**

— Open dumps of refuse decrease aesthetic value
— Rodents, flies, mosquitoes and insects act as vectors of disease carrying germs (Spread malaria, dengue, gastro and plague etc.)
— Pathogenic organisms become airborne and inhaled
— Production of bad odours and toxic gases like, $H_2S$, $NH_3$, $CH_4$
— Accumulation of toxic chemicals in soil by use in agriculture or fall-out
— Leaching of toxic chemicals into ground and surface waters
— Entry into food chains especially radioactive substances and heavy metals

**Fig. 1.7 :** Environmental consequences and health effects of solid wastes.

## Noise Pollution

Noise is treated as a sound without agreeable musical quality or as an unwanted sound. The effects of noise on Man can be auditory (related to hearing) or nonauditory, and may be related to physiological, behavioural and psychological responses (Fig.1.8). The immediate nonauditory reactions to noise at relatively low levels (70-75 dB) include constriction of peripheral blood vessels with a consequent increase in blood flow to the brain, a change in breathing rate, change in muscle tension and gastrointestinal mobility. If the exposure is continuous for long, loss of some hearing acuity may result with increasing age.

At slightly higher noise levels pulse rate and blood pressure increase and the body experiences a fear reaction due to excess production of adrenalin. Greater effort is required to maintain the concentration at work, and the onset of fatigue is quicker. Noise also leads to the annoyance and irritation which can impair the quality of life. Very high level of noise above 125 dB can also interfere with vision.

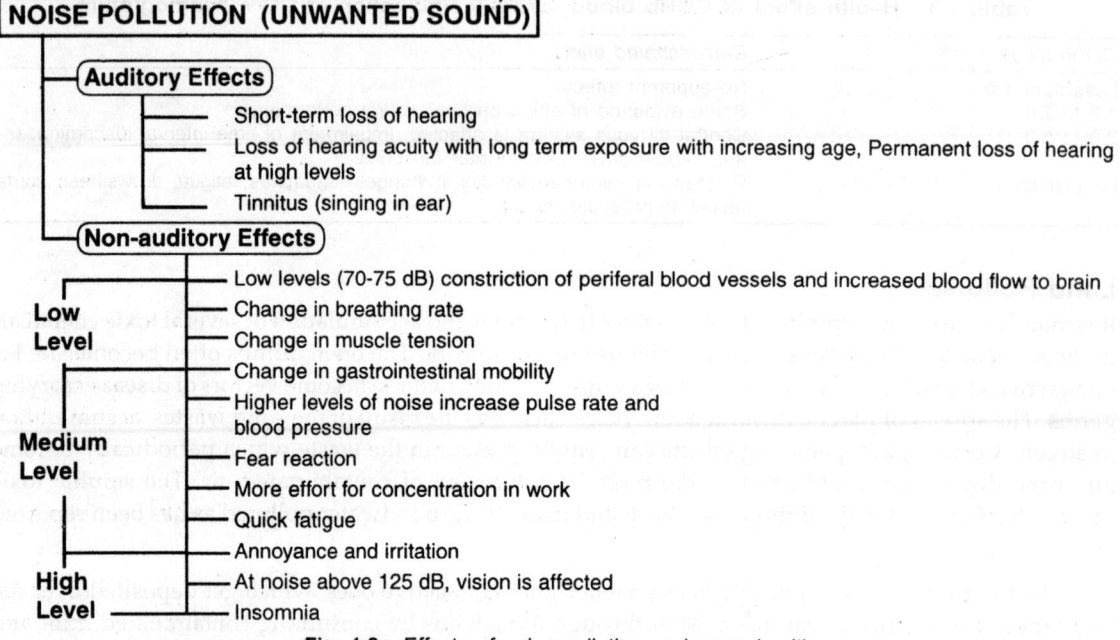

Fig. 1.8 : Effects of noise pollution on human health.

The short-term auditory effects of noise include some temporary loss in hearing at high noise levels. Explosions or other high intensity sounds may cause immediate deafness. Exposure to continuous noise levels above the threshold of discomfort may cause some permanent damage and result in insomnia (sleepnessless).

## Radiation Effects

The human population can be exposed to radiation from a variety of sources. The natural sources can be in the form of naturally occurring radioisotopes and cosmic-rays. The man-made sources include atomic explosions and nuclear fall-out, wastes from nuclear power plants, processing of radioactive chemicals, and otherwise use of radioactive chemicals in laboratory and research. The radiation emitted from these substances is composed of $\alpha$, $\beta$ and $\gamma$ radiations which can cause severe damage to the body. The summary of the radiation doses and the effects caused by them on Man are given in Fig.1.9. A radiation dose of 650 rads or above can cause death in few hours or days. The sublethal symptoms

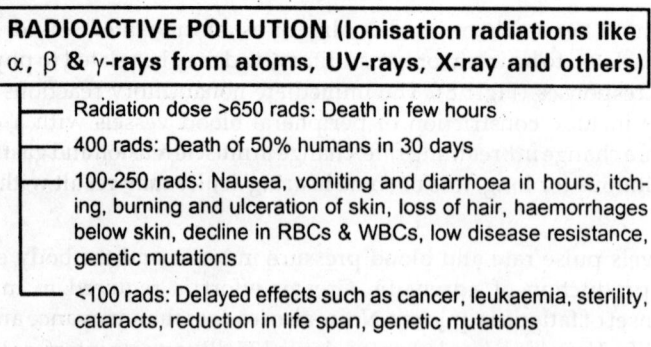

Fig. 1.9 : General effects of radiation on human health.

of radiation include nausea, vomiting, diarrhoea, itching, burning, ulceration of skin, loss of hair, decline of RBCs and WBCs in blood, reduction of disease resistance and mutations. The delayed effects of the radiation include cancers, leukaemia, sterility, cataracts, genetic mutations and reduction of life span.

## General Health Risk from Everyday Chemicals and Other Materials

Today, each house is a mini-chemical store, consisting of a variety of chemicals used in our day to day life (Table 1.4). Accidental intake or exposure to lethal doses usually leads to painful death. Overdoses of certain medicines or sometimes their permissible doses in sensitive persons may result in severe problems. A number of wild as well as cultivated plants are in use in various forms of medicines. Active ingredients in them are alkaloides, amines, glucosides, steroids and saponins etc. The excessive doses of these can also result in adverse body responses. Certain wild plants species are also very poisonous resulting in death after accidental intake.

Toxic substances can also develop in our food products due to poor storage quality as well as cooking. Intake of such food often becomes fatal as commonly encountered in the village feast, particularly in summer. A large number of chemicals and byproducts in industry are the cause of diverse occupation hazards. Indiscriminate use of some pesticides at home and in agriculture is poisoning food chains in both natural and Man-made ecosystems. The World Health Assembly held in 1953 noted new public health problems as a result of increasing use of various chemicals in the food industry. In response to this the WHO along with FAO initiated two series of annual meetings on food additives and on pesticides residues. These have resulted in the formulation of "Acceptable Daily Intake" (ADIs) and "Maximum Residue Limits" (MRLs) for chemicals in food commodities.

Besides, a large number of commonly used chemicals such as used in cosmetics, food preparation, sanitary, stationery, antirusts, cleansing solvents, fluorescent lamps, furniture paint and polish, shoe polish, hair bleach, and fireworks, etc. can also pose long term health problems. Tables 1.5 and 1.6 list some common day to day materials and the health risks associated with them.

### Table 1.4 : Common house-hold poisons

| Preparation | Toxic substance |
|---|---|
| **A DOMESTIC POISONS** | |
| **1. Cosmetics** | |
| a. Cuticle remover | Potassium hydroxide; trisodium phosphate |
| b. Depilatories | Barium sulphide; thallium |
| c. Hair wave lotions | Thioglycollate salts; perborates; bromates |
| d. Nail polish removers | Acetone |
| e. Sun-tan lotions | Denatured alcohol; methylsalicylate |
| f. Baby powder | Boric acid |
| **2. Kitchen** | |
| a. Baking power | Tartaric acid 50% |
| b. Baking soda | Sodium bicarbonate |
| c. Dish washing compounds | Sodium polyphosphates; sodium carbonate; sodium silicates |
| d. Fire extinguishing fluids | Carbon tetrachloride; sodium carbonate; methyl bromide |
| e. Matches | Antimony; phosphorus; sesqui-sulphide; potassium chlorate |
| **3. Rat Poisons** | |
| a. Rat paste | Aluminium phosphide; zinc sulphide; phosphorus; zinc phosphide; arsenious oxide; red squill; thallium sulphate |
| b. Rodine | Yellow phosphorus |
| **4. Roach Power** | Sodium fluoride |
| **5. Sanitary** | |
| a. Deodorant tablets | Formaldehyde; naphthalene |
| b. Drain cleaners | Sodium hydroxide |

*Contd....*

| Preparation | Toxic substance |
|---|---|
| c. Disinfectants | Phenol; bleaching powder |
| **6. Miscellaneous** | |
| a. Insecticide spray | D.D.T., Gammexane etc. |
| b. Moth Balls | Naphthalene |
| c. Marking ink | Aniline |
| d. Ink remover | Sodium hyphochlorite 5% |
| e. Anti-rust products | Ammonium sulphide, hydrofluoric acid, naphtha, oxalic acid |
| f. cleaning solvents | Petroleum hydrocarbons; trichloroethylene; $CCl_4$ |
| g. Fluorescent lamps | Beryllium |
| h. Furniture Polish | Turpentine; petroleum hydrocarbons |
| l. Toys (paints) | Lead |
| m. Fire works | Arsenic; mercury; antimony; lead; phosphorus; thiocyanate |
| n. Crayons (chalk) | Salts of arsenic, copper, lead |
| o. Crayons (wax) | Para-nitro-aniline |
| **B GARDEN POISONS** | |
| 1. Insecticides | Organophosphorus compounds; chlorinated hydrocarbons; nicotine; tar oils |
| 2. Fungicides | Lead arsenate; copper compounds; organic mercurials; lime; sulphur |
| 3. Weed killers | Sodium chlorate; arsenious oxide and arsenites; dinitrocresol, paraquat |
| **C THERAPEUTIC POISONS** | |
| 1. Antiseptics | Iodine, benzoin |
| 2. Tonic tablets | Iron |
| 3. Tonic syrup | Strychnine |
| 4. Sleeping tablets | Barbiturates |
| 5. Headache tablets | Aspirin |
| 6. Cough remedies | Codeine |
| 7. Throat tablets | Potassium chlorate |
| 8. Pep tablets | Benzedrine |
| 9. Others | Antidepressants; tranquilisers |

**Table 1.5 : Effect of diverse toxicants on human health (Based on Reddy (1990) and other reports)**

| Toxicants | Lethal dose | Lethal period | Remarks |
|---|---|---|---|
| Sulphuric acid | 10–15 cc | 18–24 hrs | Corrosion of mucous membranes of mouth, throat and oesophagus; teeth chalky white; tongue; swollen, sodden and black; toxamia. |
| Nitric acid | 10–15 cc | 18–24 hrs | Causes yellow discolouration of tissue due to picric acid formation; fumes inhalation results lachrymation, photophobia, irritation of air passage, sneezing, coughing and asphyxia. |
| Hydrochloric acid | 15–20 cc | 18–24 hrs | Destroys mucous membrane which at first is grey or grey white and later brown or black; fumes inhalation causes intense irritation of throat and lungs including suffocation. Constant exposure to fumes results in conjunctivitis, corneal ulcer, bronchitis, inflamation of gums and teeth loosening. |
| Oxalic acid | 15–20 g | 1–2 hrs | Destroy mucous membrane of digestive tract; results hypocalcaemia and renal damage. |
| Carbolic acid | 10–15 g | 3–4 hrs | Skin burning and eschar formation; Hot burning (Phenol) pain in mouth and stomach, speech painful and difficult, bronchitis. |
| Caustic Alkalies a. K/Na hydroxide | 5 g | 24 hrs | Acid caustic taste and sensation of burning |

*Contd....*

| Toxicants | Lethal dose | Lethal period | Remarks |
|---|---|---|---|
| b. K–carbonate | 18 g | 24 hrs | heat extending from the throat to the stomach; abrasions, blisters and brown discolouration on the lips and mouth skin; red brown, soap like swollen eschar. |
| c. Na–carbonate | 30 g | 24 hrs | |
| d. Ammonia | 30 g | 24 hrs | Inhalation of ammonia vapours results in eyes watering, violent sneezing, coughing and suffocation. |
| Phosphorus White & red form | 60–120 mg | 4–8 days | Burning pain in the throat and abdomen; convulsion and coma; skin contact produces painful penetrating second and third degree burns; frequent inhalation of fumes over a long period results fossy jaw; also causes nausea, vomiting, abdominal pain, indigestion etc. |
| Iodine | 3–4 g | 1–several days | Burning pain from mouth to stomach; intense thirst, salivation, vomiting, cramps or convulsions, movements of the limbs and lip and angus of mouth stained brown. |
| Chlorine | 1 part in 1000 | 48 hrs | Inhalation results irritation and suffocation; fatal in 5 minutes; eyes irritation; nausea; vomiting |
| Tetraethyl pyrophosphate (TEPP) | 50 mg i.m. or 100 mg orally | 1–3 hrs | Inhibit acetyl choline esterase (AChE) activity- important for maintenance of impulse transfer between nerve and skeletal muscle cells. Intake results vomiting, abdominal cramps, diarrhoea, headache, convulsion, coma and paralysis of respiratory muscle. |
| Octamethyl pyrophosphoramide (OMPA) | 80 mg i.m. or 175 mg orally | 1–3 hrs | -do- |
| Parathion (diethy nitrophenyl thiophosphate) | 180 mg i.m. or 175 mg orally (tolerance level 0.1 ppm) | 1–3 hrs | -do- |
| Hexaethyl tetraphosphate (HETP) | 60 mg i.m. or 350 mg orally | 1–3 hrs | -do- |
| Malathion | 1 g orally | 1–3 hrs | -do- |
| Diazinon | 1 g orally | 1–3 hrs | -do- |
| Endrin | 5–6 g | 1–2 hrs | Most toxic chlorinated hydrocarbon insecticides; vomiting; froth at mouth and nose; headache; hyper-irritability; death due to respiratory failure. |
| Chlorate | 20–30 g | 1–4 hrs | Vomiting, diarrhoea, abdominal pain, blood in urine and renal failure. |
| Paraquat | NA | NA | Mouth and throat burning; abdominal pain; painful ulceration of the lips and tongue; vital organs failure. |
| Dinitroorthocreson/ | NA | NA | Contact results yellow colour of the skin and hair; inhalation and ingestion result insomnia, convulsions, coma, intense respiration, burns of lips, buccal mucosa and acute renal failure. |
| Arsenic-as oxide | 0.2 g | 1–2 days | Massive doses result death from shock and peripheral vascular failure; acute poisoning resembles bacterial food poisoning; repeated small dose intake in food or drink causes anaemia and weight loss. |
| Mercury compounds as mercuric chloride, mercurous chloride, mercuric oxide, mercuric iodide, mercuric nitrite, mercuric sulphide, mercuric cyanide, amino | 1–4 g | Few hours to 1–2 weeks | Burning pain, ashen discolouration of the mucosa in mouth and pharynix; severe vomiting and diarrhoea; fumes inhalation produce nervous symptoms as restriction of visual field. |

*Contd....*

| Toxicants | Lethal dose | Lethal period | Remarks |
|---|---|---|---|
| mercuric chloride, organic componds of mercury Lead and its salts like lead acetate, lead carbonate, lead chromate, lead monoxide, lead tetraoxide, tetraethyl lead | 20–30 g | 1–2 days | Inhalation of lead dust and fumes (daily intake of 1-2 mg of lead) results chronic poisoning; result facial pallor, anaemia, and formation of stippled blue line on gums; general weakness; foul breath; headache; vertigo; loss of hairs and drowsiness; acute poisoning causes abdominal pain, nausea, vomiting, headache, coma and death. |
| Copper sulphate and copper subacetate | 30 g and 10 g respectively | 1–3 days | Metallic taste; abdominal pain; vomiting; difficulty in breathing; cold perspiration; severe headache; sometime limb paralysis, coma and death; chronic poisoning occurs among workers due to inhalation of dust or food cooked in copper vessel. |
| Potassium permanganate | 10–20 g | 20–90 hrs | Lips, gums, teeth, tongue, tonsils and pharynx discoloured; burning pain from mouth to stomach; nausea; vomiting; difficulty in speaking. |
| Zinc salts–chloride, oxide, sulphate, phosphide and stearate | 15 g ($ZnSO_4$) 1–4 g ($ZnCl_2$) 0.5–1 g (Zinc phosphide) | Few hours to few days | Metallic stypic taste; abdominal pain and vomiting; convulsions, collapse and death; volatilised zinc results chilling at the end of a day's work similar to malaria (zinc chill) and great thirst, profuse perspiration and deep sleep (industrial hazard). |
| Barium as nitrate, carbonate, sulphate and sulphide | 1 g | 12 hrs | Nausea, vomiting and diarrhoea; cramps and stiffness of muscles, paralysis of tongue and larynx, and vertigo. |
| Antimony as antimony potassium tartrate (tartar emetic) and antimony trichloride | 0.5–1 g & 0.1 0.2 g | – | Poisoning symptoms similar to arsenic. |
| Sodium nitrate | 1–2 g | NA | Toxic doses convert haemoglobin to methamoglobin; causes low blood pressure, throbbing headache, vertigo, visual disturbances, vomiting and diarrhoea. |
| Methyl isocyanate (MIC) | NA | NA | Vapour results intense irritation of the skin, eyes and mucous membranes; pulmonary oedema in acute cases and fibrosing alveolitis in chronic cases; death occurs due to exhaustion. |
| Vesicant/ Blistering gases | NA | NA | Mainly mustard gas and lewisite mustard gas results irritation of eyes, nose and respiratory passages; vomiting and abdominal pain; skin contact causes intense itching, redness and ulceration particularly of the moist areas. |
| Chlorine and phosgene | NA | 24–48 hrs | Phosgene is 10 times toxic as chlorine, inhalation results eyes watering, coughing, chest tightness, headache, vomiting, cynosis and collapse. |
| Tear gases | NA | NA | Mainly chloracetophenone (CAP) and ethyliodoacetate (KSK) and bromobenzyl cyanide (BBC). Their vapours result intense irritation of eyes and excessive tearing, eyelids spasm and temporary blindness; also irritate air passages; constant exposure causes vomiting and blistering of eyes. |
| Nasal irritants | NA | NA | These are diphenyl chlorarsine (DA), diphenylamine chlorarsine (DM) and diphenylcyanarsine (CD). Their vapours have a specific action upon vomiting centre in the brain. Results intense pain and irritation in the nose and sinuses; sneezing, headache, vomiting and chest tightness. |

*Contd....*

| Toxicants | Lethal dose | Lethal period | Remarks |
|---|---|---|---|
| Carbon monoxide | NA | NA | Strong affinity for haemoglobin; results in formation of carboxy haemoglobin. Blood saturation in children faster than adults; exposure to lower concentration results in state of complete helplesness. Exposure to 0.2% of gas results death in about 4 hrs, 0.4% in 1 hr and 10% in 20–30 minutes. The upper safety limit of CO is 0.01% in air. |
| Carbon dioxide | NA | NA | Symptoms vary with concentration of gas. More than 30% $CO_2$ in air as occasionally present in manholes, wells, silos and cellers; results discomfort, ringing in the ears, tightness in the chest, unconsciousness, coma and death. |
| Hydrogen sulphide | NA | NA | It occurs in large quantities in sewers, cess pools, privy vaults and tannery vats and in industries such as artificial silk and petroleum refinery. Weak concentration results cough, giddiness, nausea, feeling of oppression, face cyanosis, lachrymation, photophobia, convulsions or coma and finally death from asphyxia. Exposure to high concentration results immediate death from paralysis of respiratory centre. |
| Methane | NA | NA | Produced in wells after decomposition of organic matter. In diffuse daylight it combines with chlorine to form chloroform and carbon tetrachloride. Chloroform changes into carbonyl chloride slowly which is an extremely poisonous gas. |
| Ethyl alcohol | 200–300 ml of absolute alcohol | 12–24 hrs | Noticeable intoxication occurs when blood concentration exceeds 150 mg %. |
| Methyl alcohol | 60–240 ml | 24–30 hrs | Vomiting and pain or severe cramps in the abdomen; headache; dizziness; vision failure or complete blindness; effects on CNS, liver and kidney. |
| Chloroform | 30 cc/5% in | NA | Oral intake results unconsciousness within 10 minutes; inhalation causes irritation in throat, eye burning and unconsciousness in 3–4 min. |
| Ether | 30 cc | NA | Effects similar to chloroform but there is more irritation of respiratory tract. |
| Chloral hydrate | 5-10 g | 8 12 hrs | Gastrointestinal irritation, convulsions, mental degeneration and liver damage. |
| LSD (Lysergic acid diethyl amide) | 14 mg | NA | Ingetion results vomiting, headache, chills, sweating, extremely emotional behaviour and visual hallucinations. |
| Peyote - from a cactus (Peytoe) | NA | NA | Plant is a potent hallucinogen. |
| Industrial solvents | NA | NA | Excessive inhalation of fumes in a work place from a cloth or plastic bag soaked in solvents may severely damage kidneys, liver, bone marrow and nervous system. |
| Petroleum distilates, kerosene paraffin etc. | 30 cc of kerosene | 24 hrs | Ingestion of kerosene results burning pain in throat, vomiting, diarrhoea, drowsiness and coma; sometime convulsions; inhalation of moderate concentration results dizziness, headache, vomiting and unconsciousness after prolong inhalation. |
| Acetyl salicylic acid (Aspirin) | 20–30 g | Few minutes- several hours | Mild burning pain in the throat and stomach; vomiting; body temperature raised; vertigo; ringing in the ears; deafness and impaired vision; severe headache. |
| Antifebrin | 15 g | Uncertain | Vomiting, vertigo, rapid irregulr pulse, subnormal |

*Contd....*

| Toxicants | Lethal dose | Lethal period | Remarks |
|---|---|---|---|
| (acetanilide, phenylacetamide) | | | temperature, collapse and death. |
| Antihistamines | NA | NA | CNS depression characterised by drowsiness, fatigue and coma followed by CNS hyperexcitability; finally there is severe central nervous depression. |
| Tranquilisers | NA | NA | Tongue stifness; dry mouth; diplopia; drowsiness and in severe cases result in coma. |
| Methaquoline (Mandrax and Melsedine) | NA | NA | Sensitive persons become unconscious even after one tablet. Intake after meals in patients causes dizziness, sweat and a syndrome similar to hypoglycaemia; 2.5g of drug produces unconsciousness in 1/2 hr. |
| Meperidine (pethidine) | NA | NA | Results dizziness more than morphine; hallucination, dialation of pupils, dry mouth and sometime convulsions. |
| Formaldehyde | 30–90 cc | 1–2 days | Vapour inhalation irritates eyes and air passages; intake results burning pain from mouth to the stomach; vomiting and flushing of face. |
| Bromide of K and Na | 30–45 g | 6–8 hrs | Skin rashes on face and head; depression of nervous system; vomiting and fall of blood pressure. |
| Paraldehyde | 100–120 cc, blood levels over 50 mg/100 cc | Uncertain | Ingestion causes vomiting, headache and bad smells of paraldehyde, subnormal temperature, coma and death. |
| Sulphonamide | NA | NA | Vertigo, headache, abdominal colic, bluish skin, and visual disturbance. |

## Table 1.6 : Effect of diverse plants, animals and foods on human health
### [Based on Reddy (1990) and other reports]

| Toxicants | Lethal dose | Lethal period | Remarks |
|---|---|---|---|
| Ergot (dried sclerotium of fungus (*Claviceps purpurea*) | 10 g | 12–24 hrs | Powder in eyes causes lachrymation, burning pain and redness; causes irritation to skin. |
| *Scamecarpus anacardium* (Brulwal) – active principles are semecarpol and bhilawanol | 10 g | 12–24 hrs | Plant juice causes irritation and painful blister leading to eczema; oral intake results blisters in throat and severe gastrointestinal irritation, coma and death. |
| *Calotropis procera* and *C. gigantea* (Akda, Madar) | Uncertain | 12 hrs | Oral consumption of plant juice produces acrid bitter taste and burning pain in throat and stomach, vomiting, diarrhoea, tetanic convulsions, collapse and death. |
| *Plumbago rosea* (Lalchitra). *P. zeylanica* (Chitra) – Root contains plumbagin | Uncertain | Few days | Irritation and blister formation after external application of roots; oral consumption results burning pain from mouth to stomach, vomiting, thirst, diarrhoea, collapse and death. |
| *Papaver somniferum* (Afim, Opium) | Opium 2 g; Morphine 0.2g | 6–12 hrs | Morphine contact with sensitive person causes urticaria and itching dermatitis; opium intake paralyses nerve centres and patients finally pass into stage of deep coma. |
| *Ricinus communis* (Arandi) – Ricin, a water soluble glycoprotein (poison), present maximum in seed | 10 seeds | 2–several days | Seed-dust rsults eyes watering, conjunctivitis, sneezing, headache, dermatitis and bronchitis; while intake causes burning of mouth, throat and stomach, convulsions, shallow breathing and death. |

*Contd....*

| Toxicants | Lethal dose | Lethal period | Remarks |
|---|---|---|---|
| *Croton tiglium* (Jamalgota or Naepala) seeds contain crotin & crotonoside (poison) | 5–6 seeds | 4–6 hours to 3 days | Hot burning pain from mouth to stomach, vomiting, vertigo, collapse and death. |
| *Abrus precatorius* (gunchi or ratti) Seeds contain arbin, abrine, abralin (all poisonous) | 15–120 mg by infection | 3 to 5 days | Symptoms resemble with those of viperine snake bite; these are faintness, vertigo, vomiting, convulsions and death from cardiac failure. |
| *Datura alba* & *D. niger*-seeds and fruits are poisonous | 0.6–1g (50–75 seeds) | 24 hrs | Alkaloids in plant parts are highly toxic, contact with leaves or flowers results dermatitis in sensitive persons; intake causes dryness of mouth, burning pain in stomach, vomiting and difficulty in talking; affects central nervous system. |
| *Atropa belladonna* | NA | NA | 120 mg of atropine alkaloid is fatal within 24 hours. |
| *Hyoscyamus niger* (Henbane) | NA | NA | 120 mg of hyoscyamine/30 mg of hyoscine are fatal within 24 hours. |
| *Cannabis saliva indica* (Indian Hemp/hashish/ marihuna) | Charas–2 g, Ganja–8 g and Bhang – 10 g/kilo body weight | Several days | Loss of appetite, weakness, red eyes and mental deterioration; rarely become insane. |
| Cocaine - leaves of *Erythroxylum coca* | 1–1.5 g | NA | Intake results dryness in mouth; feeling of well being and loss of depression and fatigue; temporary xcitement. Cocaine addict face is pale, eyes sunken, pupil dilated, tounge and teeth black and cocaine bugs symptoms. |
| *Lathyrus sativus* (Khesari dal) | NA | NA | About 1% neurotoxic chemical B–(N) oxalyl amino alanine – BOAA is present in the seed cotyledons. Dal consumption over 6 months period result paralysis. |
| Mushrooms | Uncertain | 24 hrs | *Amanita phalloides* and A. *muscaria* are the most common poisonous fungi. Symptoms include constriction of throat, burning pain in the stomach, vomiting, convulsion, sweating, collapse and death. |
| *Argemone mexicana* (Pili kateli) | NA | NA | Loss of appetite, diarrhoea, marked oedema of the legs; myocardial damage and dilation of the heart; death results from severe heart damage. |
| *Lolium temulentum* (Damel) | NA | NA | Grains infected with fungus contain a toxin temuline. Their intake results headache, muscular weakness, tremors, gastrointestinal irritation and coma. |
| *Paspalum scrobiculatum* (Kodra) | NA | NA | Poison present in corn is destroyed by boiling; poisoning symptoms are similar to those of *Lolium*. |
| Cotton seeds | NA | NA | Contains gossypol toxin which adversely affect lysine availability to the body. |
| Groundnut | NA | NA | Fungi *Aspergillus flavus* grows over groundnuts stored under humid conditions. The fungi produces aflatoxins which have carcinogenic property. Also results hepatic damage in domestic and laboratory animals. |
| Cabbage | NA | NA | Sulphur containing compounds inhibit thyroxine secretion. |

*Contd....*

| Toxicants | Lethal dose | Lethal period | Remarks |
|---|---|---|---|
| Soyabean | NA | NA | Contains trypsin inhibitor which makes protein unavailable to the body. This toxin is destroyed by heat. |
| Sweet clover | NA | NA | Dicoumarin forms in spoiled sweet clover. It is chemically related to vitamin K and blocks its action. Cattle feeding on spoiled sweet clover develops haemorrhagic disease. |
| *Strychnos nux vomica* (Kuchilla) | 30–120 mg; one crushed seed | 1–2 hrs | Strychnine, an alkaloid from seed, is poisonous; (Kuchilla) ingestion results convulsions, discontinued sedation and release excitation. Death after 4-5 times convulsions. Uncrushed seeds have no effects. |
| *Nicotiana tabacum* (Tobacco) | 60 mg | NA | Leaves contain nicotin and anabasine – toxic nicotine alkaloids; ingestion results burning acid sensation from mouth to stomach, vomiting, headache, faintness, excessive urination, audio-visual disturbances, unconsciousness and cardiovascular collapse. |
| *Digitalis purpurea* | 1–30 mg of digitalein, 4 mg of digitoxin | 12–24 hrs | All plant parts contain digitoxin, digitalein and digitonin (steroidal glycosides); ingestion results vomiting, abdominal pain, diarrhoea, unconsciousness, slower and later faster heart rate, coma and finally death. |
| *Nerium odorum* (Kaner) | 15 g root | 24–36 hrs | Plant – a source of contact dermatitis; ingestion of plant parts particularly root results vomiting, abdominal pain, vomiting and profuse frothy salivation and diarrhoea followed by lockjaw, drowsiness, coma, respiratory paralysis and death. |
| *Cerbera thevetia* (Yellow oleander) | 8–10 seeds | 2–3 hrs | Ingestion of seeds causes burning pain in the mouth, vomiting, headache, low blood pressure, heart block and death. |
| *Cerbera odollam* (Pili Kirbir) | Kernel of one fruit | 1–2 days or more | Vomiting, abdominal pain, blurring of vision, irregular respiration, collapse and death from heart failure. |
| Quinine | 2–8 g | Few minutes to hours or even days | Tree bark contains quinine, cinchonidine alkaloids; headache, ringing in the ears, partial deafness, vision disorder and rash on the skin; cyanosis, coma and death from respiration failure. |
| *Aconitum napellus* & *A. ferox* (Aconite) | 1–2 g root, 4–6 mg of aconitine | 1–8 hours | Root most poisonous, contains aconitine alkaloid which stimulates and then depress CNS; death due to paralysis of heart or respiratory centres; pollen causes pain and swelling in the eyes. |
| Hydrocyanic acid | NA | NA | Present in many fruits and leaves as almonds, apricot, apple, cherry, peach, plum, pear, bamboo shoots, certain oil seeds and beans. Ingestion results headache, stiffness in the lower jaw, irregular respiration, bitter almonds odour in the breath or vomit, violent convulsions, paralysis, brick red skin and death from respiratory failure. |
| Curare | 30–60 mg | 1–2 hrs | Curarine – an active principle is obtained from various species of *Strychnos*; causes flaccid paralysis of skeletal muscles; used as arrow poison. |
| Hemlock-*Conium maculatum* | NA | NA | Alkaloid coniline is maximum in the unripe fruit and seeds, also in leaves at flowering and in root during summer. Ingestion results burning in mouth and throat, gastric inflamation, vomiting, diarrhoea, sometime blindness, motor paralysis, coma and death from respiratory paralysis. |
| Potato | NA | NA | Solanin develops in exposed green part of potato which results severe or fatal poisoning. |
| Fish poisoning | NA | NA | Ovaries, testes and liver of certain fishes such as herring, |

*Contd....*

| Toxicants | Lethal dose | Lethal period | Remarks |
|---|---|---|---|
| | | | porcupine, sea bass, mackerels and toad fish contain neurotoxin. This produces a syndrome known as 'icthyotoxicosis'. Symptoms like burning of throat, abdominal pain and vomiting appear in 10-30 minutes; finally death occurs from respiratory failure. |
| Shell fish | NA | NA | Muscles and Calms contain heat stable alkaloidal neurotoxin produced by planktons ingested as food. Neurotoxin is passed to human after ingestion of shell fish. It causes vomiting, convulsions and death from respiratory failure. |
| Venomous fish | NA | NA | Cat fish, muraena (eel), dragon fish, lion fish, etc. **have spine which may cause poisonous wounds.** |
| **Bacterial Food Poisoning:** | | | |
| Infectious type– Pathogenic Organisms present in food | NA | NA | *Salmonella* group most common; other groups like *Proteus*, coli group, *Streptococcus*, paratyphoid bacilli also occur; certain poisonous foods as fish, toadstools, eggs, ergots etc. are also involved. |
| Toxin type–ingestion of poisonous toxin containing food formed by bacterial growth | NA | NA | Milk, meat, fish and eggs are frequently contaminated by enterotoxin and botulinum. Food poisoning is common during summer on account of warm temperature favouring microrganisms multiplication. |
| Botulism | 0.01 mg | NA | *Clostridium botulinum* produces neurotoxin after multiplication in food. Fatal dose of toxin is 0.01 mg or even less. Toxin paralyses the nerve endings. |
| Food allergy | NA | NA | Few persons are hypersensitive to certain protein forms, e.g., meat, fish, egg, milk etc. They suffer from gastroenteritis, local urticarial rashes or asthamatic attack. |
| Ptomaines | NA | NA | Bacterial decomposition of protein results ptomaines - the alkaloid bodies. Neurine and mydaleine are toxic. Symptoms resemble with atropine. |

## SUMMARY

Increasing environmental pollution and indiscriminate use or otherwise consumption of everyday chemicals and other materials in our daily life pose severe health risks.

The major water pollutants include heavy metals, pesticides, toxic organics and inorganics, degradable organic matter, nutrients and a variety of pathogens. Many of them cause severe ailments of kidneys, liver, brain, bones, skin, gonads and other organs. Some of these have also been found to cause cancers and teratogenic effects. The pathogenic organisms present in water are responsible for spread of several waterborne epidemic diseases like typhoid, cholera, diarrhoea, gastroenteritis, poliomyelitis, jaundice and intestinal colitis.

Air pollution is caused mainly by gaseous and particulate matter of different nature. The major effects have been reported on eye and respiratory system. The common diseases of respiratory tract induced by air pollution include chronic bronchitis, pulmonary emphysema, bronchial asthma, pulmonary oedema, silicosis, asbestosis, cancers of skin and lung, and accelerated ageing.

Land pollution is caused by accumulation of unnecessary chemicals in soil and dumping of solid wastes in open. The solid waste dumps can serve as the sites for breeding of vectors and other organisms which can spread diseases like malaria, dengue, gastro and plague. The pathogenic organisms may also be present in the dumps which can spread certain diseases through air or water. The toxic substances can leach into water resources and pose the danger of water pollution.

Noise pollution can result in auditory and non-auditory effects. Long term low exposure to noise causes loss of hearing acuity, while high levels of noise may result in permanent loss of hearing. Other effects of noise on humans include change in breathing rate and gastrointestinal mobility, increase in pulse rate and blood pressure, fear reaction, annoyance, irritating behaviour, quick fatigue, impaired vision and insomnia.

While higher levels of radiation above 400 rads result in death in few hours to 30 days, the radiation of lower doses result in several sublethal effects. These may include nausea, vomiting, diarrhoea, itching, burning and ulceration of skin, decline in blood corpuscles, genetic mutations, cancers, leukaemia, sterility, cataracts and reduction in life span.

A large number of chemicals and other materials are used in our daily life. These may belong to the cosmetics; kitchen chemicals like washing chemicals, fire estinguishing compounds, matches and food additives; rat poisons; sanitary chemicals; insecticide sprays; moth balls; marking inks; anti-rust products; cleaning solvents; furniture polish; shoe polish; hair bleach; fire works; children crayons of chalk and wax; garden chemicals; and common medicinal chemicals. Most of these, while have deleterious effects on the body in lower concentrations, can be lethal at higher concentrations when consumed accidentally or otherwise. Besides, several plants or their products, animals and foods can also have adverse effects after consumption and even may result in death at certain concentrations.

## BIBLIOGRAPHY AND REFERENCES

- Goel, P.K. (1997) *Water Pollution: Causes, Effects and Control,* New Age International (Pvt.) Ltd., Publishers, New Delhi.
- Goel, P.K. and Sharma, K.P. (1996) *Environmental Guidelines and Standards in India.* Technoscience Publications, Jaipur.
- Liptak, B.G.(1974) *Environmental Engineers' Handbook: Air Pollution,* Vol. 2, Chilton Book Company, Pennsylvania
- Liptak, B.G.(1974) *Environmental Engineers' Handbook: Land Pollution,* Vol. 3, Chilton Book Company, Pennsylvania.
- Painter, D.E. (1974) *Air Pollution Technology,* Reston Publishing Company, Inc., Reston Virginia.
- Reddy, K.S.N. (1990) *The Essentials of Forensic Medicine and Toxicology.* 12th Ed., K.Suganabai Publishers, Hyderabad.
- Trivedy, R.K. and Goel, P.K.(1998) *An Introduction to Air Pollution,* 2nd Ed., Technoscience Publications, Jaipur.

# 2

# Ecohydrological Features
# of the Ganga River

*R. J. Rao, B. K. Sahu, Sandeep K. Behera and Ravi K. Pandit*

The Ganga River, which drains different Northern States of the country has been under constant threat of pollution due to various human activities like sewage and industrial wastes disposal, dead bodies disposal, deforestation, excessive use of fertilizers and pesticides, bathing, pilgrimage and water development programmes. The pollution of the river has become a matter of concern for all. The Govt. of India has taken up an Action Plan for prevention of pollution. The principal thrust of the Ganga Action Plan is immediate reduction of the pollution load on the river Ganga and establishment of treatment systems, which are technically and financially self-sustaining. To control the pollution in the Ganga River several agencies like the Central Ganga Authority, several research establishments, Government and non-Government organizations have done considerable work under various projects. It is necessary to monitor the impact of various projects on the river quality. In order to assess the river quality various approaches have been identified. One of the best-suited approaches is study of indicator species in the Ganga River.

The presence of potential human health hazards from persistent bioaccumulative chemicals may be more readily detected by analysis of aquatic organisms than by analysis of water samples. Any change in environment will alter the structure and perhaps composition of the community (Chawla and Viswanathan, 1989). Presence of pollution is apparent when human interference alters river chemistry or temperature enough to alter the biota.

For proper management of aquatic ecosystem and water resources, the biological monitoring is essential. According to Cairns (1982) biomonitoring often needed as a support to chemical monitoring because toxicity can not be tested without biota and chemicals below analytical detection limits may elicit biological response. The biota reacts to the pollution by translating chemical dosage to well defined biological response. Thus biological assessment techniques lead to information on the quality, condition and quantity of the streams. Since chemical analysis of water or sediments alone cannot give a quantitative idea of amount, history and consequences of pollution biomonitoring is all the more important (Chawla and Vishwanatham, 1989).

Life evolved in water, with water and with the physical and chemical characters of natural water (Haslam, 1991). The natural river bears a natural balance of plants and animals, some interdependent, some competing, some independent. It is the responsibility of man to maintain and conserve life forms in the ecosystem. River quality is measured both chemically and biologically, although the former is time-consuming and ecologically inaccurate (Haslam, 1991). Presence of organisms indicates the habitat quality of the animal, which experiences the change of the environment, if any. If an animal of different age groups is present in the river, it shows that the animals have survived the change of aquatic ecosystem, thus indicate the water quality status. Although each chemical parameter show permissible or non-permissible limits, which have an impact on the water quality for varied purpose, the organism face effects of all such parameter irrespective of their nature. So studying an organism will indicate pollution status of the river.

Success of any environmental quality maintenance programme depends on the satisfactory restoration of the diversity of biota and productivity of the ecosystem to normalcy. The density of organisms is an index of the production potentialities of aquatic environments. To understand the status of restoration of any managed ecosystem it is essential to study the biotic components of the ecosystem, especially on the indicator species.

Ideas about pollution indicator species are almost as numerous and diverse as are the people concerned with them. In order to measure the water quality a number of factors are to be considered including the studies of species composition, population sizes, and the physico-chemical environments to which they are exposed. While considerable work has been done on individual species or species communities, which indicate degree of pollution, concern has been with relatively few organisms, mostly of lower vertebrates and invertebrates (Krishna Murti, *et al* 1991).

Studies on large aquatic fauna such as dolphins, otters, crocodiles and freshwater turtles, which are also considered as indicator species for determination of water quality, are surprisingly lacking. The present study is carried out to identify the status of higher vertebrates in the river, which will enable to indicate the quality and the biological restoration of the Ganga River.

## Study Area

The present study has been carried out in the Ganga river in a stretch between Rishikesh and Kanpur in Uttar Pradesh. The total length of the river under study is 645 km (Fig. 2.1). The general features of the study area are shown in Table 2.1.

### Table 2.1 : General information of the study area

| Road bridges | Railway bridges | Barrages | Purpose | Tributaries |
|---|---|---|---|---|
| Laxman Jhula Ram Jhula, Rishikesh | Balawali Brijghat | Pasulok barrage, Rishikesh | Hydro Electricity | *Rishikesh-Haridwar* |
| | | Bhimgoda barrage, Haridwar | Irrigation | - Sushwa river<br>- Song river |
| Bhimgoda barrage, Haridwar | Rajghat Kachlaghat | Madhya Ganga barrage, Bijnor | | |
| Chandighat, Haridwar | Sukhlaganj | Lower Ganga barrage, Narora | Irrigation Irrigation and Atomic power station | Haridwar-Bijnor - Banganga river |
| Brijghat | | | | - Malin river |
| Phantoom bridge, Anupsahar canal | | | | - Sonali river<br>*Bijnor-Brijghat*<br>- Kalagarh feeder |
| Kachla Ghat | | | | |
| Ghatia Ghat | | | | *Narora-Kachla* |
| Mahandi Ghat | | | | - Mohawa river |
| Nanamau Ghat | | | | *Kachla-Ghatia Ghat* |
| Phantoom bridge, | | | | - Sol river |
| Bittor | | | | *Ghatia ghat-Kanpur* |
| Sukhalaganj, Kanpur | | | | - Ramganga river<br>- Isan river - Kalinadi<br>- Kalyani river |

## Geography

The Ganga rises at 7010 meters in Gangotri, Uttar Kashi District, (U.P.), India, on the Southern slopes of the Himalayan range. It flows through three different States-Uttar Pradesh, Bihar and West Bengal covering a distance of 2525 km. before it joins the Bay of Bengal. During its long course it embraces many small torrents and tributaries of varied origin.

The river after passing through Rishikesh enters Haridwar, which is situated on the right bank of the river. The Chilla sanctuary is situated on the left bank. At Nagal, the river makes a sweep towards

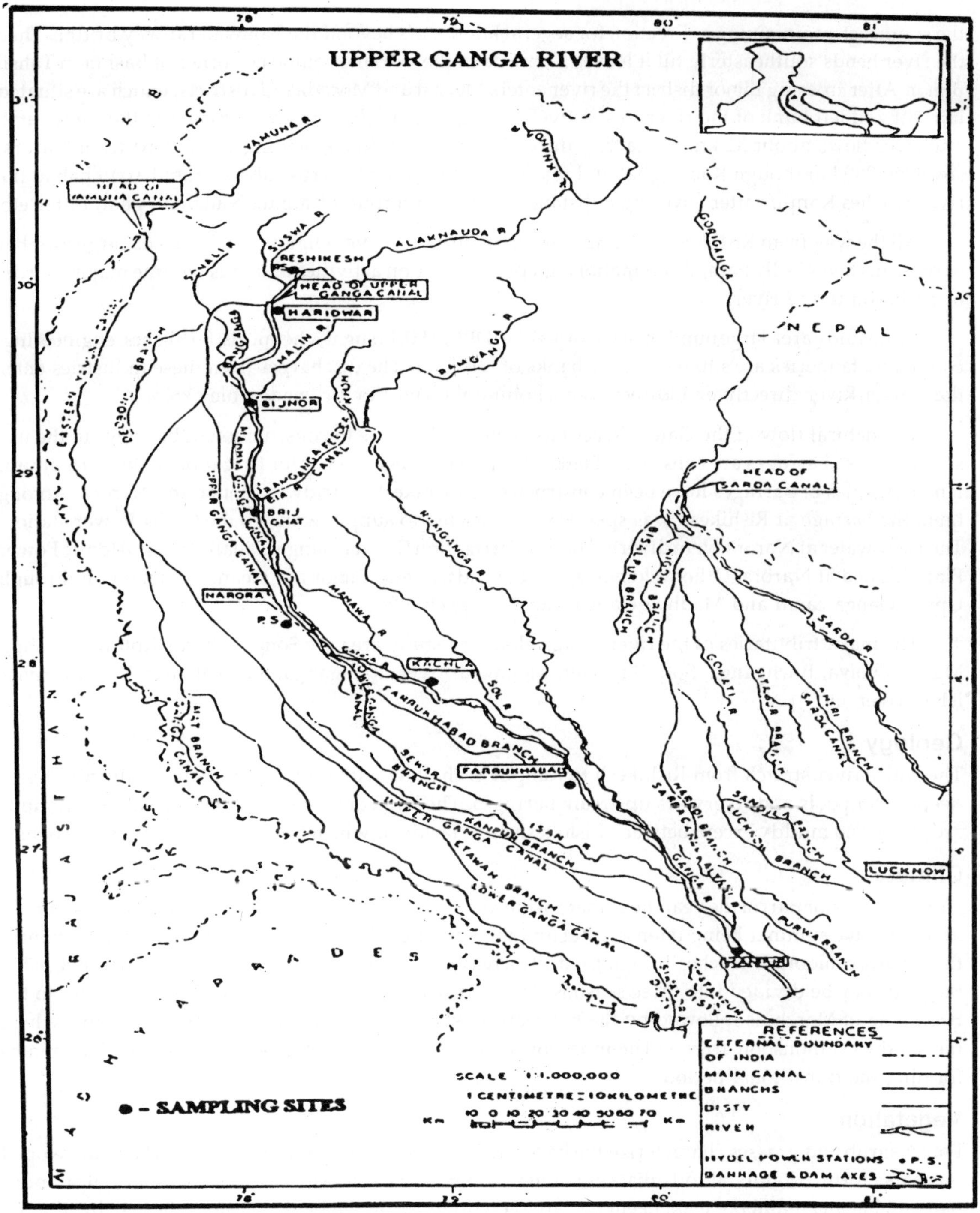
UPPER GANGA RIVER
YAMUNA R
HEAD OF JAMUNA CANAL
SUSWA R
ALAKNANDA R
RESHIKESH
HEAD OF UPPER GANGA CANAL
HARIDWAR
MALIN R
RAMGANGA R
BIJNOR
BRIJ GHAT
UPPER GANGA CANAL
NARORA
P.S.
KACHLA
SOT R
MAHAWA R
FARRUKHABAD BRANCH
FARRUKHABAD
KANPUR BRANCH
ETAWAH BRANCH
LOWER GANGA CANAL
UPPER GANGA CANAL
ISAN R
N E P A L
HEAD OF SARDA CANAL
SARDA R
SARDA CANAL
GOMATI R
LUCKNOW
KANPUR
PURWA BRANCH
REFERENCES
EXTERNAL BOUNDARY OF INDIA
MAIN CANAL
BRANCHS
DISTY
RIVER
HYDEL POWER STATIONS • P.S.
BARRAGE & DAM AXES
SCALE 1:1,000,000
1 CENTIMETRE = 10 KILOMETRE
• - SAMPLING SITES

**Fig. 2.1** : Map showing upper Ganga river.

the southeast, maintaining a direction for several kilometers beyond the Balawali railway bridge. Then the river bends southeasterly till it leaves Kumhria in the extreme southeast corner of Bashta in Tahsil Bijnor. After crossing Bijnor district the river enters Meerut and Moradabad districts, which are situated in right and left bank of the river, respectively. Brijghat is a religious ghat situated at the right bank. The river flows about 82 km to reach Narora. The river continues flowing southward from Narora, covering 200 km though Kachlaghat and reaches Ghatia ghat at Farrukhabad. From Farrukhabad the river reaches Kanpur after covering a distance of 160 km through Kannuj. Nanamau ghat, Bittor etc.

All the way from Rishikesh to Kanpur most of the ghats have religious importance. Large number of pilgrims takes holly bath, do cremation and post cremation activities and thus become major sources of pollution to the river.

In the study area large number of factories like IDPL, BHEL, sugar, chemicals, fertilizers, engineering, cotton and tanneries are situated on the banks of the river. The discharges from these industries enter the Ganga River directly or indirectly and pollute the river to a considerable extent.

The natural flow of the Ganga River has been checked due to construction of barrages in the up-stream. These barrages are constructed either for power generation or for irrigation to the agricultural lands. A series of barrages have been constructed at Rishikesh, Haridwar, Bijnor and Narora. Among them the barrage at Rishikesh was specially constructed to supply water to the Chilla Power station. The river water at Narora were diverted both for irrigation (Lower Ganga Canal) and for Atomic Power Plant located at Narora. Other two barrages at Haridwar and Bijnor are meant for irrigation through Upper Ganga canal and Madhya Ganga Canal, respectively.

The major tributaries of the river Ganga along the study area are Song, Pali rao, Kotawali, Lahpi, Malin, Choiya, Burhganga, Soti, Bia river, Mohawah river, Ramganga, Sol, Kalinadi, Kalyani river, Ishan river, etc.

## Geology

The entire river stretch from Rishikesh to Kanpur is shallow with only intermittent small stretches of deep-water pools and reservoirs upstream barrages. The bank of the entire river stretch up to Kanpur are sandy and muddy except between Rishikesh and Haridwar which has riffle areas with rocky banks.

## Climate

During the major part of the year the climate of the total study area is influenced largely by the prevalence of dry air, the summer being intensely hot and the winter cold. It is only during the monsoon months that air of oceanic origin reaches, bringing with it increased humidity, cloudiness and rain. Climatologically, the year may be divided into three seasons. The cold season, from about the end of November to the beginning of March, is followed by the hot season, which continues till about the end of June where the southwest monsoon arrives. The monsoon season lasting till September and the next two months forming the transitional period.

## Vegetation

Forest shrub and grasses characterize the banks of the study area. These communities have developed on coarse textured alluvial soil adjacent to the riverbank. The trees such as seesam, asoka, eucalyptus, banyan, banana, bamboo, teak, neem etc. are seen dominating the banks. Besides these babwai grass and some aquatic flora like *Eichhorina* etc. are also seen dominating many of the bank vegetation along the river stretch.

## Fauna

Aquatic mammals like dolphins and otters dominate the faunal resources; aquatic reptiles like crocodiles and turtles; fishes; migratory birds and other bank-side wildlife.

## Zones

The river stretch in the study area is divided into 7 zones depending on the presence of barrages and bridges (Table 2.2). The barrages separate the river into different stretches that restrict the free movement of different aquatic animals.

### Table 2.2 : Different zones in the study area

| Zone | Area | Km. |
|------|------|-----|
| I | Rishikesh – Haridwar | 29 (0–29) |
| II | Haridwar – Bijnor | 100 (29–129) |
| III | Bijnor – Brijghat | 84 (129–213) |
| IV | Brjghat – Narora | 82 (213–295) |
| V | Narora – Kachlaghat | 67 (295–362) |
| VI | Kachlaghat – Ghatia ghat | 123 (362–485) |
| VII | Ghatia ghat – Kanpur | 160 (485–645) |

## Sampling stations

The stretch of the Ganga river under investigation is divided into North and South Ganga river. The North Ganga river is from Rishikesh to Narora (0-295 km.) and the South Ganga river is from Narora to Kanpur (295 to 645 km.). At Rishikesh, Laxman Jhula is considered as 0 km of the present study area. The study area is extended up to Sukhlaganj in Kanpur, which is the termination point of the study area.

For monitoring of the river water quality a total of 8 sampling stations have been selected depending on various land markings (Table 2.3). While selecting the sampling stations various human activities, which have impact on the water quality have been taken into consideration. The sampling stations are as follows:

1. Rishikesh
2. Haridwar
3. Bijnor
4. Garmukteswar (Brij ghat)
5. Narora
6. Kachla ghat
7. Farrukhabad (Ghatia ghat)
8. Kanpur (Sukhlaganj)

### Table 2.3 : Details of sampling stations in the study area

| Sampling station | District | Distance (km)+ | Sampling point | Activities of concern* |
|------------------|----------|----------------|----------------|------------------------|
| Rishikesh | Dehradun | 0 | Downstream Muni ki Reti | CB, CR, DM, WR |
| Haridwar | Haridwar | 29 | Upstream barrage | CB, CR, WR |
| Bijnor | Bijnor | 129 | Upstream Barrage | CR, AG, WR |
| Brijghat | Gaziabad | 213 | Below Road bridge | CB, CR, DM, AG |
| Narora | Bulundsahar | 295 | Upstream barrage | CB, CR, DM, AG, WR |
| Kachlaghat | Badaun | 362 | Below Rail/Road bridge | AG, CB, CR, DM, ID |
| Ghatia ghat | Farrukhabad | 485 | Below Road bridge | CB, CR, DM |
| Kanpur | Kanpur | 645 | Below Sukhlaganj Rail bridge | AG, CB, CR, DM, ID |

AG : Agricultural runoff  CB : Community bathing  CR : Cremation & post–cremation

DM : Point/Non-point domestic sewage  ID : Point/non-point industrial effluents  WR : Water regulation activity

+ Laxman Jhula in Rishikesh is taken as 0 km.
* Criteria for human activities are modified after Mathur (1991)

# WATER QUALITY

## Introduction

Freshwater habitat may be defined as the place where an organism lives. Water has several unique qualities from ecological point of view, which render it as the most suitable medium for the living beings. The source and nature of freshwater, its motion and changing conditions as it flows to the sea and the life it support along the way, are now the subject of limnology. Due to fast growing need of water for irrigation, municipal, industrial and other uses, water has become or is fast becoming an extremely limited resource. Today, quality of many of the aquatic ecosystem has deteriorated considerably, which affected the habitat conditions of the aquatic organisms (Chakraburthy *et al.*, 1959; Rajan, 1963; Vass *et al.*, 1977). Different physiological systems of these animals will be disorganized if there is any disturbance in their environment. The rivers and other aquatic bodies are important areas of conservation for a large and varied pattern of aquatic lives.

Starting from the prehistoric Indus civilization to the modern Ganga-Jamuna many cities were and still are situated at or near river banks and water bodies, first as centres of cultivation and later as areas of mass colonization due to factories, mass production, export-import trading and the vast resources, generated by these (Das and Nath, 1988). The increasing pollution of natural aquatic environment is related and caused by increasing population and their demands and the limited nature of both renewable and non-renewable natural resources, including water. The discharge of large scale effluents from factories and domestic sewage into the water is causing irreversible changes in the quality of the water. Prevention of such aquatic pollution is a complex problem requiring co-organisation between the Scientists, the Technologist and the Administrator. The growing demand for understanding the water quality status of the Ganga River prompted to take up various studies on the Ganga river.

## Present Status of Water Quality

The physico-chemical, biological and microbiological characteristics of the Ganga river have been analyzed during 1993-95 by following standard methods (APHA, 1989; Trivedy and Goel, 1986).

## Hydrology

The river Ganga originating from Himalayas passes through the States of Uttar Pradesh, Bihar and West Bengal and drains an area of about 861 thousand square kilometers in India (Vats and Dalwani, 1992). According to Krishna Murti *et., al.,* (1991) "the average annual rainfall over the Ganga basin varies from 78 cm in the upper part, 104 cm in the middle course and 182 cm in the lower delta of Bangladesh. Most of rainfall occurs during the Southwest monsoon season. The present surface water availability in the Ganga basin is about 446 million acre feet (MAF) in India".

The detailed information on localities, elevations above sea level, estimated flow rates and river situation at different sampling stations are shown in Table 2.4.

The hydrological parameters of different sampling stations are as follows:

**Rishikesh** : Laxman Jhula at Rishikesh is the 0-km in the present study. Rishikesh is situated at an elevation of 348. above Mean Sea Level (MSL) in between 30° 07′ 21″ N latitude and 78° 19′ 10″E. longitude. The river water is checked by Chilla barrage (Fig. 2.1). The river water is diverted to Chilla Hydro Electrical Power Station. The major tributary of Ganga river at this point is Song river, which joins the Ganga at Satyanarayana, 12 km downstream. Community bathing, cremation and post cremation, point and non-point domestic and industrial effluents from IDPL, water regulation activities are marked in this station.

**Table 2.4 : Data on hydrological parameters of different sampling stations in the Ganga river between Rishikesh and Kanpur**

| S. No. | Sampling stations | Longitude | Latitude | MSL (m) | Water current (M/min) | | Water depth (m) | | River width (m) | |
|---|---|---|---|---|---|---|---|---|---|---|
| | | | | | Min | Max | Min | Max | Min | Max |
| 1 | Rishikesh | 78°19'10" | 30°07'21" | 348 | 19.8 | 40.2 | 7 | 9 | 25 | 100 |
| 2 | Haridwar | 78°10'23" | 29°57'24" | 288 | 18.9 | 31.5 | 5.2 | 6.8 | 650 | 750 |
| 3 | Bijnor | 78°04'35" | 29°22'55" | 205 | 12.9 | 26.8 | 2.2 | 2.8 | 100 | 400 |
| 4 | Brijghat | 78°08'40" | 28°45'40" | 195 | 25.7 | 34.9 | 11.1 | 14.0 | 100 | 600 |
| 5 | Narora | 78°21'51" | 28°14'32" | 176 | 12.0 | 22.4 | 13.0 | 13.5 | 950 | 950 |
| 6 | Katchla ghat | 78°12' | 27°57' | – | 9.39 | 26.1 | 2.1 | 2.9 | 50 | 200 |
| 7 | Ghatia ghat | 79°37' | 27°24' | – | 11.6 | 10.6 | 1.0 | 1.5 | 50 | 400 |
| 8 | Kanpur | 80°24' | 26° 28' | 123 | 10.6 | 23.9 | 1.9 | 6.3 | 175 | 600 |

**Haridwar :** Haridwar is situated 29 km from Rishikesh at an elevation of 288 m above MSL in between 29° 57' 24" N. latitude and 78° 10' 23" longitude. The river water is diverted at Haridwar from the Bhimgoda Barrage (Fig. 2.1). The diverted water is used for irrigation purpose through Upper Ganga Canal. Cremation, post cremation, community bathing and water regulation are the chief activities marked at this station.

**Bijnor :** It is 129 km down from Rishikesh and is situated at an elevation of 205 m above MSL in between 29° 22' 55" N latitude and 78° 04' 35" E longitude. Its importance is due to the presence of Madhya Ganga Barrage, the third one in continuation from Rishikesh (Fig. 2.1). The water is diverted to Madhya Ganga Canal, which provides irrigation for the 'rabi cultivation'. The barrage is situated 10 km South of Bijnor town.

**Garmukteswar (Brijghat) :** The Brijghat is 213 km down of Rishikesh and is situated at an elevation of 195 m above MSL. The sampling station is situated in between 28° 45' 40" N latitude and 78° 08' 40" longitude. The minimum water current during summer is 25.7 m/min with a maximum current of 34.9 m/min. Water from Ramganga feeder canal is coming into the Ganga river upstream of Brijghat at Tigrighat.

**Narora :** Narora is 295 km from Rishikesh with an elevation of 176 m above MSL in between 28° 14' 32" N latitude and 78° 21' 51" longitude. The fourth and last barrage in the study area is located here (Fig. 2.1). The water is diverted to Lower Ganga Canal for irrigation purpose. The river water is also supplied to Narora Atomic Power station for cooling purpose. The heated waters from the Atomic power station are released back into the canal. The maximum width of the river above barrage is 950 m with a maximum depth of 13.5 m.

**Kachla Ghat :** This station is 362 km down from Rishikesh. It is located between 27° 57' N latitude and 78° 12". longitude. The Mahwa river, major tributary of the Ganga River joins 2 km above this station. This tributary drains large quantities of Industrial effluents from factories located at Gajroula, Moradabad and Babrala. It is a major source of pollution to the Ganga River. Due to the industrial discharges through the tributary the water in Ganga river sometimes turn into red colour. The maximum water current during summer at this station is 26.14 m/min.

**Farrukhabad (Ghatia Ghat) :** It is 485 km down from Rishikesh and lies between 27° 24' N latitude and 79° 37" longitude. The maximum river current during summer is 10.69 m/min with a maximum depth of 1.5 m. Community bathing, point and non point domestic effluents and cremation and post-cremation activities are marked at this station.

Kanpur (Sukhlaganj) : This is the last sampling station in the present study. It is 645 km down from Rishikesh with 123 m above MSL. The sampling station lies between $26^0 28^{"}$ N latitude and $80^0 24^{"}$ E. longitude. The Ramganga a major tributary is joining the Ganga River upstream of Kanpur. Major sources of industrial and domestic pollutants are recorded at this station.

## General Features

The MSL is gradually decreased from 348 at Rishikesh to 123 at Kanpur. The flow rates (m/min) were also decreased from Rishikesh (40.2) to Kanpur (23.9). The river becomes wider at different sampling sites either due to the presence of barrages (Haridwar and Narora) or due to joining of tributaries (Kanpur) or feeder canal from the Ramganga (Brijghat). The water level in up-stream of Bijnor barrage is very low during summer as the purpose of the barrage is to store water during monsoon only. Water level at Rishikesh and Haridwar during June increases due to melting of snow in the high altitudes. These waters are diverted to several purposes. After the blockage of water at Rishikesh barrage water is still added from different sources like tributaries up to Haridwar. So the water level is almost maintained at a constant level. The gradual increase of water level in the Ganga river during summer is a typical hydrological feature of the Himalayan fed river system. This increase of water is also considered as summer floods of the river. The river is naturally flooded very high during monsoon. The mean annual rainfall recorded at Narora during 1993 was 642 mm. The climatic parameters recorded at Narora during 1993-94 are shown in Fig. 2.2.

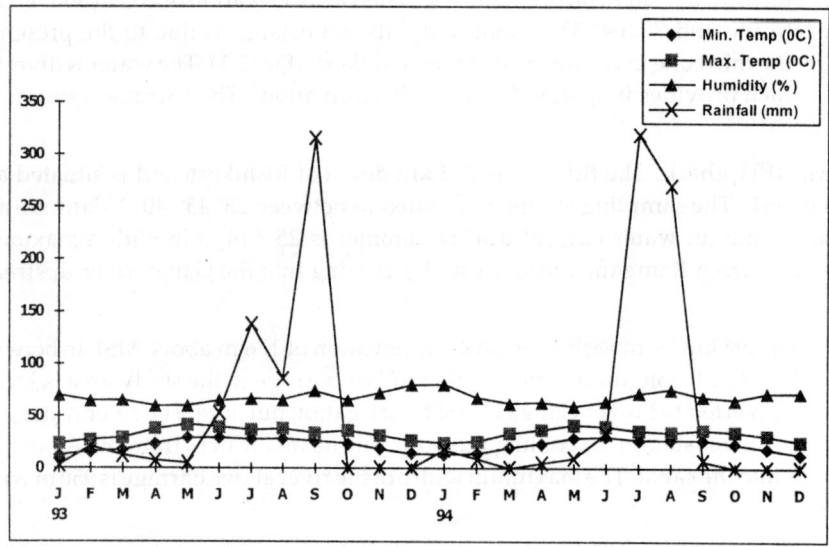

**Fig. 2.2** : Climatological parameters at Narora during 1993-1994

## Macrophytes

The macrophytes comprised aquatic and semi-aquatic vegetation. The macrophyte vegetation keeps on changing due to floods (Bilgrami, 1991). It is apparent that the most polluted sites will not bear macrophytes. River changes induce macrophyte changes slowly (Haslam, 1991). To assess the macrophyte composition in the study area macrophyte samples were collected from various sampling stations. The samples were identified with the help of Botany Dep. of Jiwaji University, Gwalior. The plants identified were mainly aquatic and some were semi-aquatic in nature. The macrophytes collected from the Ganga River between Rishikesh and Kanpur are:

*Chara* Sp., *Vallisneria spiralis, Hydrilla verticelata, Ceratophyllum, Potamogeton crispus, Potamogeton perfoliatus, Potamogeton pectinatus, Nymphoides cristatum, Monochoria hastata, Rannunclus ascliratus, Herestis monniera, Eclipta alba, Vandalia cristata, Oldenlandia corimbosa, Polygonum glabrum, Echhornia* Sp, *Typha* Sp, *Trapa bispinosa, Lemna paucicostata, Equisetum* Sp.

## Water Pollution

The Ganga River was polluted due to many human activities like sewage and industrial wastes disposal, dead bodies disposal, deforestation, excessive use of fertilizers and pesticides, bathing, pilgrimage etc. (Sinnarkar *et al.*, 1987). Under the Ganga Action Plan various programmes have been taken to control the pollution in the river (Krishna Murti *et al,* 1991).

At Rishikesh various measures like renovation of pumping station at Mayakund, setting up additional septic tanks and rising sewer mains at Laxman Jhoola, Swarg Ashram and Muni-ki-Reti, and effluent treatment by IDPL were taken (Sinnarker, *et al*, 1987). To control pollution at Farrukabad and Kanpur remedial measures were recommended which include adequate effluent treatment by various industries like textile mills, tanneries and other small industries, adequate sewage treatment before discharge into the river, connecting sewage outfalls to main sewer, and enforcement of pollution control laws (Sinnarker, *et al*, 1987).

Surveys have been conducted in the study area between Rishikesh and Kanpur to identify various point and non-point domestic sewage, industrial discharges and agricultural run off areas. Major human activities at different sampling sites are given in Table 2.3. The data on current pollution sources are given in Table 2.5.

**Table 2.5 : Survey results of pollution sources in the Ganga river between Rishikesh and Kanpur**

| Sources of pollution | Location |
|---|---|
| Domestic sewage | Rishikesh, Haridwar, Brijghat, Anupsahar, Narora, Kachalaghat, Ghatiaghat, Kannauj, Bitthor, Kanpur<br>*Note:* Sewage treatment plants are available at Rishikesh and Haridwar. |
| Industrial waste disposal | Satyanarayan (Rishikesh), Kachlaghat, Farrukhabad, Kanpur.<br>*Note:* IDPL has effluent treatment plant (but not effective?)<br>Untreated industrial effluents are released from Moradabad and Badaun Districts through Mohawa river before Kachlaghat<br>Treated and untreated Industrial effluents are released through different nalas at Sukhlaganj |
| Dead bodies disposal | Rishikesh, Haridwar, Kachlaghat, Farrukhabad, Bittor, Sukhlaganj<br>*Note:* Maximum human dead bodies disposed in the Ganga river were noted after Kachlaghat, with a record disposal at Sukhlaganj. |
| Mass bathing | Rishikesh, Haridwar, Brijghat, Narora, Kachlaghat, Ghatiaghat, Mahandighat, Bittorghat, Kanpur.<br>*Note:* Regular activity at Rishikesh, Haridwar and Brijghat<br>Other places during various important festival period and also during Full moon and New moon days. |
| Pilgrimage | Rishikesh, Haridwar, Brijghat, Narora, Kachlaghat, Ghatiaghat, Bittorghat, Kanpur.<br>*Note:* Regular at almost all places. Major religious places are at Rishikesh, Haridwar, Brijghat and Bittorghat. |

In each sampling stations point and non-point domestic wastes are still discharged to the river on both the banks. The waste disposal from IDPL is still being released into the Ganga River through Song river at Satyanarayana. Although domestic sewage from Rishikesh and Haridwar is diverted into sewage treatment plants for necessary treatment before releasing into the Ganga River large quantities of domestic sewage from these two cities are still diverted into the river through many drainages without treatment of the effluents. The sugar factory effluents are discharged into the Ganga

River indirectly through small rivulets between Bijnor and Garmukteswar. The municipal sewage of Anupsahar is discharged to the river before Narora and two kilometers away from the barrage of Narora. The wastes water of National Atomic Power Plant (NAPP) colony is also discharged into the river. The industrial effluents of Gajroula and Babrala as well as many industrial effluents of Moradabad and Badaun districts are discharged into the Ganga River in between Narora and Kachlaghat through Mohawa river. The river water at Kachlaghat turns into brownish red colour, regularly due to the mixing of sugar factory effluents. The domestic as well as tannery effluents are regularly released at Kanpur.

Naturally the carrying capacity of rivers would depend on the rate of flow, mixing and dilution of the pollutants. The flow of the Ganga river in the study area is very much reduced due to the diversion of river waters at barrages of Rishikesh, Haridwar, Bijnor and Narora. So the river, perhaps lost its carrying capacity to receive large amount of sewage effluents.

Due to discharge of industrial as well as domestic sewage major wetlands including the Ganga river are polluted to an extent that fish resources are dwindling to a considerable extent (Das and Nath, 1988). The disposal of organic wastes like molasses and acids by sugar factories and tannery effluents by leather factories along the Ganga river has been recorded in the present study. The sudden release of effluents from these factories may have adverse impact on the aquatic animals like fish, turtles, otter etc. The higher predators in the rivers like otters are greatly affected by the organic pollution through food chain.

To assess the water quality of the Ganga River, which is a major habitat for large number of animals, physico-chemical and biological analyses at different sites were carried out during 1993-94. The results of various studies are given in the following sections. Sinnarkar, et al., (1987) gave the major physico-chemical parameters, which are essential for monitoring of pollution status. These parameters were monitored every month. The results are shown in Table 2.6.

The concentrations of the BOD, COD, total hardness and total alkalinity of the river in the present study were slightly higher whereas the concentrations of total solids were comparatively lesser than the earlier studies between Rishikesh and Narora (Sinnarkar et. al. 1987). But at Kanpur the COD, total hardness and total alkalinity values were comparatively lesser than earlier studies. The present studies revealed that the river at Kanpur is less polluted in comparison with previous studies.

## Physico-chemical Properties of Water

To evaluate water quality in the habitats of various animals limnological studies were carried out at 8 sampling sites. Physico-chemical properties were analysed at monthly intervals from September 1993 to August 1994. The description of various parameters has been given below:

**Temperature** : Ambient temperature near the sampling stations and water temperature in the study area varied from 11.5 to $39.2^0$ C and 10.2 to $34.4^0$ C, respectively. Ambient temperature was always higher than water temperature during rainy and summer seasons. But in most of the months during winter season water temperatures were higher than ambient temperatures except at Rishikesh and Haridwar.

**Transparency** : Transparency values varied from 2 cm to 500 + cm in the whole study area. Lower and higher transparency values were recorded during rainy and winter season, respectively. The low transparency during rainy season was due to presence of soil particles. At Kanpur always lower values were observed due to discharge of municipal, domestic and industrial wastes before the sampling station.

**Table 2.6. : Summary of some important physico-chemical parameters to show pollution status in different sampling stations in the Upper Ganga river**

| Stations / Parameters | Pollution Domestic/Industrial | pH | DO (mg/l) | BOD (mg/l) | TDS (mg/l) | COD (mg/l) |
|---|---|---|---|---|---|---|
| Rishikesh | Domestic | 7.48 (7.04–8.01) SD 0.27 | 8.36 (6.52–10.26) SD 1.23 | 2.34 (0.64–4.50) SD 1.49 | 84.7 (46.3–140.0) SD 27.3 | 13.9 (4.6–25.6) SD 7.0 |
| Haridwar | Domestic / Industrial | 7.86 (7.05–8.52) SD 0.44 | 8.19 (6.40–10.32) SD 1.11 | 2.75 (1.76–5.0) SD 1.08 | 75.8 (52.5–93.5) SD 14.6 | 14.5 (5.6–31.6) SD 8.6 |
| Bijnor | – | 7.7 (7.05–8.65) SD 0.40 | 7.12 (5.50–8.60) SD 0.82 | 2.27 (0.32–5.55) SD 1.35 | 111.5 (61.0–169.5) SD 38.5 | 21.6 (6.0–58.8) SD 18.1 |
| Brijghat | Domestic | 7.86 (7.10–8.70) SD 1.69 | 7.04 (4.85–9.56) SD 1.66 | 1.98 (0.32–3.60) SD 1.07 | 85.8 (65.0–110.0) SD 13.2 | 19.1 (6.4–43.2) SD 11.7 |
| Narora | Domestic | 7.66 (7.00–8.30) SD 1.22 | 6.80 (4.60–9.09) SD 1.53 | 2.45 (0.68–6.00) SD 1.64 | 90.0 (67.0–111.3) SD 33.5 | 18.7 (6.4–31.8) SD 8.2 |
| Kachla ghat | Domestic/Industrial | 7.73 (6.90–8.20) SD 0.41 | 6.83 (4.77–8.52) SD 1.29 | 2.70 (0.60–9.60) SD 2.41 | 100.0 (75.0–131.3) SD 33.3 | 27.0 (4.8–66.2) SD 20.0 |
| Ghatia ghat | Domestic/Industrial | 7.66 (6.36–8.63) SD 3.31 | 6.83 (5.04–8.46) SD 1.04 | 1.99 (1.00–3.50) SD 0.85 | 114.8 (80.6–154.3) SD 24.1 | 20.7 (4.0–38.8) SD 11.6 |
| Kanpur | Domestic/Industrial | 7.66 (6.86–8.50) SD 0.68 | 5.24 (3.00–7.01) SD 1.35 | 6.36 (2.32–18.5) SD 5.48 | 188.0 (101.0–357.6) SD 76.1 | 36.0 (8.0–61.8) SD 15.7 |
| **The tolerance limits of pollution discharge :** | | | | | | |
| | WHO | 6.5–9.2 | – | 6.0 | 500 | 10 |
| | ISI standards | 6–9 | 3.0 | 3.0 | – | – |

pH : pH varied from 6.36 to 8.50. All the values were found within the highest desirable and maximum permissible limit prescribed for drinking water standard (WHO, 1971). Only at Farrukhabad in the month of July it had crossed the lower boundary of these limits i.e. 7.0 and 6.5, respectively, which may be due to heavy discharge of industrial wastes before the sampling station through Mohawa river.

Conductivity : Conductivity varied from 0.088 to 0.714 m.mho/cm. The lowest and highest values were observed at Rishikesh and Kanpur, respectively. The values were gradually increased from upstream stations to downstream stations.

Total solids : Total solids varied from 100 to 2600 mg/l. Normally during rainy season highest values were recorded in all sampling stations which were found above the highest desirable limit of drinking water standard (WHO. 1971). These may be due to soil erosion. The occasional higher value at Kachla Ghat and Farrukhabad may be due to heavy discharge of industrial wastes before Kachla Ghat in the month of January. At Kanpur always higher values were recorded than other stations. It was apparent that such higher values are due to discharge of municipal, domestic and industrial wastes. The values in almost all months at Kanpur were above the highest desirable limit of drinking water standard (WHO, 1971).

Total dissolved solids : Total dissolved solids varied from 46.3 to 357.6 mg/l. The lower and higher values were observed in the upstream and downstream, respectively. All the values were found within the limit of 500 to 1500 mg/l prescribed by different agencies (WHO, USPHS, ICMR) for drinking purposes.

Total suspended solids : Suspended solids had been varied from 12 to 1021 mg/l. There were no regular pattern of increased or decreased values in the sampling stations of upstream and downstream. The values higher than 100 mg/l are considered as harmful. Throughout our study area in almost all months the values were above 100 mg/l. This indicated that the river water should be used only after proper treatment or filtration.

**Free carbon dioxide :** Free Carbondioxide was varied from 0.00 to 16.5 mg/l. There was no regular pattern of variation in the upstream stations to downstream stations. In the month of March at Narora and in the months of January, May and August at Kanpur the values crossed the limit of 6 mg/l prescribed for fish culture (Kudesia, 1990); but this range of free $CO_2$ is not harmful for drinking purposes. Highest values of free carbondioxide were observed regularly at Kanpur.

**Dissolved oxygen :** Dissolved oxygen varied from 3.00 to 10.32 mg/l. Highest values were observed at Rishikesh and Haridwar, whereas lowest values were recorded at Kanpur. The dissolved oxygen concentrations were gradually decreased from Rishikesh to Kanpur, which is an indication of degradation of water quality from Rishikesh to Kanpur. All the values were found well above the limit 3.0 mg/l prescribed for fish culture (Kudesia, 1990). At Kanpur the concentrations just touched the margin during April, May and June.

**BOD :** The BOD values varied from 0.32 to 18.5 mg/l. There were no systematic pattern of variation from upstream and downstream stations. The values crossed the limit of 3.0 mg/l prescribed for bathing ghat (Kudesia, 1990) during some months from Rishikesh to Farrukhabad. However, in almost all months the BOD values had crossed the desired limit at Kanpur. Occasionally, the values were crossed the limit of 5.0 mg/l (International Standard for drinking water -WHO) during different months at various stations. The highest values at Kanpur is a clear indication of highest amount of organic pollutants as well as contamination by microorganisms.

**COD :** COD values varied from 4.6 to 61.8 mg/l. There were no such systematic pattern of variation in upstream and downstream sampling stations. The values were suddenly increased at Kachla Ghat and Kanpur, which may be due to discharge of oxygen demanding chemicals through industries before the sampling station. In other stations the values had crossed the limit of 4.0 and 10.0 mg/l of International Standard for drinking purpose (De, 1993).

**Calcium hardness :** Calcium hardness varied from 28 to 110 mg/l. Values were increased from upstream to downstream except some interruption at Rishikesh and Bijnor. All the values were found within the drinking water standard (250 mg/l) (De, 1993).

**Chloride :** Chloride values varied from 3.90 to 52.2 mg/l. From Rishikesh to Farrukhabad it varied within a narrow range. At Kanpur its concentration was always higher than other sampling stations, which may be due to heavy discharge of municipal and domestic wastes. At all sampling stations the values were always found to be within the drinking water standards (WHO, 1971).

**Total alkalinity :** Total alkalinity values varied from 48 to 325 mg/l. Lower and higher values were observed in the upstream and downstream sampling stations, respectively. Less alkalinity shows better taste of the water. Alkaline waters have no health hazards.

**Total hardness :** Total hardness varied from 52 to 194 mg/l. The values had crossed the highest desirable limit of 100 mg/l prescribed for drinking water standard. However, the values are within the maximum permissible limit (500 mg/l) prescribed for drinking water standard (WHO, 1971). Although a systematic pattern was not seen in the values of different stations still the upstream stations were shown lower values in comparison with downstream stations.

**Hydrogen sulphide :** Hydrogen sulphide values varied from 0.17 to 53.3 mg/l. The values were shown fluctuating in different sampling stations. The hydrogen sulphide has some toxic effects on the aquatic organisms. In all sampling stations the hydrogen sulphide values were higher than 0.05 mg/l (USEPA limit).

**Magnesium hardness** : Magnesium hardness was varied from 9 to 118 mg/l. It did not show any systematic pattern of variation. The values have shown fluctuations in different sampling stations. However, all the values were within the International Standard for drinking water (123-617 mg/l) (De, 1993).

**Calcium** : Calcium was varied from 11.22 to 44.08 mg/l. Lowest and highest values were observed at Haridwar and Kanpur, respectively. The values were increased from upstream to downstream except at Rishikesh and Bijnor. All the values were found within the limit of International Standard for drinking water (100 mg/l) (De, 1993).

**Magnesium** : Magnesium was varied from 2.18 to 28.83 mg/l. There was no systematic pattern of variation in this parameter from upstream to downstream. The quantity of magnesium was very less in comparison with the International Standard for drinking water 30-150 mg/l (De, 1993).

**Residual chlorine** : Residual chlorine values were varied from 0.00 to 73.66 mg/l. Chlorine is primarily added to the waters for destroying the harmful microorganisms. In this range it is not harmful to use the water for drinking. But the water having more than 1.0 mg/l residual chlorine is harmful for aquatic animals if they come in contact with such water for long period (Kudesia, 1990). The average values from Garmukteswar to Kanpur had crossed the limit 1.0.

## BIOLOGICAL PARAMETERS

### Introduction

The presence of potential human health hazards from persistent bio-accumulative chemicals may be more readily detected by analysis of aquatic organisms than by analysis of water samples (NRTC, 1984 in Hirethota and Ringler, 1993). Knowledge on the species availability and their habitat ranges elucidates the habitat conditions. Pollution makes it possible for some species to extend their distribution, but some disappear from the specific habitats due to pollution. During the present study in addition to hydrological and limnological studies, aspects related to biological material have also been analysed to assess the water quality in terms of biological components. Using standard methods mentioned earlier collected monthly samples of phyto and zoo planktons, and coliforms. In addition different invertebrate and vertebrate animals were also collected from the Ganga river to gather information on species diversity and habitat conditions

### Zooplankton

The density of zooplankton was varied from 24 to 280 no./l. Lowest number was observed at Rishikesh and the number was increased towards the downstream. The number of species of the family Difflugiidae and Branchionidae were occupied the highest position in comparison with others in the river Ganga from Rishikesh and Kanpur. Species like *Arcella discoides*, *Difflugia sp.* and *Cypris sp.* were found in all the sampling stations (Table 2.7).

### Phytoplankton

The density of phytoplankton varied from 36 to 2116 no./l. Highest and lowest number of phytoplankton was observed during summer season and rainy season respectively. But the river Ganga is a snow-fed river. In the month of June 1994 the river Ganga received a huge amount of water from Himalayan region by melting of ice. The increase in water level of the river was blocked completely at Narora barrage after passing through different barrages at Rishikesh, Haridwar and Bijnor.

Due to high water level in the first five sampling stations lowest values of phytoplankton were observed in the month of June. The number of phytoplankton were gradually increased from Rishikesh to Kanpur except some minor differences at Haridwar and Narora which may be due to discharge of municipal wastes in the upper Ganga River *i.e.,* at Haridwar and Anupsahar, respectively.

**Table 2.7 : Distribution of Zooplankton in different sampling stations of the river Ganga**

| Zooplankton | Species | Zooplankton | Species |
|---|---|---|---|
| **Protozoa** | | | B. q. mirabilis |
| Arcellidae | Arcella discoides | | Keratella tropica |
| Difflugidae | Difflugia oblonga | | Platyias quadricornis |
| | Difflugia sp. | Colurellidae | Lepadella ovalis |
| | Centrophyxis ecornis | Lecanidae | Lecane luna |
| | Centrophyxis aculeata | | L. bulla |
| | Centrophyxis constricta | Dicranophoridae | Dicranophorus dolerus |
| Amphileptidae | Litonatus fasciola | Filiniidae | Filinia opoliensis |
| Parameciidae | Paramoecium sp. | | F. longiseta |
| Vaginicolidae | Epistylis sp. | **Arthropoda** | |
| Vorticellidae | Vorticella sp. | Daphniidae | Daphnia sp. |
| Euplotidae | Euplotes sp. | | Simocephalus exspinosus |
| **Aschelminthes** | | Moinidae | Moina brachiata |
| Epihanidae | Epiphanes clavulata | Chydorinae | Chydorus sp. |
| Brachionidae | Anuraeopsis fissa | | Chydorus sphaericus |
| | Brachionus angularis | Aloninae | Alona rectangula |
| | B. bidentata | Diaptomidae | Diaptomus sp. |
| | B. caudatus | | Neodiaptomus sp. |
| | B. calyciflorus | Cyclopidae | Cyclops sp. |
| | B. patulus | Cypridae | Cypris sp. |
| | B. quadridentatus | | Cypris subglobosa |
| | B. urceolaris | | |

## Invertebrate Fauna

In the present study surveys have been made to collect various aquatic Invertebrates, which may indicate pollution status of the river. Animals like insects, freshwater prawns and molluscs were collected from the sampling sites by using different techniques. The molluscans and crustaceans were identified with the help of Zoological Survey of India, Kolkata. The details of these animals are as follows:

From the study area a total of 51 species of insects belonging to 8 orders were identified. The list of insects collected in different stations is given in Table 2.8. In the entire study area the insects belonging to order hemiptera, odonata and coleoptera were dominated. *Bactis* sp., *Corixa hieroglyphica*, *C. promonotoria*, *Micronecta* sp. *Chironomous* sp. *and Monopelopia* sp. were well dominated in most of the stations. According to Bilgrami (1991), these species can be used as organic pollution indicators. A total of 42 and 22 species of insects were identified at Narora and Rishikesh, respectively. The low species diversity at Rishikesh and Haridwar may be due to high water current, high wind velocity and scarcity of macrophytes. Out of 40 insect species at Kanpur, 7 species are indicators of organic pollution.

In the study area a total of 15 species of molluscs were identified (Table 2.9). Most of the specimens collected in our study area were after monsoon. The specimens were collected from the bank as well as from the shallow waters.

**Table 2.8 : List of aquatic insects found in the Ganga river between Rishikesh and Kanpur**

| Order/Family | Type | Order/Family | Type |
|---|---|---|---|
| **Ephemeroptera** | | | Laccophilus sp. |
| Bactidae | Bactis sp. | | Canthydrus sp. |
| | Ephemerella sp. | Hydrophilidae | Hydrochus sp. |
| | Cloeon sp. | | Hydrocanthus sp. |
| | Epeorus | | Hydrophilus olivaceous |
| | Heptagenia | | Amphiops sp. |
| **Odonata** | | | Regimbartia attenuata |
| Cordulegusteridae | Cordulegaster sp. | Hylipidae | Haliplus pulchellus |
| Gomphidas | Mesogemphus sp. | **Diptera** | |
| Coenagriedae | Ischura sp. | Chironomidae | Chironomous sp. |
| Labellulidae | Potomarcha obsura | | Monopelopia sp. |
| | Anisopteran larva | Culicidae | Anopheles larvae |
| **Hemiptera** | | | Culex larvae |
| Belostomatidae | Belostoma | **Zygoptera** | Lestes |
| Notonectidae | Notonecta sp. | | Zygopteran larvae |
| | Antisops sp. | | |
| Nepidae | Ranatra filiformis | **Plecoptera** | Neoperia |
| | Laccotrephes griseus | | Isoperia |
| Corixidae | Corixa hieroglyphica | | Alloperia |
| | C. promontoria | **Trichoptera** | Limephilus |
| Pleidae | Plea sp. | | Leptocella |
| Gerridae | Gerris ossarum | | Triaenodes |
| | G. spinole | | Glossosoma |
| | Sphaenoderma sp | | Hydropsyche |
| | Lethocerus sp. | | Hesperophylax |
| | Hydrometra sp. | | |
| **Coleoptera** | | | |
| Dytiscidae | Cybistar tripunctatus | | |
| | Dytiscus sp. | | |

**Table 2.9 : List of freshwater molluscs in the study area**

| Phylum: | Mollusca | Phylum: | Mollusca |
|---|---|---|---|
| Class : | Gastropoda | | L. (P). acuminata f. rufescens Gray |
| Order: | Mesogastropoda | Family: | Planorbidae |
| Family: | Viviparidae | | Indoplanorbis exusstus (Deshayes) |
| | Bellamya bengalensis f. typica (Lamarck) | Family: | Physidae |
| Family: | Pilidae | | Physa acuta (Draparnaud) |
| | Pila globosa (Swainson) | Class: | Bivalvia |
| Family: | Bithyniidae | Order: | Unionoida |
| | Digoniostoma cerameopoma (Benson) | Family: | Unionidae |
| Family: | Thiaridae | | Lamellidens corrlanus(Lea) |
| | Thiara (Thiara) scabra (Mueller) | Family: | Amblemidae |
| | T.(Melanoides) tuberculata (Mueller) | | Parreysia favidens deltae (Benson) |
| | T.(Tarebia) lineata (Gray) | | P. (Radiatula) caerulea (Lea) |
| Order: | Basommatophora | Order: | Veneroida |
| Family: | Lymnaeidae | Family: | Corbiculidae |
| | Lymnaea (Pseudosuccinea) acuminata f. chlyamys Benson | | Corbicula striatella |

The crustaceans identified in the study area are *Macrobrachium altifrens* (Henderson), *Macrobrachium lamarrei lamerrei* (H.M. Edw.), *Macrobrachium henderso dayanum* and *Caridina* sp.

## Fish Fauna

The fishes forms the largest group of living natural resources in the Ganga River (Ghosh 1991). During the present study a total of 83 species of fishes belonging to 20 families have been collected from the study area (Rishikesh to Kanpur). The list of fishes identified during the present study is shown in Table 2.10.

**Table 2.10 : List of fishes identified from the Ganga river during 1993-94**

| | | | |
|---|---|---|---|
| **Family: Clupeidae** | *D. rerio* | *N. zonatus* | *M. bleekeri* |
| *Gudusia chapra* | *Gara gotyla* | *N. scaturingina* | *Rita rita* |
| **Family: Notopteridae** | *Gara prshadi* | *N. multifasciatus* | **Family: Sisoridae** |
| *Notopterus chitala* | *Labeo rohita* | *N. savena* | *Bagarius bagarius* |
| *N. notopterus* | *L. boga* | *Lepidocephalichthys guntea* | *Nangra nangra* |
| **Family : Cyprinidae** | *L. calbasu* | **Family: Anabautidae** | **Family: Chascidae** |
| *Amblypharyngodon mola* | *L. pangusia* | *Colisa lalius* | *Chaca chaca* |
| *A. melettinus* | *L. gonius* | *C. fasciata* | **Family: Schilbeidae** |
| *Barilus bola* | *Osteobrama cotio* | *Anabas testudineus* | *Ailia colia* |
| *B. barila* | *Oxygaster bacaila* | **Family: Centropomidae** | *Clupisoma garua* |
| *B. modestus* | *O. boopis* | *Chanda ranga* | *Eutropiichthys vacha* |
| *B. vagra* | *Puntius sophore* | *C. nama* | **Family: Pangasidae** |
| *Chela laobuca* | *P. ticto* | **Family: Nandidae** | *Pungasium pungasius* |
| *Catla catla* | *P. chola* | | |
| *Tor tor* | *P. sarana* | *Nandus nandus* | **Family: Heteropneutidae** |
| *Tor putitora* | *Laubuca atper* | | |
| *Cirrhinus reba* | *Rasbora daniconius* | **Family: Badidae** | *Heteropneustes fossilis* |
| *C. mrigala* | **Family: Siluridae** | *Badis badis* | **Family: Clariidae** |
| *Crossocheilus latius* | *Ompok bimaculotus* | **Family: Mastacembelidae** | *Clarias batrachus* |
| *Danio devario* | *O. pabda* | *Mastacembelus armatus* | *C. magur* |
| *D. dangila* | *Wallago attu* | *M. puncalus* | **Family:** |
| **Family: Gobitidae** | **Family: Bagridae** | **Ophiocephaledae** | |
| *Botia dario* | *Mystus vittatus* | *M. acculatus* | *Channa gachua* |
| *Nemochilus botia* | *Mystus seenghala* | **Family: Belonidae** | *C. marulius* |
| *N. corica* | *M. cavasius* | *Xenentodon cancila* | *C. punctatus* |
| *N.bevasni* | *M. oar* | **Family: Gobiidae** | *C. striatus* |
| *N. montanus* | *M. tangara* | *Glossogobius giuris* | *C. slewartii* |

## Turtle Species

Based on collection of shell and live specimens eight species belonging to four genera and one family of hard-shell turtles (66.6%), and 4 species belonging to three genera and one family of soft-shell turtles (33.3%) were identified in the Ganga river (Table 2.11).

**Table 2.11 : Freshwater turtles in the Ganga River between Rishikesh and Kanpur**

| Family | Genus | Species | English Common Name |
|---|---|---|---|
| Emydidae | Geoclemys | hamiltonii | Spotted pond turtle |
| | Hardella | thurjii | Crowned river turtle |
| | Kachuga | kachuga | Red-crowned turtle |
| | Kachuga | dhongoka | Striped roof turtle |
| | Kachuga | smithii | Brown roofed turtle |
| | Kachuga | tecta | Indian roofed turtle |
| | Kachuga | tentoria | Indian tent turtle |
| | Melanochelys | trijuga | Indian black turtle |
| Trionychidae | Lissemys | punctata | Indian flapshell turtle |
| | Aspideretes | gangeticus | Indian soft-shell turtle |
| | Aspideretes | hurum | Indian peacock soft-shell  turtle |
| | Chitra | indica | Narrow headed soft-shell turtle |

## Crocodiles

The crocodile species identified from the Ganga River between Rishikesh and Kanpur were *gharial* and *mugger*. Many taxonomists studied the crocodiles in India. These two species were included in two separate families: Gavialidae (gharial) and Crocodylidae (mugger).

## Bird Species

A list of bird species found in different areas along the Ganga River between Rishikesh and Kanpur is given in Table 2.12. A total of 48 species of wetland birds in 36 genus and 14 families were identified in the present study area. The species composition along different sampling sites indicates that more number of migratory water fowls visit upper Ganga River. The number of species and the population are decreased in the lower Ganga River. It is observed that in the Ganga River maximum visiting birds are carnivores (66%).

**Table 2.12 : Avifauna along the Ganga River between Rishikesh and Kanpur**

| Family | Phalacrocoracidae |
| | *Phalacrocorax carbo, P. fuscicollis, P. niger, Anhinga rufa* |
| Family | Ardeidae |
| | *Ardeola grayii, Ardea cinerea, Bubulcus ibis, Ardea alba, Egretta garzetta, Nycticorax nycticorax* |
| Family | Ciconiidae |
| | *Mycteria leucocephala, Anastomus oscitans, Ciconia episcopus, C. ciconia, Ephippiorhynchus asiaticus* |
| Family | Theskiornithidae |
| | *Pseudibis papillosa, Platalea leucorodia* |
| Family | Amatiade |
| | *Anser indicus, Tadorna ferruginea, Anas acuta, A. crecca, A. poecilorhyncha, A. platyrhynchos, A. strepera, A. penelope, A. clypeata Neeta rufina, Sarkidiornis melanotos* |
| Family | Accipitridae |
| | *Elanus caeruleus, Gyps bengalensis, Neophron percnopterus* |
| Family | Gruidae |
| | *Grus antigone* |
| Family | Rallidae |
| | *Amaurornis phoenicurus, Porphyrio porphyrio, Fulica atra* |
| Family | Jacanidae |
| | *Hydrophasianus chirurgus* |
| Family | Recurvirostridae |
| | *Himantopus himantopus* |
| Family | Charadriidae |
| | *Vanellus indicus, V.spinosus, V.malabaricus, Tringa totanus* |
| Family | Laridae |
| | *Sterna aurantia, Rynchops albicollis* |
| Family | Alcedinidae |
| | *Ceryle rudis, Alcedo atthis, Halcyon smyrnensis* |

## Aquatic mammals

In the study stretch of the Ganga River two species of aquatic mammals have been identified. They are smooth coated otter, *Lutra perspicillata* and Gangetic dolphin *Platanista gangetica*. Poaching and habitat destruction were the major threats for continued survival of these mammals. The series of barrages on the river have also contributed for the damage of habitat.

## Habitat Requirements

In India most of the rivers including Ganga River have a wide range of biotic resources. The aquatic animals in the rivers have specific requirements. The presence of one species shows the availability of such specific factors. Since each animal live in a possible range of habitat requirements in which it is expected the other associated animals, which have similar requirements, may also live in those specific habitats. It is necessary to study the group of animals rather than studying an individual animal in an ecosystem to understand the quality of the habitat. Various species identified in the Ganga River inhabit in a similar habitat conditions with minor specific requirements. The summary of ecological parameters required for different vertebrate species in the Ganga River are shown in Table 2.13.

**Table 2.13 :  Summary of ecological parameters of aquatic vertebrates in the Ganga between Rishikesh and Kanpur (1993-94)**

| S.No. | Study area | Habitat parameters | Species available |
|---|---|---|---|
| 1. | Upper Ganga river (Rishikesh–Bijnor) | Riffle area, Rocky, sandy and muddy river banks, reservoirs in up-stream barrages at Rishikesh, Haridwar and Bijnor, <br><br> river depth 2.2–25.0 m <br> river width   200–1000 m <br> river flow 12.9 m/min (minimum) <br> Air temp.1.0–37.5 °C, <br> Water temp.11.3–26.1 °C, <br> pH 7.04–8.65, DO 5.50–10.32 mg/l, <br> BOD 0.32–5.55 mg/l, <br> TDS 46.3–169.5 mg/l | Fish including Mahseer, turtles, crocodiles wetland birds, otters? |
| 2. | Middle Ganga river (Bijnor–Narora) | Sandy and muddy banks, deep pools, sandy peninsulas, very shallow river after Bijnor barrage, Reservoir upstream Narora barrage, <br><br> river depth 0.5–20.0 m <br> river width 200–1000 m <br> river flow 11.1 m/min (minimum) <br> Air temp. 4.0–45.5 °C <br> Water temp.12.0–34.5 °C <br> pH 7.0–8.7, DO 4.6–9.56 mg/l <br> BOD 0.32–6.0 mg/l <br> TDS 65.0–111.3 mg/l | Fish, (stray cases of  mahseer) turtles, crocodiles, wetland birds, Gangetic dolphins |
| 3. | Lower Ganga river (Narora–Kanpur) | Shallow river after Narora barrage, sandy and muddy banks, sandy peninsulas, <br><br> river depth 0.5–15.0 m <br> river width 150– 1000 m <br> river flow   10.0 m/min (minimum) <br> Air temp.10.0–46.0°C <br> Water temp 15.0–39.0 °C <br> pH 6.3–8.6, DO 3.0–8.5 mg/l <br> BOD 0.60–18.5 mg/l <br> TDS 75.0–357.6 mg/l | Fish, Turtles, crocodiles, wetland birds, Gangetic dolphin (stray cases) |

Biomonitoring of the Ganga River was carried out in a stretch between Rishikesh and Kanpur during 1993-94. During the present study various aspects of water quality like physico-chemical and biological analyses were carried out. The following are the major conclusions drawn from the results obtained in the present study.

The physico-chemical parameters of the Ganga water in 8 sampling stations were analysed. From these studies it was concluded that the Ganga river from Rishikesh to Farrukhabad water is slightly polluted as the parameters like BOD, COD, suspended solids, residual chlorine, hydrogen sulphide, total coliform and faecal coliform were crossed, irregularly, the tolerance limits prescribed by different agencies for different purposes. Occasionally, the river water at Kachla Ghat and Farrukhabad were acidic in nature which may be due to discharge of acidic industrial effluents before Kachla Ghat through Mohawa river. All the water quality parameters were lesser in the upstream stations in comparison with downstream stations except dissolved oxygen and net primary productivity (NPP) which were decreased towards Kanpur from upstream stations. The concentrations of dissolved oxygen as well as quantity of NPP at Kanpur were lowest and the concentrations of all other parameters were found highest here. The river water at Kanpur is moderately polluted as all the above parameters and total solid concentrations here crossed the tolerance limits prescribed by different agencies for different purposes. These may be due to heavy discharge of domestic wastes, municipal sewage and industrial effluents. The free carbondioxide values had also occasionally crossed the limit of 6 mg/l prescribed for fish culture here and at Narora which is an indication of high amounts of pollutants in the river water; but not harmful for other purposes. All the values of different water quality parameters observed from Rishikesh to Farrukhabad can classify the river water as class B to C in this zone. So in this zone the river water can be used for different purposes after proper treatment followed by disinfection. But at Kanpur all the observed values of water quality parameters always crossed the limits prescribed for class C type of water. So it was advised to the authority of Kanpur municipality and different industries in and around the Kanpur City that they should properly treat the sewage and effluents before discharge into the river.

In the present study area a rich biodiversity has been identified. The study on freshwater turtles in the Ganga River is first of its kind. A total of 12 species of freshwater turtles occur in this stretch. Both species of crocodiles, mugger and gharial are still present. Presence of different age group indicate that natural breeding of turtles and crocodiles is going in the study stretch of the Ganga River. Although one of the aquatic mammal, the otter is not found during the study period, Gangetic dolphin occur in the stretch from Bijnor.

The survey results during the present short study period may not indicate the population status of higher animals like turtles, crocodiles and dolphin. However, from the data gathered it is apparent that all the species are facing threats like exploitation and habitat degradation. The populations of fishes including Mahseer were reduced and according to fishermen it was very hard to catch large sized fish in this stretch. After considering the Ganga River as a good habitat, captive reared gharial have been released in the upstream of the river. However, due to lack of protection these animals might have killed in the fishing activities. Due to heavy human activities animals like crocodiles and dolphins are not getting suitable habitats. River otters might have been totally extinct in this stretch. While large number of migratory birds are visiting the upper stretch of the river but their numbers are very low in the lower stretch. This may be due to rich  food sources in the upstream than in the downstream, which is comparatively polluted than the upstream. Large scale exploitation of aquatic resources are still continuing. Freshwater turtles are illegally caught for sale in turtle markets. Shooting of wetland birds is a normal practice in some villages along the study area of the Ganga river. Gangetic dolphins were also killed in fishing nets.

Looking into the various problems it is concluded that unless urgent and strict measures are taken to protect the animals in the Ganga river most of the species, especially turtles, crocodiles and dolphin, will soon become extinct.

## SUMMARY

Biomonitoring of the Ganga River was conducted (1993-95) between Rishikesh and Kanpur to determine the water quality and biodiversity. The study area was comprised of a 645 km (approx.) of the Ganga River from Rishikesh, after the river reaches the plains, and up to Kanpur in Uttar Pradesh. The study area was situated between 30°07'-26°28' N latitude to 78°19'-80°21' E longitude. The study. area experiences typical tropical monsoon climate with three distinct seasons viz. summer, rainy and winter. May was recorded as the hottest month during summer when the average maximum temperature reached up to 46°C during 1994. During the study period maximum annual rainfall was recorded as 86.0 cm during 1994. In winter the temperature came down to 2°C at Rishikesh and 6°C at Kanpur.

Intensive studies were conducted to investigate the water quality by analyzing physico-chemical, bacteriological and other biological parameters. Species diversity of higher vertebrates was identified from the study stretch of the Ganga River. The eco-hydrological information of the Ganga River in the study stretch is provided in this paper.

## GLOSSARY

**Ecohydrology** : Integration of Ecology and Hydrology
**Biodiversity** : All the Different Forms of Life that share Our Biosphere
**Habitat Degradation** : Loss of Suitable Habitat for Species Survival
**Biomonitoring** : Use of Bioindicators for Monitoring Habitat Quality

## ACKNOWLEDGMENTS

We are grateful to the Ganga Project Directorate, Ministry of Environment and Forests, Govt. of India for providing financial assistance to carry out the present study. Thanks are due to Vice Chancellor, Jiwaji University, Gwalior for permitting to conduct the study.

## REFERENCES

- APHA, AWWA, WPCF, (1989). *Standard Methods for Estimation of Water and Waste Water.* 17th ed., Washington, D.C.
- Bilgrami, K.S. (1991). Biological Profile of the Ganga: Zooplankton, Fish, Birds and Other Minor Fauna. In: *The Ganga Scientific Study.* Ed. Krishnamurti *et al.* Northern Book centre, New Delhi.
- Cairns, J. (1982). *Biological Monitoring in Water Pollution.* Pergamon Press.
- Chakraburthy, R.D., Roy, P and Singh, S.B. (1959). A Quantitative Study of Plankton and the Physio-chemical Conditions of the river Jamuna at Allahabad. *Indian J. Fish.* 6(6):186-203.
- Chawla, G. and Viswanathan, P.N. (1989). Role of Predictive Ecotoxicology and Biological Monitoring in the Management of Aquatic Ecosystem. Ed. Agrawal, V.P. *et. al. Publ. Society of Bioscience,* Muzaffarnagar.
- Das, S.M. and Nath, S. (1988). *Aquatic Pollution and Fisheries in India.* Ed. Nath, S. Creative Publ. New Delhi.
- David, A. (1955). Notes on Bionomics and Some Early Stages of Mahanadi mahseer. *J. As. Soc. Bengal.* 19(2):197-289.
- De., A.K. (1993). *Environmental Chemistry,* Wiley Eastern Limited, New Delhi.
- Ghosh, A.K. (1991). *The Ganga : A Profile and Biological Resources.* Ed. Jairajpuri, M.S. Zoological Survey of India, Calcutta.
- Haslam, S.M. (1991). River Pollution and Ecological Prospective. CBS Publ. Delhi.

- Hirethota, P.S. and Ringler, N.H. (1993). Fish Population as Bioindicators of Long Term Contaminant Related Stress. In: *Advances in Limnology* p189-206. Ed. Singh, H.R. Narendra Publ. House, Delhi.
- Krishnamurti, C.R. Bilgrami, K. S. Das, T.M. and Mathur, R.P. (1991). The Ganga. A Scientific Study. Publ. Northern, Book Centre, New Delhi.
- Kudesia, V.P. (1990). Water Pollution. 3rd revised Ed. Pragati Prakashan, Meerut.
- Kulkarni, C.V. (1988). Recent Advances in Our Knowledge of the Biology and Conservation of Mahseer. *J. Indian Fish. Assoc.* 18:203-212.
- Mathur, R.P. (1991). Sampling Stations for Water Quality Monitoring. In: *The Ganga Scientific Study.* Ed. Krishnamurti *et. all* P. Northern Book Centre, Delhi.
- Rajan, S. (1963). *Ecology of the Fishes of the river Pykara and Moyar* (Nilgiris). South India. Proc. Nat. Aca. Sci. India. 58:291.
- Sinnarkar, S.N., Kesarwani, S.K. and Bhat, S.G. (1987). *River Ganga* (An overview of Environmental Research), NEERI, Nagpur.
- Trivedy, R.K. and Goel, P.K. (1986). *Chemical and Biological Methods for Water Pollution Studies,* Environmental Publ. Karad.
- Vats, V. and Dalwani, R. (1992). *Hydrological and Ecological Features of the river Ganges in India.* Seminar on Cons. of Rriver Dolphins of the Indian Subcontinent, New Delhi.
- Vass, K.K., Raina, H.S., Zutshi, O.P. and Khan, M.A. (1977). Hydrobiological Studies on River Jhelum *Geobios.* 4(6):238-242.
- World Health Organisation (WHO) (1971). *Indian Standard for Drinking Water,* 3rd Edn. Geneva.

# 3

# Microbial Contamination of Drinking Water Sources: A Real Hazard in Modern India

*S. R. Naik*

The world is reeling under the impact of expanding population and continuing neglect of environment. Although most of the rich countries have managed to reach the ideal of zero population growth, the developing countries including India have generally failed to solve this problem. These countries therefore continue to add to more numbers to their already high population and consequently to the number of people with significant health problems. On the other hand, the neglect of the environment is a more global phenomenon, of which even many advanced countries are guilty. The environmental degradation encompasses several aspects, of which air and water pollution are the major concerns of today.

Water borne diseases continue to cause significant mortality and morbidity worldwide; for instance, in 1997, diarrhea (including dysentery) ranked the sixth among the major killer diseases globally accounting for an estimated 2.5 million deaths and was the topmost cause for morbidity causing 4 billion cases (World Health Organization, 1998). Alma Ata declaration (1978) said "An estimated 80 percent of all diseases and over one-third of deaths in developing countries are caused by consumption of contaminated water and on an average as much as one-tenth of each person's productive time is sacrificed for water related diseases". This article focuses chiefly at contamination of drinking water with sewage resulting in epidemics of hepatitis virus E as an illustrative example.

## Drinking Water Sources and Pollution in Urban and Rural Areas

Water is essential to sustain life. Surprisingly, although it constitutes two-thirds of the earth, it is threatening to become the single most important scarce resource for future and therefore ways to preserve this important resource vital for all living beings has engaged global attention. Scarcity of water is compounded by the constant threat of pollution and contamination of water.

Let us first look at the sources of drinking water and how they get polluted. The sources of drinking water for the majority of India's population include rivers, watersheds, lakes, ponds, wells and springs, which constantly get polluted with undesirable matter of which human and animal excreta are the most important. The cities and small towns usually derive water supply from these surface sources after processing through water treatment plants, whereas the villages derive their water supply directly from surface water sources. In recent times, ground water has become available as an alternative source of drinking water through hand pumps, which have been popularized by the Indian government both in the cities and the villages. These hand pumps draw ground water from deeper subsoil and hence are generally much safer microbially. Their wider use however have caused significant ecological disturbances and therefore calls for greater regulatory efforts of the government. To understand how the waterborne diseases differ epidemiologically between urban and rural areas, it is important to understand the differences in their water resources and the mode of contamination. These will be examined separately below:

Contamination of urban drinking water sources : Urban water supply is usually derived from large surface water sources like rivers or lakes from which water is channeled through water treatment plants. Water is subjected here to purification procedures such as flocculation, sedimentation, filtration and chlorination and then stored in large reservoirs in different parts of the city. Water treatment in urban areas frequently becomes ineffective because of unimaginably high pollution levels of surface water particularly in rainy seasons or when water sources become relatively drier as in hot summers.

Most water supply authorities also treat purified water stored in reservoirs to a round of secondary chlorination before final supply to the periphery. Contamination in urban water supply occurs at multiple points.

First and perhaps the most common, is pollution of raw water due to contamination through city sewage drains. City sewer drains are normally diverted to meet the river water downstream of water treatment plants, so that raw water is protected from contamination. Frequently this arrangement breaks down as occurs in rapidly increasing population and as the city limits expand. In such situations, sewage drains pass through haphazardly through the city and open upstream of the water treatment plant. This was the cause of a major epidemic of hepatitis E in the city of Kanpur in 1991. Constant monitoring of water contamination indices like biological and chemical oxygen demand, chloride and nitrate levels as also the coliform and noncoliform bacterial counts is necessary to detect early signs of contamination, so as to check its cause and take remedial action to prevent further pollution. In the event of such contamination, it may be essential to step up chlorination so that the treated water stays free of high coliform court and has adequate free chlorine levels. *Second*, water authorities fail to maintain the level of residual free chlorine in the treated water, which is supplied to the city. Often, the quantities of chlorine required to keep this level within permissible limits are much higher than normal, particularly when raw water contamination has already occurred.

*Third*, the water in the pipes carrying treated and chlorinated water may get contaminated at any point while they traverse the city to reach the water reservoirs and from there to the peripheral points of supply. Such contamination often occurs due to breaks in the pipes due to high pressures inside them and through faulty joints especially at points where the sewage drains run in close proximity or even cross water pipes. Contamination does not occur if water supply is continuous because higher pressures within the water pipes prevent contamination. In most cities of the developing world however, water supply is intermittent, which makes it possible for sewage to contaminate the water through a process of reverse osmosis when water pipes are dry. If such contamination occurs prior to the pipes reaching the reservoir, secondary chlorination takes care of it and the health hazards from such contamination are not as widespread as when contamination occurs at source or there is failure of chlorination. However, if contamination occurs distal to the reservoirs, it may be totally undetected and no warning may be available to the population; fortunately, the health hazards of such contamination are limited to small population like those residing in a small area or a building.

The above described situations are extremely common in our country and can be ascribed to poor work culture prevailing in government controlled water supply agencies, which additionally also suffer from chronic administrative and financial malaise. These finally lead to intermittent or sometimes continuous supply of contaminated water to the public. Water-borne diseases are therefore endemic in our cities, which also suffer seasonally from large scale epidemics of these diseases.

*Contamination of rural water supply* : The people of rural areas, on the other hand derive water directly from surface sources and drink water which goes through no purification processer unless they on their own use domestic filters or other methods like boiling. The villagers use peripheral surface water sources, which too are often contaminated. However, due to lower population density, although water borne diseases are endemic are rare in villages large outbreaks.

## Transmission of Waterborne Diseases

Waterborne diseases may occur due to (a) direct transmission to the host through water of viruses (hepatitis A and E, rotavirus, poliomyelitis, etc), bacteria (cholera, enterobacteriaceae, leptospira, etc) and parasites (amebiasis, giardiasis), or (b) transmission through an aquatic host like cyclopes (guinea worm, fish tape worm) or snails (schistosomiasis). Of those who get infected, only a few suffer from disease, which becomes clinically manifest after a variable incubation period. Most infections are transmitted from person to person, the infected person thus serving as a source of infection and water a vehicle. Other infections like mentioned above require another host like an aquatic host. Life of infection is thus maintained in nature.

## Prevention of Water borne Diseases

Water borne diseases can be prevented by maintaining drinking water sources clean within permissible limits. This can be done with cooperation between the public and the government. The government is expected to enact adequate legislation to prevent the public from defiling these sources and to educate the public about the need for clean water and more importantly to ensure implementation of such legislation. Further, the government should find innovative ways of involving the public in guarding the water sources from the menace of pollution. The public has to reciprocate government's efforts by following the rules of hygiene and reporting promptly instances of willful or inadvertent pollution of water sources.

The water supply of the cities is handled entirely by the civic authorities, who are in charge of purifying raw water from surface sources and distributing to the public. Impact of provision of safer water supply on water borne diseases can be impressive and may bring down the death rates in a community due to different water borne diseases by one-fourth to three-fourths. In practice however, standards of maintaining, purifying and distributing clean water to the public and maintaining the water and sewage pipelines free of leaks are extremely poor in most developing countries including India. It is thus essential to improve the working of the civic agencies through tighter control by government and vigilance from a more enlightened public. There are already strong voices in favour of privatizing water supply and sanitation, which may expose the controlling agencies to more effective pressures of public and courts , since most people today believe that the government agencies continue to rece021ive immunity from actions against incompetence and other acts of commission.

## Hepatitis E

Hepatitis E is an enterically (feco-orally) transmitted RNA virus, which may represent a prototype for epidemic and endemic water-borne infection. This article will deal briefly with different epidemics of hepatitis E (HEV) in India with reference to experience of author and his colleagues with the world's largest epidemic, which ravaged the people of the city of Kanpur in Uttar Pradesh in 1991.

The first major epidemic of HEV occurred in Delhi in 1955-56 causing jaundice to an estimated 29,300 persons (1.4% of the then Delhi's population of 2.1 million) (Vishwanathan, 1957). Elegant investigations of this epidemic, then world's largest such experience, led to sound insight into transmission, pathogenesis and clinical features of HEV. The epidemic followed a bout of heavy flood in river Yamuna leading to opening of a large open sewage drain into a water pumping station, which supplied drinking water to a large part of the city. Thus the water supply was grossly contaminated during the period November 10 to 17, 1955. The epidemic began in the first week of December 1955, reached a peak in 2 weeks and then rapidly subsided within 6-7 weeks. It was estimated that 29, 300 persons (2.3% of the population receiving contaminated water) were affected during the epidemic. Attack rate was much higher in areas receiving contaminated water as compared to areas receiving water from another source (2.3% *vs.* 0.34%). The attack rate was the highest in young adults (1.2% in those aged <14 years, 2.9% in the 15-39 year age group, and 2.0% in those aged >40 years). There were no delayed cases or a secondary peak of cases. Occurrence of a single highly compressed peak of cases during the epidemic was interpreted as absence of significant intrafamilial spread.

Several subsequent large epidemics of hepatitis E have been described from the Indian subcontinent (Sreenivasan *et al,* 1978, Tandon *et al,* 1982) including the largest one in Kanpur in 1991 that we investigated (Naik *et al*, 1992), which affected an estimated 80, 000 persons. All these had the following epidemilogical features: *(i)* large outbreaks that affect several hundred to several thousand persons and follow use of fecal contaminated water; *(ii)* a high attack rate among young adults in the age group of 15-40 years with relative sparing of children; *(iii)* male-to female case ratio of 1:1 to 4:1; *(iv)* a particularly high attack rate and mortality among pregnant women; and *(v)* a course varying from single-peaked, short lived outbreaks to prolonged, multi-peaked epidemics lasting for over a year. Based on these epidemiologic features and the high prevalence among Indian adults of protective antibodies against HAV, the other enterically transmitted hepatitis virus, any large waterborne epidemic of acute viral hepatitis among adults in our country can be safely presumed as related to HEV.

The hepatitis E epidemics frequently follow heavy rains and floods which lead to contamination of water sources (Vishwanathan, 1957). On the other hand some epidemics have occurred in hot summer months when reduction of water flow rate in rivers and streams possibly leads to an increase in the concentration of fecal contaminants in water (Naik *et al*, 1992). In some outbreaks, contamination of water was shown to occur in peripheral water distribution pipes, where these pass through contaminated soil. Intermittent water supply leads to a negative pressure in the pipes and inward suction of contaminants during periods of no flow (Sreenivasan *et al*, 1978).

HEV infection has a high prevalence in Asia, in particular the Indian subcontinent. Several epidemics of this infection have been reported from India, Nepal, Pakistan and Burma. In addition, epidemics have been reported from other parts of Asia, including China and the Central Asian republics of the forme, Soviet Union, *viz.* Turkmenistan, Tajikistan and Kirghiz. Epidemics of hepatitis E have been reported from several parts of Africa, including Algeria, Ivory Coast, Sudan, Ethiopia, Ghana, Senegal, Chad, Morocco and Somalia and from Mexico. In other parts of the world, HEV disease is much less frequent and is restricted primarily to travellers to endemic areas. This infection has two main epidemiologic forms: epidemic and sporadic.

## Sporadic HEV Infection

In HEV-endemic geographical regions, this virus accounts for a large majority of patients with sporadic viral hepatitis, *i.e.* viral hepatitis occurring in the absence of a recognizable outbreak in the neighborhood. In India, HEV infection is estimated to account for 50% to 70% of all patients with sporadic hepatitis (Khuroo *et al*, 1983, Arankalle *et al*, 1993). Patients with sporadic HEV infection have demographic and clinical features that closely resemble those of epidemic hepatitis E; these include male preponderance, higher prevalence among young adults, severity and duration of illness, poor prognosis among pregnant women, absence of chronic sequelae, etc.

## Transmission and Routes of Spread

Transmission of HEV is predominantly fecal-oral. The most frequent mode of transmission for *epidemic* HEV appears to be through the use of fecally contaminated water. During HEV epidemics, there is usually a clear relationship between the use of contaminated water and disease attack rate. During the Kanpur epidemic, our group showed that clinical attack rate was markedly higher in areas with municipal water supply derived from water from the river Ganga, which was contaminated, than in areas not supplied with such water (Naik *et al*, 1992). Further, in the former areas, attack rate was lower among those who used an alternative water source (hand pumps) for drinking purposes. Using polymerase chain reaction, HEV has been detected in sewage (Jothikumar *et al*, 1993); heavy contamination of drinking water with such sewage may be expected to lead to spread of infection.

In contrast to hepatitis A infection, which is also enterically transmitted, intrafamilial or person-to person spread plays an insignificant role in disease transmission during HEV epidemics (Aggarwal and Naik, 1994). Secondary attack rate among household members is low.

## Reservoirs of HEV Infection

Presumably, an environmental reservoir of HEV exists in disease-endemic areas that is responsible for recurrent epidemics. However, HEV appears to be a labile virus when exposed to high concentrations of salt, freeze-thawing, and pelleting. Another potential reservoir for persistence of HEV during· interepidemic periods in disease-endemic areas may be in the form of serial transmission among susceptible individuals who have sporadic or subclinical hepatitis E. Recent data suggest that hepatitis E may be a zoonotic disease. HEV RNA has been detected in the feces of domestic swine in Nepal (Clayson *et al*, 1995), and anti-HEV antibodies have been detected in the serum of pigs, cattle, sheep, and rodents in disease-endemic areas. Furthermore, a swine HEV has recently been described in the United States (Meng *et al*, 1997); molecular studies show that this virus though genetically distinct possesses a high degree of relatedness with human HEV strains. In particular, a newly described US isolate of HEV (Schlauder *et al*, 1998) and swine HEV (Meng *et al*, 1997) have been shown to be phylogenetically related and to possess cross-species infectivity, lending further support to the zoonosis hypothesis. However, further data are required on this aspect before a definitive opinion can be made.

## Incubation Period

The incubation period of HEV infection varies between 2 and 9 weeks with a mean of 6 weeks. This estimate is based on observations during epidemics which followed a known short period of water contamination. ·

## Mortality Rates

The case-fatality rate in several reports has ranged between 0.5 percent; and 4 percent these reports, however, are based on hospital data and thus may overestimate mortality. Studies based on data obtained from population surveys during outbreaks report lower mortality rates varying from 0.07 percent to 0.6 percent. Mortality rates among pregnant women, especially those infected in third trimester, range between 5 percent and 25 percent (Kane *et al*, 1984, Myint *et al*, 1985).

## Serology and Sero-epidemiological Findings

In the last few years, serological tests for antibodies to HEV have become available leading to several seroepidemiological studies. These tests can detect either IgM or IgG antibodies directed against HEV. Presence of IgM anti-HEV in test serum indicates a recent infection with HEV, whereas that of IgG anti-HEV is taken as evidence of HEV infection in the past, recent or remote.

Frequency of IgG anti-HEV in healthy subjects has thus been used as a seroepidemiological tool to measure the extent of exposure to this virus. Using these tests, presence of anti-HEV antibodies has been shown in persons living in all continents though as may be expected, prevalence rates vary widely in various areas. In the developed countries of Europe and North America, a small proportion of subjects (<5%) have IgG anti-HEV suggesting that *(i)* HEV infection does exist in these areas, and *(ii)* the rate of transmission of HEV infection in these communities is very low. On the other hand, in endemic areas of Africa and Asia, the prevalence rates are higher. In most areas, the antibody prevalence rates are higher in older age groups than in younger age groups. Also the seroprevalence is higher in males than in females in many areas. However, in endemic areas, studies from different groups in India show widely discrepant data. The reasons for these discrepancies could be related to varying epidemiologic conditions in different populations and regions within a country, differences in serological techniques used or both.

A closer look at HEV seroprevalence in India reveals rates ranging from 5 percent among adults in Kashmir (Khuroo *et al*, 1981) to 60 percent to 100 percent in a small group of subjects in New Delhi (Panda *et al*, 1995). In the area around Pune, anti-HEV antibody prevalence has been shown to increase with age till young adulthood and became constant thereafter. On the other hand, data from Lucknow show that IgG anti-HEV prevalence was as high as 70 percent even in children in the age group of 0-5 years and did not rise thereafter with age, suggesting that exposure to HEV was very common in pre-school children (Aggarwal *et al*, 1997). Thus it is clear that epidemiology of HEV differs widely in different parts of the country and further studies are needed to clarify these differences.

## Prevention

Prevention of hepatitis E in disease-endemic areas depends primarily on the supply of clean drinking water and strict attention to sewage disposal. Steps to improve water quality can lead to rapid termination of an outbreak. Boiling of water before consumption appears to reduce the risk of transmission of HEV. During the Kanpur epidemic, failure of water chlorination was followed by a rapid rise in the number of cases and its reinstitution led to rapid abatement of the epidemic (Naik *et al*, 1992). Isolation of affected persons is not indicated since person -to-person transmission is uncommon (Aggarwal *et al*, 1994).

The role of immune globulin manufactured in hepatitis E-endemic areas in pre-or post exposure prophylaxis has been evaluated in few studies. No significant difference in disease rates was found among recipients of immune globulin preparations and placebo controls. In experimental studies, however, passively acquired anti-HEV has been shown to modify the course of HEV infection, making it milder. Cloning of HEV and subsequent availability of recombinant proteins have encouraged preliminary trials of candidate recombinant vaccines in HEV-susceptible primate hosts. Two recent studies have shown protection against hepatitis and viremia after immunization with recombinant proteins corresponding to HEV capsid protein, though fecal excretion of virus was not prevented (Purdy *et al*, 1993, Fuerst *et al*, 1996).

There are however little human data available to support the protective role of anti-HEV antibodies. The occurrence of large hepatitis E epidemics among adults in disease-endemic areas suggests either that anti-HEV antibody may not be fully protective or that antibody levels decline with time and may no longer protect. The effort to produce vaccine must however continue because even short-term protection conferred by a vaccine may be useful for travelers to disease-endemic areas and high risk groups, such as pregnant women living in HEV-endemic areas.

## SUMMARY

Microbial contamination of natural drinking water continues to pose a threat to human health. Recurrent contamination of water supplies with sewage is common in urban areas of the developing countries leading to epidemics of enterically transmitted infections. The article discusses the ways in which the drinking water sources get polluted in rural and urban settings and the role that the government agencies and the public should play in preventing pollution. The dynamics of pollution of raw river water with sewage near water treatment plants has been illustrated by accounts of hepatitis E epidemics in the country. The experience of the author's group with the Kanpur epidemics the world's largest hepatitis E epidemic to date is described and some epidemiologic and clinical aspects of hepatitis E are discussed. Hepatitis E is a common disease in India causing acute liver damage, which usually manifests as self-limiting anicteric hepatitis or jaundice of mild or moderate nature. Rarely affected patients develop fulminant liver failure and death. Infected pregnant women however suffer a much higher death rate.

## REFERENCES

- Aggarwal R, Naik SR. Hepatitis E: intrafamilial transmission versus waterborne spread. *J Hepatol* 1994; 21: 718-23.
- Aggarwal R, Shahi H, Naik S, Yachha SK, Naik SR. Evidence in favour of high infection rate with hepatitis E virus among young children in India (letter). *J Hepatol* 1997; 26:1425-6.

- Alma-Ata 1978. In : Primary Health Care, World Health Oraganization, Geneva.

- Arankalle VA, Chobe LP, Jha J, Chadha MS, Banerjee K, Favorov MO, *et al.* Aetiology of acute sporadic non-A, non-B viral hepatitis in India *J Med Virol* 1993; **40**: 121-5.

- Clayson ET, Innis BL, Myint KS, Narupiti S, Vaughn DW, Giri S, *et al.* Detection of hepatitis E virus infections among domestic swine in the Kathmandu Valley of Nepal. *Am J Trop Med Hyg* 1995; 53:228-32.

- Fuerst TR, Yarbough P, Zhang Y, McAtee P, Tam A, Lifson J, *et al.* Prevention of hepatitis E using a novel ORF-2 subunit vaccine. In: Buisson, Y, Coursage P, Kane M, editors. Enterically-Transmitted Hepatitis Viruses. Tours: La Simarre, 1996:384-92.

- Jothikumar N, Aparna K, Kamatchiammal S, Paulmurugan R, Saravanadevi, S, et al. Detection of hepatitis E virus in raw and treated wastewater with the polymerase chain reaction. *Applied & Environmental Microbiology* 1993; 59:2558-62.

- Kane, MA, Bradley DW, Shrestha SM, Maynard JE, Cook EH, Mishra PP, et al. Epidemic non-A, non B hepatitis in Nepal: recovery of a possible etiologic agent and transmission studies in marmosets. *JAMA* 1984; 252:3140-5.

- Khuroo MS, Deurmeyer W, Zargar SA, Ahanger MA, Shah MA, Shah MA. Acute sporadic non-A, non-B, hepatitis in India. *Am J Epidemiol* 1983;118: 360-64.

- Khuroo MS, Teli MR, Skidmore S, Sofi MA, Khuroo MI. Incidence and severity of viral hepatitis in pregnancy. *Am J Med* 1981; 70:252-5

- Meng XJ, Purcell RH, Halbur PG, Lehman JR, Webb DM, Tsareva TS, *et al.* A novel virus in swine is closely related to the human hepatitis E virus. *Proc Natl Acad Sci USA* 1997; **94**: 9860-5.

- Myint H, Soe MM, Khin T, Myint TM, Tin KM. A clinical and epidemiological study of an epidemic of non-A, non-B hepatitis in Rangoon. *Am J Trop Med Hyg* 1985; 34:1183-9.

- Naik SR, Aggarwal R, Salunke PN, Mehrotra NN. A large waterborne viral hepatitis E epidemic in Kanpur, India. *Bull WHO* 1992; **70**:597-604.

- Panda SK, Nanda SK, Zafrullah M, Ansari IH, Ozdener MH, Jameel S. An Indian strain of hepatitis E virus (HEV): cloning, sequence, and expression of structural region and antibody responses in sera from individuals from an area of high-level HEV endemicity. *J. Clin Microbiol* 1995; **33**: 2653-9.

- Purdy MA, McCaustland KA, Krawczynski K, Spelbring J, Reyes GR, Bradley DW. Preliminary evidence that a trpE-HEV fusion protein protects cynomolgus macaques against challenge with wild-type hepatitis E virus (HEV). *J Med Virol* 1993; **41**:90-4.

- Schlauder GG. Dawson GJ, Erker JC, Kwo PY, Knigge MF, Smalley DL, *et al.* The sequence and phylogenetic analysis of a novel hepatitis E virus isolated from a patient with acute hepatitis reported in the United States. *J Gen Virol* 1998; **79**:447-56.

- Sreenivasan AM, Banerjee K, Pandya PG, *et al.* Epidemiological investigation of an outbreak of infectious hepatitis in Ahmedabad city during 1975-76. *Indian J Med Res* 1978; 67:197-206.

- Tandon BN, Joshi YK, Jain SK, Gandhi BM, Mathiersen LR, Tandon HD. An epidemic of non-A, non -B hepatitis in north India. *Indian J Med Res* 1982; 75:739-44.

- The World Health Report 1998. In : Chapter 2, pp 39-60. World Health Organization, Geneva.

- Vishwananthan R. Infectious hepatitis in Delhi (1995-96): A critical study: epidemiology. *India J Med Res* 1957; 45 (Suppl 1) : 1-29.

# 4

# Conservation and Monitoring of Coastal and Inland Areas for Fisheries and Aquaculture

*A. S. Ninawe*

## Introduction

The oceans that cover 71 percent of the earth's surface provides a haven for a multitude of biologically diverse life forms ranging in size and complexity from the smallest known virus to the very largest blue whale. Marine environment includes the large oceans, seas, bays, fjords, backwaters and estuaries. Marine environment has unique characteristics unlike the terrestrial environments. In spite of its varying characteristics and conditions in the marine environment, in different parts of the world, it is rich in diverse forms of life. So far about 1, 80, 000 species of marine algae, animals, bacteria, fungi and viruses have been identified and characterised and estimated that more than 8,00,000 are yet to be discovered. The diversity of life found in tropical and subtropical marine waters is greater than in colder waters. These warm richly endowed waters fall mostly under the jurisdiction of developing countries and may possess potentially the most valuable marine resources (Zilinskas and Lundin 1993)

The freshwater aquatic resources of the country are huge in terms of 2.855 million hectares of ponds and tanks and 1.79 million hectares of beels, jheels and direlict waters, in addition to 0.17 lakh km of rivers and canals and 2.02 million hectares of reservoirs that could be put to different fish culture practices or even culture based capture fishery in case of large water bodies. The details of aquatic resources are given in Table 4.1.

## Available Aquatic Resources

**Table 4.1 : Inland water resources and their production potential**

| Resources | Area |
|---|---|
| Rivers and canals | 0.17 lakh km |
| Reservoirs | 2.02 million ha |
| Ponds and Tanks | 2.855 million ha |
| Bheels, Ox-bow, lakes, direlict water bodies etc. | 1.79 million ha |
| Brackish waters | 1.422 million ha |
| Present area under fish culture | 6.00 lakh ha |
| Average productivity/ha | 2.00 tonnes |
| Estimated production potential | |
| Inland sector | 4.5 million tonnes |
| Marine sector | 3.9 million tonnes |

(*Source* : Ministry of Agriculture, Government of India Handbook on Fisheries Statistics, 1996).

Marine and inland pollution have seriously affected the exploitable living resources, recreational and commercial uses of oceans and the overall integrity of the marine, coastal and inland eco-systems. Hence, protection of the seas from continuing pollution becomes most essential in management of these water bodies. A wide variety of pollutants enter the coastal marine environment are classified in different ways according to their nature, source, physical state etc. The most widely known according to the nature and sources are sewage, heavy metal, oil and pesticides. The levels of various pollutants reported along the Indian coast are given in Table 4.2.

## Table 4.2 : Levels of pollution along the Indian coast

| | |
|---|---|
| Domestic sewage added to the sea by coastal population per year | $4.1 \times 10^9 m^9$ |
| Industrial effluents added to the sea by coastal industries per year | $0.41 \times 10^9 m^9$ |
| Sewage and effluents added by the rivers to the sea per year | $50 \times 10^6 m^3$ |
| Solid waste and garbage generated by coastal population per year | $33 \times 10^6$ tonnes |
| Fertilisers used per year | $5 \times 10^6$ tonnes |
| Pesticides used per year | 75,000 tonnes |
| Synthetic detergents used per year | 125,000 tonnes |

(*Source* : Proceeding of workshop on Environmental Impact Assessment of Aquaculture Enterprises, 1997).

Most inland and coastal waters in many developing countries are heavily polluted with solid and liquid wastes from uncontrolled garbage disposals, untreated sewage discharge and unregulated factory effluents, some of which are toxic chemicals. While domestic sewage is an important nutrient source for maintaining the biological richness of estuaries and coastal waters, most industrial and domestic wastes entering riverine and coastal systems seriously affect the chemical and biological constitutents of the aquatic environment (Gomez, 1988). The net result is eutrophication, leading to loss of biological diversity, loss of primary productivity and subsequent loss of fish production. Details of marine pollution in India is given in Table 4.3.

## Table 4.3 : Details of marine pollution in India

| Locality | Sources of Pollution | Pollutants |
|---|---|---|
| **KERALA** | | |
| Veli Lake (Trivandrum) | Travancore Titanium Industries | $4000 m^3 d^{-1}$ effluent discharge. $H_2SO_4$, Fe, traces of silica, slats of titanium dioxide |
| Veli lake and Kadinamkulam | Coir retting | Polyphenols, pentosom, tannins lipids, and $H_2S$ (Coir retting) |
| Veli lake and Poonthura backwater (Trivandrum) | Sewage | Organic Matter, faecal coliforms |
| Ashtamudi estuary (Quilon) | Paper mill | |
| Cochin | Chemical enginerring, food, fertilizer, rayon, rubber, tannaries, Plywood Industries sewage Coir retting | Industrial effluents Organic matter and faecal coil forms Polyphenols, pentoson, tannins, lipids and $H_2S$ |
| **KARNATAKA** | | |
| Mangalore | Fertilizer factory, Iron ore industry | High sediment nutrient contenc |
| Mringa Bay (Karwar) | caustic soda factory | Mercury |
| **GOA** | | |
| Velsao bay | Fertilizer factory | Ar, Se, $NH_3$ and urea, waste water $(15,000\ m^2 d^{-1})$ |
| **Maharastra** | | |
| Mumbai | Industrial and sewage | Industrial effluent, organic matter and and faecal coli forms |
| Bombay harbour | Industries, Tanker traffic and refineries | Industrial effluent, oil spills in sediments |
| Ulhas river estaury | Industries | Lit of Cu, 7t of Pb, 400t of Zn, 7t of Hg and 0.5t Cr/year |
| **GUJARAT** | | |
| Par river estuary | Chemical Industries | Effluent $30,000 m^3/day$ |
| Porbandar | Soda-ash industry | High levels of inorganic suspended load and Ammonia Waste water $(3200\ m^3 d^{-1})$ |
| Damanganga river estuary | Gujarat Industrial Development Corporation | |

*Contd....*

| Locality | Sources of Pollution | Pollutants |
|---|---|---|
| Kolak river estuary | GIDC (Paper mill) | Paper mill effluent |
| **TAMILNADU**<br>Chennai | Sewage and Industrial | Industrial effluent, organic matter & faecal coliform |
| Kalpakkam (Madras) | Nuclear Power Plant | Heated Effluents |
| **ANDHRA PRADESH**<br>Visakhapatnam harbour | Petroleum, Fertilizer and Polymer Industry | $6 \times 10^5 m^3 d^{-1}$ industrial effluents<br>$3 \times 10^3 m^3 d^{-1}$ -domestic sewage |
| **Orissa**<br>Rushikulaya river estuary | Chloride alkali industry | Mercuric concentratonm (1.5mg $lit^{-1}$ to 108mg $lit^{-1}$ in water, sediment). |
| **WEST BENGAL**<br>Hoogly | Jute, Paper Mill & Sewage | 0.4 million $m^3 d^{-1}$ - Industrial<br>0.8 million m3$d^{-1}$ sewage waste |

(*Source* : Proc. Sem. Coast. Zone Manag., 1997 : 47-60).

## Environmental Problems

Many countries increase their revenue by increasing agriculture, industry and mining. These economic activities have resulted in problems of pollution in marine environment since the activities are largely confined to coastal areas in most of the countries. These problems are severe in some countries. Monitoring the health of the seas requires consideration of many contaminants and potentially toxic substances. Domestic wastewater, industrial effluents, agricultural operations etc. also lead to the anthropogenic fluxes of other contaminants such as heavy metals, toxic organic chemicals, industrial effluents, synthetic organic petroleum, trace metals and radio-nucleotides to the marine environment.

## Sewage and Industrial Effluents

Sewage is a product of municipal drainage system containing domestic wastes with or without addition of discharges from industry, storm water and surface run-off. It contains large heterogeneous elements and has variable composition. It contains large quantities of organic matter, nutrients and various micro organisms. Oil and metals are usually present from different sources and sometimes chemicals are found in industrial wastes. The coastal activities are responsible for marine pollution by discharge and disposal of untreated and partially treated domestic and industrial wastes etc. Various fishing activities such as mechanised fishing vessels movement, draining of waste oil, painting of fishing vessels, scrapping of metal linings of fishing boats, dumping of waste and trash fishes, oil exploration and oil refining activities, recreation, tourism activities also create large quantities of effluents.

Rapidly increasing population growth and development in coastal regions could be a source of even more coastal water quality problems in future. These are generating an increasing amount of municipal sewage, urban runoff, and marine debris, industrial manufacturing and processing plants, landfills, docks and littering and contribute to marine pollution. The domestic and municipal wastes from many coastal cities in India are discharged directly in the coastal waters. They are discharged into the sea from most of the urban and rural areas and untreated. The main concern of waste disposal at sea arises from possible effects on man through accumulation of substances by marine animals, tainting of seafood and reduction of amenities by dicolouration of floating debris.

The standards set by Bureau of Indian Standards of different pollutants in the effluents for discharge into sea. The minimum national standards are proposed in Table 4.4.

**Table 4.4 : Effluent Water Quality**

| No. | Pollution Parameters | BIS-7968 standards | MINAS | Reference effluent | River Coovum |
|-----|---------------------|--------------------|-------|--------------------|--------------|
| 1. | TSS mg/1 | 100 | 20 | 30 | 6343* |
| 2. | Oil & Grease mg/1 | 20 | 10 | 1.4 | — |
| 3. | BOD5 Grease | 100 | 15 | 30 | 176* |
| 4. | COD Grease | 250 | NS | 6.23 | 51# |
| 5. | Phenols Grease | 5 | 1 | — | 10# |
| 6. | Sulphide Grease | 5 | 1 | — | 120# |
| 7. | pH Grease | 5.5–9 | 6-8.5 | 7 | 7.3* |

Source : *–Somasundaram *et al.* (1987) # – Ravichandran (1987)
MINAS – Minimum National Standards Proposed.

## Heavy Metal Pollution

The natural sources of metals in coastal waters are through river run-off. The mechanical and chemical weathering of rocks serve as another major source. In addition, components washed from the atmosphere through rainfall, wind blown dust, forest fires and volcanic particles also add to this. The natural concentrations of metals in sea water are very low and the possibilities of contamination are high (Bryan, 1984). Virtually all industrial processes involving water are potential sources of metallic contamination in estuaries and coastal waters. They include wide range of heavy and trace metals. They are absorbed on the surface film or become absorbed on the suspended matter and finally settle at the bottom of the seabed along with sediments. Later, they may enter the water column by various physical, chemical and biological processes. Many industries release trace metals into the environment, which reach the sea through a variety of routes.

The essential metals, copper and zinc, showed high concentrations than non-essential metals like cadmium, lead, mercury and nickel. The biota analysed include phytoplankton, zooplankton, molluscs and fishes. The biota from various coastal water reported high values than in other places naturally due to high levels of pollutants in ambient water. Moreover, oil spills, waste discharge, cargo spills, vessel movements, maintenance dredging etc. during operation phase of a port has a high potential for chronic impacts on local flora and fauna.

## Coastal Zone Management for Fishery related Activities

Aquaculture is being promoted for its potential to compensate for the slow rate of capture fisheries. Stocking and release of hatchery reared organisms into inland and coastal water supports capture based fisheries (Larkin,1991). The Group of Experts on the Scientific Aspects of Marine Pollution (GESAMP, 1991) concluded that, while the seas and oceans are relatively clean, most coastal waters are seriously threatened with increasing sedimentation from unregulated upland deforestation, eutrophication from nutrient enrichment, chronic oil spills and industrial pollution from manufacturing industries. Coastal erosion and pollution are the major problems encountered in coastal zone management. Coastal zones in many parts of the world are subject to steadily increasing pressure from development and resource utilisation and are threatened by the long term impact of climate change and associated sea-level rise. The coastal zone of India consisting of the near-shore shallow waters and associated vast inter-tidal areas alongwith the adjacent land mass is the most affected region as well as the most vulnerable to human abuse, apart from dumping of industrial wastes, over 300 million people living in the coastal areas. A significant fraction of the domestic wastewater ($11.1 \times 10^9 \, m^3 \, y^{-1}$) generated by coastal population in India reaches the marine zone causing widespread contamination in inshore marine waters particularly around coastal cities and towns. The domestic waste is often released directly to a nearby creek, bay or an estuary frequently in excess due to absence of adequate facilities for treatment.

The coastal zone of India which contributes $2.06\times10^6$t of fish catch every year has become increasingly vulnerable to anthropogenic pressure and adversely affect the marine ecology. A large number of valuable commercial stocks such as shrimps has been affected. The inshore waters favoured by several important species of fish and shellfish for spawning and/or breeding apart from serving as nursery grounds for some of them adversely influence capture fishery. A serious consequence of eutrophication could be an increase in frequency of occurrence of red tides. These massive growth of phytoplankton, often dinoflagellates contain some toxic chemicals which can cause illness and even death to marine organisms and humans.

Compelling need for an operational integrated coastal zone management system has been recognised for sustainable development of fisheries (Singh, 1997a). Thus the coastal environment such as mangroves, coral reefs, estuaries and coastal lagoons should be preserved. The coastal aquaculture, the delicate and complex ecosystem also requires careful management programmes. In view of multiple use of coastal areas, steps have been taken by Central Marine Fisheries Research Institute (CMFRI) to bring awakening among the fisher-folk about the coastal and marine fisheries management. This will facilitate the sustainable use of coastal resources and conservation of environment. There is need to establish a mechanism in co-operation and co-ordination among national authorities involved in planning, development, conservation and management of coastal areas. Thus integrated coastal zone management would help in utilisation of potential fishing zones and help in sustainable fishery development.

The marine fisheries potential in the Indian EEZ estimated at $3.92\times10^6$t constitutes $1.93\times10^6$ t demersals, $1.74\times10^6$t coastal pelagics (neritic) and $2.5\times10^5$t oceanic tuna and allied fish stocks. Of the exploitable resource estimated at $2.69\times10^6$t, the contribution through coastal fishing (0-50 m) is $2.06\times10^6$ t; the remaining $6.3\times10^5$ t being from 50-200 m depth with negligible catch from beyond 200 m depth. Hence, clearly the resources of the coastal seas are under the pressure of exploitation (Somvanshi, 1997). The coastline fisheries resources in the form of estuaries, mangroves, backwaters, brackishwater lagoons, bheries, etc. extending to about 2.6 million ha area contribute significantly to our total inland yields. The brackishwater systems and the coastal zones are particularly important since they offer a lucrative shellfish fishery that brings more than 5000 million rupees in foreign exchange every year. The south west coast of India is one among the most productive marine zones of the world. With this right of exclusive economic zone, India has acquired a responsibility to conserve, develop and optimally exploit the fragile coastal living resources upto 200 miles of our coastline.

## Agricultural Wastes

Fertiliser, pesticides and insecticides are widely used in the country in agriculture, pest control and vector control. In some countries organochlorine pesticides are prohibited. They are not replaced by organo-phosphorus and carbonate pesticides.

## Use of Pesticides

Indiscriminate and heavy use of pesticides has contaminated the food grains, dairy products, fruits, vegetables, fodder, horticulture, drinking water and the living environment as a whole (Mehrotra, 1983). Pesticides that are transported to the aquatic environment are primarily of agriculture origin. The agriculture return flow and drainage constitutes the main pathway of transport of pesticides from arable soils to the marine environment. The impact of DDT, pesticides and chemicals affected the reproductive cycle of fish eating birds and sexual changes in gastropods caused by tri-butyrin. The anti-fouling agent employed in marine paints are also widely reported. The number of potential endocrine-disrupting chemicals is significant but there is lack of understanding world-wide about their impact on the marine organism(Colborn *et al*,1993).

Some analyses of DDT and its metabolites have been carried out. In most cases, the values have been found to be below the detection limit. Recent survey has shown that plankton in the Arabian Sea has DDT concentrations of 0.05-3.21 ppm wet weight. The concentrations of organochlorine and organophosphorus pesticides in some of the fishes of the Indian ocean, particularly in plankton feeders, may be appreciably high because of the wide use of pesticides in agricultural activities. The information is scanty for the coastal waters of India except for the levels of some chlorinated pesticides (Shailaja and Nair, 1997) and heavy metals (Sen Gupta *et al*, 1990) in few organisms. While the available results indicate the absence of bio-accumulation to objectionable level, it is considered to be ecologically degraded.

## Hazardous Substances like Petroleum Spillovers

Oil pollution arises from the exploration, extraction, stabilisation, transport, storage and refining of crude oil. The different sources for oil pollution in the marine environment are pollution by crude and refined oil arises from tanker accidents, deblasting operations and tank washings, refinery effluents, pipelines and offshore production losses. Thus the losses can arise in the operations at every stage. Oil also enters the sea from natural seepages (Johnston, 1984). The input of petroleum to the marine environment from all sources range from 2 to 20 million tonnes per annum. With domestic production of petroleum products remaining more or less stagnant at around $3.3 \times 10^7$ t y$^{-1}$, large volume import of crude oil or petroleum product is inevitable (Zindge, 1997). Maritime oil transportation including tanker operations, other shipping activities and accidental spills from ships make upto 26 percent of the total input of oil to the oceans (GESAMP, 1993). Hence, traffic of bulk carriers is expected to increase substantially at the Indian ports thereby exposing the coastal segments to oil pollution due to discharge of ballast waters and bilge washings apart from risks of tanker disasters.

Oil slicks at sea kill or affect 200 plankton including totally planktonic species like copepods, as well as planktonic eggs and larvae of fish and benthic invertebrates. Approximately 4 to 6 million tonnes of oil enter the oceans every year, of which, the largest source is the terrestrial discharge. Off-shore oil exploration to locate sub-sea reserves can kill fish while sensors of the seismic equipment interfere with commercial fishing operations. The presence of rigs and pipelines creates exclusion zones for fishing vessels while the debris associated with the offshore operations can damage fishing gear or entangle ship propellers (GESAMP, 1990).

## Radioactive and Thermal Wastes

Radioactive wastes from nuclear power plants are disposed off according to strict international conventions. However, their heat generation poses several problems. Nuclear power plants normally release the generated heat to the coastal marine environment particularly when sea water is used for cooling purpose; flora and fauna in the warm tropical waters live close to their upper lethal limits of temperature in summer months affects the marine biota.

## Habitat and Destruction

Different pollutants have different effects on fisheries and on living aquatic organisms. There has been evidences that habitat destruction has been gradually increasing destroying mangroves, coral reef, seagrass beds, mudflats etc. Corals of Lakshadeep and Gulf of Mannar are also under increasing stress due to human interference (Sharma *et al*, 1997). In India coral reefs occur along the Northwest and Southeast coasts, Lakshadweep and Andaman and Nicobar Islands. In the Gulf of Katchchh, mining of coralline sand in the past and destruction of mangroves leading to increase in suspended solids in water have imposed considerable strain on the corals and large stretches of dead corals is a common occurrence. Heavy land drainage and siltation due to deforestation, saw dust from timber factories, port activities around Port Blair and coastal pollution have increased the mortality of corals of the Andaman and Nicobar Islands. Mangroves are the most productive ecosystem after corals with high biodiversity. Many species of finfish, shrimp and other crustaceans, molluscs, habitat have been affected. In india, the yield of mangrove-cum-estuarine dependent fisheries is estimated at 30,000 t of fish and $1.3 \times 10^5$ t of prawns per year (Untawale and Wafer, 1994). The mangroves along the Indian coast are under considerable stress and their destruction may result in reduction in breeding grounds subsequently a reduced catch or production of shrimp, crab and other coastal seafood species.

## River Pollution

As urbanisation and industrialisation increased in the region, the volume of sewage and industrial waste also increased. More than 2000 crore litres of sewage water and about 5000 metric tonne of garbage are produced per day in the urban areas which are polluting the surface and ground water resources. Several countries in the world have a number of rivers flowing through their land masses. These rivers get polluted because of human activities around them. The sewage and industrial wastes are either untreated or partially treated in many of the countries. In India, only 50 cities with a population of over 100,000 have sewage treatment facilities.

The greatest pollution centres are seen in the industrial townships along the Indo-Gangetic plain. Rivers are being polluted by sewage, industrial effluents, mining wastes and runoff from farm fields and city streets. Pollution due to toxic chemicals like organo-chlorines and heavy metals and other organo-tin compounds are posing threat to aquatic species. Vast stretches of the 600 km long Ganga river continue to remain highly polluted due to industrial activity. The Ganga river basin receives 1.15 million metric tonnes of chemical fertilizers of all kinds annually (Gupta, 1984). It is estimated that 2573 metric tonnes of pesticides end up in the Ganga river system every year (Mohan, 1989). This has made the river Ganga highly polluted in the world. It is reported that the industrial effluents containing various pollutants (particularly toxic metals and pesticidal residues) are drained to nearby lands and decrease the soil fertility (Singh, 1989). They are introduced in aquatic environmental by-products of factories, sewage and sludge, household garbage, petro-chemicals and oils; dyeing industries, alcohol, fertilisers, pesticides, heavy metals, thermal pollutants, detergents and radio-active substances.

## Threat to Aquatic Life

Similar threat was reported on the ecology of Cauvery. Spawning of Mahaseer and trout is affected, as a result these fishes have dwindled. A mass fish mortality was reported in river Gomti at Lucknow due to the sudden release of effluents from a sugar and alcohol factory. These effluents had high BOD as untreated sewage, evolving methane, $H_2S$ and ammonia which are toxic to fish and rendering the water anoxic. The Narmada Valley project is a typical case of government priorities towards industries over the environment. A large area of cultivable fertile lands are being inundated and thousands of people are being displaced for the sake of hydroelectric generation. In many countries for cultivation of cash crops vast regions of virgin forest lands are cleared for the cash crops like coffee and rubber plantations of India and Malaysia; rubber, sugarcane and rice plantations of Brazil. These are the typical examples of land degradation along with fish and other aquatic resources.

Excess of nitrogen and phosphorus reduce the number of species in the aquatic environment and only those thrive which are unsuitable for fish, such as the blue-green algae. The changes in plant population cause changes throughout the ecosystem, even in organisms not directly affected by pollution. The surviving fishes are such that they are less valuable as a fishery resource from an economic and food point of view. This holds true for the disappearing fine fishes, *e.g.* Mahaseer and Salmon, Trout, and the snow-trout of Kashmir, the only pollution tolerant species being the common carps (*Cyprinus carpio*) and the small forage fishes. The water body deteriorates very rapidly due to the inflow of various substances from different industries which in turn affect the fauna and flora especially the fish fauna. Thus the polluted waterbody by industrial effluents, sewages and human wastes, etc. causes serious threat to aquatic life and affect their habitat.The fish may not always die but their reproductive capacity, breeding, spawning and development of eggs is adversely affected. Biological effects on fish include morphological and physiological changes, effects on migration as in Hilsa, which rarely comes upto Allahabad these days to spawn, behaviour, disease incidence, life cycle, nutrition, and also genetic effects. The effects of pollutants on fisheries are so multifaceted that until detailed analysis of the water is done for all harmful ingredients, it is difficult to pinpoint the causes of toxicity and mass mortality.

## Degradation of Lakes Ecology

Lakes that have been oligotrophic and clear for hundreds of years have become eutrophic and polluted with man-made effluents, rendering them repulsive and malodorous. Lakes are being lost or altered because of the disruption of natural processes by intensification of agriculture, urbanisation, pollution, construction of dams and disposals of sewage and industrial effluents. Pesticide and fertiliser use in the Krishna and Godavari delta region is heavy. Eleven major industries release about 7.2 million litres of effluents into the lake every day. The Andhra Pradesh Pollution Control Board reported that more than 17,000 tonnes of fertiliser waste enters the lake annually. The construction of roads and bridges disrupted the organic continuity of the Kolleru lake. The fish farms around the lake block water channels from the catchment area has been reduced by economic development. The freshwater fish culture activity started in the state in co-operative sector in 1976 had engulfed vast areas including highly fertile agricultural land with an extent of 1.38 acres in central coastal districts. This has resulted in habitat destruction of insectivorous and predatory fishes because of conversion of paddy fields into fish farms. The result was depletion in paddy production, destruction of Kolleru lake's ecology and fish habitat destruction and fish endemic to the lake species like murrels, cat fishes and *Anabas* were depleted. This has resulted into depletion of fish stock from 35 million tonnes to 7 million tonnes. Bird fauna came down from 165 to 60 species. Studies reported that the presence of pollutants in the lake sediment supports the growth of fast-growing weeds. The sewage and discharge from factories have also affected the growth of water-borne organisms that the fish consume. The reduced catchment area has led to eutrophication, loss of drinking water and declining fish catches. In some incidences fishes are reported to be blind yielding less production and bird egg shells are becoming more fragile. The obstructions of the lake's periphery resulted in flooding of agricultural land even during normal rainfall.

The coastal lakes such as Chilka and Pulicat were dynamic few years ago, thriving highly productive brackish water production centres. These lakes on the west coast are now silting and become shallow and is full of weeds in which freshwater fishes dominate. The northern mouth of the brackish water lake, reported to be India's largest inland lake, has been choked by heavy siltation and traces of toxic metals like cadmium and mercury. This has threatened the lake's marine life in the lagoon-bed and its connecting channel with the sea, profuse weed infestation, decrease in salinity as well as quantitative decline in the fishery. Aquatic living species die as the pesticides washed down from the fields of rivers, tanks and other water reservoirs. The survey of Chilka lagoon in 1995-96 by CIFRI (Banerjee *et al.*, 1996) has indicated that regulated discharge from incoming rivers, siltation and anthropogenic pressure have made considerable negative impact on its fishery. The water area of Chilka (Orissa) has been reduced from 1165 sq. km. to 620 sq. km. in 1995. Loktak lake, the largest freshwater inland lake has been reduced from 495 sq km. to 390 sq km in the last ten years causing a serious ecological problem in Kashmir valley.

## Biotechnological Interventions

Apart from the environmental pollution impact, aquaculture may also have some other ecological impacts such as, pressure on natural stock, problems in the introduction of new species, disease transmission in culture organisms, generation of drug-resistant strains of pathogens, etc. Thus urbanisation, industrialisation and intensive farming wastes need adequate disposal and treatment. Environmental biotechnology offers specific application of biotechnology of the management of environment and environmental related socio-economic and developmental issues. With the emergence of the concept of sustainable development, there is need to address the issues like environmental monitoring, restoration of environmental quality, resources/residue/waste recovery/utilisation, treatment and substitution of renewable resources.

The naturally occurring micro-organisms such as bacteria and fungi break down complex substances into simpler forms to harmless or less toxic end products by feeding directly on the organic pollutants or by breaking down the pollutant while they catabolize a primary source of carbon, or by secreting enzymes to breakdown the pollutant (Portier and Ahmed, 1988). Deliberate attempts are needed to employ endogenous micro-organisms to clean up polluted and waste water as suggested by (Martello, 1991). Chakrabarti (1992) has pointed out that micro-organisms are well known for their adaptability to extreme environments. There are increasing evidence to know about micro-organisms in learning to cope with the multitude of toxic, man made chemicals released into the environment in massive amounts. A number of bacteria, viz, *Pseudomonas, Vibrio, Enterobacter, Azotobacter Iwoffi, Moraxella* etc., have been found to volatilise various forms of mercury. Use of these bacteria and the micro algae like *Isochrysis galbana* with the capacity to volatilise mercury would be of immense importance in the abatement of mercury pollution of the aquatic systems(Anon, 1996). Hence isolation and development of indigenous bacteria from such polluted environments to degrade the pollutants is necessary for successful bio-remediation.

To conserve and monitor the coastal and inland resources and preserve our biodiversity, it is proposed to take the following measures:

1. Proper management of existing aquatic resources are extremely important, especially since new fishing grounds and new resources are not easily discovered. Thus we need to identify and locate the economically important marine resources/fishing grounds and develop appropriate methods for their sustainable use. Also there is need to evaluate and monitor various pollution aspects and take necessary preventive measures to promote sustainable fishery development in the country for ecological and economic benefits.

2. We need to conduct surveys of aquatic pollution to estimate the economic loss on a national basis. There is need to assess the endangered and threatened marine animals and plants and protect their habitats and update their status for conservation measures.

3. We need to create a mechanism for public awareness for the sustainable use of our marine and inland ecosystem. Various aspects of research on marine pollution, biodiversity should be given due emphasis. There is need to give emphasis on taxonomy, ecosystems, species diversity, ecological advantages, etc.

4. Strengthening of legislation and stricter implementation of regulation should be undertaken for preservation of marine and inland biodiversity. For this, we need to prepare inventory of all known aquatic fauna and flora and their habitats.

## SUMMARY

India's biodiversity is very vast having rich resources which are not fully and profitably utilised. These resources are under constant threat because of the population pressure. As a consequence, the resources both in coastal and inland areas are increasingly utilised resulting into a loss of habitats, over-exploitation of fishing grounds, pollution and eutrophication due to increasing load of nutrients, pathogens, introduction of exotic species and disposal of litter at sea. Increasing inland and coastal water pollution affects not only the composition and abundance of plants and animals in the aquatic environment, but also poses serious health hazards to consumers. Due to intense human activity especially in coastal areas, there are signs of habitat loss resulting in the decline of fishery resources and nursery habitats. We need to take proper management measures to save our existing resources from their exploitation since new fishing grounds and new resources are not easily discovered. The need is also felt to evaluate the ecological and economic status and benefits of marine diversity and create better awareness for preserving marine habitat. In the present paper various aspects of pollution and environmental threats to aquatic species have been critically examined. Appropriate strategic measures have been suggested for preservation and conservation of our coastal and inland areas for aquaculture and fishery production by improving our catch levels and production systems.

## REFERENCES

- Anon, 1996. Handbook on fisheries statistics. Publication of Department of Agriculture and Fisheries, Govt. of India, 217p.
- Anon, 1996. Abatement of mercury pollution in aquatic systems: A biotechnological approach. *Fishing Chimes* vol. 16 (4), p.35-36.
- Anon, 1997. Environmental impact assessment of aquaculture enterprises. Proceedings of the workshop held at Rajiv Gandhi Centre for Aquaculture, Chennai during December 10-12, 1997 ,188 p.
- Anon, 1997. Proceedings of the seminar on coastal zone management held at Nagercoil, Tamil Nadu during December 30-31, 1997, 123 p. IACS Publication No. 1.
- Banerjee, R. K., P. K. Pandit and M. Sinha., 1996. Chilka-Now & Then. *Sci. Cult.*, **62** p.5-6.
- Bryan, G. W., 1984. Pollution due to heavy metals and their compounds. In: Marine Ecology,(Ed. O. Kinne), John Wiley & Sons, New York, Vol. V part 3: p.1289-1432
- Chakrabarty, A.M., 1982. Biodegradation and detoxification of environmental polluants (Ed.), C.R.C. Press, Inc. Florida, 127p.
- Colborn T., F. S. Vom Saal and A.M. Soto, 1993. Developmental effects of endocrine - disrupting chemicals in wildlife and humans. *Environmental Health Perspective* **101** : p.378-384.
- GESAMP, 1990. IMO/FAO/UNESCO/WMO/WHO/IAEA/UN/UNEP. Joint Group of Experts on the Scientific Aspects of Marine Pollution: The state of the marine environment. Reports and Studies GESAMP No. 39: 111 p.
- GESAMP, 1991. IMO/FAO/UNESCO/WMO/WHO/IAEA/UN/UNEP. Joint Group of experts on the scientific aspects of Marine pollution). 1991. Reducing environmental impacts of coastal aquaculture. Report and Studies GESAMP No. 47: 35 p.
- GESAMP, 1993. IMO/FAO/UNESCO/WMO/WHO/IAEA/UN/UNEP. Joint Group of Experts of the Scientific Aspects of Marine Pollution. Report and Studies GESAMP No. 50: p.16-65.
- Gomez, E.D.,1988. Overview of environmental problem in the East Asian seas region. *Ambio* 17(3) : p.166-169
- Gupta, D.(ed.), 1984. The Ganga Basin. Basin sub-basin inventory of water pollution. Part II L ADSORB 5/7/1982-83. Centre for study of man and environment. Central Board for the Prevention and Control of Water Pollution, New Delhi.

- Johnston, R., 1984. Oil pollution and its management. In: Marine Ecology, (Ed. O. Kinne) John Wiley & Sons. New York. Vol. V. Part 3: p.1433-1582.
- Larkin, P. A., 1991. ICES Marine Science Symposium 192: p.6-14.
- Martello, A., 1991. The Scientist (51), P. 18-19..
- Mehrotra, K.N.,1983. Benefits and hazards of pesticides to society, *Pesticide Information*, **38**.
- Mohan, R.S. Lal,1989. Conservation and management of the Ganges River dolphin, Platanista gangetica, in India. In : Biology and Conservation of river Dolphins (Eds.W.F.Perrin, R.L.Brownell, Jr.Zhou Kaiya and Liu Jiankang), Occasions papers of the IUCN Species Survival Commission No.3.
- Portier, R. J. and S. I. Ahmed., 1988. *Marine Technology Society Journal* 22 (2), P. 6-14.
- Ravichandran, S., 1987. Water quality studies on Buckhingham canal (Madras, India)- A discriminant analysis. *Hydrobiologia*, **154**: p.121-126
- Sen Gupta, R., M Ali, A. L. Bhuiyan, M. M. Hussain, P. M Sivalingam, S. Subasinghe and N. M. Tirmizi, 1990. State of the marine environment in the South Asian Seas region. UNEP Regional Seas Reports and Studies No. 123, P. 42
- Shailaja, M. S. and M. Nair, 1997. Seasonal difference in organochlorine pesticide concentrations of zooplankton and fish in the Arabian Sea. *Marine Environmental Research* 44: p.263-274.
- Sharma, V. K., P. Tiwari and R. Jaiswar, 1997. Environmental and socio-economic problems of the coastal ecosystem in India- A focus on Mumbai. In: Coastal Cities in India: Responding to Environmental and Socio-economic Issues of Concern (Ed) (Ed. V.K. Sharma), Indira Gandhi Institute of Development Research, Mumbai, p.17-35.
- Singh V. V., 1997a. Incorporation of integrated coastal zone management (ICZM) in fisheries course curricula at different levels, p 184-190 In: N. K. Thakur, R.S.Biradar and B. S. Sontakki (Eds.) Proceedings of the National Seminar on Fisheries Education organised at CIFE, Mumbai on 23-24 May 1996:273 p.
- Singh, K.M., 1989. Problems and prospects of environmental pollution in India. Mittal Publ., New Delhi.
- Somasundaram, M. V., G. Ravindran and A. Ramasamy., 1987. Pollution in Coovum estuary and adjoining wells. In: Proc.Natl. Seminar on Estuarine Management. Govt. of Kerala, Trivandrum (In press).
- Somvanshi, V. S., 1997. Deepsea fishing and its impact on coastal fishing. In: Proceedings of National Seminar on Coastal Ocean Regime and Developing Countries (Ed. H.P. Rajan ); Department of Ocean Development, New Delhi. p.38-46
- Untawale, A G. and S. Wafar, 1994. Impact of conversion of mangrove ecosystem for aquaculture purposes. In: Proceedings of Seminar on Ocean and Industry - Realities and Expectations (Ed. P.S. Srivastava) Society of Ocean Scientists and Technologists, Gaziabad: p.89-92.
- Zilinskas R A and G. S. Lundin., 1993. Marine Biotechnology and Developing Countries: World Bank Discussion papers, No.210.
- Zingde, M. D., 1997. Marine pollution - What are we heading for? In: Proceedings of Seminar on Present Trends and Future Directions in Ocean Science, (Ed. B.L.K. Somayajulu) Indian National Science Academy, New Delhi (In press).

---

* *The views expressed are the author's and not necessarily those of the Department of Biotechnology.*

# 5

# Acid Rain and Plants

*Bhoomika Singh and Madhoolika Agrawal*

Air pollution was earlier considered as a local problem around the large point sources. But due to use of tall stacks and long range transport of pollutants, it has become a regional problem. The transboundary nature of transport of pollutants was clearly evident when areas remote from sources of air pollution also showed higher concentrations of air pollutants. Uncontrolled use of fossil fuels in industries and transport sector has led to increase in concentrations of gaseous pollutants such as sulphur dioxide ($SO_2$), nitrogen oxides (NOx), etc. These air pollutants are known to be phytotoxic at short-term high concentrations as well as low-level exposures for longer duration. Gases and particles injected into the atmosphere by natural or anthropogenic sources are returned to the earth's surface through wet and dry removal processes. In cloud and below cloud, scavenging processes are the prime mechanisms by which gaseous and particulate pollutants are removed from the atmosphere. Scavenging of air pollutants affects the chemical composition and pH of rainwater. Acidification of rainwater is considered as one of the most serious environmental problems facing the industrialized nations today.

Acid rain, the term was first used by Robert Angus Smith in 1872 to describe the acidic nature of rain around industrial town of Manchester, U.K. Subtle but lethal, acid rain is rising up as the most crucial ecological issue, particularly in Europe and North America. It is a modern post industrial form of ruination.

Acid rain refers to any precipitation, which has a pH less than 5.6, the pH of uncontaminated rainwater. The normal rainwater is weakly acidic due to dissolution of atmospheric $CO_2$ to form carbonic acid (Likens and Bormann, 1974). Sweden was one of the first countries to observe the adverse environmental effects of acid rainfall in the early sixties. By 1965 the annual average pH of rainwater in Sweden was 4 or less. Such observations were reported in the UN conference on the human environment held at Stockholm in 1972 citing specific deleterious effects such as massive fish killing, lake acidification, crop and forest damage, corrosion of cultural properties, etc. After the reports of Sweden, various other countries also set up individual committee/ review groups to look into the problem of acid precipitation. The Canadian Network for Sampling Precipitation (CANSAP) in Canada, National Atmospheric Deposition Program (NADP) in USA and UN Economic Commission for Europe have assumed responsibility for monitoring the long range transport of air pollutants in Europe.

Earlier acid rain has been considered as an European and North American problem, but now it is spreading to the developing countries of the world (Khemani *et al.*, 1989b). The developing countries consume only one fifth of the world's commercial energy but it's share is growing (Khemani *et al.*, 1989b). In India the annual $SO_2$ emissions have tripled since the early 1960s (Naik *et al.*, 1988). The fossil fuel consumption has increased from 75 million tonnes per year in 1964 to 245 million tonnes per year in 1990 (Shrestha *et al.*, 1996). The number of vehicles has increased from 1.86 million in 1971 to 32 million in 1996 and is expected to increase further to 53 million by the year 2000 (Varshney *et al.*, 1997). According to a report of NEERI (1980) the air pollution has already become very severe in the metropolitan cities like Kolkata, Delhi, and Mumbai.

## Occurrence of Acid Rain Events

**In India :** Studies on rain water of India showed a range of pH from alkaline to acidic (Tables 5.1 and 5.2). Occurrence of acid rain problem in India is often ruled out due to abundance of alkaline particles in the atmosphere. But the strict rule of maintaining air quality at source has reduced the particulate emissions. The gases responsible for incorporating sulphate and nitrate ions into the precipitation are, however, not reduced. The world meteorological organization has predicted substantial increase in acidity in cities like, Hyderabad, Chennai, Pune and Kanpur (Banerjee, 1997). TEERI has also predicted heavy acid rain problem in Bihar, West Bengal, Orissa and southern coastal India, which may lead to infertile soil (TOI, 1998).

**Table 5.1 : Range of rainwater pH in different parts of India**

| Coastal | | Urban | |
|---|---|---|---|
| Trivendrum | 5.30 | Pune | 6.30 |
| **Industrial** | | Delhi | 6.10 |
| Kalyan | 5.70 | **Non-Urban** | |
| Chembur | 4.80 | Sirur | 6.70 |
| **Power Plant** | | Muktsar | 7.30 |
| | | Goraur | 5.30 |
| Indraprastha | 5.0 | **Forest Region** | |
| Koradi | 6.70 | Masingudi | 6.04 |

*Source*: Khemani (1993); Sequeira (1976)

**Table 5.2 : Mean pH of rainwater in Indian BAPMoN stations (1974-1990)**

| STATIONS | OBSERVED pH | STATIONS | OBSERVED pH |
|---|---|---|---|
| Allahabad | 6.93 | Nagpur | 5.97 |
| Jodhpur | 7.42 | Port Blair | 6.15 |
| Kodaikanal | 6.28 | Pune | 6.43 |
| Minicoy | 6.58 | Srinagar | 7.22 |
| Mohanbari | 5.98 | Visakhapatnam | 6.01 |

*Source*: Datar *et al.* (1996).

Chandrawanshi *et al.* (1997) have analyzed the rainwater samples in Korba during March to November 1995, and found average pH of rainwater to be 4.8. Sulphuric acid was found in high amount in the precipitation. The coal burning operations were found to be the main source for the contribution of high amount of sulphuric acid in rainwaters, whereas aluminium plant was mainly contributing F ions. Korba is an industrial area having coalmines, thermal power plants, aluminium factory and several small scale industries using coal as the energy source. In India, acid rain was first reported in Chembur, Trombay area of Mumbai with a pH of 4.8 (Sequeira, 1976) and the trend continued up to 1980. The Chembur-Trombay area is a highly industrialized area and loads of gaseous and particulate pollutants are released from the refineries, power plants, fertilizer plant and many chemical industries which are located in this area. Burman (1985) reported the rainfall with a pH of 3.5 in Mumbai. In the metropolitan cities like Kolkata, Delhi and Mumbai air pollution levels are steadily rising (Khemani *et al.*, 1987). The pH has decreased from 9.1during 1963 to 6.2 in 1984 in Agra and from 7.0 during 1965 to 6.1 in 1984 at Delhi (Khemani *et al.*, 1989a). Rao *et al.* (1993) reported a pH below 5.0 in the silent valley forests.

Kulshrestha *et al.* (1995) studied the individual rain events at New Delhi during monsoon, 1994. They observed higher pH (*i.e.* in alkaline range) of rain water occurred after a longer antecedent period, causing higher loading of atmosphere with components like Ca and Mg which have higher acid neutralizing capacity. Rain water showed acidic pH when the antecedent period was very short.

**In Other Countries :** There are reports from many developed countries of rain with pH less than 5. The past and current monitoring data revealed that Scandinavia, the northeastern U.S. and southern Canada received the highly acidic rain fall (Bubenick, 1984). During the past, there are several reports of rainwater with pH values below 5.6 *e.g.* pH 4 at Cumbria, U.K. (Gorham, 1958), 3.8-4.2 at Liverpool, U.K., 3.0 at Hubbard Brook, New Hampshire (Likens *et al.*, 1972) and 2.8 in Scandinavia (Likens *et al.*, 1972, Walker, 1963). There are records of very low pH of 2.0 for fog and pH 2.1 for rain also (Likens and Bormann, 1974).

Acid rain occurs over much of the eastern United States (Brezonik *et al.*, 1980), from Maine to Florida (Haines, 1979; Likens and Butler, 1981) and Europe (Breakke, 1976; Likens *et al.*, 1979; Abrahamsen, 1980). A strong acidification of rainwater by air pollution from oil fields and petrochemical plants in Venezuela is reported (Sanhueza *et al.*, 1988). In China, rainwater pH mainly occurred less than 5.0 throughout the provinces of southwest China and also in area around southeast of Anhui province and northeast of Shanghai and Hanghou provinces (Hongfa, 1989). Rainwater in thirteen cities in the south of China has an annual average pH less than 4.5 (Wei *et al.*, 1988). The pH values in industrialized nations in 1978 had been recorded between 4 and 6, by Background Air pollution Monitoring stations (BAPMoN) (Mohan and Kumar, 1998).

Data from the National Atmospheric Deposition Program (NADP) for 1978 and 1979 clearly showed that the mean pH of precipitation in portions of New York, Ohio, and Pennsylvania was less than 4.2, while most of the north-eastern portion of the United States had mean pH below 4.4 (NADP, 1978 & 1979). Waldman *et al.* (1985) had reported the average pH of cloud water as 2.9 for 1982 and 1983 at Henninger Flats (USA). Table 5.3 describes the range of rainwater pH observed in different regions of the world.

**Table 5.3 : Rain water pH values in different regions of the world**

| | |
|---|---|
| Japan | 4.7 |
| Europe | 4.1-5.4 |
| China acid rain area | 4.1-4.9 |
| China non-acid rain affected area | 6.3-6.7 |
| US North west | 5.1-5.2 |
| US West-middlewest | 5.0-5.5 |
| US North west | 4.1-4.2 |

*Source*: Khemani *et al.*, 1994

## Constituents of Acid Rain

The acid rain is mainly a mixture of $H_2SO_4$ and $HNO_3$ and the ratio of these two vary depending on the relative quantities of oxides of sulphur and nitrogen emission. These oxides are mainly produced by combustion of fossil fuel, smelters, power plants, automobile exhausts, domestic fires, etc. On an average 60-70 percent of the acidity is ascribed to $H_2SO_4$ and 30-40 percent to $HNO_3$ (Fowler *et al.*, 1982).

Burning of fossil fuel for power generation contributes to almost 60-70 percent of total $SO_2$ emitted globally. Relatively stable in the atmosphere, $SO_2$ acts either as a reducing or an oxidising agent. Reacting photochemically or catalytically with other components in the atmosphere, $SO_2$ can produce $SO_3$, $H_2SO_4$ droplets and salts of sulfuric acid. $SO_2$ reacts with water to form sulphurous acid. The most probable reactions involve highly reactive hydroxyl ($O°H$) free radicals formed from $O_3$ or monatomic oxygen (reactions 1&2). These radicals react readily with $SO_2$ (reaction 3) to form $HSO°_3$ radicals which are then oxidized to peroxyl radicals ($HO°_2$) and $SO_3$ (reaction 4). The predominance of this mechanism of acidification involving $O°H$ radicals means that warm, bright summer days, which favour $O_3$ and monatomic oxygen formation (and hence $O°H$ radicals), promote dry-phase acidification, while wet phase reactions are more important in winter and rainy season. Similar dry gas-phase mechanisms exist for the formation of nitric acid from $NO_2$, but gas-phase oxidation of $NO_2$ by $O°H$ proceeds 10 times faster than the equivalent reactions involving $SO_2$.

| | | | | |
|---|---|---|---|---|
| $O_3$ + light | $\Rightarrow$ | $O + O_2$ | (1) |
| $O + H_2O$ | $\Rightarrow$ | $2\ O°H$ | (2) |
| $O°H + SO_2 + M$ | $\Rightarrow$ | $HSO°_3 + M$ | (3) |
| $HSO°_3 + O_2$ | $\Rightarrow$ | $HO°_2 + SO_3$ | (4) |

Gas phase reactions also generate organic acids. For example, reactions of peroxyl radicals ($HO°_2$) with aldehydes ($HCHO$, $CH_3CHO$, etc.) lead to the formation of formic and acetic acid and higher organic acids which contribute between 5 and 20 percent towards the total acidity of tropospheric atmosphere (Wellburn, 1994). Other constituents of acid rain are those of pollutants, which are transported in the atmosphere and deposited with precipitation. Some complex organic compounds are also potentially important, but they are not well understood. Such organic compounds of anthropogenic origin are alkanes, polycyclic aromatic hydrocarbons (PAHs), Pthallic acid esters, fatty acid ethyl esters, pesticides and a diverse group of common industrial chemicals, such as polychlorinated biphenyls, benzaldenyde, tri-n-butylophosphate and diphenylamine. According to Haines (1981), these compounds are either produced by fuel combustion or are introduced into the atmosphere by combustion processes and thus are likely to be related to acidic precipitation. In areas of acidic rain, concentrations of metal are also higher in the precipitation (Hanssen et al., 1980). Lead, zinc, copper, iron, manganese, nickel, mercury and cadmium exhibited this trend (Haines, 1981). Sulphur content of Indian coal varies between 0.5 to 2 percent by weight whereas natural oil has 0.1 to 3 percent S content (Kleber, et al., 1986). Natural gas has less than 0.1 percent of sulphur content. In India oil consumption has increased approximately 50 times from $1.1 \times 10^3$ metric tons in 1952 to $54.3 \times 10^3$ in 1995. Thermal power plant's capacity has also increased from 2.6 billion kWh in 1950-51 to 247.7 billion kWh in 1993-94 (Aggarwal, 1996). It means an estimated 2500 tons of sulphur are being released in the atmosphere due to thermal power plants alone as per data available for 1993-94 thermal power generation (Mohan and Kumar, 1998).

## Effects of Acid Rain on Soil

Soils are known to be well-buffered system against chemical change. Soil acidification increases the mobility of nutrients resulting in its leaching consequently nutrient deficiency. On the other hand acidity of soil releases the toxic heavy metals such as Al, Mn, Fe, which on availability to plants cause deleterious effects. Acidification affects the biological activity of soil, reduces rates of litter decomposition and restricts consequent nutrient release, which can affect plant growth. The release of metals such as Al forms can be toxic to both soil organisms as well as the plant root. With acidification, toxic heavy metals become freely available and thus easily absorbed by the plant roots. In general acidity in soil lowers the species diversity and activity of soil biota. Accumulation of organic matter due to decrease in litter decomposition rate is often an observation due to increase in acidity of soils (NRC, 1986). This is particularly important for forest soils where decomposition of litter on the forest floor is a major source of nutrients for the trees. Soil acidity is also found to disturb the symbiotic relationships between fungus and host referred to as mycorrhizae assisting the trees in uptake of nutrients.

Deficiency of Ca, K and Mg is often linked with increasing soil acidity (Mackenzie and Ashry, 1989). Increasing H ions leach cations from soil especially those near the surface and Ca and Mg are found to be more heavily leached than K. Such negative effects may be neutralized due to increasing fertilizing effects of nitrates and sulfates. However, with continued deposition, forest productivity may be affected by lack of nutrients other than nitrogen leading to forest decline (Eriksson et al., 1992). Both wet and dry deposition transfer sulfates and nitrate to soils, but deposition of protons has the effect of increasing soil acidity. This mobilizes and leaches away nutrient cations, which then reduces soil fertility.

There is a matter of debate whether acid rain helps or harms the terrestrial and aquatic ecosystems as acid rain contains several nutrients like N, K and also trace elements, often in a form readily available for plants use. The sulphur content in the deposition is beneficial to S-deficient soils. But too much nutrients are toxic for the soil.

A 30 years study conducted at New Hampshire experimental forest, USA showed serious acid rain damage to the soil and trees. The analysis for calcium showed that organically bound calcium level of soil had dropped to about half the value observed 20 years back. Calcium has alkaline property so less Ca in the soil means less acid rain neutralizing capacity.

Forests of central and eastern European forests have been more severely damaged than that in the USA from acid rain. Water and soil acidification is up to three times greater. A German study indicated that the nitrogen had posed a greater problem than sulphur. Excess nitrogen may also be harmful due to many synergistic actions between plant's environments. In presence of excess nitrogen in acid rain, trees grow abnormally fast. Already weakened by ozone and other pollutants, the trees were further weakened by rapid growth and eventually became unable to handle ordinary stresses like weather extremes or insect attacks. Also the excess nitric acid leaches the alkaline calcium and magnesium from the soil. After the soil looses alkaline Ca and Mg, it has less ability to neutralize acid rain so tree roots are damaged. Until recently sulphur in acid rain was the major concern, but as sulphur dioxide emissions are scheduled to be controlled, the less well controlled nitrogen oxides become an increasing concern with respect to soil.

Acid rain accelerates the leaching of Ca and Mg through soil (Overrein, 1972; Haman, 1977; Abrahamsen et al., 1977). Strayer and Alexander (1981) did an experiment on forest soils by exposing the soil samples to SAR of pH 3.2 – 4.1 three times a week for 7 weeks. The major effects were lower pH values, higher total and exchange acidity, higher exchangeable Al and lower rates of heterotrophic activities in the surface than in subsurface soil. Changes in soil pH associated with agricultural practices are known to influence individual N transformations e.g. the liming of acid soils has been shown to stimulate nitrification (Dancer, et al., 1973; Nyborg and Hoyt, 1978) and N – mineralization (Ishaque and Cornfield, 1972). Labeda and Alexander (1978) have shown that acid precipitation in form of dry deposition also inhibits nitrification in certain soils.

## Effects of Acid Rain on Forest Species

Forest decline is a complex phenomenon of different appearances and different types of decline have been defined depending on symptoms and geographic occurrences (Blank *et al.*, 1988). Effects of acid rain on plant growth are often species specific. Some plants show enhanced growth (Wood and Bormann, 1977; Evans and Lewin, 1981; Lee *et al.*, 1981; Raynal *et al.*, 1982; Troiano *et al.*, 1982), some no effect (Lee *et al.*, 1981) and others reduced growth (Lee *et al.*, 1981; Evans *et al.*, 1981b; Raynal *et al.*, 1982; Johnston *et al.*, 1982) under acidic precipitation.

Tree growth is a result of multiple interacting physiological processes influenced by an inherited genetic constitution and the ambient environment (Back *et al.*, 1995). In several experiments interactions between acid rain and the chemical and biological characteristics of the soil have been found to be connected to the growth response of conifer seedlings (Ashenden and Bell, 1988; Reich *et al.*, 1988; Payer *et al.*, 1990; Shipley *et al.*, 1992). Increased acidity of the rain water predisposes tree seedlings to a number of environmental stresses, which affect the seedling germination, growth and survival (Percy, 1986; Jacobson *et al.*, 1990a; Sheppard *et al.*, 1993a and b). The erosion of epicuticular waxes by acid rain was first reported by Shriner (1974) in *Quercus prunus* and *Liriodendron tulipifera* at pH 3.2.

There were many studies conducted in Europe, USA and Canada to assess the effect of acid rain on forests. In USA from 1980-1990 a National Acid Precipitation Assessment Program (NAPAP) was conducted. One of its results showed harmful effects of acid fog on the needle of red spruce trees growing along the main coast (NAPAP, 1988). The wax on spruce needles was degraded by acid rain and damaged needles turn brown during the winter and fall from the trees. It has been proposed that the forest decline syndrome in central Europe is a consequence of an interaction between predisposing effects of air pollutants and a cold or dry climate (Brown *et al.*, 1987; Barnes and Davison, 1988). In Germany a hypothesis was developed according to which photooxidants cause deterioration of cell membranes and cuticular waxes, making them more permeable to ions and solutes (Magel and Ziegler, 1986; Mengal *et al.*, 1987). Nutrients leach out of leaves (Scherbatskoy and Klein, 1983; Reich *et al.*, 1988) of the trees exposed to acid mists. Mycorrhizal and fine root deterioration also occur due to low pH of the rain (Blaschke, 1986), so nutrient deficiency is induced in the roots and leaves, which in turn leads to a decreased state of hardening and a lowering of cold tolerance (Prinz *et al.*, 1985).

Increase in growth and the needle nitrogen concentration of conifer seedlings have been reported after exposure to acidic deposition containing nitrate or ammonium ions (Billen *et al.*, 1990; Jacobson *et al.*, 1990b; Dean and Johnson, 1992; Shelburne *et al.*, 1993; Sheppard *et al.*, 1993a). Nitrogen deposited by acid rain may prolong the growing period and delay cuticular development, thus causing a decrease in the degree of hardening (Friedland *et al.*, 1984). Sulphate containing precipitation causes decrease in growth parameters (Leith *et al.*, 1989; Jacobson *et al.*, 1990a and b; McLaughlin *et al.*, 1993; Sheppard *et al.*, 1993a). Apart from these trends, the individual conifer species showed varied response to acid rain (Lee and Weber, 1979; Percy, 1986; Abouguendia and Baschak, 1987; Billen *et al.*, 1990). White spruce was found to be more susceptible to visible injuries and sulphur accumulation than Jack pine, which did not show any symptoms of disturbances in physiology during 7 weeks exposure (Abouguendia and Baschak, 1987). Percy (1986) found conifer seedlings to be more susceptible to acid treatment than deciduous forest trees. It was found that post germination development of seedlings of sugar maple might be retarded by simulated rain of pH 3.0 (Raynal *et al.*, 1982; Dustine and Raynal, 1988).

During biochemical study of needles of Scots pine at 10 sites in Norway with different levels of acid deposition, Spidso and Korsmo (1993) found that the concentrations of N and P were highest in needles from the area receiving most acidity and the level of resin and tannin decreased significantly with increasing acidification. While Jordon *et al.* (1991) and Shumejko *et al.* (1996) did not find any effect of SAR on tannins in loblolly pine (*Pinus teada* L.) foliage, Shumejko *et al.* (1996) did not find any significant change in total phenolics, soluble proanthocyanidins and individual low molecular weight phenolics upon exposure to acid rain..

Tree damage due to acidification showed variety of symptoms :

1. **Yellowing in stands:** Tip yellowing starts in the older needles of the lower and middle crown area. After sometimes, they become necrotic showing sub top dying symptom. This happens in combination with frost, drought, insect or fungal interactions.

2. **Crown thinning:** It generally occurs on nutrient poor sites at middle elevations. There is pronounced crown thinning due to death of crown having different visible symptoms on leaves.

3. **Needle necrosis:** In older needles particularly in the lower and middle lower area, orange yellow symptoms start which then turn into reddish brown and then fell off. This type of damage occurs in stands more than 60 years old.

4. **Storknest development:** Due to reduced height of firs, the treetop becomes flattened.

5. **Development of secondary branches:** Adverse growth of apical portion leads to growth of secondary lateral branches reducing the timber quality of affected trees.

## Effects of Acid Rain on Crop Plants

Acid rain is widely believed to be harmful to vegetation either by direct deposition on the foliage or indirectly by leaching of nutrients from the soil (Rathier and Frink, 1984). Although forests are thought to be particularly endangered, agriculture crops may also be damaged. A report by EPA (1980) expressed concern for the future food supply due to acid rain problem. Detrimental effects of increased rain acidity on crop plants may include visible necrosis of foliage (Ferenbaugh, 1976; Evans *et al.*, 1977a and 1978; Evans and Curry, 1979), reduced symbiotic nitrogen fixation by legumes (Shriner and Johnston, 1981) and reduced growth and yield (Lee *et al.*, 1981; Ashenden and Bell, 1987; Ashenden and Bell, 1989; Singh and Agrawal, 1996). The acid deposition not only changes the growth pattern of individual plants, but also changes the species composition and diversity due to its direct impact on plants and indirect impact on soil acidification (Falkengren – Grerup, 1990).

**Foliar Injury by Acid Rain** : Injury to leaf by acid rain largely depends on the effective dose, determined by the contact time of an individual water droplet or film with the foliage surface, to which the leaf tissue is exposed (Evans *et al.*, 1981a; Shriner, 1981). The extent of contact time depends on wettability of leaf and its morphological features that affect the run off of water from the surface (Martin and Juniper, 1970). The damage to foliage by acid rain first causes effects at the cellular level (Swanson *et al*, 1973; Dixit, 1988). Inside the tissues of leaves, the cells undergo parallel changes in physiology and morphology (Olszyk *et al*, 1987). Johnston *et al.* (1986) found visible foliar injury symptoms on radish leaves at 4.0 and 3.0 pH. Injury symptoms include adaxial and bifacial interveinal necrosis and marginal bleached necrotic areas. The leaves of plants exposed to simulated acid rain at pH 3.0 were often puckered due to continued leaf expansion and often marginal necrosis occurred.

Evans *et al.* (1982a) in an experiment on radish, lettuce, wheat and alfalfa observed visible foliar injury on radish at pH below 3.4 at the beginning of exposure and at pH 4.2 at latter stage. In lettuce, visible foliar injury was present in plants exposed to rainfalls of pH 3.1 and 2.7, in alfalfa below 4.0, and very little visible foliar injury was observed in case of wheat. Foliar injury was also reported in case of soybean leaves (Evans and Curry, 1979) and in pinto beans, sunflower and spiderwort (Evans and Curry, 1979 and Evans *et al.*, 1977a) at low pH. Rathier and Frink (1984) observed visible injury near the midrib and veins of leaves in tobacco plants treated with SAR of pH 2.0 and 2.5. Evans (1980) and Evans and Curry (1979) showed that the foliage of herbaceous dicotyledonous plants may be the most sensitive of all angiosperms and gymnosperms.

The cuticle of plants provides the primary barrier from infection and chemical and physical injuries. Rain with a low pH has the potential to affect the cuticle since it contacts the leaf surface directly. Evans *et al.* (1977a, b) and Evans and Curry (1979) reported leaf surface injuries due to simulated acid rain of pH 2.3 to 3.1. Most injury occurred near vascular tissue, stomatas and trichomes. Haines *et al.* (1985) found that acidic rain injury occurs in more wettable leaves that had greater water holding capacity. Cotyledons of cabbage plants were found more affected by simulated acid rain than true leaves (Caporn and Hutchinson, 1986). Epicuticular waxes on leaf surfaces of higher plants are an important barrier to ion and water movement across the cuticle. Percy and Baker (1987) reported that the species with crystalline wax on foliar surfaces were more susceptible to acid rain damage than the species with amorphous wax in response to simulated acid rain. Cuticles with crystalline wax showed injury near trichomes and more injury overall, whereas amorphous wax surfaces were injured near veins and to a lesser extent across the leaf surface. Hongfa *et al.* (2000) studied the responses of twelve crop plants to different levels of SAR (pH 5.6, 4.6, 4.2, 3.6 and 2.8). The threshold of visible injury was pH 3.0 for wheat, maize, barley and spinach; pH 2.5 for cabbage, soybean, bean, rape, cucumber, tomato and cotton and pH 2.0 for rice.

**Effects of Acid Rain on Physiological Parameters** : Physiological studies conducted to evaluate the effects of acid rain on soybeans have produced in consistent results. Norby and Luxmoore (1983) found reduction in $CO_2$ fixation, when soybeans were treated with rain of pH 2.6. This decrease was ascribed to reduction in leaf area. Porter and Sheridan (1981) also found reduced $CO_2$ fixation in alfalfa. Norby *et al.* (1985) didn't find any decrease in $CO_2$ fixation when soybeans were treated with simulated acid rain at pH 3.4. In laboratory and green house studies, photosynthesis was decreased at pH 2.0 and 3.0 in *Platanus occidentalis* (Neufeld *et al.*, 1985) and *Cladina stellaris* (Lechowicz, 1982), respectively. Photosynthesis rate was also found to increase in *Phaseolus vulgaris* (Ferenbaugh, 1976) and Davis soybean (Norby *et al.*, 1985) at comparable rain acidities. Smith *et al.* (1991) and Takemoto *et al.* (1987) did not find any significant effect of low pH of rain on $CO_2$ fixation, leaflet chlorophyll content, leaf water potentials of soybean (Smith *et al.*, 1991).

**Effects of Acid Rain on Growth and Productivity** : The effect of acid rain on plants is not always well defined. Several workers have reported that simulated rain at high levels of acidity (pH below 3.0) may reduce primary production in plants (Harcourt and Farrar, 1980; Amthor, 1984; Evans and Lewin, 1981; Evans *et al.*, 1983). With higher pH most researchers have found little effect on plant growth responses. Evans *et al.* (1982b, 1983) found reduction in the yield of field grown crops with simulated acid rain at pH 4. Ashenden and Bell (1987) found 9 – 17% yield reductions in winter barley grown on a range of British soils in response to the normal ambient pH range of rainfall of 3.5 – 4.5. Ashenden and Bell (1989) reported yield reductions in seedlings of *Vicia faba* L. exposed to SAR at pH 4.5 in comparison to rain at pH 5.6.

Plant sensitivity may differ during different stages of plant development (Caporn and Hutchinson, 1986). In corn, Banwart *et al.* (1987) reported cultivar differences in response to acid rain and observed no significant effect on grain yield down to pH 3.5. Lee *et al.* (1981) demonstrated interspecific differences in crop response to acidic rain. Out of 28 crop species exposed to SAR at pH 5.6, 4.0, 3.5, 3.0, marketable yield was reduced for five crops, increased for six, ambiguously affected for one and unaffected for 15. Evans *et al.* (1982a) found no significant effect on yield of wheat plants exposed to simulated acid rain at pH levels between 5.7 and 2.7. Irving and Miller (1981) did not find any harmful effect on soybean productivity in response to SAR. Irving (1983) studied the effect of simulated acid rain on 14 crop cultivars in field conditions and 34 in controlled environment. He found maximum plants showed no effect on growth or yield after exposure to SAR. Few crops showed negative effect on growth and yield, others exhibited positive response. Nine percent reduction in the yield of field corn exposed to pH 4.0 was found. Reduction in root mass was demonstrated by Lee et al. (1981) after simulated acidic rainfalls. Evans et al. (1982a) found reduction in fresh mass and yield of lettuce at and below 4.0 pH. Evans et al. (1983) reported reduction in number of pods per plant, seeds per plant, mass of seeds per plant and also in the seed yield of the soybean. In experiments in which natural rain was not excluded from research plots, Heagle et al. (1983) showed no significant effect of SAR at pH levels between 5.5 and 2.4 on field grown Davis soybeans. Irving and Miller (1981) found no effect of SAR of pH 3.1 on yield of Wells soybeans in a similar situation. In those experiments where natural rain was excluded from research plots, Evans et al. (1984 and 1985) found no significant effects on the yield of Williams soybean at pH of rain between 5.6 and 2.8. Singh and Agrawal (1996) reported reduction in shoot height, root length, biomass accumulation and yield of two cultivars of wheat exposed to SAR pH from 4.5 to 3.0. Acid rain was also found to affect the pollen germination and growth in corn and other plants (Cox, 1984; Wertheim and Craker, 1988).

## Effects of Acid Rain on Lower Plants

Acid rain not only affects the higher plants, but also affects the lower plants, fungi and other micro organisms. Changes caused in the chemical and biological characteristics of soil due to acid rain, including a variety of soil borne micro organisms and microbial processes, have been reported (Strayer and Alexander, 1981; Francis, 1982; Killham et al., 1983; Johnson and Reuss, 1984; Will et al., 1986; McColl and Firestone, 1987).

Microorganisms that are closely associated with plant roots can strongly affect plant growth and function. Studies showed that simulated acid rain has altered interactions of plants with a soil borne pathogenic fungus (Shafer et al., 1985), Rhizobia (Porter and Sheridan, 1981; Shriner and Johnston, 1981) and ectomycorrizal fungi (Brewer and Heagle, 1983; Killham and Firestone, 1983). Acid depositions could affect rhizosphere microorganisms directly as acidic solution percolates through the soil or indirectly following responses by plant foliage or roots. Shafer (1988) showed that simulated acidic rain increased some bacterial populations in the rhizosphere of a hybrid of sorghum – sudan grass.

Lichens form the major portion of the total biomass and productivity in arctic and subarctic systems (Ahti and Oksanen, 1990; Longton, 1992). Lichens are also important for the maintenance of normal soil humidity (Tenhunen et al., 1992). The changes in the frequency of lichen species containing cyanobacteria during the last decades indicate that they may be more sensitive to acid pollution than the species containing green algae (Wetmore, 1989). Nitrogen fixation by lichens was found sensitive in some cases at acid rain of pH 4 (Englund, 1978; Fritz–Sheridan, 1985) and in some cases no adverse effect even at pH 3.4 (Gunther, 1988) or pH 3 (Hallingbäck and Kellner, 1992). Since wet deposits are probably important sources of nutrients for lichens (Crittenden, 1989), elevated concentrations of acidic ions in polluted rain might be expected to have an adverse impact on lichen growth. Acid rain causes changes in composition and distribution of communities (Scott et al., 1989; Farmer et al., 1991) and disturb or affect adversely the physiological activities of microorganisms (Sigal and Johnston, 1986; Scott and Hutchinson, 1987; Gunther, 1988; Roy- Arcand et al. 1989; Hallingbäck and Kellner, 1992; Kyotoviita and Crittenden, 1994). Due to this, reduced growth rates are found (Lechowicz, 1987; Scott and Hutchinson, 1990; Hallingbäck and Kellner, 1992).

There were many experiments done to assess the impact of acid rain on mycorrhizae. This includes mycorrhizal associations in Betula papyrifera (Kaene and Manning, 1988), Picea abies (Blaschke, 1988;

Blaschke and Weiss, 1990), *Picea rubens* (Meier *et al.*, 1989) and *Pinus thunbergii* (Maehara *et al.*, 1993). Honrubia and Diaz (1996) did not find any negative effect of acidity on mycorrhization. Instead, ectomycorrhizae were slightly increased in the most acidic treatments (pH 3). McAfee and Fortin (1987), Meier *et al.* (1989), Blaschke and Weiss (1990) and Edwards and Kelly (1992) found no effect on ectomycorrhizal fungi. While Shafer *et al.* (1985) reported inhibition of mycorrhization of *Thelephora terrestris* and *Lacearia laccata*. Blaschke (1988) in natural soil and Rudawska *et al.* (1996) in acid soil reported reduction in mycorrhizae. So, it can be concluded that responses to acidity may vary depending on host plant fungus species and soil characteristics and duration of exposure.

## Effects of Acid Rain on Fresh Water Biota

**Phytoplankton:** Oligotrophic lakes of temperate region are dominated by Chrysophyceae and Bacilliarophyceae members, whereas acidified lakes may be dominated by Cyanophyceae, Chlorophyceae and Dinophyceae members (Yan and Stokes, 1978; Kerekes and Freedman, 1988). Smol and Glew (1992) have suggested that species of diatoms and golden brown algae are very sensitive to change in water chemistry and hence can be used as indicators of acidity of water. Dixit *et al.* (1991) found 3 indicator groups of diatoms in a study of 72 lakes in Sudbury.

1. **Indicators of low pH:** *Eunotia pectinatus, Fragilaria acidobiontica, Pinnularia subcapitata, Tabellaria quadriseptata.*

2. **Indicators of low pH and high metals (Cu, Ni):** *Eunotia exigua, E. tenella, Frustulina rhomboides saxonica, Pinnularia hilseana.*

3. **Indicators of high pH:** *Achnanthes lewisiana, Cyclotella meneghiniana, Fragilaria construens, F. crotonensis.*

Lake acidification was found to divert the community domination of golden brown algae to those of chlorophytes especially by *Chlorella mucosai* (Findlay and Kasian, 1986). When the pH of lake increased from 5.0 to 5.5, species of preacidification phytoplankton community reappeared (Schindler, 1990). In Lake 223, the whole phytoplankton biomass was estimated as 1465 kg compared with 2410 kg following acidification (Findley and Saesura, 1980). The data clearly shows that acidification has relatively small effect on primary production compared to large changes in species diversity.

**Periphyton :** This group of microalgae can remain constant in acidified lakes. Periphytons often form felt like mats at littoral zone of lakes. Filamentous green algae Mongeotia sp. was found to be an indicator after the pH of lake decreased to less than 5.6 (Schindler *et al.*, 1985).

**Macrophytes :** Decline in abundance of certain species of macrophytes has been found associated with decline in pH of lake water (Grahn, 1986). Such decline was accompanied by abundance of acidophilous peatmoss *Sphagnum subsecundum*. Acidophilous mosses were also found abundant in acidic volcanic lakes in Japan (Yoshimura, 1933), water bodies affected by acid mine drainage (Hargreaves *et al.*, 1975) and acidic lakes near Sudbury. Acidified lakes have a much more restricted distribution of macrophytes. Plants are only found in a shallow littoral fringe and only 15 percent of the bottom of the lake is vegetated.

## Interaction of Acid Rain with Other Pollutants

Acid rain has been found to modify the response of plants to other air pollutants. The effects of a combination of air pollutants and acid rain may be considerably worse than the sum of the component effects of each pollutant if applied singly (Ormrod, 1978; Thompson *et al.*, 1972). Jacobson *et al.* (1980) found that ozone caused greater yield depression at the pH 2.8 rain treatment and that acid rain caused a shift in dry matter partitioning from vegetative to reproductive organs in the charcoal filtered air treatment.

The relative sensitivity of crop species to combined effects of $SO_2$ and SAR treatment showed bean to be most sensitive, tomato, soybean and rape to be midsensitive and rice, wheat and cotton to be tolerant (Hongfa *et al.*, 2000). The combined treatment of $SO_2$ and SAR on yield reduction of pinto bean, tomato and carrot were antagonistic and for cotton was synergistic.

Physiological functions, levels of metabolites, biomass accumulation and yield components showed unfavourable alterations in response to individual and combined treatments of SAR and $SO_2$. For yield response to SAR, vegetable crops were found to be most sensitive followed by cash crops and then cereal crops. The effects of SAR with a chemical composition similar to that of Cubatao, Brazil on soybean cultivated either in sand or in acid soil from Mogi valley or in acidity corrected soil reduced the amount of epicuticular wax and caused a decrease in photosynthetic activity and chlorophyll content. These effects were more severe at plants cultivated in acid soil (Alves *et al.*, 1990).

Treatment of eight cultivars of soybean with SAR containing different amount of F modified the response of cultivars in relation to the development of visible symptoms. The most sensitive cultivar to SAR accumulated more F and resulted in necrosis mainly to younger leaves of soybean, and the area near to the trichomes being the most sensitive part of the leaves (Bustamante *et al.*, 1993).

Shan *et al.* (1995) did not find any significant interactive effect of $O_3$ and SAR on chlorophyll contents as well as on biomass accumulation of above ground parts, below ground parts and whole seedling and carbon allocation of the Armand pine seedlings. Shan *et al.* (1996) again did not find any significant interactive effect of $O_3$ and SAR on dry weight, dark respiration rate, transpiration rate and water use efficiency of *Pinus armandi* French seedlings. Net photosynthetic rate, leaf dry weight and chlorophyll $a + b$ content were also not significant, however, the interactive effects of $O_3$ and SAR on net photosynthetic rate on a whole plant basis were significant.

Wet and dry scavenging processes are the prime mechanisms by which gaseous and particulate pollutants are removed from the atmosphere. In Western Europe and North America, the wet process in cloud scavenging modified the chemical composition and pH of rainwater. The extent of acidity was dependent on the neutralization potential of rainwater components. In the Indian subcontinent the nature of rainwater is mostly alkaline due to influence of soil derived particulate matter. The pH in industrialized nations, however, showed values ranging from 4 to 6. Predominance of sulphate and nitrate ions in precipitation has been attributed as cause of increasing acidity of rainwater. Acidification affects the biological activity of soil, reduces rates of litter decomposition and restricts constituent nutrient release. Acidity also helps releasing toxic heavy metals which on availability cause deleterious effects on growth. Forest decline has often been correlated with acid rain problem. Tree damage symptoms may vary from yellowing of stands to needle necrosis, abnormal canopy development to crown thinning in forest stands due to acidity in rainfall. Crop plants may also be affected in form of visible injury, unfavourable changes in growth pattern, physiology, growth and yield. Lower plants also showed their sensitivity to acid rain. Acid rain also influences the effects of other stresses such as air pollution by modifying the response pattern. There is a need to establish a network of measuring acidity in precipitation throughout the country to identify the risk zones in view of increasing industrialization and urbanization of the country.

## SUMMARY

Acidification of rainwater is identified as one of the most serious environmental problem of transboundary nature. The rainwater pH of many developed countries has shown values less than 5. The Scandinavia, northeastern US and southern Canada received highly acidic rainfall which had specific deleterious effects such as fish killing, acidification of fresh water bodies, crop and forest damage and corrosion of cultural property. The acid rain is mainly a mixture of $H_2SO_4$ and $HNO_3$ depending upon the relative quantities of oxides of sulphur and nitrogen emission. Wet and dry depositions of protons increase the soil acidity which mobilizes and leaches away nutrient cations, increases availability of toxic heavy metals and reduces soil fertility. Changes in soil characteristics have been found to influence the growth and productivity of forest trees unfavourably. Conifers have been shown to be particularly sensitive to acid rain. Crop plants also show a wide variety of sensitivity to acidity of rain. Crop plants are generally hampered below pH 4. Fresh water biota showed variable response to lake acidity. Change in species composition of lake biota was reported due to lowering of pH. Some important acid indicator species of phytoplanktons have been identified. The present article reviews the literature on acid rain problem and its impact on plants.

## ACKNOWLEDGEMENT

The authors thankfully acknowledge the financial assistance from the Ministry of Environment and Forests, Government of India, New Delhi.

## REFERENCES

- Abouguendia, Z. M. and Baschak, L. A. (1987). Responses of two western Canadian conifers to simulated acid precipitation. *Water, Air and Soil Pollut.* **33**: 15–22.
- Abrahamsen, G. (1980). Acid precipitation, plant nutrients and forest growth. In: Ecological Impact of Acid Precipitation (Eds. Drablos, D. and Tollan, A.) pp. 58–63, Proc. Int. Conf., SNSF Proj. Aas, Norway.
- Abrahamsen, G., Horntvedt, R. and Tveite, B. (1977). Impacts of acid precipitation on coniferous forest ecosystems. *Water, Air and Soil Pollut.* **8**: 57–73.
- Aggarwal, J. C. (1996). Human development in India since independence. Shipra Publications, Delhi.
- Ahti, T. and Oksanen, J. (1990). Epigeic lichen communities of taiga and tundra regions. *Vegitatio.* **86**: 39–70.
- Alves, P. L. C. A., Oliva, M. A., Cambraia, J. and Sant'anna, R. (1990). Efeitos, da chuva ácida simulada e decrease um solo decrease Cubatão (SP) sobre parâmetros relacionados com a fotossíntese e a traspiraçã o decrease plantas decrease soja. *Rev. Bras. Fisiol. Veg.* **2**: 7.
- Amthor, J. S. (1984). Does acid rain directly influence plant growth? Some comments and observations. *Environ. Pollut. Ser. A.* **36**: 1–6.
- Ashenden, T. W. and Bell, S. A. (1987). Yield reductions in winter barley grown on a range of soils exposed to simulated acid rain. *Plant and Soil.* **98**: 433–437.
- Ashenden, T. W. and Bell, S. A. (1988). Growth responses of birch and sitka spruce exposed to acidified rain. *Environ. Pollut.* **51**: 153–162.
- Ashenden, T. W. and Bell, S. A. (1989). Growth responses of three legume species exposed to simulated acid rain. *Environ. Pollut.* **62**, 21–29.
- Bäck, Jaana, Satu Huttunen, Minna Turunen and Jukka Lamppu (1995). Effects of acid rain on growth and nutrient concentrations in scot pine and Norway spruce seedlings grown in a nutrient rich soil. Environ. Pollut. **89**: 177–187.
- Banerjee, T. (1997). Acid rain: The danger ahead. *Momentum* (Feb.97). Vol. II (issue 7): 29–30.
- Banwart, W. L., Porter, P. M., Hassett, J. J. and Walker, W. M. (1987). SAR effects on yield response of two corn cultivars. *Agron. J.* **79**: 497–501.
- Barnes, J. D. and Davison, A. W. (1988). The influence of ozone on the winter hardiness of Norway spruce (*Picea abies* (L.) Karst.). *New Phytol.* **108**: 159–166.
- Billen, N., Schätzle, H., Seufert, G. and Arundt, U. (1990). Performance of some growth variables. *Environ. Pollut.* **68**: 419–434.
- Blank, L. W., Roberts, T. M. and Skeffington, R. A. (1988). New perspectives on forest decline. *Nature.* **336**, 27–30.
- Blaschke, H. (1986). Einfluss von saurer Beregnung und kalkung auf die Biomasse und Mykorrizierung der Feinwurzeln von Fichten. *Forstwissenschaftliches Centralblatt* (Hamburg). **105**: 324–329.
- Blaschke, H. (1988). Mycorrhizal infection and changes in fine root development of Norway spruce influenced

by acid rain in the field. In: Ectomycorrhiza and acid rain. Proceedings of the workshop on ectomycorrhiza/ expert meeting (Eds. Jansen, A. E., Dighton, J., and Bresser, A. H.) *Air Pollut. Res. Rep.* **12**: 113–115.

- Blaschke, H. and Weiss, M. (1990). Impact of ozone, acid mist and soil characteristics on growth and development of fine roots and ectomycorrhiza of young clonal Norway spruce. *Environ. Pollut.* **64**: 255–263.

- Braekke, F. H. (1976). Impacts of acid rain precipitation on forest and fresh water ecosystems in Norway. Fragrapport FR6/76, SNSF Project AS- NLH, Norway.

- Brewer, P. F. and Heagle, A. S. (1983). Interactions between *Glomus geosporum* and exposure of soybean to ozone or simulated acid rain in the field. *Phytopathol.* **73**: 1035–1040.

- Brezonik, P. L., Edgerton, E. S. and Hendry, C. D. (1980) Acid precipitation and sulphate deposition in Florida. *Science.* 208: 1027–1029.

- Brown, K. A., Roberts, T. M. and Blank, L. W. (1987). Interaction between cold sensitivity in Norway spruce: A factor contributing to the forest decline in central Europe? *New Phytol.* **105**: 149–155.

- Bubenick, D.V. (1984). Acid rain information book, 2$^{nd}$ edition. USA: Noyes Publications.

- Burman, S. (1985). Environmental impact of acid rain. *Yojana.* **29**: 15-18.

- Bustamante, M. N., Oliva, M. A., Sant'anna, R. and Lopes, N. F. (1993). Sensibilidade da sojo ao fl or. *Rev. Bras. Fisio. Veg.* **5**: 151.

- Caporn, S. J. M. and Hutchinson, T. C. (1986). The contrasting response to simulated acid rain of leaves and cotyledons of cabbage. *New Phytol.* **103**: 311–324.

- Chandrawanshi, C. K., Patel, V. K. and Patel, K. S. (1997). Acid rain in Korba city of India. In. *J. Environ. Protec.* **17**: 656–661.

- Cox, R. M. (1984). Sensitivity of forest plant reproduction to long range transported air pollutants: *in vitro* and *in vivo* sensitivity of *Oenothera parviflora* L. pollen to simulated acid rain. *New Phytol.* **97**: 63–70.

- Crittenden, P. D. (1989). Nitrogen relations of mat forming lichens. In: Nitrogen, phosphorus and sulphur utilization by fungi (Eds. Boddy, L., Merchant, R. and Read, D. J.) pp. 243–268, Cambridge: Cambridge University Press.

- Dancer, W. S., Peterson, L. A. and Chesters, G. (1973). Ammonification and nitrification of N as influenced by soil pH and previous N treatments. *Soil Sci. Soc. Am. Proc.* **37**: 67–69.

- Datar, S. V., Mukhopadhyay, B. and Srivastava, H. N. (1996). Trends in background air pollution parameters over India. *Atmos. Environ.* **30**: 3677–3682.

- Dean, T. J. and Johnson, J. D. (1992). Growth responses of young slash pine trees to simulated acid rain and ozone stress. *Can. J. For. Res.* **22**: 839–848.

- Dixit, A. B. (1988). Effects of particulate pollutants on plants at ultrastructural and cellular levels. *Annals of Bot.* **62**: 643–651.

- Dixit, S. S., Dixit, A. S. and Smol, J. P. (1991). Multivariate environmental inferences based on diatom assemblages from Sudbury (Canada) lakes. *Fresh Water Biol.* **26**: 251–266.

- Dustin, C. D. and Raynal, D. J. (1988). Effects of simulated acid rain on sugar maple seedling root growth. *Environ. Exp. Bot.* **28**: 207–213.

- Edwards, G. S. and Kelly, J. M. (1992). Ectomycorrhizal colonization of loblolly pine seedlings during three growing seasons in response to ozone, acidic precipitation and soil Mg status. *Environ. Pollut.* **76**: 71–77.

- Englund, B. (1978). Effects of environmental factors on acetylene reduction by intact thallus and excised cephalodia of *Peltigera aphthosa* Willd. *Ecological Bulletins (Stockholm).* **26**: 234–246.

- EPA (US Environmental Protection Agency, 1980). Acid rain. EPA 600/9-79-036. *Washington,* pp. 36.

- Eriksson, E., Karlun, E. and Lundmark, J. E. (1992). Acidification of forest soils in Sweden. *Ambio.* 21: 150–154.

- Evans, L. S, Hendry, G. R., Stenstand, G. J., Johnson, D. W. and Francis, A. J. (1981a). Acidic precipitation: Considerations for an air quality standard. *Water, Air and Soil Pollut.* 16: 469–509.

- Evans, L. S. (1980). Foliar responses that may determine plant injury by simulated acid rain. In: Polluted rain (Eds. Toribara, T., Miller, M. and Morrow, P.) pp. 239-257. 12$^{th}$ Ann. Rochester International Conference on Environmental Toxicity, Plenum Press, New York.

- Evans, L. S. and Curry, T. M. (1979). Differential responses of plant foliage to simulated acid rain. *Am. J. Bot.* 66: 953–962.

- Evans, L. S. and Lewin, K. F. (1981). Growth development and yield response of pinto beans and soybeans to hydrogen ion concentrations of simulated acidic rain. *Environ. Exp. Bot.* **21**: 103–113.
- Evans, L. S., Curry, T. M. and Lewin, K. F. (1981b). Responses of leaves of *Phaseolus vulgaris* L. to simulated acidic rain. *New Phytol.* **88**: 403–420.
- Evans, L. S., Gmur, N. F. and Da Costa, F. (1977a). Leaf surface and histological perturbations of leaves of *Phaseolus vulgaris* and *Helianthus annus* after exposure to simulated acid rain. *Am. J. Bot.* **64**: 903–913.
- Evans, L. S., Gmur, N. F. and Da Costa, F. (1978). Foliar response of six clones of hybrid poplar to simulated acid rain. *Phytopathol.* **68**: 847–856.
- Evans, L. S., Gmur, N. F. and Kelsh, J. J. (1977b). Perturbations of upper leaf surface structures by simulated acid rain. *Environ. Exp. Bot.* **17**: 145–149.
- Evans, L. S., Gmur, N. F. and Mancini, D. (1982a). Effects of simulated acid rain on yields of *Raphanus sativus, Lactuca sativa, Triticum aestivum* and *Medicago sativa*. *Environ. Exp. Bot.* **22**: 445–453.
- Evans, L. S., Lewin, K. F. and Patti, M. J. (1984). Effects of simulated acidic rain on yields of field grown soybeans. *New Phytol.* **94**: 207–213.
- Evans, L. S., Lewin, K. F., Cunningham, E. A. and Patti, M. J. (1982b). Effects of simulated acid rain on yields of field grown crops. *New Phytol.* **91**: 429–441.
- Evans, L. S., Lewin, K. F., Patti, M. J. and Cunningham, E. A. (1983) Productivity of field grown soybeans exposed to simulated acid rain. *New Phytol.* **93**: 377–388.
- Evans, L. S., Lewin, K. F., Santucci, K. A. and Patti, M. J. (1985). Effects of frequency and duration of simulated acidic rainfalls on soybean yields. *New Phytol.* **100**: 199–208.
- Falkengren – Grerup, U. (1990). Distribution of field layer species in Swedish deciduous forests in 1929 – 54 and 1979 – 88 as related to soil pH. *Vegitatio*. **86**: 143–150.
- Farmer, A. M., Bates, J. W. and Bell, J. N. B. (1991). Comparisons of three woodland sites in NW Britain differing in richness of the epiphytic *Lobarion pulmonariae* community and levels of wet acidic deposition. *Holarctic Ecology*. **14**: 85–91.
- Ferenbaugh, R. W. (1976). Effects of simulated acid rain on *Phaseolus vulgaris* L. (Fabaceae). *Am. J. Bot.* **63**: 283–288.
- Findlay, D. L. and Kasian, S. E. M. (1986). Phytoplankton community response to acidification of Lake 223. Experimental lakes area, northeastern Ontario. *Can. J. Fish. Aquat. Sci.* **44**: 35–46.
- Findlay, D. L. and Saesura, G. (1980). Effects on phytoplankton biomass, succession and composition in Lake 223 as a result of lowering pH levels from 7 to 5.6. Data from 1974 to 1979. Fish Mar. Serv. Manuscr. Rep. No. 1585. Department of Fisheries and Oceans, Winnipeg, Manitoba.
- Fowler, D., Cape, J. N., Leith, I. D., Paterson, I. S., Kinnaired, J.W. and Nicholson, J. A. (1982). Air pollutants in agriculture and horticulture. In: Proc. 32nd School in Agricultural Sciences, University of Nittingham, 1980. Butterworths.
- Francis, A. J. (1982). Effects of acidic precipitation and acidity on soil microbial processes. *Water, Air and Soil Pollut* **18**: 375–394.
- Friedland, A. J., Gregory, R. A., Kärenlampi, L. and Johnson, A. H. (1984). Winter damage to foliage as a factor in red spruce decline. *Can. J. For. Res.* **14**: 963–965.
- Fritz-Sheridan R. P. (1985). Impact of simulated acid rains on nitrogenase activity in *Peltigera aphthosa* and *P. polydactyla*. *Lichenologist* **17**: 27–31.
- Gorham, E. (1958). Free acid in British soils. *Nature*. **181**: 106.
- Grahn, O. (1986). Vegetation structure and primary production in acidified lakes in southwestern Sweden. *Experientia*. **42**: 465–470.
- Gunther, A. J. (1988). Effect of simulated acid rain on nitrogenase activity in the lichen genus *Peltigera* under field and Laboratory conditions. *Water, Air, and Soil Pollut.* **38**: 379–385.
- Haines, B. (1979). Acid precipitation in southeastern United States: A brief review. *Georgia J. Sci.* **37**: 185–191.
- Haines, B. L., Jernstedt, J. A. and Neufeld, H. S. (1985). Direct foliar effects of simulated acid rain II. Leaf structure characteristics. *New Phytol.* **99**: 407–416.
- Haines, T. A. (1981). Acid precipitation and its consequences for aquatic ecosystems: A review. Transactions of Am. *Fisheries Soc.* **110**: 669–707.

- Hallingback, T., and Kellner, O. (1992) Effects of simulated nitrogen rich acid rain on the nitrogen fixing lichen *Peltigera aphthosa* (L.) Willd. *New Phytol.* **120:** 99-103.

- Haman, F. (1977). Effects of percolating water with graduated acidity upon the leaching of nutrients and the changes in some chemical properties of mineral soils. *J. Sci. Agric. Soc. Finl.* **49:** 250–257.

- Hanssen, J., Ramback, J., Semb, A. and Steinnes, E. (1980). Atmospheric deposition of trace elements in Norway. In: Proceedings of International Conference on the Ecological Impact of Acid Precipitation (Eds. Drablos, D. and Tollan, A.) pp. 116–117, Aas, Norway.

- Harcourt, S. A. and Farrar, J. F. (1980). Some effects of simulated acid rain on the growth of barley and radish. Environ. *Pollut. Ser. A.* **22:** 69–73.

- Hargreaves, J. W., Lloyed, E. J. H. and Whitten, B. A. (1975). Chemistry and vegetation of highly acidic streams. *Fresh water Biol.,* **5,** 563–576.

- Heagle, A. S., Philbeck, R. B., Brewer, P. F. and Ferrell, R. E. (1983). Response of soybean to simulated acid rain in the field. *J. Environ. Qual.* **12:** 538–543.

- Hongfa, C. (1989). Air pollution and its effects on plants in China. *J. Applied Ecology.* **26:** 763–773.

- Hongfa, C., Shu, J., Shen, Y., Gao, Y., Gao, J. and Zhang, L. (2000). Effects of Sulphur dioxide and acid deposition on Chinese crops. In: Environmental Pollution and Plant Responses (Eds. Agrawal, S. B. and Agrawal, M.) pp. 295–305, Lewis Publishers, Boca Raton, Florida, U.S.A.

- Honrubia, M. and Diaz, G. (1996). Effects of simulated acid rain on mycorrhizae of Aleppo pine (*Pinus halepensis* Miller) in calcareous soil. *Ann. Sci. For.* **53:** 947–954.

- Irving, P. M. (1983). Acid precipitation effects on crops: A review and analysis of research. *J. Environ. Qual.* **12:** 442–453.

- Irving, P. M. and Miller, J. E. (1981). Productivity of field grown soybeans exposed to acid rain and sulphur dioxide alone and in combination. *J. Environ. Qual.* **10:** 473–478.

- Ishaque, M. and Cornfield, A. H. (1972). Nitrogen mineralization and nitrification during incubation of East Pakistan "tea" soils in relation to pH. *Plant Soil.* **37:** 91–95.

- Jacobson, J. S., Bethard, T., Heller, L. I. and Lassoie, J. P. (1990b). Response of *picea rubens* seedlings to intermittent mist varying in acidity and in concentrations of sulphur and nitrogen containing pollutants. *Physiol. Plant.* **78:** 595–601.

- Jacobson, J. S., Heller, L. I., Yamada, K. E., Osmeloski, J. F., Bethard, T. and Lassoie, J. P. (1990a). Foliar injury and growth response of red spruce to sulphate and nitrate acidic mist. *Can. J. For. Res.* **20:** 58–65.

- Jacobson, J. S., Troiano, J., Colavito, L. J., Heller, L. I. and McCune, D. C. (1980). Polluted rain and plant growth. In: Polluted rain (Eds. Toribara, T. Y., Miller, M. and Morrow, P.) pp. 291–299, Plenum Press, New York.

- Johnson, D. W. and Reuss, J. O. (1984). Soil mediated effects of atmospherically deposited sulphur and nitrogen. *Phil. Trans. R. Soc. Lond. B,* **305:** 383–392.

- Johnston, J. W. Jr., Shriner, D. S., Klarer, C. J. and Lodge, D. M. (1982). Effect of rain pH on senescence, growth and yield of bush bean. *Environ. Exp. Bot.* **22:** 329–337.

- Johnston, J. W., Shriner, Jr. D. S., and Kinerley, C. K. (1986). The combined effects of simulated acid rain and ozone on injury, chlorophyll and growth of Radish. *Environ. Exp. Bot.* **26:** 107–113.

- Jordan, D. N., Green, T. N., Chappelka, A. H., Lockaby, B. G., Meldahl, R. S. and Gjerstad, D. H. (1991). Response of total tannins and phenolics in loblolly pine foliage exposed to ozone and acid rain. *J. Chem. Ecol.* **17:** 505–513.

- Keane, K. D. and Manning, W. J. (1988). Effects of ozone and simulated acid rain on birch seedling growth and formation of ectomycorrhizae. *Environ. Pollut.* **52:** 55–65.

- Kerekes, J. and Freedman, B. (1988). Physical, chemical and biological characteristics of three watersheds in Keijmkujik National Park, Nova Scotia. Arch. Environ. Contam. *Toxicol.* **18:** 183–200.

- Khemani, L. T. (1993). Air pollution and acid rain problem in the Indian region. Indian J. *Radio and Space Physics.* **22:** 207–214.

- Khemani, L. T., Momin, G. A. and Naik, Medha S. (1987). Influence of atmospheric pollutants on cloud microphysics and rainfall. *Boundary Layer Met.* **41:** 367–380.

- Khemani, L. T., Momin, G. A., Rao, P. S. P., Pillai, A. G., Safai, P. D., Mohan, K. and Rao, M. G. (1994). Atmospheric pollutants and their influence on acidification of rain water at an industrial location on the west coast of India. *Atmos. Environ.* **28**: 3145–3154.

- Khemani, L. T., Momin, G. A., Rao, P. S. Prakas, Safai, P. D., Singh, G., Chatterjee, R. N. and Prakash, Prem (1989a). Long term effects of pollutants on pH of rain water in north India. Atmos. *Environ.* **23**: 753–756.

- Khemani, L. T., Momin, G. A., Rao, P. S. Prakas, Safai, P. D., Singh, G. and Kapoor, R. K. (1989b). Spread of acid rain over India. *Atmos. Environ.* **23**: 757–762.

- Killham, K. and Firestone, M. K. (1983). Vesicular arbuscular mycorrhizal mediation of grass response to acidic and heavy metals deposition. *Plant Soil.* **72**: 39–48.

- Killham, K., Firestone, M. K. and McColl, J. G. (1983). Acid rain and soil microbial activity: Effects and their mechanisms. *J. Environ. Qual.* **12**: 133–137.

- Kleber, E., Dasti, A. and Gakner, A. (1986). In: Energy and Environmental Chemistry (Ed. H. K. Lawrence) pp. 8–12, Ann Arbor Science Publishers, The Butterworth Group, Michigan.

- Kulshrestha, U. C., Sarkar, A. K., Srivastava, S. S. and Parashar, D. C. (1995). A study on short time sampling of individual rain events at New Delhi during monsoon, 1994. *Water, Air and Soil Pollut.* **85**: 2143–2148.

- Kytöviita, M. M. and Crittenden, P. D. (1994). Effects of simulated acid rain on nitrogenase activity (acetylene reduction) in the lichen *Sterocaulon paschale* (L.) Hoffm., with special reference to nutritional aspects. *New Phytol.* **128**: 263–271.

- Labeda, D. P. and Alexander, M. (1978). Effects of $SO_2$ and $NO_2$ on nitrification in soil. *J. Environ. Qual.* **7**: 523–526.

- Lechowicz, M. J. (1982). The effects of simulated acid precipitation on photosynthesis in the Caribou lichen. *Water, Air and Soil Pollut.* **18**: 421-430.

- Lechowicz, M. J. (1987). Resistance of the caribou lichen *Cladina stellaris* (Opiz.) Brodo to growth reduction by simulated acidic rain. *Water, Air and Soil Pollut.* **34**: 71–77.

- Lee, J. J. and Weber, D. E. (1979). The effect of simulated acid rain on seedling emergence and growth of eleven woody species. *For. Sci.* **25**: 393–398.

- Lee, J. J., Neely, G. E., Perrigan, S. C., and Growthaus, L. C. (1981). Effects of simulated sulphuric acid rain on yield, growth and foliar injury of several crops. *Environ. Exp. Bot.* **21**: 171–185.

- Leith, I. D., Murray, M. B., Sheppard, L. J., Cape, J. N., Deans, J. D., Smith, R. J. and Fowler, D. (1989). Visible foliar injury of red spruce seedlings subjected to simulated acid mist. *New Phytol.* **113**: 313–320.

- Likens, G. E. and Bormann, F. H. (1974). Acid rain: A serious regional environmental problem. *Science.* **184**: 1176–1179.

- Likens, G. E. and Butler, T. J. (1981). Recent acidification of precipitation in North America. *Atmos. Environ.* **15**: 1103–1109.

- Likens, G. E., Bormann, F. H. and Johnson, N. M. (1972). Acid rain. *Environment.* **14**: 33–40.

- Likens, G. E., Bormann, F. H., Pierce, R. S. and Reiners, W. A. (1979). Recovery of a deforested ecosystem. *Science.* **199**: 492–496.

- Longton, R. E. (1992). The role of bryophytes and lichens in terrestrial ecosystems. In: The role of bryophytes and lichens in a changing environment (Eds. Bates J.W, and Farmer A. M.) pp. 33–76, Oxford: Oxford University Press.

- Mackenzie, J. J. and El-Ashry, M. T. (1989). Tree and crop injury: A summary of the evidence. In Air Pollution's Toll on Forests and Crops (Eds. Mackenzie, J. J. and El-Ashry, M. T.) pp. 1-21, Yale University Press, New Haven, CT.

- Maehara, N., Kikuchi, J. and Futai, K. (1993). Mycorrhizae of Japanese black pine (*Pinus thunbergii*): protection of seedlings from acid mist and effect of acid mist on mycorrhiza formation. *Can. J. Bot.* **71**: 1562–1567.

- Magel, E. and Ziegler, H. (1986). Einfluss von Ozon und saurem Nebel auf die Struktur der stomatärem Wachspropfen in den Nadeln von *Picea abies* (L.) Karst. Forstwissenschaftliches Zentralblatt (Hamburg). **105**: 234–238.

- Martin, J. T. and Juniper, B. E. (1970). The cuticle of plants. St. Martin's Press, New York.

- McAfee, B. J. and Fortin, J. A. (1987) The influence of pH on the competitive interactions of ectomycorrhizal mycobionts under field conditions. **Can. J. For. Res.** 17: 859–864.

- McColl, J. G. and Firestone, M. K. (1987). Cumulative effects of simulated acid rain on soil chemical and microbial characteristics and conifer seedling growth. *Soil Sci. Soc. Am. J.* **51**: 794–800.

- McLaughlin, S. B., Tjoelker, M. G. and Roy, W. K. (1993). Acid deposition alters red spruce physiology: Laboratory studies support field observations. *Can. J. For. Res.* **23** : 380–386.
- Meier, S., Robarge, W. P., Bruck, R. I. and Grand, L. F. (1989). Effects of simulated acid rain on ectomycorrhizae of red spruce seedlings potted in natural soil. *Environ. Pollut.* **59**: 315–324.
- Menzel, K., Lutz, H. J. and Breininger, M. Th. (1987). Auswaschung von Nährstoffen durch sauren Nebel aus jungen intakten Fichten (*Picea abies*). *Zeitschrift für Pflanzenernährung und Bodenkunde.* **150**: 61–68.
- Mohan, Manju and Kumar, Sanjay (1998). Reviews of acid rain potential in India: Future threats and remedial measures. *Current Sci.* **75**: 579–593.
- NADP (1978 and 1979). National Atmospheric Deposition Program Data Reports. Vol. II (1–3). Available from NADP Coordinator's office, Natural Resource Ecology Laboratory, CSU, Fort Collins, CO.
- Naik Medha S., Khemani, L. T., Momin, G. A. and Rao, P. S. Prakas (1988). Measurement of pH and Chemical analysis of rain water in rural area of India. *Acta Meteorologica Sinica.* **2**: 91–100.
- NAPAP (1988). Annual Report 1987 to the President and Congress. National Acid precipitation Assessment Program, office of the Director, 722, Jackson Place, NW, Washington D. C. 20503, USA.
- NEERI (National Environmental Engineering Research Institute, 1980). Air quality in selected cities in India, 1978–1979.
- Neufeld, H. S., Jernstedt, J. A. and Haines, B. L. (1985). Direct foliar effects of simulated acid rain. I. Damage, growth and gas exchange. *New Phytol.* **99**: 389–405.
- Norby, R. J. and Luxmoore, R. J. (1983). Growth analysis of soybean exposed to simulated acid rain and gaseous air pollutants. *New Phytol.* **95**: 277–287.
- Norby, R. J., Richten, D. D. and Luxmoore, R. J. (1985). Physiological processes in soybean inhibited by gaseous pollutants but not by acid rain. *New Phytol.* **100**: 79–85.
- NRC (1986). Aid deposition. Long term trends. Committee on monitoring and assessment of trends in acid deposition. National Research Council. National academy Press, Washington D.C., U.S.A.
- Nyborg, M. and Hoyt, P. B. (1978). Effects of soil acidity and liming on mineralization of soil nitrogen. *Can. J. Soil Sci.* **58**: 331–338.
- Olszyk, D. M., Bytnerowicz, A., Fox, C. A., Kats, G., Dawson, P. J. and Wolf, J. (1987). Injury and physiological responses of *Larrea tridentata* (DC) Coville exposed *in situ* to sulphur dioxide. *Environ. Pollut.* **48**: 197–211.
- Ormrod, D. P. (1978). Pollution in horticulture. Elsevier, New York.
- Overrein, L. N. (1972). Sulphur pollution patterns observed; leaching of calcium in forest soil determined. *Ambio.* **1**: 145–147.
- Payer, H. D., Pfirrmann, T., Kloos, M. and Blank, L. W. (1990). Clone and soil effects on the growth of young Norway Spruce during 14 months exposure to ozone plus acid mist. Environ. *Pollut.* **64**: 209–227.
- Percy, K. E. (1986). The effects of simulated acid rain on germinative capacity, growth and morphology of forest tree seedlings. *New Phytol.* **104**: 473–484.
- Percy, K. E. and Baker, E. A. (1987). Effects of simulated acid rain on production, morphology and composition of epicuticular wax and on cuticular membrane development. *New Phytol.* **107**: 577–589.
- Porter, J. R. and Sheridan, R. P. (1981). Inhibition of nitrogen fixation in alfalfa by arsenate, heavy metals, fluoride and simulated acid rain. *Plant Physiol.* **68**: 143–148.
- Prinz, B., Krause, G. H. M. and Jung, K. D. (1985). Responses of German forests in recent years: causes for concern elsewhere? In: Effects of Acid Deposition on Forests, Wetlands and Agricultural Ecosystems. Proceedings of NATO Advanced Research Workshop, Toronto, May 1985, Springer- Verlag.
- Rao, P. S. P., Momin, G. A., Safai, P. D., Pillai, A. G. and Khemani, L. T. (1993). International Conference on Sustainable Development, New Delhi.
- Rathier, T. M. and Frink, C. R. (1984). Simulated acid rain: Effects on leaf quality and yield of broadleaf tobacco. *Water, Air and Soil Pollut.* **22**: 389–394.
- Raynal, D. J., Roman, J. R. and Eichenlaub, W. M. (1982). Response of tree seedlings to acid precipitation. II. Effects of simulated acidified canopy throughfall on sugar maple seedling growth. *Environ. Exp. Bot.* **22**: 385–392.
- Reich, P. B., Schoettle, A. W., Stroo, H. F. and Amundsen, R. G. (1988). Effects of ozone and acid rain on white pine (*Pinus strobus*) seedlings grown in five soils. III. Nutrient relations. *Can. J. Bot.*, **66**, 1517–1531.
- Roy-Arcand, L., Delisle, C. E. and Briere, F. G. (1989). Effects of simulated acid precipitation on the metabolic

activity of *Cladina stellaris*. *Can. J. Bot.* 67: 1796–1802.

- Rudawska, M., Kieliszewska-Rokicka, B. and Leski, T. (1996). Effect of acid rain and aluminium on the mycorrhizae of *Pinus sylvestris*. In: Mycorrhizae in integrated systems from genes to plant development (Eds. Azcon-aguilar, C. and Barea, J.) pp. 469–471, Brussels, Belgium.

- Sanhueza, E., Cuenca, G., Gomez, M. J., Herrera, R., Ishizaki, C., Marti, I. and Paolini, J. (1988). Characterization of the venezuelan environment and it's potential for acidification. In: Acidification in Tropical Countries (Eds. Rodhe, H. and Herrera, R.), SCPOE 36, John Wiley & Sons, Chichester, U.K.

- Scherbatskoy, T. and Klein, R. M. (1983). Response of spruce and birch foliage to leaching by acidic mists. *J. Environ. Qual.* 12: 189–195.

- Schindler, D. W. (1990). Experimental perturbations of whole lakes as tests of hypothesis concerning ecosystem structure and function. *Oikos.* 57: 25–41.

- Schindler, D. W., Mills, K. H., Malley, D. F., Findlay, D. L., Shearer, J. A., Davies, I. J., Turner, M. A., Linsey, G. A. and Cruinkshank, D. A. (1985) Long term ecosystem stress: The effects of years of experimental acidification on small lake. *Science.* 228: 1395–1401.

- Scott, M. G. and Hutchinson, T. C. (1987). Effects of a simulated acid rain episode on photosynthesis and recovery in the caribou – forage lichens, *Cladina stellaris* (Opiz.) Brodo and *Cladina rangiferina* (L.) Wigg. *New Phytol.* 107: 567–575.

- Scott, M. G. and Hutchinson, T. C. (1990) The use of lichen growth abnormalities as an early warning indicator of forest die back. *Environ. Monitoring and Assess.* 15: 213–218.

- Scott, M. G., Hutchinson, T. C. and Feth, M. J. (1989). Contrasting responses of lichens and *Vaccinium angustifolium* to long term acidification of a boreal forest ecosystem. *Can. J. Bot.* 67: 579–588.

- Sequeira R. (1976). Monsoonal deposition of sea salt and air pollutants over Bombay. *Tellus.* 28: 275.

- Shafer, S. R. (1988). Influence of ozone and simulated acidic rain on micro organisms in the rhizosphere of Sorghum. *Environ. Pollut.* 51: 131–152.

- Shafer, S. R., Grand, L. F., Bruck, R. J. and Heagle, A. S. (1985). Formation of ectomycorrhizae on *Pinus taeda* seedlings exposed to simulated acidic rain. *Can. J. For. Res.* 15: 66–71.

- Shan, Y., Feng, Z., Izuta, T., Aoki, M. and Totsuka, T. (1995). The individual and combined effects of ozone and simulated acid rain on chlorophyll contents, carbon allocation and biomass accumulation of Armand pine seedlings. *Water, Air and Soil Pollut.* 85: 1399–1404.

- Shan, Y., Feng, Z., Izuta, T., Aoki, M. and Totsuka, T. (1996). The individual and combined effects of ozone and simulated acid rain on growth, gas exchange rate and water use efficiency of *Pinus armandi* Franch. *Environ. Pollut.* 91: 355–361.

- Shelburne, V. B., Reardon, J. C. and Paynter, V. A. (1993). The effects of acid rain and ozone on biomass and leaf area of shortleaf pine (*Pinus echinata* Mill.). *Tree Physiol.* 12: 163–172.

- Sheppard, L. J., Cape, J. N. and Leith, I. D. (1993a). Influence of acidic mist on frost hardiness and nutrient concentrations in red spruce seedlings. 1. Exposure of the foliage and the rooting environment. *New Phytol.* 124: 595–605.

- Sheppard, L. J., Cape, J. N. and Leith, I. D. (1993b). Influence of acidic mist on frost hardiness and nutrient concentrations in red spruce seedlings. 2. Effects of misting frequency and rainfall exclusion. *New Phytol.* 124: 607–615.

- Shipley, B., Lechowicz, M., Dumont, S. and Hendershot, W. H. (1992). Interacting effects of nutrients, pH – Al and elevated $CO_2$ on the growth of red spruce (*Picea rubens* Sarg.) seedlings. *Water, Air and Soil Pollut.* 64: 585–600.

- Shrestha, R. M., Bhattacharya, S. C. and Malla, S. (1996). Energy use and sulphure dioxide emmissins in Asia. *J. Environ. Manag.* 46: 359–372.

- Shriner, D. S. (1974). Effects of simulated rain acidified with sulphuric acid on host – parasite interactions. Ph. D. thesis, North Carolina State University, Raleigh NC.

- Shriner, D. S. (1981). Terrestrial vegetation – air pollutant interactions: Non gaseous pollutants, wet deposition. In: Proceedings of the International Conference on "Air Pollutants and their Effects on Terrestrial Ecosystem". Banff. Alta. May 10–17, 1980, (Eds. Krupa, S. V. and Legge, A. H.) John Wiley & Sons, New York.

- Shriner, D. S. and Johnston, J. W. (1981). Effects of simulated, acidified rain on nodulation of leguminous plants by *Rhizobium* spp. *Environ. Exp. Bot.* 21: 199–209.

- Shumejko, Pavel, Ossipov Vladimir and Neuvonen Seppo (1996). The effect of simulated acid rain on the biochemical composition of scots pine (*Pinus sylvestris* L.) needles. *Environ. Pollut* **92**: 315 – 321.
- Sigal, L. L. and Johnston, J. W. (1986). Effects of simulated acidic rain on one species each of *Pseudoparmelia, Usnea* and *Umbilicaria. Water, Air and Soil Pollut.* **27**: 315–322.
- Singh, A. and Agrawal, M. (1996). Response of two cultivars of *Triticum aestivum* L. to simulated acid rain. *Environ. Pollut.* **91**: 161–167.
- Smith, C. R., Vasilas, B. L., Banwart, W. L. and Walker, W. M. (1991). Physiological response of two soybean cultivars to simulated acid rain. *New Phytol.* **119**: 53–60.
- Smol, J. P. and Glew, J. R. (1992). Paleolimniology. In: Encyclopedia of Earth System Science (Ed. Nirenberg, W.) pp. 95–107, Taylor and Francis, London.
- Spidso, T. K. and Korsmo, H. (1993). Effect of acid rain on pine needles as food for capercaillie in winter. *Oecologia* **94**: 565-570.
- Strayer, R. F. and Alexander, M. (1981). Effects of simulated acid rain on glucose mineralization and some physicochemical properties of forest soils. *J. Environ. Qual.* **10**: 460–465.
- Swanson, E. S., Thomson, W. W. and Mudd, J. B. (1973). The effect of ozone on leaf cell membranes. *Can. J. Bot.* **51**: 1213–1219.
- Takemoto, B. K., Shriner, D. S. and Johnston, J. W. Jr. (1987). Physiological responses of soybean (*Glycine max* L. Merr.) to simulated acid rain and ambient ozone in the field. *Water, Air and Soil Pollut.* **33**: 373–384.
- Tenhunen, J. D., Lange, O. L., Hahn, S., Siegwolf, R. and Oberbauer, S. F. (1992). The ecosystem role of poikilohydric tundra plants. In: Arctic ecosystems in a changing climate: an ecophysiological perspective (Eds. Chapin, F. S. III, Jefferies, R. L., Reynolds, J. F., Shaver, G. R. and Svoboda, J.) pp. 213–237, Academic Press Inc., San Diego.
- Thompson, C. R., Kats, G. and Hensel, E. (1972). Effects of ambient levels of ozone on navel oranges. *Environ. Sci. Technol.* **6**: 1014–1016.
- TOI (The Times of India, 1998). Scientists predict acid rains by 2020. News Digest, Front Page, 22nd Jan, 98.
- Troiano, J., L. Heller and J. S. Jacobson (1982). Effects of added water and acidity of simulated rain on growth of field grown radish. *Environ. Pollut. (Series A).* **29**: 1–11.
- Varshney, C. K., Agrawal, M., Ahmad, K. J., Dubey, P. S. and Raza, S. H. (1997). Effect of air pollution on Indian crop plants. Final report, ODA Project Imperial College of Sci., Tech. And Med., UK, pp. 2.
- Waldman, J. M., Munger, J. W., Jacob D. J., and Hoffmann, M. R. (1985) Chemical characterization of stratus cloud water and its role as a vector for pollutant deposition in a Los Angeles pine forest. *Tellus.* **35**: 91–108.
- Walker, R. E. (1963). Acid droplets in town air. *Int. J. Air Water Pollut.* **7**: 773-778.
- Wei, F. S., Wang, M. X. and Wang, R. B. (1988). Distribution characteristics of time and space of chemical compositions and acidity of precipitation in China. Proceedings of symp. of effects of acid precipitation on comprehensive agriculture and its counter measures, pp. 24–30. China Association for Science and Technology.
- Wellburn, A. (1994). Air pollution and climate change: The Biological Impact. pp. 97–122. Longman Scientific and Technical, John Wiley & Sons Inc., New York.
- Wertheim, F. S. and Craker, L. E. (1988). Effects of acid rain on corn silks and pollen germination. *Environ. Qual.* **17**: 135-138.
- Wetmore, C. M. (1989). Lichens and air quality in Cuyahoga Valley National Recreation Area, Ohio. *Bryologist.* **92**: 273–281.
- Will, M. E., Graetz, D. A. and Root, B. S. (1986). Effect of simulated acid precipitation on soil microbial activity in a typic quartzipsamment. *J. Environ. Qual.* **15**: 399–403.
- Wood, T. and Bormann, F. H. (1977) Short term effects of simulated acid rain upon the growth and nutrient relations of *pinus strobus* L. *Water, Air and Soil Pollut.* **7**: 479–488.
- Yan, N. D. and Stokes, P. M. (1978). Phytoplankton of an acidic lake and its response to experimental alterations of pH. *Environ. Conserv.* **5**: 93–100.
- Yoshimura, S. (1933). Kata-numa, a very strong acid water lake on volcano Katanuma, Miyagi Prefecture. Japan. *Arch. Hydrobiol.* **26**: 197–202.

# 6

# Environmental Problems in and around Opencast Coal Mines

*R. S. Yadav, Madhoolika Agrawal and P. R. Yadav*

The challenge of creating and maintaining a sustainable environment is probably the most pressing issue of our times throughout the world. As humans increasingly alter earth's land, water and atmosphere on local, regional and global levels, the resulting environmental problems can seem insurmountable. Technological civilization uses the atmosphere and lithosphere both as resource and medium for discharge of waste products. This results in the physcio-chemical change in the quality of air, water and soil. That have harmful biological consequence.

Human society depends on energy. We use it to grow and cook our food, to warm our homes in winter and cool them is summer, to extract and process natural resources, to manufacture items of daily use, to power various forms of transportation. Energy supplies us many of the convenience of modern living. Currently energy consumption is increasing worldwide with most of the increase occurring in developing countries.

Energy is obtained from a variety of sources. Earth is the storehouse of various minerals and sources of energy. Today most of the energy required is supplied by fossil fuels, coal oil and natural gas. Coal is composed of the remains of prehistoric plants. The national energy policy, accepted by the Government of India in May 1981 recognises coal as the principal source of energy. Most of the coal consumed in India is burned at thermal power plants, which contributes 85 percent of the total installed electric generating capacity in the country. In China, the contribution of coal to total energy has increased from 71.8 percent in 1980 to 76.03 percent in 1986. Coal, the most abundant fossil fuel in the world, is found mainly in the Northern Hemisphere. North America, Russia and China have the largest coal deposits, but large deposits are also found in the arctic island, Western Europe, India, South Africa, Australia and eastern South America.

Coal generally occurs in the geological basins which are covered by the hills and forests. Coal is found in underground layers called seams that vary from 2.5cm to more that 30 m in thickness. Coal mines are of two types, surface, or open pit or opencast or strip mines and subsurface (underground) mines. When the coal bed is within 30 m of the surface, open pit mining is usually done. Coal resources is estimated to be 110 billion tons in India. The total coal production for India during 1989-1990 was 226 million metric tons which is likely to reach a level of 400 million metric tons by the end of the century. In India, opencast coal mining contributed about 56 percent of the current coal production and will contribute about 70 percent by 2000 A.D.

Exploration, mining and benefaction of coal is associated with variety of environmental hazards. Coal mining especially strip mining, has substantial effects on the environment (Chandwick *et al*, 1987). In opencast mining, vegetation and topsoil are completely removed, causing a loss of habitat for plants and animals and increasing soil erosion and air and water pollution. Opencast coal mining results in serious disruption of surface topography and water courses due to digging of huge open cast pits and massive overburden dumps.

The impact of mining activities on the environment may be summarized as follows:

## Land

Surface mining in the area drastically changes the landscape. All the land actually used for mining gets spoiled. During surface mining a vast quantity of soil, overburden and bed rocks from mining site are removed and dumped at adjoining non coal bearing areas. The pre exisitng ecosystems are, thus destroyed at both the sites. Surface coal mining results in the dumping of huge amounts of overburden materials in adjacent unmined land leading to serious land degradation. The overburden originates from the consolidated and unconsolidated materials haphazardly mixed during mining activity. This is also called mine spoil. These drastically disturbed mine spoil ecosystems ae usually physically, chemically, biologically and nutritionally recalcitrant media for plant growth (Meyer, 1973). Mine spoils present undesirable conditions for both plant and microbial growth because of low organic matter content unfavourable pH, coarse texture, low water retention, poor water drainage and compacted structure.

## Forests (Flora and Fauna)

Due to opencast mining, forest land and consequently flora and fauna would get disturbed. Forest plays an important role in maintaining rainfall and temperature of area besides having many other economic utilities. Extensive damage to this national wealth without any compensatory afforestation would disturb the ecosystem greatly. Most of the coal mines are in the forest land. Blasting of hill tops and stripping of land is a routine operation in the coalfield area. This result in a complete destruction of tree cover and other vegetation. Distraction of forest is a major threat to wild life. Loss of habitat due to large scale changes in land use and likely poaching by the growing population drawn to the area due to variety of other developmental activities result in total loss of wild life in mining and adjoining areas.

## Noise Pollution

The various sources of noise pollution in opencast mining and allied operations are: blasting for coal and overburden, operations of heavy duty vehicles, drilling operations, etc. The workmen associated with operation of drills, shovels, dumpers and pay loaders generally experience a noise level above 90 dB for more than 4 to 4.5 hours per shift. The impact of noise on exposed workmen is generally of two types *i.e.* physiological and biochemical. However, suitable control measures adopted during various operations reduces the impact of noise to minimum.

## Villages and Settlements

Due to mining and allied activities population in the area would increase. So the new settlements would come up in the area to accommodate them. Further village falling in the area would be displaced, Rehabilitation of the land oustees in terms of occupation as well as housing amenities, etc. would be a major impact in the area. Operation of coal mining project and allied activities have direct and indirect impact on the socioeconomic condition of the exisitng inhabitants.

Although projects have created ample job opportunities, but are not sufficient enough to employ all the affected one with the impact that major proportion of the population has been shifted from this region. The public amenities like educational institutions, health care, communication facilities, markets etc. have increased but its major share goes to project personnels, while huge tertiary service population are left out. This has created a chaotic and unco-ordinated development at the fringes of colonies, colliery and power plants. The cause of the problem is influx of outsiders for livelihood and other necessities making tremendous impact on the demographic and behavioural pattern in the area.

## Water Quality

The operation of open cast mines would generally affect the natural drainage network, underground aquifers and also the water quality. Effluent from mine colony and mining area besides the surface runoff passing through coalpiles and overburden dumps pollute the nearby surface water. The water has objectionable odour, colour and pH and may not be fit for drinking purpóse. The water generally has high turbidity and affect the aquatic life due to poor oxygenation of water body. In some cases, it may contain certain pathogenic bacteria causing helath hazards. Further high oil and grease in water may affect the aquatic life.

# Air Quality

Due to blasting, drilling, loading and conveying of overburden and coal in opencast mines dust and gases are produced leading to air pollution in and around the opencast mining areas. Mining is a very ancient and one of the most useful industrial activity though it is dirty and dangerous. Opencast mining can be hazardous to the environment as the dust and gases are emitted directly into the atmosphere. Particulates, $SO_2$, $NO_x$, CO and hydrocarbons are considered major air pollutants in mining areas. The particulates may be released into the atmosphere from point source such as centralised vent system to exhaust dust laden air from crushing and screening plants. The important non point sources of particulates and other gaseous pollutants are:

1. Operation of various coal mining and overburden removal equipments such as shovel, front end loaders, draglines, bucket wheel excavators, bulldozers, drilling machines etc.
2. Haul roads bothe of the paved and unpaved types, wind erosion from coal stock piles, benchs and oever burden dumps.
3. Blasting operations
4. Trailing dumps
5. Transportation activities on poorly maintained roads
6. Coal burning activities.

Particulate pollutants are the major threat in the vicinity of coalmines. These pollutants, when released into the atmosphere, remain suspended for varying lengths of time depending upon their size, weight, chemical nature and atmospheric conditions. Particulates may be distinguished as quickly sedimenting coarse particles (diameter>63 μm) and slowly sedimenting coarse particles (diameter>10μm but<63 μm.) These factions of particulates are designated as sedimentation or settled dust. The other category of dust is suspended dust (diameter<10μm) with a very light weight and low sinking period. The particle larger than 10um in size quickly settle under the force of gravity on surface of vegetation, aquatic systems and soil, but smaller ones remain suspended in air for longer time and get dispersed, distributed and diffused by wind motion and eddy currents in accordance with aerodynamic resistance. The particles suspended in the air ultimately form aggregates through agglomeration, coalescence and water vapour deposition and settled down or exposed surfaces in due coarse of time or may be washed down by rain. Settled dust are mainly responsible for unfavourable changes in plants and soil whereas suspended dust which is composed of 20-80 percent breathable dust (below 1-2 um particle diameter) can get into the respiratory tract of animals and humans. Dust of silica and coal particles are very harmful to lungs and a large number of mine workers suffer from solicosis, tuberculosis chronic bronchitis, pneumoconiosis, lung cancer etc.

Mc Crone *et al,* (1967) have categorized particulate pollutants into three broad groups; *(i)* wind eroded particles; *(ii)* industrial dust, and *(iii)* combustion products. The first group belongs to biological materials, soil particles and mineral particles relatively less toxic to plants. The second group includes metal refining products, mining activities cement dust etc. which have potential phototoxic influence. The third group of combustion products get readily absorbed into the plant tissues, and relatively more toxic. The particles between 1μ and 10μ size mostly reflect industrial and combustion product with some local wind eroded particles.

Waste dumps in case of coal mines contaminate the air by emitting smoke and foul gases due to spontaneous combustion. Blasting and diesel equipments are the important sources that generate harmful gases like $CO_2$, $NO_x$, CO, $CH_4$, $SO_2$ etc.

The present study is mainly emphasized on the air pollution problem in the area and its impact on vegetation and soil. Air pollution has long been recognized to cause unfavourable changes on plants. Measurement of air pollution removal rates by vegetation indicates that plants are very effective pollution sink. Therefore air environment is one of the vital and critical component of environment on which plants depend. Primarily, the air pollution damage was studied through the measurements of acute visible injury symptoms. Studies on the effects on London 'fog' on chlorophyII (Oliven, 1894) and influence of sulphurdioxide on photosynthesis (Cohen and Ruston, 1925) were amongst the pioneer work of physiological aspects of air pollution impact. The first report on biochemical basis of air pollution damage was due to Wisticenees (1914). Later, Stoklasa (1923), Katz (1949) and Thomas *et.al.* (1950) have investigated various physiological and biochemical processes of plants responsible for the visible injury symptoms.

Air pollution was largely considered a local problem around industries and cities until the middle of the present century. But due to long range transport of pollutants, significant concentrations of pollutants were recorded even in areas distant from industrial centers.

Mining activities result in the emission of various gaseous and particulate pollutants in the area. There is dearth of information regarding the impact of air pollution on plants in and around opencast mining areas. Studies have, however, indicated deterioration of air quality due to minig (Bose *et al*, 1986; Sahoo, 1981; Sharma and ingh, 1990; Singh *et al*, 1990). Variety of particulates are known to affect the vegetation adversely under field (Darley, 1966; Rao, 1971; Mccune *et al* 1965; Khanam and Agrawal, 1988; Nandi *et al*, 1987; Agrawal and Khanam, 1989) and laboratory conditions (Singh and Rao, 1978; Borka, 1980; Singh, 1991). Rao (1971) studied the effects of coal dust on the growth and fruiting behaviour of *Mangifera indica* (Mango) and *Citrus lemon* (lemon) near a gravity transshipment yard in Varanasi, where during unloading of coal from broad gauge to meter gauge railway wagons pulverized coal fell out on the surfaces of soil and vegetation. The qantity of dust deposition was more on mango leaves compared to lemon leaves. The dust covered leaves showed necrotic lessions starting at the tip and progressing down the lamina. Due to dust deposition and subsequent death on terminal buds, the lateral buds became activated leading to the development of asymetrical trees canopy. Significant reduction in the fruit yield of the two species of palnts affected by coal dust was reported. Rao (1979) has shown significant reduction in growth of *Delburgia sissoo* a leguminous tree species growing around coal depot, in Chandasi, Varanasi.

It has long been believed that vegetation can filter out dust and fine particulate matter present in the air. Hyde park, a green area in the centre of London reduced the smokl concentrations by 27%. From a study in erstwhiti Soviet Union, it is estimated that Lilac, Maple, Lindon and Popular trees can filter 2.33, 1.11, 0.61 and 0.26 mg dust m-2 leaf surface, respectively (Back, 1972). The dust collecting effectiveness of plants is governed by morphological traits of leaves such as epidermal and cuticular features, surface geometry, phylotaxy, orientation, size and area of leaf, etc. Evergreen plants with horizontally oriented leaves were found to be good dust catcher as compared to deciduous vertically suspended leaves (Shetye and Chaphekar, 1980), Trees with needle like leavs also exertes a filtering effect when air current passes through them.

The threshold value or tolerance limit of a plant species with regard to a particular type of particulate pollutant is not the same to all species, it is variable under different environmental conditions and with the age of plant. (Rao, 1980; and Das *et al*, 1981). Particulates can interfere with the energy exchange processes of the leaf due to dust layer (Rao, 1971; Bohne, 1963) on leaves which changes the quality and quantity of solar radiation impinging on the leaf surface. Das and Pattnayak (1978) has shown disturbance in gaseous exchange due to shading of cuticle and clogging of stomata by dust. Cement dust deposition on foliar surface has been shown to reduce chlorophyll content and led to chloroplast injury (Czaja, 1962). Particulates also interfere with the pH and other physico-chemical properties of the soil supporting the plant growth (Singh *et al*, 1995).

Sulphur has been recognised as a major gaseous air pollutant around coal burning operations (Agarwal and Agrawal, 1989); Singh, *et al*, 1993; Rao and Dubey, 1990). Several reviews and books have been published on the effect of sulphurdioxide ($SO_2$) on plants (Mudd, 1975; Hallgreen, 1978; Unsworth and Ormarod, 1982; Bell, 1984; Treshow, 1984; Treshow and Richardson, 1989). Sulphur dioxide is known to cause serious perturbations to natural forests, and grasslands and yield of agronomically important crops around the $SO_2$ emitting sources such as thermal power plants, smelters, etc. (Gordon and Gorham, 1963; Treshow, 1968; Tomlinson, 1983).

After emission, $SO_2$ disperses in the atmosphere and is transported to the distant places along with the wind. the residence time of $SO_2$ in air may vary from an hour to several days, depending upon the level of moisture and reaction potential of the atmosphere (Georgi, 1978). Chemical reactions of $SO_2$ during long range transport is major contributor to acidic precipitation (Heck, 1989).

Plants have been described as efficient scavangers of atmospheric $SO_2$ (Posthumus 1983). $SO_2$ enters the leaf interior through stomata and gets oxidised to $SO_3^{2-}$ or $HSO_3^-$ and finally to $SO_4^{2-}$ Sulphate is either consumed metabolically for organic- S formation or stored. During oxidation of $SO_2$ free radicals are produced which are responsible for various adverse effects of $SO_2$ on different metabolic processes of plants, (Black, 1982; Tomlinson, 1983; Treshow, 1984; Winner et al, 1985; Darrall, 1989).

Several laboratory and field experiments have confirmed the adverse impact of $SO_2$ on the morphological characters of plants Davies (1980), Sharma (1975) and Garg and Varshney (1980) have observed reduction in stomatal size and density and increase in trichome size and number in plants growing in the polluted area. Following the entry of $SO_2$ to mesophyll cells, visible injury symptoms in the form of chlorosis and necrosis appear. The pattern and the intensity of the injury depend upon the exposure concentration and duration. These lesions are bifacial and interveinal. The chronic injury appears as yellowing or chlorosis, which later on changes to brown or black necrotic areas. Furukawa et al. (1980) correlated the degree of necrosis or damage to the quantity of $SO_2$ absorbed.

Many workers have shown reduction in various morphological, physiological and biochemical processes without appearance of visible injury symptoms. A considerable reduction in the leaf area without any visible foliar injury symptoms has been reported by Rao et al. (1990) in the plants growing near the coal-fired thermal power plants. Similarly, Steubing and Fengmuer (1987) observed a reduction in productivity and leaf area index of Allium Ursinum plants treated with $SO_2$ pollutants, without appearance of any visible injury symptoms. Tingey (1977) and Hallgren (1978) suggested that the $So_2$ induced disruption of metabolic processes of plants are responsible for reduction of growth and development of plants. There are many report demonstrating the influence of $SO_2$ on various physiological processes; Farooq et al, (1985) Darral, (1986, 1989).

Inhibition of plant photosynthesis due to $SO_2$ has been well established (Darrall, 1989). There are also reports that photosynthesis enhances at sub-inhibitory concentrations (winner and Mooney, 1980). The role of stomata in contributing to the changes in photosynthesis has been discussed by Darrall (1989). Increased $CO_2$ concentration in the leaf, leads to stomatal closure and this inhibition of photosynthesis (Muller et al., 1979; Sij and Swanson, 1974; Winner and Money, 1980; Winner et al, 1985; Taylor et al, 1986). Photosynthetic pigments have been found very sensitive to $SO_2$ (Agrawal et al, 1983). Shimazaki et al. (1980) suggested photo-oxidation of chlorophyll molecule by the active oxygen ($O_2^-$; OH and $H_2O_2$) species formed during $SO_2$ oxidation in foliar tissue

Khan and Malhotra (1977) reported alteration in lipid composition of pine needle chloroplast after $SO_2$ exposure. These structural changes can disrupt the enzyme systems invloved in carbon dioxide fixation. Several reports suggest that biochemical loci are the primary site of alteration during $SO_2$ exposure leading to ultrastructural and cellular changes (Jager and Klein, 1977; Beg and Farooq, 1988). $SO_2$ induced alterations in carbohydrate and nitrogen metabolism of plants have been reported (Koziol and Jordan, 1978; Pahlsoon, 1989). The concentrations of sugar, starch and certain amino acids were found to increase while the protein concentration reduced (Malhotra and Sarkar, 1979; Koziol and Cowling, 1980; Grunhage and Jager, 1982). Beg and Farooq (1988) suggested that in sensitive plants, the process of metabolism is activated towards synthesis after $SO_2$ exposure and therefore most of the biochemical constituents get accumulated in higher amounts. In contrast, Constantinidou and Kozlowski (1979) observed a decrease in the carbohydrate content of the various plant parts exposed to $SO_2$. Black and Unsworth (1979) suggested that the inhibition of photosynthetic $CO_2$ fixation by $SO_2$ is a primary cause of carbohydrate reduction. Changes in the activity of various enzymes due to $SO_2$ pollution have been well documented (Peters et al, 1989). Keller and Schwager (1971) and Nandi et al, (1984) observed a positive correlation between the pollutants concentration and peroxidase activity. Mehlorn and Kunert (1986) suggested that the increased amount of phenolic compounds stimulate peroxidase activity.

Inorganic sulphur has been reported as the main product in the plant cells resulting due to the absorption of $SO_2$ (Weigl and Ziegler 1962; Jagar et al, 1972). Thus, sulphates quantification may be considered as an important parameter to characterise the effect of $SO_2$ in plants.

High concentrations of Nitrogen oxides may occur in mining areas, depending upon the meteorological conditions and density of road traffic. Coal burning alone is believed to account for high $NO_2$ in the atmosphere (Morrison, 1980). Nitrogen dioxide can affect the plants directly and can cause visible plant injury. There are several reports of $NO_2$ fumigation promoting plant responses such as increase in chloophyII and darker green leaves, leaf number, area and dry weight have been reported (Whitmore and Freer-Smith, 1982; Singh, 1980). These promotive effects are usually associated to gaseous $NO_2$ functioning as aerial fertilizers under conditions of nutrient deficiency. Decrease in productivity due to $NO_2$ exposure has also been reported (Singh, 1980; Sinn and Pell, 1984). Response of tree species to chronic $NO_2$ doses is also quite variable. Kresh and Skelly (1982) have shown significant reduction in root and total dry weight of sweet gum, while seven other species were found unaffected. Freer-Smith (1984) reported that shoot growth of some tree species initially stimulated due to $NO_2$ exposure but latter on these effects were lost, when renewed growth of deciduous tree occurred.

Nitrogen oxides also play an important role in the complex phytochemistry of smog formation. $NO_2$ also contributes to acid precipitation during wet deposition, which consequently damage aquatic life, forestry and agriculture. Furthermore $NO_2$ may lead to additive or more than additive effects with other atmospheric pollutants like $SO_2$, $O_3$ and particulates (Bull and Mansfield, 1974; Karlson, 1983; Welburn, 1982).

A wide range of sensitivity in plant both within and between species has been documented for $SO_2$, $NO_2$ and particulates (Heath, 1988; Darall, 1989). This suggests an adoptive metabolic mechanism among plants to keep balance in response to air pollution damage. Stomatal response was often correlated with the level of plant sensitivity (Black, 1982). Stomatal closure is a resistance mechanism referred to as avoidance response to pollutants (Natori and Totsuka, 1984). Antioxidants such as catalase (Sarkar et al, 1986), Superoxide dismutase (Agrawal et al, 1987), Peroxidase (Nandi et al, 1986; Sarkar et al, 1986), Polyamine (Pierre and Querioz, 1981) and Glutathione (Chiment et al, 1986; Alscher et al, 1987) have been suggested to activate defence mechanism in plants against oxidative damage caused by pollutants.

Since independence, India have made tremendous technological advancement and ranks among the first ten industrialised nations. Evidently, such major industrial trasformation has caused air pollution as one of the major environmental problem in the country. The steadly growing demands of coal for energy production in India have led to the fast expansion of coal mines. It is therefore important to establish monitoring network over large area around coal mines

## SUMMARY

Open cast mining creats numerous environmental problems. It drastically changes the landscape. Pre-existing ecosystems are destroyed due to removal of vast quantity of soil. Surface coal mining results in the dumping of huge amount of overburden materials in adjacent unmined land leading to serious land degradation. These overburden materials after mixing activities form mine spoils are usually poor for plant growth because of low organic matter, unfavourable pH, low water retention, poor drainage and compacted structure. Due to open cast mining forest land and consequently flora and fauna would get disturbed. Blasting of hill tops and stripping of land is a routine operations results complete destruction of tree cover and other vegetation.

The operations of opencast coalmines also leads water air and noise pollution in the area. Effluents from coalmines pollute the fresh water bodies in the area. Mining operations such as blasting, drilling, loading and conveying of overburden and coal produce gaseous and particulate pollutants. These gaseous and particulate pollutants directly or indirectly affect the growth and performance of the plants growing in the vicinity of coalmines. These gaseous and particulate pollutants reduces the morphological, physiological and biochemical processes with or without appearance of visible injury symptoms.

# REFERENCES

- Agarwal, M. and N. Khanam. 1989. Impact of cement factory emission on vegetation and soil. In: *Man and His Ecosystem*. Elsevier Sci. Pb. B.H. Amsterdam, The Netherlands G.J. Brasser and W.C. Mulder (eds). 2:53-60)
- Agarwal, M. and S.B. Agrawal, 1989. Phytomonitoring of air pollution around a theral power plant. *Atmos. Environ.* **23**: 763-769.
- Agrawal, M., D.N. Rao, P.K. Nandi and S.B. Agrawal. 1987. Responses of plant to particulate pollutant: A review. In : Ecology of Urban India. Ed. 1. Mohan Pramila Publications (India). 93-114.
- Agarwal, M., P.K. Nandi and D.N. Rao. 1983. Ozone and sulphur dioxide effects on Panicum miliaceum plants. *Bull. Torrey Bot.Club.*, **110**: 435-441.
- Beg, M.U. and M. Farooq. 1988. Sulphur dioxide resistance of Indian tress. II Experimental evalution of metabolic profile. *Water, Air & Soil Pollut.*, **40**:317-326.
- Bell., J.N.B. 1984. Air pollution problems in western Europe.In: *Gaseous Air pollutants and plant Metabolism*, M.I. Koziol and F.R. Whatley (eds.), Butterworths Publications, London.
- Black, V.J. 1982. Effects of sulfur dioxide on physiological precesses in plants. In : *Effects of Gaseous Pollutant in Agriculture and Horiulture*, M.H. Unsworth and D.P. Ormrod 9eds.), Butterworths, London, pp.67-91.
- Black, V.J. and M.H. Unsworth. 1979. Effects of low concentrations of sulphur dioxide on net photosynthesis and dark respiration if vicia faba. *J. Exp. Bot.*, **30**: 473-483
- Bohne, H. 1963. Schadlichkeit von staubaus zemenlwerken fur waldbestande Allg. *Forstz.*, **18**: 107-111
- Borka, G. 1980 The effect of cement dust pollution on growth and metabolism of Helianthus annus. *Environ. Pollut., Ser. A.* **22**:75-80
- Bose, A.K., P.K. Mullick, B.N. Dalal, A.K. Mukerjee, J.K. Sinha and P.K. Gangopadhyaya. 1983. Air pollution study in Jharia coalfield. *Ind J. Air Pollut. Contr.*, **4**:56-61.
- Bull, J.N. and T.A. Mansfield. 1974. Photosynthesis in leaves exposed to $SO_2$ and $NO_2$ *Nature*, **250**:443-444
- Chandwick, M.J., N.H. Highton and N. Lindma. 1987. Enviornmental impacts of coal mining and utilization. Pregamon Press, Oxford, Great Britain.
- Chiment, J.J., R. Alscher and P.R. Hughes. 1986. Glutathione as an indicator of $SO_2$ induced stress in soyabean. *Environ. Exp. Bot.*, **26**:147-152
- Cohen, J.B. and A.G. Ruston. 1925. Smoke: A study of town air, Edward Arnold, London.
  Constantinidou, H.A. and T.T. Kozlowski. 1979. Effect of sulphur dioxide and ozone on *Ulmus americana* seedlings II. Carbohydrare, protein and lipids. *Can J. Bot.*, **57**: 176-184.
- Czaja, A.T. 1962. Uber des proble, *der zementstaubwirk ungen auf pflanzen staub.*, **22**: 228-232
- Darley, E.F. 1966. Studies on the effect of cement kiln dust on vegetation. *J.Air Pollut. Contr. Assoc.*, **16**:145-150.
- Darrall, N.M. 1986. The sensitivity of net photosynthesis in several plant species to short term fumitgation with sulphurdixoide. *J. Exp. Bot.*, **37**: 1313-1322.
- Darrall, N.M. 1989. The effect of air pollutans on physiological process in plants, *Cell and Environ.*, **12**: 1-30.
- Das, T.M., A. Bhaumik, A.ghosh and A. Chakraborty. 1981. Trees as dust filters. *Science Today*, **19**:19-21.
  Davies, T. 1980. Grasses more sensitive to $SO_2$ pollution in condition of low irradiance and short days. *Nature*, **284**: 483-485
- Farooq, M., A. Masood and M.V. Beg. 1985. Effect of acute exposure of sulphur dioxide on the metabolism of *Holoptelea integrifolia* plants. *Environ. Pollut.*, **39**: 197-205.

- Freer Smith, P.H. 1984. The response of six broadleaved trees during long-term exposure to SO2 and NOx. *New Phytol.*, **97**: 49-61.
- Furukawa, A.T. Natori and A. Totsuka. 1980. the effect of $SO_2$ on net photosynthesis in sunflower lead. In: *Studies on the Effects of Air Pollutants on Plants and mechanism of Phytotoxicity*. Research Report from the National Institute for Environmental Studies, No. 11, pp. 1-8
- Garg, K.K. and C.K. Varshney. 1980. Effects of air pollution of the leaf epidermis at the submicroscopic level. *Experimentia*, **36**: 1364- 1366.
- Georgii, H.W. 1978. Globale aspekte der liftveruneiningung. In : Naturu. Umweltschutz in d. Budesrepublik Deutschland G. Olschowy (ed.),
- Verlag Paul Parey, Hamburg, Berlin, pp. 216-224.
  Gordon, A.G. and E. Gorham. 1963. Ecological aspects of air pollution from an iron sintering plant at Wawa, Ontario. *Can. J. Bot.*, **41**:1063-1078.
- Grunhage, L. and H.J. Jager. 1982. Kombination swirkungen von $SO_2$ and cadmium auf Pisum sativum L.2 Enzyme, freie Aminosaurev organische Saurea and Zucker. *Angew. Bot.*, **56**: 167-178.
- Hallgren, J.E. 1978. Physiological and biochemical effects on sulphur dioxide on plants. In : *Sulphur in the Environment* Part II. Ecological Impacts, J.O. Nriagn (ed.) John Wiley & Sons, Inc. Londoa, pp. 164-209.
- Helath, R.L. 1988. Biochemical mechanism of pollutant stress. In. Assessment of Crop Loss from Air Pollutant,
- W.W. Heck, O.C. Taylor and D.T. Tingely (eds), Elsevier applied Science, London, pp. 259-286.
  heck, W.W. 1989. Assessment of crop losses from air pollutants in the United States. In Air pollution Toll on forest and Crops, J.J. Mackenzie and M.T. EI. Ashry (eds.) Yale Univ. Press, London, pp. 235-315.
- Katz, M. 1949. Sulphur dioxide in teh atmosphere and its relation to plant life. *Ind. Engg. Chem.*, **41**: 2450-2465.
- Keller, T. and H. Schwager. 1977. air pollution and ascorbic acid. *Eur. J. Forest Pathol.*, **7(6)**: 338-350.
- Khan, A.A. and S.S. Malhotra. 1977. Effects of aqueous sulphur dioxide on pine needle gycolipids. *Phytochem.*, **16**: 539-543.
- Koziol, M.J. and C.F. Jordan. 1978. changes in carbohydrate leveles in red kidney bean (Phaseoluus vulgaris L.) exposed to sulphur dioxide. *J. Exp. Bot.*, **29**: 1037-1043.
- Koziol, M.J. and D.W. cowling. 1980. Growth of rye grass (Lolium perrennel L.) exposed to SO2 III effects on free and storage carbohydrate concentrations. *J. Exp. Bot.*, **31**: 1687-1699.
- Kress, L.w. and J.M. Sketly. 1982. Response of several eastern forest tree species to chronic doses of ozone and nitrogen dioxide. *Plant Dis.*, 228.
- Mayer, R. 1983. Interaction of forest canopies with atmospheric constituents : Aluminium and heavy metals. In : *Effects of Accumulation of air Pollutant in Forest Ecosystems*, B. Ulrich and J. Pankrath (eds.), d. Reidel Publishing Comp., Holland/USA/England, pp. 47-55.
- McCune, D.C., A.E. Hitchcock, J.S. Jacobson and L.H. Weinstein. 1965. Flouride accumulation and groth of plants exposed to particuae cryolite in the atmosphere. Contrib. *Boyce Thombson Inst.*, **23**: 1-22.
- McCrone, W.C., R.G. Draftz and J.G. Delly. 1967. The particle atlas. Ann. Arbor Sci. Publ. Inc., Ann. Arbor. Mich., pp. 406
- Mudd, J.B. 1975. Sulfur dioxide. In : *Responses of Plants to Air Pullution*, J.B. Mudd and T.T. Kozlowski (eds, Academic Press, New York. pp. 9-22.
- Muller, R.N., J.E. Miller and D.G. Sprugel. 1979. Photosynthetic response of field grown soybean to fumigations with sulphur dioxide. *J. Appl. Ecol.*, **16**: 567-576.
- Nandi, P.K., M. Agrawal and D.N. Rao. 1984. $SO_2$ induced enzymatic changes and ascorbic acid oxidation in Oryza sativa. *Water, Air and Soil Pollut.*, **21**: 25-32.
- Nandi, P.K., M. Agrawal and D.N. Rao. 1986. Effects of fumigating rice plants with sulphur dioxide on photosynthetic pigments and non-structural carbohydrate. Agric. *Ecos. and Environ.*, **18**: 53-62.
  Nandi, P.K., M. Agrawal and D.N. Rao. 1987. Monitoring of cement kiln emission through plants : A case study. Proceedings EPA/APCA. Symposium on Measurement of Toxic and Related Air Pollutants. EPA/SPCA Publication, pp. 671-676.
- Natori, T. And T. Totsuka. 1984. Effects of mixed gas on transpiration rate. Research Report No. 15, National Institute for Environmental Studies. Ibaraki, Japan.

- Oliver, F.W. 1894. On the effect of urban for cultivated plants. *J. of the Royal Horticultural Society,* **13**: 139-151.
- Pahglsson, A.B. 1989. Effects of heavy metal and So₂ pollution on the concentrations of corbohydrates and nitrogen in treees leaves. *Can. J. Bot.,* **67**: 2106-2113.
- Peters, J.L., F.J. Castillo and R.L. Heath. 1989. Alteration of extracellular enzymes in pinto bean leaves upon exposure to air pollutants, ozone and sulphur dioxide. *Plant Physiol.,* **89**: 159-164.
- Pierre, M. and O. Querioz. 1981. Enzymic and metabolic changes in bean leaves during continuous pollution by subnectrotic leaves of SO₂ *Environ. Pollut.,* **25**: 41-51.
- Posthumus, A.C. 1983. Higher plants as indicators and accumulators of gaseous air pollution. envrion. *Monitor. Assess.,* **3**: 263-272.
- Rao, D.N. 1971. Study of the air pollution problem due to coal unloading in Varanasi, India. Proceedings of the wnd Inter. Clean Air Cong. N.M. Englud and W.T. Berry (eds.), Academic Press Inc., New York, pp. 273-276.
- Rao, D.N., 1980. Ecological implications of urban industrial pollution. In : *Rural habitat Transformation in World Frontiers* R.L. Singh and Rana P.B. Singh (eds.), Varanasi, pp. 84-95.
- Rao, D.N., M. Agarwal and J. Singh. 1990. Study of pollution sink officiency, growth response and productiivity pattern of plants with respect to flyash and SO₂. Final Technical Report submitted to Ministry of Envrion. & Forest, India, DOE/141/266/85.
- Rao, M.V. and P.S. Dubey. 1990. Biochemical aspect (antioxidants) for development of tolerance in plants growing at different low levels of ambient air pollutants. *Environ. Pollut.,* **64**: 55-56.
- Sharma, G.K. 1975. Leaf surface effects of environmental pollution on sugar maple (Acer saccharum) in Montreal. *Can. J. Bot.,* 53 2312-2314.
- Shetye, R.P. and S.B. Chaphekar. 1980. Some estimates on dust fall in the city of Bombay using plants. In : *Progress in Ecology,* New Delhi, Today and Tomorrow Publications, 4: 61-69.
- Shimazaki, K., T. Sakaki and K. Sugahara. 1980. Active oxygen participation in chlorophyll destruction and lipid peroxidation in SO2-fumigated leaves of spinach. In ; Studies on the Effects of air Pollutants on Plants and Mechanism of Phytotoxicity. *Res. Rep. Natl. Inst. Envrion. Stud. Japan,* **11**: 91-101.
- Sij, J.W. and C.A. swanson. 1974. Short term kinetic studies on inhibition of photosynthesis by sulphur dioxide. *J. Environ. Qual.,* **3**: 103-107.
- Singh, J. 1991. Responses of plants to thermal power plant emission. Ph.D. Thesis, Banaras Hindu University, Varanasi.
- Singh, J., M. Agrawal and D. Narayan. 1995. Changes in soil characteristics around coalfired power plants. *Environmental International,* **21** (1) 93-102.
- Singh, J.S., K.P. Singh and M. Agrawal. 1990. Envrionmental degradation of Obra-Renukoot-Singrauli area and its impact on natural and derived ecosystems. Final Tech. of a MAB Project sponsored by Ministry of Environment and Forest, Govt., of India. 14/167184-MAB/En-2 RE.
- Singh, S.N. 1980. Synergistic action of particulate and gaseous pollutants on the growth of Triticum aestivum L. *J. Exp. Botany.,* **31**: 1701-1705.
- Singh, S.N. and D.N. Rao. 1978. Effect of cement dust pollution on soil properties and on wheat plants. *Indian J. Environ. and Health,* **20**: 258-267.
- Steubing, L. and A. Fangmeier. 1987. SO2 sensitivity of plant community in a beech forest. *Environ. Pollut.,* **44**: 197-306.
- Stoaklasa, J. 1923. Die Bescliadigungen der vegetation durch rauchgase und fabrik-exhalationen. Veriag Urban and Schauarzenberg, Berlin, Wien.
- Taylor, G.E. Jr., D.T. Tingey and C.A. Gunderson. 1986. Photosynthesis, carbon allocation and growth of sulfur dioxide ecotypes of *Geranium Carolinamum L. Oecologia,* **68**: 350-357.
- Thomas, M.D., R.H. Hendricks and G.R. Hill. 1950. Sulfur metabolism of plants, effects dioxide on vegetation. *Ind. Engg. Chem.,* **42**: 2231-2235.
- Tingey, D.T. 1977. Ozone-induced lalteration in plant growth and metabolism. *Intern. Conf. Photo. Chem. Oxidant Pollut. and its Control.,* **2**: 601-609.
- Tomlinson, G.H. 1983. Air pollutants and forest decline. *Environ. Sci. Tech.* 17: 246A-256A.

- Treshow, M. 1968. Impact of air pollutants on plant populations. *Phytopathol.,* **58**: 1108-1113.
- Treshow, M. 1984. air Pollution and Plant Life. John Wiley & Sons, New York, pp. 479.
- Treshow, M. and Anderson, F.K. 1989. Plant Stress from Air Polluttion. John Wiley and Sons, New York, pp. 270
- Unsworth, M.H. and D.P. Ormrod. 1982. Effect of Gasoeous air Pollution in Agriculture and Horticulture. Butterworths Scientific, London.
- Weigl, J. and H. Aiegler. 1962. de raumliche vertiel ung von 35s und die art der markeierten verbindun gen in spinatblattern nach Begasung mit 35 $SO_2$. *Plants.,* **58**: 435-447.
- Wellburn, A.R. 1982. Effects of $SO_2$ and $NO_2$ on metabolic function. In : *Effect of Gaseous Air Pollution in Agriculture and Horticulture,* M.H. Unworth and D.P. Ormrod (eds.), Butterworth Scientific London, pp. 169-187.
- Whitmore, M.E. and P.H. Freer Smith. 1982. Growth effects of $SO_2$ and for $NO_2$ on woody plants and grasses during spring and summer. *Nature,* **300**: 55-56.
- Winner, W.E. and H.A. Mooney. 1980. Ecology of $SO_2$ resistance. II. Photosynthetic changes of shrubs in relation to $SO_2$ absorption and stomatal behaviour. *Oecologia,* **44**: 296-302.
- Winner, W.E., H.A. Monney and R.A. Goldstein. 1985. Sulphur Dioxide and Vegetation. Physiology, Ecology and Policy Issues. Stanform Univ. Press, Stanform California.
- Wislicenus*, H. 1914 Uber die au Beren and inneren vorgang der einwirkung stark ver dunn ter saurer gases and sourer nobel auf die pflanzen (versuche uber kunstilche rauchschanden im neuen rauchversuchshows in Tharandt). Mitt. a.d. Kohigl Sachs. forstl. versuchsanstalt Tharndt. **1**: 85-176.

# 7

# Plant Growth and Development in Arid Environment of NW India

*R. S. Singh*

Life demands food. Production of food depends upon the effect of four factors mainly plant and genetic material, weather, soil and water. Many factors contribute to the success or failure of agricultural production but weather and environment play more decisive role. India is a vast country covering the entire climatic spectrum. The amount of rainfall received in different parts of the country is highly variable. Particularly in arid NW India, rainfall is erratic, uncertain and unevenly distributed. In addition, extreme variations in seasonal and diurnal air and soil temperatures, long sunshine hours, intense radiation and high wind regime and evaporation make it difficult to grow any crop in the arid region. This climatic mosaic also leads to frequent occurrence of meteorological and agricultural drought situations in this part of the country.

Understanding the mechanism of crop production in relation to weather remained a complex problem for a long time. India is bestowed with favorable thermal and radiation regimes throughout the year, which makes it possible to grow several crops on the same plot of land in a year, provided water is not the limiting factor. Generally periods of maximum solar radiation coincides with period of minimum or no rainfall which calls for investment in irrigation. If other factors (including water availability) are not restricted, crop growth mainly depends on availability of radiation at a particular place. The major environmental factors influencing phenological development are ambient temperature (thermal time) and day length (bright sunshine hour). Impact of some of these environmental factors on growth and development of pearl millet and jujube fruit crops in arid areas have been described in this chapter.

## Solar Radiation and Crop Plants

The solar radiation is generally high in the arid regions. The radiation records in the arid region of Jodhpur indicate that even in the coldest month of January incoming solar radiation varies between 8.0 and 16.2 MJ m$^{-2}$ day$^{-1}$ with a mean of 14.7 MJ m$^{-2}$ day$^{-1}$. During the summer months of April and May, the daily values of incoming solar radiation ranges from 12.6 to 27.3 MJ m$^{-2}$ day$^{-1}$ with a mean of 22.1 MJ m$^{-2}$ day$^{-1}$. The lower values of daily solar radiation recorded in the winter months, during periods of western disturbance while those in the summer months are due to occurrence of dust storms.

The mean duration of bright sunshine hours in the region remain above 10.0 in May and reduces to 6.6 to 6.7 in July and August due to prevailing cloud cover and are above 8.8 hours day$^{-1}$ in the winter season. This indicates that sunshine is not a limiting factor for vegetative growth in this region.

It is established that a plant leaf strongly absorbed blue and red wavelengths, less strongly the green. Several studies have been conducted to find out plant responses to solar radiation. It has been and very weakly the near infrared and strongly the far infrared wavelengths. The Dutch Committee on Plant Irradiation has divided the solar spectrum into the following eight divisions or bands on the basis of the physiological response of plants to the incident radiation.

**Band one** : Wavelength greater than 1.000µ. No specific effects of this radiation are known. It is acceptable that this radiation, as far as the plants absorb it, is transformed into heat without interference in biochemical processes.

**Band two** : Wavelength 1.000 to 0.700µ. This is the region of specific elongation effects on plants.

**Band three** : Wavelength 0.700 to 0.610μ. This is almost the spectral region of the strongest absorption of chlorophyll and of the strongest photosynthetic activity in the red region. In many cases, it also shows the strongest photoperiodic activity.

**Band four** : Wavelength 0.610 to.510μ. This is the region of low photosynthetic effectiveness in the green and of weak formative activity.

**Band five** : Wavelength 0.510 to 0.400μ. This is virtually the region of strong chlorophyll absorption by yellow pigments. It is also·a region of strong photosynthetic activity in the blue violet and of strong formative effects.

**Band six** : Wavelength 0.400 to 0.300μ. It produces fluorescence in plants and strong response by photographic emulsions.

**Band seven** : Wavelength 0.400 to 0.315μ. It produces antirachitic effects in the production of vitamin D from ergosterol. This radiation has significant germicidal action. Under natural conditions, practically no solar radiation of shorter than 0.29μ wavelength reaches the earth's surface.

**Band eight** : Wavelength shorter than 0.280μ. No such radiation reaches the earth's surface. This radiation has strong germicidal action. It is injurious to eyesight and below 0.26mm has killing effects on some plants.

## Net Radiation

The balance of energy after gain and loss of both short wave and long-wave radiation fluxes is known as net radiation. Net radiation ($R_n$) represents the amount of energy, which is used for various kinds of activities within a crop. It is dispensed as sensible heat flux (H), latent heat flux (LE), soil heat flux (G) and also in physiological processes such as photosynthesis and respiration (P). The radiation energy utilized by vegetation in photosynthesis processes are very small and can be considered negligible in comparison to the energy utilized by the vegetation in evapotranspiration (latent heat flux) and in other processes.

Bare soil had the lowest $R_n$ because of higher soil temperatures and higher albedo in comparison to the canopies of jujube or any green vegetation. The $R_n$ (Watt m$^{-2}$) was available more over Gola cultivar (539) than over local Tikadi cultivar (498) of jujube. Thus Gola cultivar had more energy to utilize or to dispose of than did Tikadi cultivar during fruit maturity stage (Singh *et al.* 1999). Decker (1959) in his study over annual crops also reported higher net radiation than over the bare soil.

Ramakrishna *et al.*, 1991 reported in their energy balance study over field crops under arid environmental conditions that pearl millet crop maintained at potential irrigation rate exhibited lower values of soil heat flux (G) due to lower gradients in soil temperatures and higher energy utilization in evapotranspiration (Table 7.1).

### Table 7.1 : Day time energy balance (W m$^{-2}$) in pearl millet

| Crop stage | $R_n$ | LE | H | G | Advection (%) |
|---|---|---|---|---|---|
| **Rainfed** | | | | | |
| Vegetative | 298 | −68 | −105 | −125 | 0 |
| Reproductive | 268 | −236 | +11 | −44 | 4 |
| Physio. maturity | 222 | −68 | -82 | −72 | 0 |
| **Irrigated** | | | | | |
| Vegetative | 300 | −281 | −1 | −18 | 0 |
| Reproductive | 295 | −623 | +338 | −10 | 114 |
| Physio. maturity | 327 | −530 | +211 | −8 | 64 |

Advection was significantly high in the irrigated crop due to the high evaporative demand of the atmosphere and free water availability to the crop.

## Environmental Temperature and Crop Plants

*Temperature:* It is a measure of degree of hotness. Temperature is therefore the intensity aspect of heat energy. Solar radiation is the main source of heat energy to the biosphere. Temperature is of paramount importance for organic life because of the following factors:

Physical and chemical processes within the plants are governed by the temperature and these processes in turn control biological reactions that take place within the plants:

1  The diffusion rate of gases and liquids changes with temperature;
2  Solubility of different substances is dependent upon temperature;
3  The rate of reaction varies with variations in temperature;
4  Equilibrium of various systems and compounds is a function of temperature; and
5  Temperature effects the stability of the enzyme system.

## Air Temperature

Air temperature is the most important climatic variable, which affects plant life. The growth of higher plants is restricted to a temperature between 0 and 60°C and crop plants are further restricted to a narrower range of 10 to 40°C. However, each species and variety of plants and each age group of plants has its own upper and lower temperature limits. Beyond these limits, a plant gets considerably damaged, and even gets killed. In another range, growth of the plant stops and it becomes dormant, but remains alive. There is also a third range of temperature in which the growth of the plant at a particular stage of development is optimal. Thus it is the amplitude of variations in temperature, rather than the mean values of it, which is more important to plant growth.

## Growing Degree Days

Growing degree days (GDD), also called heat units, effective heat units or growth units, are a simple means of relating plant growth development and maturity to air temperature (Vittum *et al.*, 1965). The heat unit or growing degree-day concept assumes that there is a direct and linear relationship between growth and temperature. It starts with the assumption that the growth of plants is dependent on the total amount of heat to which it is subjected during its lifetime. A degree day or a heat unit, is the departure from the mean daily temperature above the minimum threshold temperature. This minimum threshold is the temperature below which no growth takes place. The threshold varies with different plants and for the majority ranges from 4.5 to 12.5°C., there being higher values for tropical plants and lower value for temperate plants. The growing degree days are calculated with an equation written as:

$$\text{Thermal time} = \sum \frac{T_{max} + T_{min}}{2} - T_t \qquad \qquad \dots (1)$$

where $T_{max} + T_{min}/2$ is the average daily temperature and $T_t$ is the minimum threshold temperature for a crop. The simplicity of the degree day method has made it widely popular in guiding agricultural operations and planning land use. Most applications of the growing degree day concept are for the forecast of crop-harvest dates, yield, and quality. It helps in forecasting labour needs for factory and to reduce harvesting and factory cost. The concept is also applied to plants other than crop plants and to the problems of growth and development of insects, plant pathogens, birds and other animals (Hord and Spell, 1962). A potential area of its application lies in estimating the likelihood of the successful growth of a crop in an area in which it has not been grown earlier. The growing degree concept can also be applied to the selection of one variety from several varieties of plants to be grown in a new area. Another application of the concept can be to change or modify the microclimate in such a way as to produce the nearly optimum conditions at each point in the developmental cycle of an organism. This application is however, still to be evaluated. Though the degree day concept is very simple and useful, it lacks theoretical soundness and has a number of weaknesses. In spite of the weaknesses and limitations, the degree day or heat unit concept, with a slight modification, seems to answer a number of questions in forecasting crop growth and maturity.

## Crops and Unfavorable Temperatures

The mid day high temperature increases the saturation deficit of the plants. It accelerates photosynthesis and ripening of fruits. The maximum production of dry matter occurs when the temperature ranges between 20 and 30$^0$C, provided moisture is not a limiting factor. When high temperature occurs in combination with high humidity, it favors the development of many plant diseases. High temperature also affects plant metabolism. High night temperature increases respiration and also affects plant metabolism. Crops will have a threshold temperature below which no growth takes place. The threshold temperature for most of the crops is about 5°C. The difference between the mean daily temperature and the threshold temperature of the crop will indicate the number of heat units available to the crop on the particular day. The number of heat units required for completion of phenophases of the crop growth can be obtained by adding the average daily temperature over the threshold value during a particular phase. The total heat unit requirements from sowing to harvest for many particular variety of crop will be faster in regions with higher temperature than in regions with lower temperature. During the periods of drought and moisture stress, the temperatures will be comparatively high accelerating the process of crop development to early maturity. High temperature increases the evapotranspiration demand. The evaporation will be high from the soil due to excessive heating because of low specific heat of the dry soil.

Most crop plants are injured and many killed when night temperature is very low. Tender leaves and flowers are very sensitive to lower temperature and frost. Plants that are rapidly growing and flowering are easily killed. Low temperature interferes with the respiration of plants. If low temperature coincides with wet soil, it results in the accumulation of harmful products in the plant cells. Frost also interferes with plant metabolism. When the temperatures fall below freezing point during the winter season in association with cold waves, there will be frost injury to the crops. The low temperatures dampen the growth and development of crops.

## Sowing Date and Thermal Time Requirements of Pearl millet Crop

Pearl millet grown under optimal moisture and rainfed conditions behaved differently in different growing seasons (Table 7.2) due to variation in natural sowing time linked with arrival of the SW monsoon in the region (Singh *et al.*, 1998). The crop, when sown early during the 1993 season, took more thermal time to reach flowering as compared to normal and late sowing seasons. This delay in the flowering seems to be due to availability of longer photo-period (9.5 h day$^{-1}$ ) during the crop vegetative phase (August, 1993) in comparison to 4.2 h day$^{-1}$ in 1994 and 6.6 h day$^{-1}$ in 1995 (Table 7.3) during the same period (Muchow and Carberry 1990).

**Table 7.2 : Thermal time (degree days) taken by pearl millet at Jodhpur in relation to rainfall and sowing time under arid environment**

| Year | Date of sowing | Rainfall (sowing to harvest) mm | Rainy days | Thermal time for maturity ($^0$Cd) taken by the crop | |
|------|----------------|-------------------------------|------------|------------------|---------|
| | | | | Optimal Moisture | Rainfed |
| 1993 | 28 June (Early) | 206.2 | 11 | 1675 | 1794 |
| 1994 | 04 July (Normal) | 486.9 | 28 | 1714 | 1560 |
| 1995 | 21 July (Late) | 266.5 | 12 | 1552 | 1490 |
| Mean | | | | 1647 | 1615 |
| Sem | | | | 10.3 | 15.3 |

| Growing | Mean air temperature ($^0$C) | | | | Photoperiod (hrs day$^{-1}$) | | | |
|---------|------|------|------|------|------|------|------|------|
| Season | Jul | Aug | Sep | Oct | Jul | Aug | Sep | Oct |
| 1993 | 31.5 | 31.2 | 30.2 | 29.7 | 7.0 | 9.5 | 9.4 | 9.5 |
| 1994 | 29.9 | 28.2 | 27.2 | 26.1 | 4.9 | 4.2 | 8.4 | 9.8 |
| 1995 | 32.0 | 30.0 | 30.4 | 29.1 | 7.5 | 6.6 | 10.0 | 9.2 |

## Dry Biomass of Pearl millet and Thermal Time

The relationship between total dry biomass (Y) and cumulative thermal time (X) for the crop maintained under optimal moisture condition was:

$$Y = 4.83*10^{-17}*0.996^X*X^{6.5}; R^2 = 0.96 \qquad \text{... (2)}$$

And for the rainfed crop was:

$$Y = 4.43*10^{-16}*0.997^X*X^{6.1}; R^2 = 0.93 \qquad \text{... (3)}$$

The fitted relationship (Fig. 7.1) was of the type of $Y = A*B^X*X^C$ which is the product of the power and exponential type of function and known as hoerl function. This explained that biomass accumulation (growth rate) was generally linear with respect to thermal time between 900$^0$Cd and 1500$^0$Cd after emergence under both moisture conditions. However, growth gradient was significantly higher under optimal moisture condition (0.13 g plant$^{-1}$ $^0$Cd$^{-1}$) than under rainfed condition (0.08 g plant$^{-1}$ $^0$Cd$^{-1}$).

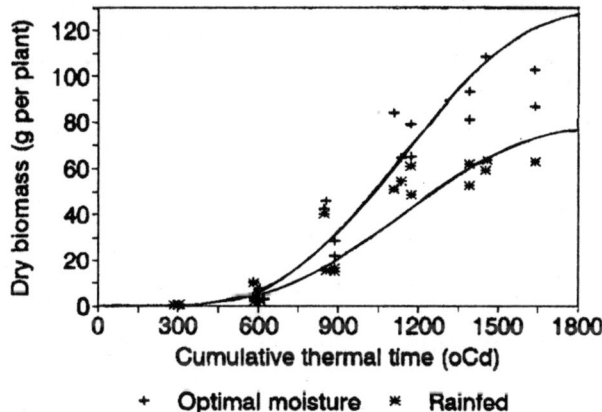

+   Optimal moisture   *   Rainfed

**Fig. 7.1** : Pearl millet growth curve in relation to thermal time ($^0$Cd after emergence)

## Moisture Availability, Canopy Temperature and Thermal Time

The reproductive phase and maturity of pearl millet grown under optimal moisture required more thermal time than the rainfed crop except some exception. Crop development was also slightly affected due to variation in soil moisture availability in the field conditions during different growing seasons. The reproductive phase of the crop under optimal moisture conditions was slightly prolonged in comparison to the rainfed crop irrespective of sowing date. This yields higher biomass and grain under optimal moisture in comparison to the rainfed conditions. The difference in the requirement of thermal time for the physiological maturity between the crop under optimal moisture and rainfed condition irrespective of growing seasons and sowing dates is indicative of the role if other environmental factors for completion of various phenophases. It is likely that the crop is more affected by canopy temperature ($t_c$) than ambient temperature ($t_a$), which is not considered in the calculation of thermal time.

Cumulative values of stress degree days (SDD's) calculated from measured $(t_c-t_a)$ temperature for both the optimal and the rainfed plots of pearl millet as a function of day after emergence (DAE) are presented in Fig. 7.2 The SDD values for the crop raised under optimal moisture was lower than the rainfed crop (Singh *et al.*, 1998). This is because of the fact that under optimal moisture plants maintain temperature below ambient air due to a high transpiration rate and under rainfed conditions the reduced availability of water limits the transpiration rate and the canopy temperature is increased (Idso *et al.* 1977, Jackson *et al.* 1981). The afternoon fluctuation of $(t_c-t_a)$ followed irrigations and rainfalls. The rainfed crop experienced stress and recorded positive values of $(t_c-t_a)$ during the grain filling and maturity periods. Therefore, the change in the thermal time required for the completion of different phenophases from one growing season to another season, could be due to the impact of day to day crop micro-climate and associated moisture availability (*viz*: canopy temperature, radiation interception, wind turbulence, vapour pressure deficit and soil moisture), on the crop phenological development.

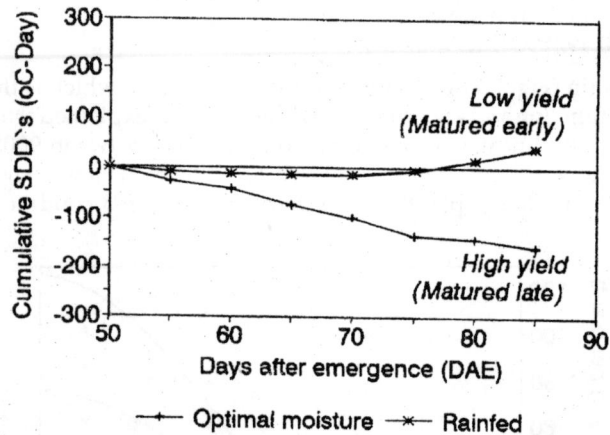

Fig. 7.2 :   Seasonal progression of stress degree days (SDD'S) for the pearl millet maintained at the different moishere availability conditions

As long as crop is provided with adequate water to meet its evapotranspiration requirements, the crop canopy maintains the same temperature as the ambient air or less than it. Whenever there is inadequacy of water and moisture stress for the crop, its canopy will be at higher temperature than the ambient air. Therefore a positive difference is a clear indication of moisture stress. A negative correlation of 0.91 was observed between the accumulated stress degree days and productivity of wheat grown at Anand (Anonymous, 1986a) thereby indicating that higher canopy temperatures will result in low productivity of crops unless adequate water is applied to the crop. Therefore, information on the difference in crop canopy temperature and ambient air is very useful in scheduling of irrigation.

Studies conducted on the effect of shelterbelts on crop micro-climate and productivity of tomatoes grown in the winter season at Ludhiana have brought out that the crop canopy temperatures remain higher by 2°C in sheltered crop compared to the crop grown in open. Significant increase in productivity per plant is well indicated under the influence of shelterbelt, as a protective measure against cold weather conditions (Anonymous, 1986b).

Canopy temperatures $(t_c)$ of four cultivars of jujube in an orchard were studied (Singh *et al.*, 1998). Canopy temperature of Gola cultivars were lower by at least 0.5 to 2.0°C from the flowering to fruit maturity stages in comparison to local Tikadi cultivar of jujube, particularly during afternoon (Table 7.4). The higher $t_c$ of Tikadi is because of the higher absorption of incoming radiation as well as lower albedo (23%) in comparison to cultivars Gola and Seb (26%).

**Table 7.4 : Canopy temperature (t$_c$) and canopy air temperature difference (t$_c$-t$_a$) of various jujube cultivars during afternoon at Jodhpur (1990-91)**

| Cultivars | Temperature (°C) | | | | | | | | | |
|---|---|---|---|---|---|---|---|---|---|---|
| | Sep | | Oct | | Nov | | Dec | | Jan | |
| | $t_c$ | $t_c$-$t_a$ | $t_c$ | $t_c$-$t_a$ | $t_c$ | $t_c$-$t_a$ | $t_c$ | $t_c$-$t_a$ | $t_c$ | $t_c$-$t_a$ |
| Tikadi | 30.8 | −6.1 | 32.4 | −5.2 | 26.5 | −7.2 | 23.8 | −4.6 | 20.8 | −5.7 |
| Seb | 30.4 | −6.5 | 31.7 | −6.9 | 25.8 | −8.2 | 23.2 | −5.6 | 21.4 | −6.0 |
| Gola | 30.3 | −7.2 | 31.2 | −7.5 | 24.5 | −8.9 | 23.0 | −6.4 | 20.6 | −6.7 |
| Umran | 29.7 | −6.8 | 32.0 | −7.1 | 25.6 | −8.6 | 23.7 | −5.2 | 20.3 | −6.4 |

The relative stress (indicated by the difference between canopy and air temperatures), measured $t_c$-$t_a$ indicated that all cultivars were able to maintain $t_c$ lower by at least 4.6°C than the surrounding ambient temperature during all growth stages during the year 1990-91. This suggested that no cultivar were under stress during the year. However, this difference ($t_c$-$t_a$) was comparatively more in case of Gola than in other cultivars, favourable better growth and higher fruit yield of Gola variety during the year.

## Phenological Development in Jujube in relation to Thermal Time

Studies conducted by Singh *et al.*, 1999 on jujube orchard of different cultivars grown in arid Rajasthan indicated that Seb cultivar requires the lowest accumulation of thermal time (2595±10°Cd) during pruning to the stage of bud formation. This cultivar followed by Gola and Tikadi, with the latter requiring the highest heat summation units (3044°Cd). It was observed that fruit setting in the Seb cultivar occurred about two weeks earlier than that in Tikadi and Gola cultivars in this region (Table 7.5). However, Gola cultivar matured earlier than all other cultivars (Vashistha and Pareek, 1989). It needs only 1689°Cd accumulation from fruit setting to first harvest of fruit whereas Seb cultivar require much accumulation of thermal time (2191°Cd), followed by Tikadi cultivar (1954°Cd).

**Table 7.5 : Heat unit accumulation for the completion of different growth stages of jujube cultivars in hot arid climate at Jodhpur**

| Growth stages | Cultivars | | | | |
|---|---|---|---|---|---|
| | Tikadi | Seb | Gola | SEm | CD at 5% |
| Pruning to bud formation | 3044 | 2595 | 2874 | 10 | 29 |
| Budding to fruit setting | 763 | 938 | 928 | 9 | 27 |
| Fruit setting to maturity | 1954 | 2191 | 1689 | 19 | 54 |

## Jujube Fruit Development and Thermal Time

Singh *et al.*, 1999 have worked out relationship between jujube fruit growth size (cm) and accumulated thermal time after fruit setting for two contrasting cultivars (Tikadi and Gola). In both cases linear regression (Fig. 7.3) was the best fit with high correlation coefficients, significant at 1% level. The regression equation fitted between fruit size (Y) and accumulated thermal time (X) in case of Tikadi and Gola cultivars maintained under rainfed conditions, respectively, were

$$Y = 1.11 + 0.0003X; R^2 = 0.81 \qquad \text{.... (4)}$$
$$Y = 0.78 + 0.0011X; R^2 = 0.94 \qquad \text{.... (5)}$$

This indicates that inspite of taking almost similar time for fruit setting by both the cultivars, the fruits of local Tikadi cultivar, thereafter, grow slowly and need more heat units (around 335°Cd) per mm of growth, in comparison to the fruits of Gola cultivar, which grows rapidly and requires less heat units (88°Cd) per mm of growth.

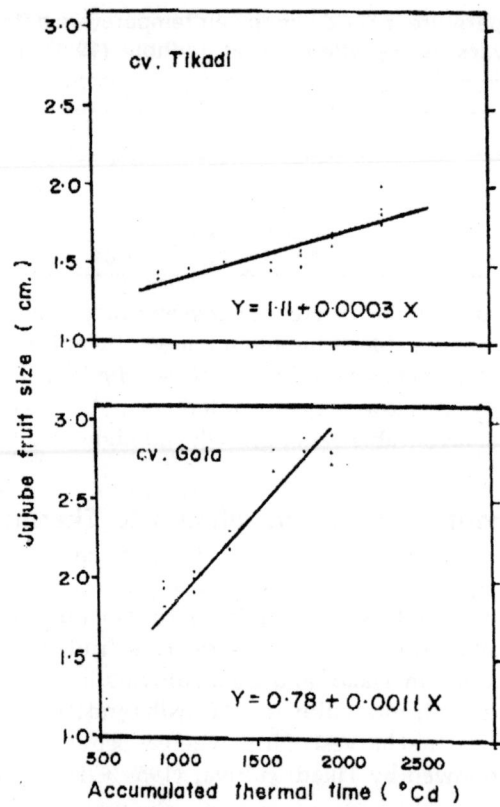

**Fig. 7.3 :** Relationship between jujube fruit growth size and accumulated thermal time under and conditions.

## Prediction of Maturity Time for Jujube Fruits

Thermal time is widely used for predicting the maturity time of annual crops as well as fruit crops. Thermal time worked out by Central Arid Zone Research Institute, Jodhpur for the maturity time of fruits of different cultivars of jujube was tested to predict the maturity of the fruits in subsequent years, 1993-94 and 1994-95. It was reported that the actual thermal time required by the fruits of Gola cultivar for maturity were 1656 and 1729°Cd during the year 1993-94 and 1994-95, respectively. These thermal time values are almost close to the predicted thermal time (1689°Cd) for the fruit maturity of Gola cultivars. Similarly, the predicted time for fruit maturity of Seb and Tikadi cultivars were also comparable to the actual thermal time taken during the year 1993-94 and 1994-95 in the region. In general, different jujube trees took more (104 to 137) days for their fruit maturity during the season 1994-95 in comparison to days (85 to 116) taken in 1993-94 season. The likely reason for this could be the considerably lower ambient temperature (20.8°C) regime during the fruit development period (October-January) in 1994-95, in comparison to the same period in 1993-94 (23.2°C). The rainfall was much higher in 1994-95, which had favoured the growth of the jujube tree canopy and ultimately high fruit yield was recorded (Table 7.6). But, in the same year, cropping season was prolonged due to low temperature regime and finally, fruit maturity was delayed by 12 to 21 days during the season.

**Table 7.6 : Rainfall and mean air temperatures during different growing seasons of jujube**

| Year | Annual Rainfall (mm) June–May | Mean air temperature (°C) | | | | Fruit yield (kg tree⁻¹) | | |
|------|------|------|------|------|------|------|------|------|
| | | Jun–Sep | Oct–Jan | Feb–May | Annual | Tikadi | Seb | Gola |
| 1990-91 | 788.9 | 30.6 | 21.6 | 27.6 | 26.6 | 20.0 | 24.2 | 27.0 |
| 1991-92 | 241.0 | 31.5 | 22.1 | 26.8 | 26.8 | 17.4 | 18.1 | 21.6 |
| 1992-93 | 419.8 | 31.3 | 21.9 | 27.6 | 26.9 | 19.0 | 20.6 | 28.5 |
| 1993-94 | 345.1 | 31.7 | 23.2 | 28.1 | 27.7 | 5.5 | 5.4 | 8.6 |
| 1994-95 | 547.0 | 29.1 | 20.8 | 27.7 | 25.9 | 15.0 | 30.8 | 35.1 |

## Relative Humidity (RH) and Vapour Pressure Inside the Jujube Orchard

In general, the RH inside jujube orchard is higher by 6 to 40 percent in comparison to the humidity in outside field (Table 7.7). This difference in RH was maximum during fruit setting stage (October), which may be beneficial in fruit setting (Kretchman, 1968; Picken, 1984). Vapour pressure was also higher by 14 to 34 percent inside the orchard in comparison to that measured in the open. Vapour pressure deficit (vpd) varied between 22 and 41 mb during the different growth stages inside the orchard. This larger vpd may be responsible for higher leaf transpiration rate from different cultivars (Rosenberg, 1974).

**Table 7.7 : Monthly variation of RH and vapour pressure during afternoon (3 p.m.) period inside and outside the orchard at CAZRI, Jodhpur (1990-91)**

| Month | RH (%) | | Vapour pressure (mb) | |
|-------|--------|---------|------|---------|
| | Inside | Outside | Inside | Outside |
| Oct. | 42 (31) | 32 | 15.5 (14) | 13.6 |
| Nov. | 28 (40) | 20 | 8.3 (34) | 6.2 |
| Dec. | 14 (17) | 12 | 3.6 (16) | 3.1 |
| Jan. | 19 (06) | 12 | 3.9 (15) | 3.4 |
| Feb. | 19 (27) | 15 | 6.7 (22) | 5.5 |

Figures in parenthesis indicate percentage increase over outside.

## Winds and Vegetation

Strong wind blows during the months from April to August in most parts of the country. Wherever the wind speed exceeds 10kmph, wind erosion takes place from open and dry soils. Wind causes increased evapotranspiration losses due to advection. Stormy winds cause lodging of the crops.

Tree shelterbelts (Gupta et al., 1983) reduce the wind speed on leeward side thereby controlling wind erosion as well as loss of soil fertility. Tree shelterbelts were also found to be very effective in reducing the evaporative demand of the air by minimizing the advection effects both during the summer and monsoon seasons. Higher water use efficiency and better productivity can be achieved for irrigated crops grown in isolated patches during summer season by providing wind breaks across the predominant wind direction.

## Turbulence

Turbulence in the atmosphere is another environmental factor that strongly affects the intake of carbon dioxide. The intake of carbon dioxide depends on its concentration in the atmosphere and on its delivery to the leaf. When the atmosphere is calm, carbon dioxide reaches the leaf by the slow process of diffusion. Under these conditions, after a short while, the availability of carbon dioxide to the leaf becomes restricted. When the air is in turbulence, the transfer of carbon dioxide to the leaf is quite rapid.

To begin with, it can be said that the rate of photosynthesis is less when it is calm and is greater when the wind is blowing. However, a positive correlation is not always observed between the speed of wind and photosynthesis. On the other hand, a decrease in the rate of assimilation has been recorded as the speed of wind increases. This may, however, be attributed to an inadequate water supply to plants growing in sandy soils. Different workers have given various values for the maximum wind velocity up to which the rate of assimilation increases. These values range from 0.3 to more than 1 metre per second.

## SUMMARY

Vegetation growth in relation to arid environment is described based on the data recorded at Central Arid Zone Research Institute (CAZRI), Jodhpur from 1990 to 1995. Pearl millet and jujube (ber) crop development is discussed in terms of changes in photoperiod and ambient temperature. It is world wise established that availability of solar radiation over any place decides crop growth (accumulation of dry matter) subjected to no shortage of water supply to root zone of the crop field. However, crop phenological development is mainly governed by ambient temperature and photoperiod over the crop field. Experimental study on pearl millet conducted at CAZRI, Jodhpur revealed that the crop required 1490-1794 degree Celsius days ($^0$Cd) thermal time to reach physiological maturity. In another study, relationships between phenological growth stages in three promising cultivars of jujube (viz., Tikadi, Seb, and Gola) and ambient temperature were worked out under rainfed arid conditions. It was observed that Gola fruits mature early and required about 1689$^0$Cd thermal time (growing degree days, GDD) after fruit setting. The thermal time calculated for jujube (ber) is successfully tested for predicting the fruit maturity (harvesting) time in the region.

## GLOSSARY

**Advection** : The process of transfer of an air-mass property by virtue of motion. The term is however, often used to signify horizontal transfer only.

**Albedo** : A measure of the reflecting power of a surface.

**Amplitude** : For a true wave variation, the magnitude of the maximum departure of the quantity concerned from its mean value. For a more complex type of oscillation, the amplitude is usually taken as being half the mean difference between maxima and minima.

**Arid** : A climate in which the rainfall is insufficient to support vegetation is termed arid.

**Biosphere** : That part of the earth's envelope, comprising the seas, lower atmosphere and surface layer of the earth's crust in which living organisms exist in their natural state.

**Diffusion** : Molecular diffusion is the process by which contiguous fluids mix slowly, despite differences in their density. The process follows laws similar to those of thermal conduction (heat diffusion).

**Evapotranspiration** : The combined processes of evaporation from the earth's surface and transpiration from vegetation.

**Microclimate** : The physical state of the atmosphere close to a very small area of the earth's surface, often in relation to living matter such as crops or insects. In contrast to climate, microclimate generally pertains to a short period of time.

**Phenology** : The study of the sequence of seasonal changes in nature. All natural phenomena are included, seed time, harvest, flowering, ripening and etc.

**Sandstom or duststorm** : An ensemble of particles of dust or sand energetically lifted to great heights by a strong and turbulence wind.

**Solar radiation** : The transmission of energy by electromagnetic waves (the term is also used to signify the emission of particles by a source, as in 'cosmic radiation' and 'solar particle radiation').

**Turbulence :** It is generally taken to comprise the complex spectrum of fluctuating motion which is superimposed on a 'mean flow'. Small scale atmospheric turbulence is evident in the fluctuation of windspeed and direction recorded by an anemograph.

# REFERENCES

- Anonymous (1986a). Annual report of the All India Coordinated Research Project on Agrometeorology for 1986. Gujarat Agricultural University, Anand. pp 56.
- Anonymous (1986b). Annual report of the All India Coordinated Research Project on Agrometeorology for 1985. Central Research Institute for Dryland Agriculture, Hyderabad, India. pp 59.
- Decker, W. (1959). Variations in the net exchange of radiation from vegetation of different heights. *J. Geophys. Res.* **64**: 1617-1619.
- Gupta, J.P., Rao, G.G.S.N., Gupta, G.N. and Raman Rao, B.V. (1983). Soil drying and wind erosion as affected by different types of shelterbelts planted in the desert region of Western Rajasthan, India. *J. Arid Environ.* **6**: 53-58.
- Hord, H.H.V. and Spell, O.P. (1962). Temperature as a basis for forecasting banana production. *Trop. Agric.* **39**: 219-233.
- Idso, S.B., Reginato, R.J. and Jackson, R.D. (1977). Remote sensing of crop yields. *Science* **196**: 19-25.
- Jackson, R.D., Idso, S.B., Reginato, R.J. and Pinter Jr., P.J. (1981). Canopy temperature as a crop water stress indicator. *Water Resources* **17**: 1133-1138.
- Kretchman, D.W. (1968). A preliminary report of several aspects of fruit setting of green house tomatoes. *Research Summary of the Ohio Agricultural Research and Development Centre* **26**: 5-8.
- Muchow, R.C. and Carberry, P.S. (1990). Phenology and leaf-area development in a tropical grain sorghum. *Field Crops Res.* **23**: 221-237.
- Picken, A.J.F. (1984). A review of pollination and fruit set in the tomato (*Lycopersicon esculentum* Mill.). *J. Hort. Sci.* **59**: 1-13.
- Ramakrishna, Y.S., Rao A.S., Singh, R.S. and Joshi, N.L. (1991). Studies on water and energy use efficiency of pearl millet (*Pennisetum americanum* (L) Leeke). In: *Proceedings of the National Seminar on Hydrometeorology* (Eds. Varshneya, M.C. and Bote, N.L.) pp. 13-17, MPKV Res. Pub. No. 8, Mahatma Phule Krishi Vidyapeeth, Rahuri-413 722, India.
- Rosenberg, N.J. (1974). *Microclimate: The Biological Environment.* Wiley-Inter-Science Publication, NewYork.
- Singh, R.S., Vashishtha, B.B. and Prasad, R.N. (1999). Micro-climatic impact on productivity of jujube cultivars under arid conditions. In : *Management of Arid Ecosystem* (Eds. Faroda, A.S., Joshi, N.L., Kathju, S. and Kar A.) pp. 369-378, Arid Zone Research Association of India and Scientific Publishers, Jodhpur, India.
- Singh, R.S., Prasad, R.N., Gupta, J.P., Vashishtha, B.B. and Ramakrishna, Y.S. (1999) Thermal time requirement for fruit development and maturity of jujube (*Zizyphus mauritiana*) grown under rainfed conditions in Indian hot desert. *Annals of Arid Zone* **38**: 161-166.
- Singh, R.S., Joshi, N.L. and Singh, H.P. (1998) Pearl millet phenology and growth in relation to thermal time under arid environment. *J. Agronomy & Crop Science* **180**: 83-91.
- Singh, R.S., Vashishtha, B.B. and Prasad, R.N. (1998) Micrometeorology of ber (*Zizyphus mauritiana*) Orchard grown under rainfed arid conditions. *Ind. J. Hort.* **55**: 97-107.
- Vashishtha, B.B. and Pareek, O.P. (1989) Identification key for the cultivars of Indian jujube. *Ind. J. Hort.* **46**: 183-188.
- Vittum, M.T., Dethier, B.E. and Lesser, R.C. (1965) Estimating growing degree days. *Proc. Am. Soc. Hort. Sci* **87**: 449-452.

# 8

# Insects and Environment

*T. C. Narendran*

## Introduction

Insects form the largest group among animals. Their great diversity of form and colour and their biological intricacy and specialization combine to make them one of the most marvelously rewarding groups of animals to study. Insects and its environment mutually interact. The insect have inter-relations with plants and animals. They show diverse adaptations to various environmental factors. They have seasonal and geographical variations. Ecoclimate and micorclimate affect their populations. They interact with the living environment in various ways. The activities of man greatly affect insects in several ways. The man made conditions in the environment such as deforestation, monoculture, indiscriminate use of pesticides, habitat destruction, industrialization etc. cause biodiversity crisis and extinction of several species. While many species are endangered, some are coming under 'threatened' category. Hence it is high time for us to take appropriate steps not only to study them but also to create conditions for preserving their diversity.

## Faunal Diversity and Systematics

Insects constitute approximately three-fourth of the total number of organisms known. This shows that all the other groups of organisms are comparatively small in number. Today about one million insects are described and this forms only one-tenth of the total estimated fauna of insects of the world. Thus the majority of insects persent in the world remain undescribed and not yet discovered. Though India is a paradise as far as the faunal diversity of insects are concerned, only about 60000 species are named and described. This shows the need for undertaking detailed taxonomic studies on the insect fauna of India inorder to know their actual faunal diversity.

The insects are classified into 28 orders as follows:

Class **Insecta**

Sub class: **Apterygota**-Primitive wingless insects

Order 1. Protura
   2. Collembola
   3. Diplura
   4: Thysanura

Subclass: **Pterygota**-Winged and Secondarily wingelss insects

Division: **Exopterygota** (Heterometabola) Insects with simple metamorphosis

| | |
|---|---|
| 5. Ephemeroptera | 13. Embioptera |
| 6. Odonata | 14. Plecoptera |
| 7. Grylloblattoidea | 15. Zoraptera |
| 8. Orthoptera | 16. Psocoptera |
| 9. Dictyoptera | 17. Pthiraptera |
| 10. Phasmida | 18. Thysanoptera |
| 11. Dermaptera | 19. Hemiptera    sub order: Heteroptera |
| 12. Isoptera | sub order: Homoptera |

Division: **Endopterygota** (Holometabola) insects with complete metamorphosis.

20. Neuroptera
21. Coleoptera
22. Strepsiptera
23. Mecoptera
24. Trichoptera

25. Lepidoptera
26. Diptera
27. Siphonaptera
28. Hymenoptera

**Protura:** These are rare soil inhibiting insects with less than 2mm in body length. About 99 per cent of India is unexplored as far as Protura is concerned. So far only 20 species belonging to 8 genera and three families are known from India (Hazra et.al. 1998).

**Collembola:** They are commonly known as spring tails since they jump using their caudal furca. Their size varies from 0.25 - 6mm in length. There are approximently 212 species and about 85 genera. They live in terrestrial and aquatic conditions. Collembola are useful insects for biodegradation of leaf litter etc. for increasing the fertility of soil.

**Diplura:** Diplurans are small, blind whitish insects measuring less than 7mm (but rerely upto 50mm in length). They live in soil. About 400 species and about 80 genera are known from the world. Among these, 16 species under 7 genera are known from India (Hazra et. al 1998). They are good bioindicators of rich organic soil.

**Thysanura:** The members of this order are known as bristletails. Members of the genus *Lepisma* are known as Silver fishes. The thysanurans occur under stones, fallen leaves, decaying barks, in caves, in mammal burrows or some, in the nests of ants. The silver fish eats paper, painting etc. The thysanurans are omnivorous. Very little systematic studies have been done on Indian fauna which consists of approximately 32 species and 21 genera.

**Ephemeroptera:** Members of this order are known as mayflies. Their size varies from 10-40mm in length. They live near streams, ponds and lakes. Since most of them have a very short life span of a few hours they got the name Ephemeroptra. About 1500 species are known from the world. So far no detailed information is available regarding the exact number of species occurring in India. The mayflies form food for fresh water fishes and other aquatic animals. They are also indicators of aquatic conditions.

**Odonata:** The odonates are commonly known as Damselfly or Ddamselfly. There are approximately six thousand species described in the world and approximately 500 species are recorded from India. The order Odonata is divided into two suborders *viz.* Anisoptera (Dragonflies) and Zygoptera (Damselflies). The odonates are predators on other smaller insects and the immature stages of odonates are aquatic in habit. since odonates are predators of other insects including mosquitoes, flies etc. they are of economic value. Several species are intermediate hosts of helminth parasites which cause diseases in poultry and other birds.

**Grylloblattoidea:** It is believed that the crickets and roaches have evolved from the common ancestral stock of Grylloblattoidea. There is only one family which contains about 20 species in the world. None is so far reported from India. The insects are secondarily apterous and are usually found beneath stones and high altitudes. They are reported from Palearctic and Nearctic Regions.

**Orthoptera:** The grasshoppers, locusts and crickets belong to this order. About 17500 species are known from the world and out of this about 10 percent of species occur in India. They are widely distributed in the tropical areas. These orthopterans are economically very important since many species are major pests of crops. They are also important as food for several species of birds and reptiles.

**Dictyoptera:** The cockroaches and mantids constitute Dictyoptera. It contains two subfamilies, *viz.* Blattaria and Mantoidea. In the world 2310 species are known and out of which 162 species occur in India (Hazra & Mukerjee, 1998). The mantids are predators of other insects and they play an important role in preventing the populations of many insects from reaching the economic injury level. The Blattaria contains about 5000 species in the world and 186 species are known from India (Mandal 1998).

**Phasmida:** This order is comprised of leaf and stick-insects. They are very curious looking insects resembling plant leaves and twigs. Some species of stick-insects may exceed 30cms in length. There are 2500 species known from India. Very few species are reported to reach pest status occasionally. They feed on plant leaves.

**Dermaptera:** Members of this order are known as Earwigs. They possess a pair of pincer like cerci at the tip of their abdomen. Earwigs represent somewhat a middle status between Apterygota and Pterygota. This order contains both winged and wingles insects. Some species emit foul smelling liquid as a defensive action against enemies. There are 2000 species known from the world (Steinmann, 1989) and 320 are known from the Indian sub-continent (Srivastava, 1998).

**Isoptera:** Members of this order are known as Termites or whiteants. They are social insects living in communities having division of labour among individulas. About 2000 species are known from the world and about 253 species are reported form India (Maiti and Saha, 1998). Many species are serious pests. However they play a vital role in the biodegradation of soil material and in increasing soil fertility.

**Embioptera:** Embiopterans are known as webspinners since most species live in silken tunnels. They are small insects of 4-7mm in length. They feed on dead plants materials, fungi, lichens, moss and bark. They are beneficial insects in keeping the soil layers humid. There are 200 species known from the world and only 33 species are known from India (Mitra 1998).

**Plecoptera:** The members of this order are known as stoneflies, salmon flies and perlids. They are medium-sized or small, soft-bodied insect found near streams or rocky lakes. They are poor fliers. The naiads are phytophagous feeding on algal slime or predaceous on immatures of other insects. 2100 species are known from the world and among these 113 species are known from India (Varshney 1998).

**Zoraptera:** The Zorapterans are rare insects measuring less than 3mm in length. They resemble termites. They may be winged or wingless. Only very few (about 30 species) are known from the world and they are found in all regions except the Palearctic. They live under barks, rotten logs and in saw dust. They feed on fungal spores and dead arthropods. Their economic value has not so far been ascertained.

**Psocoptera:** The members of this order are known as Psocids. They are delicate insects with length lesser than 6mm. Most species feed on molds, fungi, cereals, pollen, dead insects, etc. There are 2500 species known from the world and out of these 90 species are reported from India (Ray, 1998). Psocopterans are economically very important since they damage stored cereals, herbarium, zoological specimens etc. The species *Ectopsocus maindrini* Badonnel is a very important pest of stored products, and this species have posed a threat to rubber industry by damaging rubber infected with moulds in India.

**Pthiraptera:** This order comprises the chewing lice and sucking lice. They are parasites of birds and mammals. The order contains 3 suborders *viz.* Mallophaga, Anoplura and Rhynchophthirina. There are 3000 species of Pthiraptera known to occur in the world and out of these 400 are known from India. (Varshney, 1998).

**Thysanoptera:** The thrips are slender insects measuring 0.5mm to 2mm in length. Both winged and wingless forms are present. The wings are with peculiar long fringes. Majority of species are phytophagous and a few are predaceous on other small insects and mites. A few live as inquilines in galls. About 6000 species are known from the world and 693 species are serious pests of crops. They are economically very important. Some species are useful in pollination of flowers and others are useful in destroying weeds.

**Hemiptera:** The members of this order are known in general as bugs. It is divided into two suborders *viz.* Heteroptera and Homoptera. The length of the members of this order vary from extremely small insect to 145mm in length. Several species are serious pests of agricultural crops. Some are useful predators of pests. A few are harmful to man and animals through their painful bites. About 80000 species are known form the world and out these about 6500 are reported from India (Varshney. 1998). The members of this order have sucking mouth-parts. They are widely distributed all over the world. The aquatic bugs play a prominent role in water pollution. Many bugs are useful insects such Lac insects.

**Neuroptera:** The Neuropterans are known as Nerve-winged insects. The other commonly known antlions, lacewings, snakefiles, alderflies and dobsonflies also belong to this order. The order contains two suborders *viz.* Megaloptera and Planipennia. Nearly all neuropterans are predaceous in both the immature and adult stages on sects. They are terrestrial or aquatic or semi-aquatic in habit. There are 5000 known species of Neuroptera in the world and 335 species are known from India (Ghosh, 1998). The benefical neuropteras are predatory on harmful insects.

**Coleoptera:** The coleopterans are known as beetles. It is the largest order of Insecta containing about 3,50,000 species in the world. From India 15500 species are reported. (Sengupta and Pal, 1998). Most species have their front pair of wings modified into a hard covering, called as elytra. The order is divided into 100 families. While some are useful predators of noxious insects, many others are serious pests of agricultural importance. The activities of dung beetles increases soil fertiity.

**Strepsipteas:** Members of this order are known as 'twisted winged insects' or 'twisted wing parasites' or 'stylopids' or 'stylops'. The length of these insects are 3 mm or shorter than 3 mm. They are endoparasites of many other insects of Diptera, Hymenoptera, Hemiptera, Orthoptera and Thysanura. They are cosmopolitan in distribution. Over 554 species of Strepsipteran are known from the world (Kathiarithamby, 1993). From India 18 species are known. These insects are found in all zoogeorgraphical regions (Choudhari, 1998).

**Mecoptera:** Mecopterans are commonly known as 'scorpionflies' since the posterior of abdomen of males of many species are raised upwards as in the case of scorpions. Most species are scavengers, feeding on dead insects and other organic debris. However the adults of a few species are predators. They are mostly in subtropical and temperate regions, but some genera like *Panorpa* and *Bittacus* have world wide distribution. Over 350 species are known from the world and out of these 15 species are known from India (Prasad, 1998).

**Trichoptera:** This order include the "caseworms" and "caddisflies". They look-like microlepidopteran moths. The development of immature stage take place in water. The immature stages of some species build portable cases with silk secreted by their modified salivary glands. Some other species make their cases using grains, bits of leaves, twigs, shells, debris etc. 7000 species are reported from various parts of the world and out of these 812 species are known from India (Ghosh, 1998). Caddisflies are beneficial insects since they form food for fishes.

**Lepidoptera:** This order include Butterflies and Moths. This include some of the most beautiful species of insects and some of the most serious pests of agricultural crops. Some species of moths of the genus

*Pionea* frequent eyes of man and other animals in India and adjacent countries. The caterpillars of many species produce irritant dermatitis. A recent estimate shows about 1,42,500 species of Lepidoptera occur in the world and out of these over 15,000 species occur in India.

**Diptera:** This order comprises the true 'flies'. The order includes both beneficial and harmful insects. They occur in every conceivable terrestrial and aquatic habitats in all continents. The dipterans can be easily separated from all other groups of insects on the basis of their wings. The dipterans have only a pair of well- developed forewings. The hind wings are reduced and known as halters which are balancing organs. Over a lakh species are reported from the world and out of these 6093 are known from India (Datta, 1998).

**Siphonaptera:** The members of this order are known as Fleas. They are small parasitic, blood-sucking, jumping insects with body flattened from side to side. They are external parasites of birds and mammals. A few act as vectors of diseases. *Xenopsylla cheopis* is the common Indian rat flea which is a vector of bubonic plague caused by *Bacillus pestis* in man. More than 1200 species are known from the world.

**Hymenoptera:** Hymenopterans do not have a common name. Wasps and saw flies belong here. This is the most beneficial order among all orders of Insecta since they help in pollination of plants and in keeping the population of several insect pests under check by parasitising on them. More than one lakh valid named species are known from the world and over 10,000 species are reported from India. Among the insect parasitoids used in biological control programmes all over the world, parasitic hymenoptera is found to be most successful. The hymenopterans are cosmopolitan in distribution, but more abundantly found in tropical and neotropical areas.

## Scope of Systematic Studies

According to a recent rough estimate, 20,717 species and 2500 genera of insects are endemic to India (Varshney, 1998). This is much below the actual number of endemic species and genera of insects existing in India. In order to understand the species diversity of insects it is absolutely essential to know their systematics. Sound systematics is absolutely essential for knowing the faunal diversity. Unfortuantely, though India is blessed with great diversity and variety of fauna and flora, very little efforts are made so far to study them taxonomically. This is primarily because of lack of sufficient knowledge on the part of the authorities of various funding agencies of the country regarding the scope of systematic research in India.

## Insects and the Living Environment

In the environment there is an interrelation between insects and all other living organisms. This interrrelationship can be resolved into two components. *viz.* 1. Interrelation with plants and 2. Interrelations with animals.

## 1. Interrelations with Plants

Insects depend on plant for their food, shelter and for various other activities. Insects do both good and evil to plants. They damage or destroy plants parts by chewing the foliage or other parts, by sucking the sap, by boring and tunneling inside stems, by mining the leaves, by causing galls, by using parts of plants for nest construction, by bringing other injurious insects such as coccids to plants, by spreading pathogens to plant (such as *Nilparvata lugens* the Brown plant Hopper of Paddy, acting as vectors of the mycoplasma disease "Grassy stunt' in Paddy and the rice jassid, Nephotettix *virecescens* causing the viral disease "tungro" in rice).

Some plants also cause destruction and damage to insects. Carnivorous plants have various mechanisms to trap and digest insects. There are active trappers such as *Dionaea* and passive trappers such as *Drosophyllum*. Fungi and bacteria cause diseases in insects. The fungi belonging to Entomophthoraceae, Ascomycetes, Eumycetes and *Phycomycetes* are common microorganisms which cause death and destruction of insects. The mycelial threads penetrate the body and the insects often become mummified and die. *Metarrhizium anisioliae* infects the sugarcane leafhopper *Pyrilla perpusilla* and *Oryctes rhinoceros* of Coconut. Fungi also attack preserved insects and destroy them. The bacteria *Bacillus thuringiensis* (commonly known as "BT) is an efficient biological control agent against various pests including mosquitoes. Thus it is seen that not only insects become enemies of plants but plants also become enemies of insects. Apart from these interrelations, there exists another phenomen viz. mutualism between plants and insects. Many plants depend on insects for pollination of their flowers and the insect inturn get nectar and honey as their food. The honey bee is a typical example. The fig trees depend upon their specific figwasp of the family Agaonidae of Chalcidoidea for pollination. A fig tree cannot exist without its specific pollinator agaonid. A very interesting mutualism exists between some species of ants and plants. These ants build their nests in the plants without destroying them, but at the same time protect them from other phytophagous pests. The Red tree *ant Oecophylla smaragdina* Fabr. build nests on Mango tree and Cashew tree and prevent many phytophagous insects from feeding these plants, Symbiosis occur between many insects and many microorganisms such as fungi, protozoa, bacteria etc. In this symbiosis, the metabolic products of these microoganisms are utilized by the insects and inturn the insect serve as a nutritive media for the symbiote.

## 2. Interrelations with Animals

The interrelations with animals can be resolved into two components *viz.* Intraspecific relations and interspecifi relations.

(a) *Intraspecific relations:* Crowding is commonly found by several groups of insects such as beetles, butterflies, dragonflies, aphids and other insects for feeding, hibernating and for various other activities. These intraspecific associations are normally in the interest of the species and a firm homeostasis exist in the ecosystem.

Parental care is another aspect of interspecific relations. Many insects show this phenomenon by caring their immature stages or brood nests. Solitary wasps like *Eumenes, Sceliphron* etc. construct mud nests for the development of their immature stages. The wood boring Ambrosia or timber beetles cultivate particular type of fungus inside the tunnels in wood for their larvae to feed. There are several other examples for parental care among insects. In several cases many insects brood over their eggs (e.g Scutellarids) or carry them (e.g. Belostomatids).

Brood parasitism is another interesting feature of interrelations of insects in the environment. Many species of insects make use of the brood nests of other solitary wasps of *Eumenes, Scelephron* etc. and lay eggs on the provision of these wasps and develop on them.

Many groups of insects show social life. Those insects which show social life are known as social insects. Termites, many species of bees and wasps are social in their behavior and development. There occurs division of labour among the various members of a colony.

(b) *Interspecific relations:* The main aspects coming under interspecific relations of insects in the environment are predatism, parasitism, insects as vectors of diseases and insects as food for other animals.

Many species of insects predate on other animals. Dragonflies, most carabids (ground beetles), tiger beetles, dyticid beetles, praying mantids, neepids etc. are predators on other insects. Insects which attack other insects are known as Entomophagous insects. The parasitic Hymenotpera contains parasitoids which kills their insect hosts. The parasitoid differs from parasite in having its host as usually of the same taxonomic class (in the case of parasite it may not be so), the adults of the parasitoids are free living (whereas the adults of the parasites are not usually free living), and in destroying the host by the development of immatures (whereas it may not destroy immediately in the case of parasite.)

Several species of insects of *Triatoma, Glossina,* several dipterans such as mosquitoes, tabanids etc. are blood sucking parasites of man and other animals in the environment. It is a well known fact that many species of insects are vectors of diseases of man and other animals. *Sipunculina funicola* (Diptera: Chloropidae) is a vector of conjunctivitis (Eye disease) in man in India. Some species of the blood sucking *Triatoma* are vectors of the Chagas disease (Trypanosomiasis) in South America. Similarly the Tsetse fly is a vector of sleeping sickness caused by Trypanosomes in Africa. There are innumerable other examples of insect vectors which spread diseases in man and other animals.

Symbiotic relationships between two groups of insects is also met with in the ecosystem. Myrmecophiles are those insects and other creatures which inhabit the nests of ants either as true guests, fed and tended by the ants or as scavengers. Similarly termitophiles are those insects and other creatures which inhabit in termitarium.

Many insects are inquilines which live in the home of other insects or of another animal and shares its food. Many species of Eurytomidae (Hymenoptera) are inquiliness of galls of Cynipidae (Hymenoptera). There are innumerable such species of inquilines in other families of Insecta.

## Interrelations with Non-living Environment

The natality, mortality, development and population fluctuations of insects are greatly influenced by several factors of non-living environment such as temperature, humidity, light, rainfall, microclimate, macroclimate etc.

*Temperature* has a profound influence on the survival and behaviour of insects. The optimum conditions for the survival and development of insects varies from species to species. While a few species can live at a relatively high temperature of $60^0$ C (some species of Praying mantids and a few desert insects), some others can live in very low temperature (*e.g.* Some collembolans, some beetles etc. live in snow mountains of Himalayas).

The activities of insects depend upon the external temperature of the environment. Respiration, circulation, digestion, reproduction, development and various other metabolic and behavioral activities are directly depended upon the external temperature. It is a known fact that with the rise of external temperature, the insects become more and more active until it reaches a critical point known as a 'vital temperature maximum' at which insect just lives and further rise of temperature results in the death of the insect. Similarly there is 'vital temperature minimum' which is the lowest temperature at which an insect can live, (though it may be inactive). The mating behavior of many uninuptial insects are found to be increased when they are artificially kept at low temperature for a critical period of time. (Narendran, 1975). The experiments conducted by the present author of this paper on a parasitic hymenopteran *Brachymeria lasus* (Walker) have clearly shown that female *Brachymeria* reduced her activities by a decrease in temperature but its readiness for copulation were found increased. Normally the female *B. lasus* is uninuptial, mating only once in life-time in natural conditions, while a male mates more than 4 or 5 times. In the experiments conducted by the present author, females of *Brachymeria lasus* which were subjected to low temperature of 0-5 for 30-60 seconds and then brought to normal room temperature of 20-26 C each female mated 5-9 times during a period of 5 to 15 days, when these experiments were repeated, each day on the same individuals.

*Light* has a major role in the life of insects. While many are diurnal, others are nocturnal in habit.

Experiments have shown that longer exposure to light (photoperiod) may induce non-sexual reproduction in many species of insects, and when photoperiods are shorter sexual reproduction occur. The photoperiod also has profound influence on the emergence rhythms in many species of insects. Apart from this, many other motor activities of insects such as feeding behaviour, mating and oviposition behaviour are also influenced by photoperiods. Photoperiod provide environmental information in the form of signals to which insects responds (*Nair et al 1983*). Low energy laser pulses of 0.6 joules 12 milliseconds cause burning superficially or to drying up injuriously, appendage extirpation, distortion etc. (Mani, 1982) in *Trialeurodes vaporariorum*. Reasearches have shown that immature stages of some species of butterflies when exposed to more than 16 hours per day, dark coloured forms resulted and when exposed to less than 12 hours light coloured forms appeared.

*Humidity:* The atmospheric humidity is very important in the life of insects. Some insects are adapted to highly humid and saturated atmosphere while others are adapted to any dry conditions in the atmosphere. When the moisture content of the wheat is below 9 percent the stored grain pest *Rhizopertha* did not oviposit and fecundity is found to be greater at a moisture content of 12 to 20 percent. Atmospheric humidity influence the fecundicity of migratory locusts. They did not lay eggs if the relative humidity in the atmosphere is less than 40 percent. At 76 and 52 percent relative humidity the number of progeny of *Callosobruchus chinensis* increased. Contrary to this the speed of development is found to be reduced in migratory locust at high atmospheric humidities (Nair et.al 1983).

## Environment and Insect Pest Outbreak

Organisms in nature commonly exhibit a stability in their space-time relationship. This stability exisitng between various populations of organisms is an ecosystem in known as "homeostasis" or balance of nature (Doutt and Debach 1964). Several biotic as well as abiotic factors interact with each other for this stability. When one or more of these factors are prevented by any reason, the equlibrium in nature upset and opportunities offer themselves for the abnormal increase in population of the insect species to become a pest.

Deforestation over wide areas affect several of weather conditions *viz.* temperature, diurnal variations, humidity, rainfall, wind velocity etc., in that locality and thus set conditions favourable for some insects to reproduce enormously and become pests. The insects which feed on trees and plants in the forest may be forced to migrate to nearly cultivated areas where they may become pests.

The natural enemies keep the population of several insects under check from reaching economic injury level. Indiscriminate use of pesticide destroy destroy these natural enemies and as a result both pest resurgence and secondary pest out break result.

By intensive and extensive cultivation of crops limitation of food gets nullifies and there is no competition for food. This affords conditions favourable for the increase in insect population.

New plants or trees introduced into a new area where it was not previously present may serve as new hosts for some insects species and this in turn may result in pest outdreaks. Improved agronomic practices such as application of synthetic chemical fertilizers may improve the growth of a plant but often predisposes the crop to insect attack. When an insect gets introduced into a favorable new area without its natural enemies it becomes more abundant. Accidental introduction of foreign pests into a country where it was not previously present may give chances for the introduced pest to become a major pest in the country of introduction in the absence of its natural enemies. There are innumerable examples for such outbreaks of pests.

The modern method of speedier transport have brought about wide dispersal of many insect pests.

## Climate and Insects

Insects become dormant under various climatic conditions. The nature of dormancy in insects depends upon the complexity of bichemical and physiological conditions. In most cases dormancy is the result of variations of atmospheric temperature. Dormancy can be classified mainly into Hibernation, Aestivation, Quiescence and Diapause.

*Hibernation* is known as the "Winter-sleep". During hibernation metabolism slows down and the temperature drops. In the absence of moisture, hibernation of most insects is prolonged. Similarly abundance of moisture may prevent hibernation in some insects. However artificial increase in temperature has not found very effective in preventing hibernation of several species in insects, but at the same time hibernation may be shortened by the artificial increase of temperature. The role of cold condition in winter along with presence of adequate moisture content of the atmosphere and normal required temperature are necessary for normal hibernation in insects. During hibernation insects survive by developing a resistance to freezing by lowering the temperature and at the same time developing a tolerance for survival. These two phenomena are known as 'Supercooling ' and 'Freezing tolerance' respectively (Pedigo, 1996)

*Aestivation:* During extreme summer of tropical climate, many insects un dergo aestivation or "Summer Sleep". It resembles hibernation having the metabolism very much slowed down. Feeding and other body movements are very much reduced or temporarily stopped during this period. This hibernation is an inherited phenomenon which cannot be broken within a single generation, some insects have both aestivation and hibernation in their life cycle and this is known as aestivo-hibernation. Larvae of species of *Delia* (Diptera) undergo aestivation during summer and go directly into hibernation in winter.

*Quiescence:* This is a condition where growth is retarded by the environmental conditions. Quiescence differs from other types of dormancy such as hibernation, aestivation etc. in resuming growth and reproduction immediately upon return of favourable conditions. Quiescence may occur at any stage of an insect due to short changes of environmental factors. Oligopause is an advanced type of quiescence which covers conditions between quiescemce and true diapause.

Diapause represent a type of dormancy for overcominmg long unfavourable environmental conditions. However diapause is not immediately referable to the unfavourable conditions of the enviornment and this differ from Quiescence which is directly referable to conditions of the environment (Nair *et al.* 1983). The onset of diapause occurs well before the change of environmental conditions and continues even when favourable environmental conditions prevail. The diapuse occurs at a specific stage in the life-cycle of an insect and this stage is genetically fixed. The influence of external factors on some vulnerable stage of development usually decides whether diapause shall occur or not in such species. Diapause in insects can be obligatory or facultative. Usually four phases are met with in diapause. They are; (1.) Preparatory phase; (2.) Induction phase; (3.) Refractory phase; and (4.) Termination phase (Mani, 1982). In the preparatory phase there is an accumulation of metabolic reserves. The induction phase is associated with the neurosecretory activities. In the refractory phase cessation of synthesis of DNA and RNA take place along with cessation of mitosis in all tissues except in the gonads and haemocytes. In the termination phase diapause ends but mere return of favorable environmental conditions does not terminate the diapause and termination seems to be related to biochemical changes in the diapausing insect.

Diapause in the larval and pupal stages of insects are controlled by the hormòne ecdysone which when become deficient results in the arrestation of moulting and growth. The diapause in adult insects is due to the stopping of production of juvenile hormone by the corpora allata preventing growth of eggs.

## Effect of Climate on Insects

The ecoclimate of an insect is the microclimate or the climate of the immediate environment surrounding the insect. In nature not only temperature, light, humidity, rainfall etc. individually affect the activities of insects but also climate as a whole affect them. In nature the abiotic factors affect the biotic factors profoundly and the combined action of abiotic and biotic factors affect the population of insect pests to fluctuate below economic injury level.

## Seasons and Insects

It is an interesting phenomenon that many species of insects show various morphological and behavioural variations in different seasons. The colour changes from winter to summer in many species. Insects with wide geographical distribution vary in size, colour and size from colder to warmer regions or *vice versa*. This is undoubtedly due to the changes in climate in different geographical areas.

In the climate of hot deserts, insects are usually active during night at the summer season. During day many orthopterans, beetles, digger wasps, some species of butterflies etc. can be seen resting above ground attached to desert plants. The cave dwelling insects have a different climate without much variations. The cavernicolous insects mainly depend upon fungi, cadavers and other organic matters carried by rivers etc. The absence of sunlight make the cavernicolous insects without deep body pigmentation.

The climate of high altitude above 3000 m is quite different from those of the low land. In high altitude insects, colour is more pronounced than in the ground forms. Body and wings are reduced. Body is hardened. Prolonged hibernation is also met with in high altitude insects. The darker colour or heavy melanism is due to the effect of extreme cold condition, high ultraviolet radiation etc. Heavy pigmentation protect the insects from the cold and ultraviolet radiation to some extent. The cold condition of high altitude also affect the flight activity in insects so that their wings are reduced or wanting. Thus flightlessness and reduced condition of wings are related to the cold condition of the high altitude. In the North-west Himalayas above 3000m and 4000m, several species of insects are flightless.

All aquatic insects are possessed with swimming appendages or other structures for locomotion in water. In some of the rivers of evergreen forest of Malabar area, the present author has observed once, a species of acridid swimming under the water using their legs and wings. There are several structural adaptaions among aquatic insects for locomotion, respiration etc.

## Effect of Insecticides on Environment

A WHO report shows that 25 million cases of occupational pesticide poisoning is reported every year among agricultural workers in the developing world. Another study shows, that , of the 204 samples of cereals, pulses, milk, eggs, meat and vegetable analysed, 108 were found to contain insecticides and several cases of insecticide residues above permissible limits were observed. Many of the insecticides such as malathion, endosulphan, BHC, DDT etc. which are banned in many developed countries are indiscriminately and profusely used in India.

Insecticides contaminate soil and water, they also cause residue problems in the soil. Heavy clay soils retain pesticides more than alkaline sols. Acidic soils retain pesticides more than alkaline soils. Insecticides affect soil fauna and birds which feed on the soil fauna such as earthworms. The insecticides also upset the natural balance of soil fauna. The organochlorine insecticides are most persistent insecticides. They may link up with the organic matter in the soil and thus persist longer in soils. Insectieides affect useful organisms such as nitrogen fixing bacteria.

Insecticides reach water in lakes, ponds, rivers, tanks etc. from deposit from aerial spraying, as surface run off from treated soils and plants and from disposals old unwashed insecticide containers. As a result fishes and other aquatic organisms are affected and this in turn affect man when he eats these fishes or other aquatic organisms. Insecticides also reach ground water. Large number of insecticides including organochlorines, organophosohates, etc. have been detected in ground water (Cohen 1986). Some of these chemicals are found to be potential carcinogens.

It is estimated that 55 percent of the applied pesticide may leave the treated area due to spray drift, volatilization, percolation, run-off and soil erosion. Some of this drift may move to adjacent areas and contaminate residences, water-bodies, other crops, forest tress and wild life (Perry *et al* 1998).

## Keystone Species and Cascade Effect

In an ecosystem there will be diversified species of organisms including insects. However not all species have the same influence in the ecosystem. Species which have disproportionately large influence on the structure of ecosystem are called keystone species and when keystone species are removed there is profound detrimental effect on the system and that is known as cascade effect. (Reid and Miler, 1989). Solbring (1991) divided keystone species of insects into three categories. They are (1.) Predators, parasitoids, herbivores and pathogens _ that contribute to the maintenance of diversity by reducing the abundance of dominant competition and thus prevent competitive exclusion. (2.) Mutualists (3.) Species that provide resources which are critical to the survival of dependent populations. Insect predators such as several species of ants play a major role in controlling the excessive increase of many insect pests and help to maintain a natural balance in nature. Removing such predators may cause the excessive increase of some phytophagous pests and this in turn will destroy the host plants and along with the destruction of such host plants several species of insects and other organisms associated with the host plants will be destroyed. Parasitic hymenoptera is an important group which contain many keystone species which will help to maintain the natural balance of organisms in nature. In the case of keystone mutualists, loss of one species may cause the loss of a second species. It is well known that certain plants or trees will lose the ability for fertilization without their specific pollinators. Examples are many species of bees and fig wasps. Keystone resource species are species which provide some resource critical to the survival of dependent populations. (LaSalle Gauld, 1993). Many species of ants operate as keystone resource species for many vertebrates. In addition to being a food item for some mammals like ant-eaters and birds, the army ants disturbs the arthropod fauna of the soil so that they get exposed and preyed upon by a variety of other species.

## Conservation of Diversity of Insects

Insects reproduce much faster than many higher organisms. As mentioned elsewhere in this chapter, a state of homeostasis' exists in nature and the population fluctuation of each species is always under a stable value which is known as "Equilibrium position". Disrupting this 'equilibrium' will end in the destruction of some species and excessive increase of some others. As a result extinction or depletion of some species result. In other words HABITAT destruction is the main cause for a species of insect to be rarer or extinct. This habitat destruction occurs in several ways. A few are the following:

- Loss and reduction of insect species will result from loss and reduction of plant species which are direct source of food or habitat. Species most valuble to localized loss are clearly those which are the most specialized with respect to their habitat requirements. Clearly loss of habitat diversity will result in a loss of alpha diversity (Gess and Gess, 1993) of organisms.

- Overgrazing and deforestation are two important factors for the loss of species diversity of insects in nature. Species composition of the vegetation also get seriously affected by these two factors.

● Field experience have repeatedly demonstrated that in the Nilambur forest reserve of South Malabar in Kerala (India) the South American weed *Chromolaena odorata* has become excessively abundant. This plant is unproductive of both phytophagous insects and flower visiting insects including many insect parasitoids. In areas where it has become a dominant plant, there will be a reduction of insect species consequently. As a result of such loss of insect species diversity including pollination species, there occur a reduction of seed fertilization resulting in further loss of plant species diversity.

● Crop farming may change natural habitat of many insect species. Ploughing, clearing of natural vegetation and replacement with a limited range of group of plants including exotic varieties, result in localized extermination of entire communities of several insects. Similarly stock farming, excessive trampling, water pollution by stocks, extensive removal of dry wood etc. will also result in the loss of diversity of several species of insects.

● Indiscriminate use of insecticides is a major factor for the loss of many species in nature. As a result many keystone species become endangered or threatened or on the verge of extinction. Although destruction of natural habitats of insects and other organisms occur in global level, tropical environments are the most affected. Further, most of the world's diversity of insects is tropical. Raven (1988) stated that tropical forests contain atleast two-thirds of the world's organisms. As many species show a high level of habitat speciality, they are not adaptable to change. Hence continued overexploitation and consequent destruction of natural ecosystems is expected to end in total loss, atleast of many endemic species. Many species of insects are on the road to extinction before their existence is known. Indiscriminate use of pesticides, deforestation, inundation of forest land by establishing hydel and irrigation reservoirs, conversion of forest land into manmade plantations of monoculture and other so called 'developmental' programs are all destroying the natural habitats of several species of insects resulting in the depletion of abundance of these species. Preserving merely national parks and reserves does not ensure that all habitat species survive (La Salle & Gauld, 1993). It has been estimated that a 90 percent reduction in habitat will mean a 50 percent loss in species. (Myers, 1983, Reid and Miller 1989).

Along with taking necessary steps to conserve the natural habitats, it is absolutely essential to undertake an inventory of the insect and other fauna of the concerned area. For this taxonomic experts are necessary to undertake detailed monographic or reversionary work along with the population studies of these species in the region. Unless this is done, it may not be possible to know which species of insect is endangered or threatened. Herein lies the importance of systematic or taxonomic studies. Since the alpha taxonomy of majority of Indian taxa is yet to be worked out, concerted efforts at intensive exploration of various ecosystems is the need of the hour (Cherian, 1998).

Hence in order to conserve the faunal diversity of insects the following steps would be taken by the appropriate authorities:

1. Authorities for granting funds for research, may set apart sufficient funds year marked for undertaking taxonomic research on insects. Students can be encouraged to take up taxonomic research for their doctoral and post doctoral researches by giving fellwships, grants etc.

2. Theory and practice of taxonomy should be incorporated in detail in the syllabi and curriculum of graduate and postgraduate courses of Biology, Agriculture etc.

3. *Insitu* and *Exsitu* conservation may be implemented and steps should be taken to prevent habitat destruction of insects.

4. Scientists and students of our country should not be prevented from collecting insects from parks,

and forest regions for taxonomic studies, since such collection will never affect the depetion of fauna. Only habitat destruction can affect the population of insects and not the collection work of taxonmists as some gnorant forest officials believe.

## SUMMARY

Insects constitute approximately three-fourth of the total number of organisms known. They are divided into 28 orders. The majority of insects present in the world remain undescribed and not yet discovered. Sound systematics is absolutely essential for knowing the faunal diversity.

Insects exhibit both interspecific and intraspecific relations among themselves and with other animals. The abiotic factors influence the natality, mortality, development and population fluctuations of insects. Organisms in nature commonly exhibit a stability in their space-time relationship. When this stability is disturbed, there emerges a set of conditions favourable for some insects to reproduce enormously and become pests. The natural enemies keep the population of several insects under check from reaching economic injury level. Indiscriminate use of pesticde may result in both pest resurgence and secondary pest outbreak. In nature climate have profound influence on insect life. They become dormant under various climate conditions, particularly due to the variations of atmospheric temperature. Some insects show various morphological and behavioural variations in different seasons.

Species with disproportionately large influence on the structure of ecosystem, the keystone species play a key role in maintaining ecological balance and their removal is extremely detrimental to the system and result in cascade effect.

Continued overexploitation and consequent destruction of natural ecosystems is expected to end in total loss, atleast of many endemic species. Along with taking necessary steps to conserve the natural habitats, it is absolutely essential to undertake an inventory of the insect and other fauna of the concerned area. Since the alpha taxonomy of majority of Indian taxa is yet to be worked out, concerted efforts at intensive exploration various ecosystems is the need of the hour.

Insects form approximately three-fourths of total number of organisms known. Only one -tenth of total estimated fauna of insects are described and the remaining fauna of insects are still unknown. The insects are classified into 28 orders, viz. Protura, Collembola, Diplura, Thysanura, Ephemeroptera, Odonata, Grylloblattoidea, Orthoptera, Dictyoptera, Thysanoptera, Hemiptera, Neuroptera, Coleoptera, Strepsiptera, Mecoptera, Trichoptera, Lepidoptera, Diptera, Siphonaptera and Hymenoptera.

In the environment there is an interrelation between insects and other living organisms. They are: Interrelation with plants and interrelation with animals. The former include insects as pests of crops, mutualism between plants and insects, symbiosis between insects and microorganisms such as fungi , bacteria etc. The interrelation with man and insects consists of intraspecific and interspecific relations. In the interspecific category, predation, parasitism, role as vectors of diseases, insects as food for other animals etc. are involved. Insects also have interrelations with non-living enviornment. Temperature, humidity, light, rain etc. all profoundly affect the lives of insects. Conservation of the natural habitat or environment of insects is the prime requisite for conservation of faunal diversity of insects. Habitat destruction is the main cause for the loss of diversity of insects. Taxonomic studies of insects should be given as high priority research in order to know what species are endangered or threatened among various species of insects.

# GLOSSARY

**Abiotic factors** : Density independent factors: Weather, climate, rain temperature etc.etc.

**Aestivation** : Summer dormancy

**Ancestral stock** : Primitive stem of ancestors

**Biological control (biocontrol)** : The employment of any biological agent for control of a pest.

**Biodiversity** : Biological density. it is the variety of world's organisms, including their genetic diversity and the assemblage they form

**Bioindicator** : An organism which indicates the changes in population, ecological conditions etc. by their presence of various levels according to those changes.

**Biotic factors** : Density dependent factor such as parasites, predators intraspecific competition etc.

**Cosmopolitan** : Belonging to all parts of the world, worldwide

**Dermatitis** : Inflammation of the skin

**Diapause** : A physiological state that occurs at one stage in the life cycle of an organism

**Diurnal** : Belonging to the daytime

**Ecoclimate** : Climate described from standard metereological observation

**Econimic injury level (EIL)** : The lowest number of insects that will cause economic damage

**Ecosystem** : An assemblage of interacting plant and animal communities and non-living environmental components

**Elytron (Pl: Elytra)** : A thickened front wing of insects, such as of beetles bugs etc.

**Endemic** : Prevalent or regularly found in an area or district or country

**Entomophagy** : Insect eating

**Equilibrium position** : Population fluctuation of an organism around a stable value

**Facultative** : Optional, incidental

**Fecundity** : Reproductive potential as produced by the quantity of gametes, particularly eggs produced.

**Gall** : An abnormal growth of plant tissue usually induced by the presence or activities of insects or mites

**Helminth** : a worm of Platyheminthes, nematode

**Hemocyte** : A cell of the hemolymph

**Hibernation** : Winter dormancy

**Homeostasis** : Balance of nature

**Herbivore** : Plant feeding organisms

**Inquiline** : An animal that lives in the nest or abode of another species (not usually harmful)

**Keystone species** : Species that have disproportionately large influence on the character or structure of an ecosystem are called keystone species

**Macroclimate** : A climate of a locality

**Melanism** : More than normal development of dark colouring matter.

**Microclimate** : The climate of the immediate surrounding of an organism, such as inside a burrow, inside soil nest, inside the nest of any organism etc.

**Mutualism** : Symbiosis, association benefiting bothe organisms involved

**Myrmecophily** : The utiliztion by other insects (myrmecophile ) mostly beetles, of ants colonies as a domicile and source of food.

**Nocturnal** : Belonging to night time

**Obilgatory** : Compulsory,binding

**Parasite** : An organism that lives in or on the body of another organism (host) during a portion of its life cycle.

**Parasiloid** : Wasps and flies, the larvae of which parasitise and usually kill individuals of he host species of the same class.

**Parasitic Hymenoptera** : A division of the order Hymenoptera of Insects, which are mostly parastitic on other insects (a few phytophagous ones are also included here).

**Pathogen** : A disease causing microorganism

**Photoperiod** : Day length

**Phytophagy** : Feeding pf plants

**Predator** : An organism that attacks and consumes more than one animal in its life time

**Quiescence** : Inactivity induced by unfavourable environmental conditions (which causes when conditions become normal)

**Supercooling** : Resistance to freezing of body fluids begins

**Symbiosis** : A close association between two or more different organisms that benefits one or both of the organisms.

**Systematics** : The study of diversity and classification of insects

**Termitarium** : A nest or mound of termites

**Termitophile** : Organisms living in the termitarium.

**Threatened species**: A species which are likely to become endangered in ints existence and consequently become extinct if not properly conserved.

**Uninuptial** : Organism which mates only once in its life time.

## ACKNOWLEDGEMENTS

I thank Dr. G. Tripathi, Dept. of Zoology, J.N.V. University Jodhpur for inviting me to contribute a chapter in this book. I acknowledge the authorities of the University of Calicut for facilities. The help rendered by my post-doctoral research student Mrs. Rajmohana for taking floppy and computer ready copy of this article is also hereby acknowledged.

## REFERENCES

- Chaudhuri, P.K. (1998). Faunal Diversity in India. Strepsiptera In: Faunal Diversity in India (Eds. Alfred J.R.B., Sen, A.K. and Sanyal A.K) EVVIS Centre. Zoological Survey of India, Calcutta 269-278.

- Cohen, D.B. (1986). Groundwater contamination by toxic substances ; a California assessment. (EDs. Garner, W.Y., Honeycutt, R.C. and Niqq, H.N) ACS Symposium on evalution of pesticides in groundwater. American Chemical Society, Washington D.C. pp 499-529.

- Datta, M. (1998). Faunal Diversity in India: Diptera In: Faunal Diversity in India (Eds. Alfred J.R.B., Sen, A.K. and Sanyal A.K.) ENVIS Centre. Zoological Survey of India, Calcutta 285-293.

- Doutt, R.L. and DeBach, P. (1964). Some biological Control Concepts and Questions. In Biological control of Insect Pests and Weeds (Ed. DeBach, P.) Chapman and Hall, New York, London 118-142.

- Gess, F.W. and Gess, S.K. (1993). Effects of Increasing land utiliztion on species. Representation and Diversity of Aculeate Wasps and Bees in the Semi-arid Areas of Southern Africa. In Hymenoptera and Biodiversity (Eds. La Salle, J and Gauld I.D) CAB International 1-348.

- Ghosh, S.K. (1998), Faunal Diversity in India: Neuroptera. In: Faunal Diversity in India (Eds. Alfred J.R.B., Sen, A.K. and Sanyal A.K.) ENVIS Centre, Zoological Survey of India, Calcutta pp. 251- 258.

- Ghosh, S.K. (1998). Faunal Diversity in India Trichoptera In: In Faunal Diversity in India (Eds. Alfred J.R,B., Sen, A.K. and Sanyal A.K.) ENVIS Centre, Zoological Survey of India, Cacutta pp. 319-323.

- Hazra, A.K. Biswas, M and Mitra, S.K. (1998) Faunal Diversity in India: Apterygota (Thysanura, Diplura, Protura, Collembola). In: Faunal Diversity in India (Eds. Alfred J.R,B., Sen, A.K. and Sanyal A.K.) ENVIS Centre. Zoological Survey of India, Calcutta pp. 160-177.

- Kathirthmby J. (1993). Description and biological noes of Halictophagidae (Strepsiptera) from Australia with a checklist of the world genera and species. *Invert. Taxon.*6 (1): 159-196.

- Kevan, D.K. McE (1982). Contribution on "Orthoptera and Phasmatoptera: In: Synopsis and classification of living organisms (Ed. Parker, S.P.) McGraw Hill New york *et al.* 2: 379-383.

- LaSalle, J and Gauld, I.D,. (1993). Hymenoptera: Their Diversity and Their Impact on the Diversity of other organisms. In: Hymenoptera and Biodiversity (Eds. La Salle, J. and Gauld, I.D.) CAB International. 1-348.

- Maiti, P.K. and Saha, N. (1998). Faunal Diveristy in India: Isoptera In: Faunal Diversity in India (Eds. alfred J.R.B., Sen, A.K. and Sanyal A.K.) ENVIS Centre, zoological Survey of India, Calcutta pp. 219-228.

- Mandal, S.K. (1998). Faunal Diversity in India: Blattariae. In: Faunal Dversity in India (Eds. alfred J.R.B., Das, A.K. and Sanyal A.K. ENVIS Centre, Zological Survey of India, Calcutta pp. 215-218.

- Mani M.S (1982) General Entomology Oxford & IBH publishing Co, New Delhi 1-912.

- Myers, N. (1983). Conservation of rain forests for Scientific research, fr wildlife conservation and for recreation and tourism. In Tropical Rain Forest Ecosystems, Structure and Function (Ed. Golley, F.B.) Elsevier, Amsterdam, 325-3345.

- Mitra, T.R. (1998). Faunal Diveristy In India: Embioptera In: Faunal Diversity in India (Eds. Alfred J.R.B., Sen, A.K. and Sanyal A.K) ENVIS Centre, Zoological Survey of India, Calcutta pp. 203-208.

- Narendran T.C. (1975). Studies on biology, morphology, host-parasite relationships of *Brachymeria lasus* (Walker) (Hymenoptera: Chalcididae) Ph.D. Thesis. Calicut University.

- Nair, K.K. Ananthakrishnan, T.N. and David, B.V. (1983) General and Applied Entomology.
Tata Mc Graw-Hill Publishing Company Ltd. New Delhi 1-587.

- Pedigo, L.P. (1996) Entomology and Pest Management. Prentice-Hall of India New Delhi 1-0646.

- Perry, A.S, Yammamato, I. Ishaaya, I and R. Perry (1998). Insecticides in Agriculture and Environment Retorspects and Prospects. Narosa Publishiung House. New Delhi (1-261).

- Prasad, M. (1998). Faunal Diversity in India: Mecoptera. In: Faunal Diversity in India (Eds). Alfred J.R.B., sen, A.K. and Sanyal A.K.) ENVIS Centre, Zoological Survey of India, Calcutta pp. 279-284.

- Raven, P.H. (1988). Our diminishing tropical forests. In Biodiversity (Eds. Wilson, E.O). National Academy Press Washington, D.C. 119-122.

- Ray, K.K. (1998). Faunal Diversitty in India: Psocoptera. In: Faunal Diversity in India (Eds. Alfred J.R.B., Sen, A.K. and Sanyal A.K) ENVIS Centre, Zoological Survey of India, Calcutta pp. 229-232.

- Reid, N.V and Miller, K.R. (1989). Keeping options alive: the Scientific Bases for conserving Biodiversity. World Research Institute. Washington D.C.

- Sen. S. (1998). Faunal Diveristy in India: Thysanaptera. In: Faunal Diversity in India (Eds Alfred J.R.B., Das, A.K. and Sanyal A.K.) ENVIS Centre, Zoological Survey of India, Calcutta pp. 243-250.

- Sengupta, T. and Pal, T.K. (1998). Faunal Diversity in India: Coleptera. In: Faunal Diversity in In·'ia (Eds. Alfred J,.R.B., Sen A.K. and Sanyal A.K.) ENVIS Centre, Zoological Survey of India, Calcutta pp. 259 268.

● Solbrig O.T. (1991). From Genes to Ecosystems: A Research Agenda for Biodiversity. International Union of Biological Sciences, Paris 1-123.

● Srivastava, G.K. (1998). Faunal Diversity in India: Dermaptera. In: Faunal Diversity in India (Eds. Alfred J.R.B., Sen A.K. and Sanyal A.K.) ENVIS Centre, Zoological Survey of India, Calcutta pp. 197-202.

● Steinmann, H. 1989. World Catalogue of Dermaptera, Series Entomologica 43: 1-934, Kluwer Academic Publishers. The Netherlands and Kiado, Budapestm Hungary.

● Varshney, R.K. (1998). Faunal Diversity: Insecta. In: Faunal Diversity in India (Eds. Alfred J.R.B., Das, A.K. and Sanyal A.K.) ENVIS Centre, Zoological Survey of India, Calcutta pp. 145-158.

# 9

# Ecological Distribution of Rodents in Desert Environment

*R. S. Tripathi, Mohd. Idris and B. D. Rana*

## The Indian Desert

The Indian desert extends between 21° 25' and 30° 30' NL and 67° and 75° 25'EL covering an area of about 2,85,680 km². Considering the geological history and archeological evidences, Krishnan (1952), Wadia (1960), Prakash (1963) and Roy and Pandey (1971) concluded that Indian desert has been created due to multiple factors and the desert conditions prevailed in this region for more than 10,000 years. The climatic conditions of the Thar desert is characterised by low and erratic rainfall, most of which occurring during monsoon season, *i.e.* from July-September. The average annual precipitation ranges from 80-500 mm. There is great fluctuation in seasonal temperatures also. The mean minimum temperature varies between 3. 4°C-10°C in winters and mean maximum temperature remains between 40.8°-42.8°C in summers. The highest maximum temperature has been recorded to be 50° C. Similarly mean annual relative humidity ranges between 26-66 per cent. Winds are also very strong *i.e.*, up to 140 km/hr. During most of the year, the wind direction is south-west to north -west. The Indian desert is an undulating vast plain of sand. In certain localities out-crops of hills and large gravel plains also form part of its topography.

## Faunistic Diversity among Rodents of the Desert

Rodents constitute one of the largest mammalian group in this region, exhibiting a great plasticity in respect to their choice of wide spectrum of desert habitats. Tripathi *et al.,* (1992) has enlisted 18 rodent species belonging to 11 genera and three families (Table 9.1), which inhabit this region. A brief account of these species is as under:

Family Sciuridae : This family is represented by one species of five striped squirrel, *Funambulus pennanti,* which occurs in orchards, gardens, forest nurseries and residential premises.

Family Hystricidae : The Indian crested porcupine ,*Hystrix indica* is the only hystricid occurring in the arid regions of the country. It inhabits the hilly out crops in the crevices or the tunnels made by them.

## Family Muridae

(a) *Sub family Gerbillinae* : Four species of gerbils occur in this region. Of them three are exclusively the denizens of arid areas. They are Indian desert gerbil, *Meriones hurrianae*; hairy footed gerbil, *Gerbillus gleadowi* and Wagner's gerbil, *Gerbillus dasyrus(=nanus)*. The fourth species, Indian gerbil, *Tatera indica* also inhabits the desert biome, besides its presence in other regions of the country as well. *M. hurrianae* is a diurnal rodent and others are nocturnal.

(b) *Sub family Murinae* : In all twelve species of this group are known from Indian desert. Amongst these, two are commensal in habit *viz.Rattus rattus* and *Mus musculus* which are widely distributed in residential premises of this region too. Three more species of *Mus i.e. M. cervicolor, M. platythrix* and *M. booduga* occur as wild forms in this region. In recent years *M. musculus* has been reported in the crop fields also in Punjab and Sri Ganganagar district of Rajasthan. *M. cervicolor* and *M. platythrix* inhabit the rocky habitats and *M. booduga* in crop fields. Another mouse *Vandeleuria oleracea* (a tree mouse) has also been reported from this region.

Besides the *Rattus rattus*, three more species of *Rattus* occur in north-western arid zones. They are the Cutch rock rat, *R. cutchicus cutchicus* (rocky habitat), the soft furred field rat *R. meltada pallidior* (in irrigated crop fields and grasslands), and the sand coloured field rat, *R. gleadowi* (in sandy plains). The monotypic *Golunda ellioti gujerati* (the bush rat) occurs near the crop fields and grasslands.

The lesser bandicoot rat, *Bandicota bengalensis* is also found in arid areas (except in the extreme arid districts of the desert), however, its population have been established in Bikaner town in recent years. The changes in landuse pattern in the western districts of Rajasthan due to incoming of Indira Gandhi Canal is helping the spread and establishment of this aggressive species in the canal command areas (Sri Ganganagar and Bikaner districts). Another mole rat, *Nesokia indica*, a north Indian species has also been reported to occur in the forest plantations of arid areas. In recent years it has been found to cause serious damage to the arid forestry plantations (Tripathi and Jain, 1990 and Jain *et al*, 1998).

**Table 9.1 : Rodent species of Indian Desert**

| | |
|---|---|
| (a) Family Hystricidae | Indian crested porcupine, *Hystrix indica* Kerr |
| (b) Family Sciuridae | Northern Palm squirrel, *Funambulus pennanti* Wroughton |
| (c) Family Muridae | |
|    (i) Sub-Family Gerbillinae | Indian gerbil, *Tatera indica indica* Hardwicke |
| | Desert gerbil, *Meriones hurrianae* Jerdon |
| | Wagner's gerbil, *Gerbillus nanus indus* Thomas |
| | Hairy-footed gerbil, *Gerbillus gleadowi* Murry |
|    (ii) Sub-Family Murinae | Tree mouse, *Vandeleuria oleracea* Bennett |
| | House rat, *Rattus rattus* Linn |
| | Cutch rock rat, *Rattus cutchicus cutchicus* Wroughton |
| | Soft-furred field rat, *Rattus meltada pallidior* Gray |
| | Sand coloured rat, *Rattus gleadowi* Gray |
| | House mouse, *Mus musculus* Linn |
| | Fawn coloured mouse, *Mus cervicolor* Hodgson |
| | Brown spiny mouse, *Mus platythrix* Bennett |
| | Field mouse, *Mus booduga* Gray |
| | Bush rat, *Golunda ellioti* Gray |
| | Short tailed mole rat, *Nesokia indica* Gray & Hardwicke |
| | Lesser bandicoot rat, *Bandicota bengalensis* Gray |

## Zoogeography

Among various rodents occurring in the Indian desert, only two species and fifteen sub species are endemic to this region. These rodents are either Palaeotropical or Oriental in origin. Prakash (1974) reported that the Indian desert is inhabited by rodents of Saharan and Oriental regions (Table 9.2 ) It is believed that with the onset of severe aridity, some species of Saharan and Iranian origin migrated to this region and certain Oriental rodents advanced from east to west in the desert. Species like, *G. ellioti* and *R. cutchicus* have intered in this region from Gujarat state. Prakash (1974) has traced following four major routes of intrusion of rodent fauna into the Great Indian Desert :

1. from Sahara to Indian desert and/or further.
2. from Iran to the Indian desert and/or further.
3. from Indo-China-Malayan region to Indian desert through north India.
4. from Indian Deccan through Gujarat border into Indian desert.

**Table 9.2 : Zoogeography of rodents of Indian desert (after Prakash, 1975)**

| Palaeotropical | Saharo Rajasthani | Irano Rajasthani | Irano oriental | Sindo Rajasthani | Oriental |
|---|---|---|---|---|---|
| H. indica | G.dasyurus (=nanus) | M. hurrianae | M. musculus | G. gleadowi | T. indica |
| R. rattus | N. indica indica | | | R. m. pallidior | R. r. rufescens |
| M. musculus | | | | G. ellioti gujerati | R. meltada |
| | | | | | M. b. booduga |
| | | | | | M. c. phillipsi |
| | | | | | M. platythrix |
| | | | | | G. ellioti |
| | | | | | B. bengalensis |

## Habitat Preference

From the point of view of rodent distribution, Prakash (1962-64) classified desert biome into four distinct habitats, such as sandy, gravel plains, rocky and ruderal habitats. The sandy habitat occupies the largest area and is interspersed with stabilised and unstabilised sand dunes. The gravel plains are usually situated on the foothills of hillocks, except in Jaisalmer region where extensive gravel plains occur. The rocky habitats are found all over the desert but cover comparatively larger areas in the north eastern part. The ruderal habitat (the village complex) is scattered almost in all parts of the desert depending upon the availability of drinking water.

Rainfed crops are mainly grown in the vicinity of villages while in some areas irrigated cropping is also being practised. Rodents are found in almost all these habitats. They are more abundant in the 100 mm rainfall zone in the western most sector of Rajasthan desert. The ruderal habitat is very well inhabited by rodents due to maximum availability of food, shelter and water under the influence of man and his livestock.

A great degree of habitat specificity has been noticed in the rodent species of the Indian desert. Prakash et al., (1971a), Prakash and Rana (1970, 1972, 1973), Prakash and Jain (1971) and Prakash (1975) have studied the habitat preference of rodents in Rajasthan desert. Some species occur exclusively in a particular habitat, such as G. *nanus indus* in sandy habitat, R. *cutchicus cutchicus* and M. *cervicolor* in rocky habitat and M. *musculus* and M. *booduga* in ruderal habitat.Other rodents inhabit more than one habitat, but based on their frequency of occurrence in large numbers in a certain habitat, these rodents may be assigned a particular niche (Table 9.3).

**Table 9.3 : Habitat preference exhibited by rodents in the Indian deserts**

| Sandy habitat | | Rocky habitat | Ruderal habitat | |
|---|---|---|---|---|
| Sand dunes | Sandy plains | | Residential areas | Crop fields |
| G. gleadowi | G. nanus indus | H. indica | F. pennanti | T. indica |
| | | | R. rattus | M. hurrianae |
| | M. hurrianae | R. cutchicus | M. musculus | R. meltada |
| | R. gleadowi | M. cervicolor | | M. booduga |
| | | M. platythrix | | G. ellioti |
| | | | | B. bengalensis |
| | | | | N. indica |

For example, M. *hurrianae* and F. *pennanti* may be assigned to have greater preference for sandy and ruderal habitats, respectively, though they occur in several other habitats also. Similarly, G. *gleadowi* and R. *gleadowi* prefer sandy habitat; T. *indica*, R. *meltada pallidior* and G. *ellioti* prefer ruderal habitat and M. *platythrix* prefer rocky habitat (Table 9.4). An overall analysis of the frequency of occurrence of 14 rodent species in different desert habitats revealed that 4 species share rocky and sandy habitats; 6 species share sandy and gravel habitats; 5 species share gravel and ruderal habitats; 4 species share rocky and ruderal habitats and 7 species share sandy and ruderal habitats together.

Table 9.4 : Percentage distribution of rodents in various habitats in the desert biome of Rajasthan ( Prakash *et al.*, 1971a)

| Rodent Species | Sandy | Gravelly | Rocky | Ruderal |
|---|---|---|---|---|
| F. pennanti | 14.2 | – | 35.8 | 50.0 |
| G. n. indus | 100.0 | – | – | – |
| G. gleadowi | 56.0 | – | – | 44.0 |
| T. i. indica | 28.8 | 10.0 | 3.6 | 57.6 |
| M. hurrianae | 60.0 | 17.0 | – | 23.0 |
| R. c. cutchicus | – | – | 100.0 | – |
| R. m. pallidior | 37.0 | 1.6 | 5.0 | 56.0 |
| R. gleadowi | 66.6 | 33.3 | – | – |
| M. musculus | – | – | – | 100.0 |
| N. b. booduga | – | – | – | 100.0 |
| M. cervicolor | – | – | – | 100.0 |
| M. c. phillipsi | – | – | 100.0 | – |
| M. p. sadhu | 28.0 | 13.3 | 53.3 | 13.3 |
| G. e. gujerati | 25.0 | 12.5 | – | 62.5 |

It may be concluded that *M. hurrianae* and *T. indica* are the most abundant rodent species followed by *R. meltada pallidior, R. cutchicus cutchicus and G.gleadowi.* Other rodent species are represented comparatively in lower numbers. Prakash *et al.* (1971a ) established following sequence of rodent abundance in different desert habitats :

1. In sandy habitat: *M. hurrianae>T.i. indica>G. gleadowi>R.m. pallidior.*
2. In gravel habitat : *M. hurrianae>T.i. indica>M.p. sadhu.*
3. In rocky habitat : *R.c. cutchicus>M.p. sadhu>M.c.phillipsi>F. pennanti.*
4. In ruderal habitat : *T.i. indica>R.m. pallidior>M. hurrianae>G. gleadowi>F. pennanti*

## Population Fluctuations

The seasonal fluctuations of rodent population in Indian desert have not been extensively investigated on a long-term, year to year basis, but some information on this aspect is available for the predominant rodent species (Prakash, 1975). The trapping data on *F. pennanti* indicated a gradual decrease of its population from April to October (Prakash and Kametkar, 1969). But in case of *T. indica* a broad pattern of monthly fluctuation was noticed by Jain (1970) with two minor peaks in the population, the first one during March-April and the other during August-September. The merion gerbil, *M. hurrianae* has been reported to show a population buildup during winters which continues till spring and then their number declines during summer (Prakash *et al.,* 1971b). The data on other rodent species did not record any particular trend but bimonthly collections revealed uniform catches for *R. m. pallidior* and maximum catch of *M. C. phillipsi* and *M. p. sadhu* in July and March respectively (Prakash and Rana, 1970).

In another study, monthly trapping data indicated that maximum number of rodents were trapped in the months of March (19.19%),August (13.07%) and December (20.04%). In case of merion gerbils, maximum catch was obtained in March (66.37%) and in December (81.56%). However, in case of *T. indica* a broad pattern of monthly fluctuation were noticed. It was generally noticed that the numbers are low during summers and tend to increase after rainy season, which is their peak breeding period.

Comparison of seasonal fluctuations of predominant species revealed that (i) their number is lowest during the hot summer months due to hostile living conditions in the desert, and (ii) the population builds up during spring and soon after the monsoon. These two population build up periods coincide with that of highest breeding activity among desert rodents (Prakash and Mathur, 1987).

## Food Habits

Rodents are generally herbivorous animals and prefer seeds but may feed upon insects and other animal food occasionally. At times they may even be cannibalistic. The palm squirrel, F. pennanti consumes fruits, insects larvae and bird eggs. Studies on stomach contents analysis of desert rodents indicated a clear cyclic pattern in their food habits. T. indica prefers seeds during winters and rhizomes and insects during summers, stems, leaves, flowers etc. are eaten all the year round. The desert gerbil, M. hurrianae chiefly thrives on seeds but during monsoon, it switches over to leaves and shoots of green vegetation and to insects and rhizomes during summers (Parveen, 1992). Our observations have revealed that both these gerbils prefer the plant species, particularly during monsoon, which are the major forage for the livestock. The occurrence of grass species like, Lasiurus sindicus, Cenchrus ciliaris, C. biflorus and C. setigerus and the tree species like Prosopis cineraria, Ziziphus nummularia and Capparis sp. in the stomach of gerbils evidently reflect a competition between these rodents and our livestock for resource utilisation.

## Activity Patterns

In Rajasthan desert, 70 per cent of rodents are nocturnal and are therefore, able to avoid the extreme heat of the day. Three species viz., M. hurrianae, F. pennanti and G. ellioti gujerati are essentially diurnal. Two commensal species, R. rattus and M. musculus are basically nocturnal but are active in day hours also (Table 9.5). The diurnal species have adjusted their diet activity in such a manner so as to escape from both extremes of summer and winter seasons. For example, the diurnal M. hurrianae changes its activity on bimodal patterns during summers and ventures out of its burrows in morning and evening hours only. However, in winters, it is active throughout the day except the very cool hours during mornings and evenings (Prakash,1981). Burrowing patterns of the desert rodents is also governed by the circadian rhythms of the species. The diurnals construct highly extensive burrows whereas, the night dwellers have simple burrows. Besides beating the harsh climatic vagaries, the extensive burrows of diurnal rodents provide added safety to the inhabitants from natural enemies.

### Table 9.5 : Activity pattern of desert rodents

| Diurnal | Nocturnal | Nocturnal but active during day time also |
|---|---|---|
| F. pennanti | H. indica | R. rattus and M. musculus |
| M. hurrianae | G. nanus indus | |
| G. ellioti gujerati | T. indica indica | |
| | R. cutchicus | |
| | R. meltada pallidior | |
| | R. gleadowi | |
| | M. booduga | |
| | M. cervicolor | |
| | M. platythrix | |
| | Nesokia indica | |
| | Bandicota bengalensis | |

## Breeding Season and Litter Size

Most of the rodent species, on which quantitative data about their reproduction biology is available, breed all the year round and their production potential, is very high. The desert rodents are able to regulate their breeding activity in consonance with the prevailing climatic conditions, food availability and social interactions. The peak number of xeric rodents breed during monsoon when the climatic conditions are most conducive and the availability of green food is high. The periodicity of littering bears a relationship with day length si..ce the littering activity start during late summers when the actual temperatures are high and the day length is maximum. Generally, rodents do not breed during extreme winter months when the day length is shortest or the prevalence of pregnancy is lowest. Moreover, the litter size of rodents is largest during monsoon, as in *T. indica indica* (Jain, 1970), *M. hurrianae* (Prakash, 1964 ) ,*F. pennanti* (Prakash, 1971), *R. meltada pallidior* (Rana and Prakash, 1984) and *R. cutchicus cutchicus* (Prakash *et al.*, 1973). Peak breeding season and litter size of some desert rodent species is detailed in Table 9.6.

**Table 9.6 : Peak breeding season and litter size of desert rodents (after Tripathi *et al.*, 1992)**

| Rodent species | Peak breeding season | Litter size |
| --- | --- | --- |
| H. indica | Monsoon and December | 1–3 |
| F. pennanti | (i) | March to |
| September | | |
| | (ii) | March-April and |
| July-September | 1–5 | |
| G. nanus | April, June and December | 2–3 |
| G. gleadowi | May, June and October to January | 2–5 (summer) |
| | | 5–6 (winter) |
| T. indica | February, July-August and November | 1–9 |
| M. hurrianae | (i) February to April | 1–9 |
| | (ii) July and September to November | 2–7 |
| R. cutchicus | March to May and July | 2–8 |
| R. gleadowi | August to October | 2–3 |
| G. ellioti | March-August | 5–10 |
| R. rattus | April-September | 1–9 |
| R. meltada | Spring and Monsoon | 3–9 |
| M. musculus | All the year round | 1–8 |
| M. booduga | September-October | |
| | February and June | 6–13 |
| M. cervicolor | July and December | 2–6 |
| N. indica | January-March and August-October | 2–6 |
| B. bengalensis | All the year round | 4–12 |

## Rodents' Association with Desert Cropping Systems

Field rodents, besides exhibiting affinity with soil types, also show preference for crops in different cropping systems of the arid zone. In the rain fed cropping systems, *M. hurrianae* and *T. indica indica* are the common species. The crop fields near sand dunes harbour populations of *G. gleadowi* also. These rodents start damaging the crops right from sowing stage and continue their destructive activities up to threshing stage.Their burrows are spread all through the crop fields. In the well irrigated cropping system fields, *T.indica* and *R. meltada* are the two most common inhabitants along with *M.hurrianae*. Since these crops receive frequent irrigation and other inter culture operations, the rodent population is mostly concentrated on the bunds. As soon as these operations are stopped before harvesting ,the rodents invade the whole field causing serious losses to the maturing crops. Among *Mus* species, *M.booduga* is generally encountered in the irrigated cropping systems. In the Indira Gandhi Canal command areas of Sri Ganganagar and Bikaner districts, the irrigated crop fields are infested with *R. meltada, T. indica, M. booduga, B. bengalensis* and *N. indica*. Since rodents are omnivorous, they may not show specific preference for any crop, however, a complex of 2-3 rodent species are found to have some association with certain crops in the desert agroecosystem (Table 9.7).

**Table 9.7 : Rodent pest species complex associated with crops**

| Important crops | Rodent pests complex |
|---|---|
| Pearl millet | M. hurrianae – T. indica |
| Sorghum, maize | T. indica – R. meltada – M. hurrianae |
| Wheat, barely | T. indica – R. meltada – M. hurrianae |
| Gram and mustard | N. indica – M. booduga – M. hurrianae |
| Groundnut | M. musculus – M. booduga – R. meltada – M. hurrianae – T. indica |
| Cotton | R. meltada – T. indica – M. booduga |
| Sesame | T. indica – M.hurrianae, – R. meltada |
| Moong and moth beans | M. hurrianae – T. indica |
| Vegetables | T. indica – R. meltada – Mus spp. – F. pennanti – H. indica |
| Orchards | F. pennanti – T. indica – N. indica – H.indica |

## Ecological Takeover

During the last 100-150 years the entire Indus Basin covering the states of Punjab, Haryana and northern Rajasthan have witnessed great ecological transformation with respect to soil, vegetation and land use patterns. These changes in Punjab, and northern Rajasthan (Sri Ganganagar district) started with channelisation of river waters. Major canal system in Sri Ganganagar district of Rajasthan are Gang canal (1927-28), Bhakhra canal (1951-52) and Indira Gandhi Canal (1956-57). Prior to irrigation system, desert represented a true dry deciduous scrub jungle where sands with undulating sand dunes were the characteristic topography of this area. The climate, soil and vegetation was similar to today's arid region of western Rajasthan. Low shrubs and thorny bushes of *Acacia jacquemontii* and *Capparis decidua* and trees like *Salvadora oleoides* and *Prosopis cineraria*, the floral indicator of sandy soil were very common. Among the herbs species like *Salsola foetida* and *S. fruiticosa* on saline soil and *Crotalaria burhia, Leptadenia pyrotechnica, Sericostema pauciflorum,Calligonum polygonoides, Aerva tomentosa* etc. on sandy soils were present in vast stretches (Parker, 1924 and Saxena, 1977). It is evident from earlier reports that the Indian desert is quite rich in rodent species due to Saharan and Iranian affinities of most of the species. Since river waters are being channelised in this desert on a large scale, the vast sandy stretch comprising of grasslands are being converted into crop lands. These changes in landuse pattern have threatened xeric rodent fauna to a greater extent. The phenomenon of ecological transformation of rodent communities can be well explained on existing scenario of Punjab, which is under irrigation agriculture since last 150 years and northern Rajasthan, which is under irrigation since more than 60 years. Sri Ganganagar district in northern Rajasthan forms the south eastern limits of the Indus basin. This represents a type of transitional zone for such transformation. Prakash *et al.*, (1971a ) indicated predominance of *T. indica* (44.7%), *R. meltada* (21.1%) and *M. hurrianae* (15.8%) and grouped them under the category of abundant species. *M. musculus* and *N. indica* with 7.9 percent occurrence each were referred as common and *F. pennanti* and *G. nanus* were not observed at all. Our recent studies in this district revealed that *M. hurrianae*, another xeric species has been further driven away from irrigated crop fields to more sandy and drier areas of the district where irrigation is hardly 30-35 years old. Rana and Soni (1985) and Rana *et al.*, (1992) have observed large populations of *M. musculus* in sugarcane and cotton fields in Sri Ganganagar. *N. indica* and *B. bengalensis*, true mesic species were found in irrigated croplands and fruit orchards. *R. meltada* has acquired the predominant status in the crop fields followed by *T. indica, Mus sp., B. bengalensis* and *N. indica*.

Within a short span of 60-65 years, the desert elements (*Gerbillus* and *Meriones*) found in the xeric environment have been replaced by mesic forms (*R. meltada, Bandicota* and *Nesokia*) in irrigated croplands of Sri Ganganagar district. Another xeric species, *T. indica* has so far been successful in adapting newer environments. Diversity of rodents represented by 12 murid and one scuirid fauna recorded from true desert biome in sandy and ruderal habitats by Prakash *et al.*, (1971a ) have been reduced to nine in the irrigated croplands of Sri Ganganagar district. Among this nine, many xeric elements do not figure but include three new mesic forms.

In phase II of Indira Gandhi Canal command area in parts of Bikaner and Jaisalmer districts where irrigation is very recent, species composition of rodents is still almost similar to those reported by Prakash *et al.* (1971a). Near the canal banks where large scale afforestation of *Eucalyptus.*, *Acacia, Dalbergia sisso* and *Tecomella undulata* has been taken up, the predominance of squirrel *F. pennanti* easily noticeable even in Bajju, Nachna and Mohangarh areas.

Thus, the desert elements like *Gerbillus* ,and *Meriones* are under constant threat from the mesic elements, like *R. meltada, Bandicota* and *Nesokia* due to transformation of sandy grasslands into irrigated croplands. Changes in their relative abundance *vis-a-vis* changed land use pattern clearly indicate that faunal diversity of rodents would decrease. The species which vanish early are *G. nanus, G. gleadowi* and *M. hurrianae*.

## SUMMARY

Ecological distribution of rodents in the Indian desert presents a great faunistic diversity. However, various human interventions are creating an ecological stress for native xeric rodents, which may threaten their survival in coming years. Regular irrigation by flooding may ultimately perish the true desert elements, especially the members of subfamily "gerbillinae". Moreover, intrusion of new mesic species like *Bandicota bengalensis* may pose serious public health problems, besides causing callosal losses to the irrigated crops. The bandicoots are considered to be highly susceptible to several diseases. Serious research efforts are must for striking a balance between natural resources and human survival by evolving methods for conserving the native rodent fauna. In addition to this, the rodent control operations must be inducted as one of the regular and essential package of practice for irrigated crops, to contain the menace of pest rodents.

## REFERENCES

- Jain A.P. 1970. Body weights, sex ratio, age structure and some aspects of reproduction in the Indian gerbil, *Tatera indica indica* Hardwicke in Rajasthan desert. *Mammalia*, **34**: 415-432.
- Krishanan, M.S. 1952. Geological History of Rajasthan and its relation to present day conditions. Proc. Symp. Rajputana Desert. *Bull. Natl. Instt. Sci. India*, **1**: 19-31.
- Parveen, F. 1992. Food of the Antelope rat, *Tatera indica indica* Hardwicke. Chapt. In. *Rodents in Indian Agriculture* (Eds. Prakash, I. and Ghosh, P.K.) Scientific Publishers, Jodhpur, pp.427-431.
- Prakash, I. 1962. Ecology of gerbils of the Rajasthan desert, India. *Mammalia*, **26**: 311-331.
- Prakash, I. 1962-64. Taxonomical and ecological account of the mammals of Rajasthan desert. *Ann. Arid Zone.* **1**: 143-163, 2(2): 150-161.
- Prakash, I. 1963. Zoogeography and evoluation of the mammalian fauna of Rajasthan desert, India. *Mammalia*, **27**: 342-351.
- Prakash, I. 1964. Ecotoxicology and control of the Indian desert gerbil, *Meriones hurrianae* (Jerdon). Pt. II. Breeding season, Litter size and postnatal development. *J. Bombay Nat. Hist. Soc.*, **61**: 142-149.
- Prakash, I. 1971. Breeding season and litter size of Indian desert rodents. *Zeitsch. Zool.*, 58 : 441-454.
- Prakash, I. 1974. The ecology of vertebrates of the Indian desert. In *Biogeography and Ecology in India.* (Ed.Mani, M.S.). The Hague, Junk, pp. 369-420.

Prakash, I. 1975. The population ecology of the rodents of the Rajasthan desert, India. In *Rodent in Desert Environments* (Eds. Prakash, I. and Ghosh, P.K.). Dr. W. Junk B.V. Publishers, The Hague, pp. 75-176.

Prakash, I. 1981. Ecology of Indian desert gerbil, *Meriones hurrianae*. CAZRI, Monograph No. 10, 1-86 pp.

Prakash, I., Gupta, R.K., Jain, A.P., Rana, B.D. and Dutta, B.K. 1971a. Ecological evaluation of rodent population in the desert biome of Rajasthan. *Mammalia,* **35**: 384-423.

Prakash, I. and Jain, A.P. 1971. Some observations on the Wagner's gerbil, *Gerbillus nanus indus* Thomas in the Indian desert. *Mammalia,* **35**: 614-628.

Prakash, I. and Kametkar, L.R. 1969. Body weight, sex and age factor in population of the Northern Palm squirrel, *Funambulus pennanti* Wroughton. *J. Bombay Nat. Hist. Soc.,* **66**: 99-115.

Prakash, I. and Mathur, R.P. 1987. *Management of Rodent Pests.* (ICAR, New Delhi ). Pp. 1-133.

Prakash, I. and Rana, B.D. 1970. A study of field population of rodents in the Indian desert. *Zeit. Angew. Zool.* 57: 129-136.

Prakash, I. and Rana, B.D. 1972. A study of field population of rodents in the Indian desert. II. Rocky and piedmont zones. *Zeit. Angew. Zool.* **59**: 129-136.

Prakash, I. and Rana, B.D. 1973. A study of field population of rodents in the Indian desert. III. Sand dunes in 100mm. rainfall zones. *Zeit Angew. Zool.,* **60**: 31- 41.

Prakash, I. Rana, B.D. and Jain, A.P. 1973. Reproduction in the cutch rock rat, *Rattus cutchicus cutchicus* in the Indian desert. *Mammalia,* **33**: 102-117.

Prakash, I. Taneja, G.C. and Purohit , K.G. 1971b. Ecotoxicology and control of Indian desert gerbil, *Meriones hurrianae* Jerdon. VII. Relative number in relation to ecological factors. *J. Bombay Nat. Hist. Soc.,* **68**: 86-93.

Rana, B.D., Jain, A.P. and Soni, B.K. 1992. Bait preference. In *Rodents in Indian Agriculture.* (Eds. Prakash, I. and Ghosh, P.K. ). Scientific publishers, Jodhpur. pp. 419- 425.

Rana, B.D. and Prakash , I. 1984. Reproduction biology of the soft furred field rat, *Rattus meltada pallidior* (Ryley, 1914 ) in Rajasthan desert. *J. Bombay Nat. Hist. Soc.,* **81**: 59-70.

Rana, B.D. and Soni, B.K. 1985. Infestation of *Mus musculus* and *Suncus murinus* in the cultivation of Sri Ganganagar district, Rajasthan. *Zeit. Angew. Zool.* **4**: 497-501.

Rana, B.D., Tripathi, R.S. and Soni, B.K. 1992. Effect of irrigation agriculture to the desert rodents. *Mammalia.* **56**: 231-235.

Roy, B.B. and Pandey, S. 1971. Expansion or contraction of the great Indian desert. *Proc. Indian Natl. Sci. Acad.,* **36**: 331-344.

Saxena, S.K. 1977. Vegetation and its successons in the Indian desert.In *Desertification and its control.* Indian Council of Agricultural Research, New Delhi.160-175.

Tripathi, R.S. and Jain, A.P. 1990. Rodent damage to desert afforestation plantation. *Rodent Newsletter,* **14**: 7-9.

Tripathi, R.S., Jain, A.P., Kashyap, N., Rana, B.D. and Prakash, I. 1992. North western desert. In *Rodents in Indian Agriculture.* (Eds. Prakash,I. and Ghosh, P.K.). Scientific publishers, Jodhpur.pp. 357-375.

Wadia, D.N. The post glacial dessiccation of the Central Asia, Monograph 10. Natl. Instt. Science India. pp. 1-25.

# 10

# Pesticides

*M. Venkateshwarlu*

"Pesticides are chemicals or agents used to destroy any organism that is considered as pest". Almost any living creature can be a pest under certain circumstances. Pesticides have been used to a limited degree since ancient times. The Ebers papyrs, written about 1550 B.C, preparations to expel fleas from the house. There are records showing that by 900 A.D. the Chinese were using arsenic sulfides to control garden insects. *Veratrum album* and *V.nigrum,* two species of false hellebore were used by the Romans as rodenticides (Shepard, 1939). In 1669, the earliest known record of arsenic as an insecticide in the Western world mentioned its use with honey as an ant bait. Use of Tobacco as contact insecticide for plant lice was mentioned later in same century. Copper compounds were known since 1807 to have fungicidal value, and the Bordeaux mixture (hydrated lime and copper sulfate) was first used in France in 1883. Hydrocyanic acid, known to the Egyptians and the Romans as a poison, was used as a fumigant in 1877 to kill museum pests in insect collections (Shepard, 1939).

Until the mid 1930's, pesticides were mainly of natural origin or inorganic compounds. Earlier to that, around 1850, a fumigant property of Sulfur was recognized. Nicotine has been widely utilized as an insecticide all over the world, as has been rotenone, used as a fish poison in South America since 1725. Mercury Chloride was extensively used as fungicide since 1891, and slowly replaced by its organic forms such as phenyl mercury (1915), alkyloxyalkylmercury (1920's) and alkylmercury (1940's). Development of organochlorine insecticide took place during 1940-1950, in 1944 synthesis of *Parathion* by G.Schrader and during 1950's development of carbamates started. During 1970's development of modern *Pyrethroids* took place. Now it is the hormone analoges widely used in insect pest control.

The first synthetic organic insecticides that appeared for public use were probably the dinitro compounds and the thiooxynates in the early 1930's. Beginning in those years, significant discoveries occurred, which led to the proliferation of new synthetic pesticides including D.D.T., organophosphates and pyrethroids. The period between 1935 and 1950 was characterized by the development of D.D.T. and other chlorinated hydrocarbon insecticides. Paul Muller (1939) found that dichloro diphenyl trichloroethane (DDT) acted as a contact poison on fleas, mosquitoes and other insects. During World War II, the practical value of DDT was demonstrated when, with the aid of it, a severe epidemic of typhus in Naples was successfully controlled. This disease is transmitted by body lice, and after powdering 1.3 million people inside their clothing with DDT, the epidemic came under control. Afterwards, one of the most successful uses of DDT has been in the malaria eradication programs. But in 1962 Rachel Carson published the book *Silent Spring* in that he mentioned about the bioaccumulation of DDT and its effects on bird reproduction and on the environment. Manufacture and sale of DDT was banned in Sweden in 1970 and in the U.S.A in 1973.

Pesticides are used to increase the production of food and fiber and to promote public health. Among the pests attacking agricultural crops are insects, fungi, rodents, birds and weeds, loosely defined as any undesired plants, and also agricultural pests. The amount of manual labor necessary to control weeds without help from herbicides or machines may be difficult. So pesticides are useful in such cases.

## Origin of Pesticides

Origin of pesticides is very important aspect while studying the pesticides. On the basis of their origin the pesticides have been divided into two categories.

1.  Plant origin pesticides
2.  Chemical pesticides

# 1. Plant Origin Pesticides

These are extracted from plant parts such as flowers, roots, stems, leaves and seeds, toxicity of many of the plant derivatives used as insecticides depend on the alkaloids that they contain. Two insecticides, viz., *Nicotine* and *Pyrethrum* extracted from the plants of *tobacco*, and *pyrethrum* respectively are commonly used. A third insecticide known as *Rotenone*, manufactured from the roots of *Derris* plant is not common although it is an important insecticide.

a) **Nicotine:** Nicotine is volatile alkaloide obtained by treating byproducts of the tobacco-processing industry, *i.e.*, stems and damaged leaves, with an aqueous extract of alkali, followed by steam distillations. It has been successfully used in the control of sucking insects, *viz.* aphids, thrips, psyllids, leaf miners and jassids. Nicotine is compatible with many of the common insecticides and fungicides, including sulfur, lime-sulfur and copper preparations.

The concentrated solution of *Nicotine* is poisonous to mammals and therefore every care should be taken while preparing the spray solution.

b) **Pyrethrum:** Certain species of *Chrysanthemum* (family -Compositae) possess insect repellants. *Pyrethrins* are present in flowers, which are gathered when the disc florets are fully open. The concentration of pyrethrins in the flowers varies according to the source. For commercial extraction, the flowers are dried, ground to powder, and extracted with kerosene, petroleum - ether, ethylenedichloride, glacial acetic acid acetone or methyl alcohol. The active components of the flower bead are pyrethrin I, Pyrethrin II, cinerin I and cinerin II. The relative proportions of them are dependent on the strains, condition of cultivation, and processing methods.

Pyrethrum insecticides are generally used for the control of household pests such as mosquitoes, cockroaches, flies, bed-bugs and silver-fish, as dust or spray. For the control of various vegetable crop and cattle pests is used as spray.

c) **Rotenone ($C_{23}H_{22}O_6$):** Certain plants belonging to the family *Leguminosae* used as fish poison, contain insecticidal principles collectively designated as rotenoids. The commercial sources of rotenoids are *Derris*, *Lonchocarpus*, *Tephrosia*, and *Millettia*, the first two being important. Rotenone is prepared on a commercial scale from the roots of 2 years old Derris plants by extraction with chloroform or carbon tetrachloride. Rotenone ($C_{23}H_{22}O_6$) is soluble in most organic solvents, sparingly soluble in hydrocarbon oils, and insoluble in water. *Rotenone* is used for the control of *aphids, thrips, flea, beetles, caterpillars,* etc. on vegetable crops. The action of *Rotenone* is slower than that of *pyrithrin*. It decomposes when exposed to light and air, therefore has comparatively a limited residual effect.

d) **Ryania:** Ryania is the name of insecticide extracted from plants of Ryania species. It is extracted from roots and stems. In foreign countries, Ryania is being used against borers of corn and sugarcane. It is also used to control some of the crop pests less toxic to mammals than rotenone. Moreover some of the plant origin products like Neem oil, turmeric etc are used as pesticides.

# 2. Chemical Pesticides

(a) **Organic pesticides:** These pesticides are organic compounds. Hence these are also called as organic pesticides. The phenomenal increase in synthetic organic compounds as insecticides since the second world war has revolutionized this industry.

i. Chlorinated hydrocarbons or organochlorines
ii. Organophosphates
iii. Carbamates
iv. Synthetic pyrethroids

**(b) Inorganic pesticides:** Before the introduction of modern insecticides like D.D.T. B.H.C. parathion etc, the inorganic insecticides as well as those of plant origin were mainly used for plant protection. Their use now is greatly restricted, and that too only for the control of some specific pests. The generally used inorganic insecticides at present are lead arsentate, calcium arsenate, parisgreen and sodium fluro-silicate. The first three are mainly used for the control of some vegetable pests, and the last for grasshoppers.

1. *Calcium Arsenates:* Its principal uses are for the potato beetle and as a sulfur - combined dust against cotton insects.

2. *Lead Arsenates:* Lead arsenate is widely used, chiefly for the potato beetle and for the codling moth in apple orchards. Lead arsenate commonly used as an insecticide is an acid lead arsenate $(PbHASO_4)$. Many other lead arsenates, $Pb_2As_2O_7$ etc. are known. Calcium arsenate is also used for control of leaf feeding insects.

3. *Mercurous Compounds:* Both mercurous and mercuric chlorides are effective fungicides. The mercuric compound are still extensively used for fungicidal treatment.

4. *Paris Green:* Paris green is coarse powder having green colour, containing as on of the active ingredients. It acts as a stomach poison. Paris green is usually applied in the form of dust or spray. It is used for leaf-eating and surface-feeding insects. One per cent dust is used for spraying against mosquito larvae.

5. *Sulfur and its Compounds:* One of the most important inorganic pesticides is sulfur with its various compounds. In the finely ground condition in the form of colloidal preparations it is widely used to control plant feeding mites and powdery mildew fungi.

   For the control of plant feeding mites and as fumigant use is made of calcium polysulphide, which is known as lime sulfur. The dosage of lime sulfur with a density of $1.16 gms/cm^3$ or 13 to 150 litres per hectare is required.

6. *Compounds of copper:* Copper sulphate is applied as a fungicide to growing plants in the form of so called Bordeaux mixture. This mixture is produced by precipitation of basic copper sulphate with lime from a one percent solution of copper sulphate.

7. *Halogen Compounds:* Salts of the hydrohalogen acids such as sodium chloride, for example, have fungicidal and bactericidal effects, but at relatively high concentrations.

8. *Compounds of Phosphorous:* Two compounds of phosphorous have found practical use as pesticides zinc phosphide and aluminium phosphide. Zinc phosphide is used in baits to control mouse species and other rodents, and aluminium phosphide is used to control stored product pests.

## Classification of Pesticides

Pesticides are classified on the basis of their, target organism, mode of entry, mode of action, type of application and class of chemical

## 1. On the basis of their target organism

With respect to what they are used to control, pesticides are divided into following groups:

(a) *Acaricides*   – used to control mites
(b) *Algicides*   – used to destroy algae
(c) *Bacteriocides* – used to control bacterial growth
(d) *Fungicides*   – used to control fungal growth
(e) *Herbicides*   – used to control weeds.
(f) *Insecticides* – used to control harmful insects.
(g) *Molluscicides* – used to control molluscus (snails etc)

*(h)* *Nematicides* − used to control nematodes

*(i)* *Rodenticides* − used to control rodents. (rat, mice etc)

## 2. On the basis of mode of entry

   a. Stomach poisons

   b. Contact poisons

   c. Fumigants

   a. **Stomach poisons:** The pesticides which are most effective on the digestive system of the insect pest and bring about their death are called stomach poisons.

   b. **Contact poison:** The death of the pest species is brought about by means of contact and getting absorbed on the surface of the cuticle of the body.

   c. **Fumigants:** The toxicant which in its gaseous state, penetrates through the tracheal system and kills the pest species.

## 3. On the basis of mode of their action

   *a.* *Attractants* - Substances whose odour and taste attract insects and animals.

   *b.* *Repellents* - Gaseous substance, whose odour and taste detect and repel the insect vectors.

   *c.* *Defoliants* - Substance used to remove the leaves from the plant

   *d.* *Neurotoxic substance* - Affects the function of membrane permeability of neuron.

   *e.* *Cell toxicant* - Inhibit the cell metabolism.

   *f.* *Hormones* - Substances with a very high biological activity that are secreted into the internal medium of an organism and control its most important developmental function. (in insect, their metamorphosis).

   *g.* *Chemosterilants* - Sterilize the male vector insect or pest.

   *h.* *Systemic effect* - Very dangerous than other chemicals. First absorbed by the crop then it translocates mostly upwards into the stem, leaves etc.

   *i.* *Disinfectants* - Destroy or inactivate the harmful organisms.

## 4. On the basis of application and formulation

Formulation is the processing of a pesticidal compound by any method that will improve its properties of storage, handling, application, effectiveness or safety. The formulation is the final physical condition in which the pesticide is sold for use. Pesticides are sold in more than 35,000 formulations. Common formulations are as follows:

   *a.* *Sprays:* Pesticides have been applied as water sprays, oil sprays. Spray formaulations are prepared for insecticides, herbicides, fungicides, algicides, defoliants etc. More than 75 per cent of all pesticides are applied as sprayers. These are currently applied as water emulsions made from emulsifiable concentrates.

   *b.* *.Dusts:* These are undiluted toxic agents. Historically dusts have been the simplest formulation of pesticides to manufacture and easy to apply. Sulfur dust which is used on ornamentals and one of the older household roach dusts, sodium fluoride. In agriculture an aerial application of a standard dust formulation of pesticide will result in 10 per cent to 40 per cent of the material reaching the crop.

   *c.* *Aerosols:* To produce an aerosol the active ingredients must be soluble in the volatile petroleum solvent in its pressurized condition. The pressure is provided by propellant gas. Aerosols commonly produce droplets well below 10 mm in diameter. Aerosols are used for indoor application, like home deodorizers, shaving creams, furniture polish, window sprays etc.

d. *Granular:* The granular pesticides are small pellets formed from various inert clays and sprayed with a solution of the toxicant to give the desired content. After the solvent is evaporated, the granules are packed for use. Only insecticides and few herbicides are formulated as granules.

e. *Fumigants:* Fumigants are a rather loosely defined group of chemical substances. It can reach each and every part of the target. Moth crystals and moth balls paradichlorobenzene and naphthalene, respectively and crystalline solids that evaporate slowly at room temperature, exerting both a repellent as well as an insecticidal effect. Soil fumigants are used in horticulture greenhouse, and high value croplands to control nematodes, insect larvae and adults.

f. *Baits:* Baits can be formulated at home. These contain low-level of toxicants, incorporated into materials that are relished by the target pests.

g. *Coating:* These are used for seed treatment.

h. *Slow release insecticides:* Slow release insecticides are relatively new and only a few are available. The most recent slow release formulation appeared in 1979, a microencapsulated concentrate of diazinon for use in agriculture and for household pests. The principle of this form of slow release involves the incorporation of the insecticide in permeable covering, microcapsules or tiny sphere. They release at a reduced but effective rate. (varnishes, paints etc).

## 5. On the basis of chemical group of pesticide

Depending on the chemical group present in the pesticide they are divided into Organocohlorines, Organophosphates, Carbamates, Synthetic pyrethroids, Dinitrophenols and Botanicals.

a. *Organochlorines:* The organochlorine insecticides include the chlorinated ethane derivatives, of which DDT is the best known example. The cyclodienes, which include chlorodane, aldrin, dieldrin, hepatachlor, endrin and toxaphene and the hexachlorocyclohexanes, such as lindane. From the mid 1940s to the mid 1960s the organochlorine insecticides enjoyed wide application in agriculture, soil in insect control and in malaria control programmes. However they have as a class come into disfavor because they are very persistent in the environment and tend to accumulate in biologic as well as nonbiologic media.

b. *(i). DDT (Dichloro Diphenyl Trichloroethane)*
DDT has been best known, the cheapest and probably one of the most effective of the synthetic insecticides. It was synthesized as early as 1874 but its insecticidal effectiveness was not discovered until 1939, and it was patented for this use in 1942. DDT used extensively during world war II to control lice and other insects by dusting directly to humans and materials.

Structural Formula

DDT is available as dusting powder, water dispersible powder and emulsifiable concentrate. DDT acts both as a contact and stomach insecticide. It is white or dirty white in colour and is mainly used in the strength of one to five per cent. It is applied usually at the rate of 20 pounds per acre on a variety of crop pests namely swarming caterpillar, army worm, rice case worm, paddy gassids, cut worms, potato beetle, cotton leaf roller etc. DDT is known for its long residual toxicity and therefore, the dust formulations are commonly used soil application for controlling soil pests, especially white grubs, cutworms and weevils.

Cuccurbitacae crops such as cucumbers and melons are sensitive to stronger doses of DDT. Therefore, use on these crops may be avoided as far as possible. DDT is injurious to fishes and should not be allowed to contaminate ponds and streams. Crops for human consumption should not be harvested during the fortnight following dusting or spraying with DDT. To prevent the damage to bees this insecticide should not be used on crops during the flowering season.

DDT preparations are safe to handle in lower concentrations but care should be taken that any food material is not contaminated because DDT when swallowed tends to accumulate in the tissue and may prove harmful. Recomended limit of DDT in drinking water is 1 mg/lt.

Both field and laboratory studies have proved that reproductive success in certain species of wild birds is adversely affected by exposure to DDT or its metabolites. Additionally fish and some ldower aquatic organisms are extremely sensitive to the acute toxicity of DDT.

## Signs and Symptoms of Acute and Sub acute Poisoning

Signs and symptoms of poisoning in human and animals resulting from high doses of DDT include paresthesia of the tongue, lips and face, apprehension, irritability, dizziness, disturbed equilibrium, tremor and toxic and clonic convulsions. Symptoms appear several hours after large doses, and in animals poisoned with fatal doses death occurs in 24 to 72 hours. It has been estimated that doses of 10 mg/kg body weight will cause signs of poisoning in humans. Although the functional injury produced by high doses of DDT is referable to effects in the central nervous system. Smaller doses results in liver enlargement which in rodents is somewhat characteristic in that the cells and mitochondria themselves are enlarged.

**Distribution and storage:** DDT and one of its major metabolic derivatives DDE have high fat, water partition coefficients and therefore, tend to accumulate in adipose tissue. During the years of its most extensive use in the late 1950s, and early 1960s the average storage of DDT in fat was about 5 ppm. Total storage of DDT derived from material was about 15 ppm, this consisted primarily of DDT and its lipophilic metabolite, DDE. With declining use of DDT, there appears to have been a reduction in these levels so that the average adipose tissue level for humans in the late 1960's was 1 to 2 ppm of DDT and a total of about 9 ppm of total DDT derived materials. There is evidence that, particularly in children, high body burdens may be derived from other than dietary sources of exposure such as the private use of DDT containing insecticide preparations in and around the home and exposure to DDT contaminated dust in agricultural communities (Danis *et al.,* 1969).

Another action of DDT that may contribute to effects on wild bird populations is the capacity of DDT and related materials to enhance the metabolism of estrogens. This could create an endocrine imbalance that affects the egg-laying and nesting cycle in such a way that total reproductive success and survival of young during the nesting season may be reduced.

ii) **Methoxychlor:** Methoxychlor is a chlorinated ethane derivative that has enjoyed increasing use as an insecticide as the use of DDT has declined. The attractiveness of methoxychlor it is that is practically nontoxic to mammals and compared to DDT has relatively low persistence. Compared to oral $LD_{50}$ values for rats in the range of 100 to 250 mg/kg body weight for DDT the $LD_{50}$ for Methoxychlor is 600mg/kg. Methoxychlor is slowly bio-transformed to small extent by pathways similar to those of DDT.

iii) **Lindane:** The gamma isomer of hexachlorocyclohexane (HCH) (sometimes called benzene hexachloride (BHC) produces signs of poisonings that resemble those produced by DDT *i.e.,* tremors, ataxia, convulsions, and prostration, with stimulated respiration.

b.    *Organophosphates:* These generally have very short residual action. Consequently, the control measures remain effective only for two or three days after treatment. They control a wider range of pests than chlorinated hydrocarbons. Some of organophophates are

General formula:

$$\begin{array}{c} R^1 \\ \diagdown \\ R^2 \diagup \end{array} \overset{O(S)}{\underset{}{\overset{\|}{P}}}-X$$

R1 & R2 must be alkyl or aryl group
X- any group of aliphatic or aromatic compound or heterocyclic groups.

(i) **TEPP** : The first organophosphate insecticide was tetraethyl pyrophosphate (TEPP). It was developed in Germany as a substitute for nicotine, which was in short supply in that country during World War II.

It is used to control aphids, thirps and mites etc. It is an effective insecticide, highly toxic to mammals and rapidly hydrolyzed in the presence of moisture.

Structural formula:  $(C_2H_5O)_2-\overset{O}{\overset{\|}{P}}-O-\overset{O}{\overset{\|}{P}}-(OC_2H_5)_2$

(ii) **Parathion:** It is an organophosphorous and acts as stomach or contact poison besides exhibiting a fumigant action. It is an organic phosphate, that is five to twenty times as toxic to insects as DDT. Chemically it is 0,0 diethyl p nitrophenyl thiophosphate. It is applied in the form of dust, suspension or emulsion. It is relatively unstable and looses its insecticidal value within a few days of application because of its rather high volatility. Parathion is effective in the control of a large variety of agricultural pests, especially the mealy bugs, scale insects, mites, paddy stem borer, aphids and leaf miners. In India, it is used as spray containing 0.01 to 0.05 per cent of actual parathion. Parathion is highly toxic to human beings, and animal if inhaled or absorbed through the skin, or swallowed. It inhibits or destroys cholinesterase, an enzyme which transmits the nerve impulsion. Therefore, a careful handling while preparing the spray solution or spraying in the field should be enforced.

It causes headache, nausea, diarrhoea, giddiness, restlessness and contracted pupils.

Structural formula:  $(C_2H_5O)_2-\overset{O}{\overset{\|}{P}}-O-\langle O \rangle NO_2$

(iii) **Diazinon:** In India, it has been successfully used for the control of some scale wooly aphids, mustard aphids, thrips, bugs. It is being marketed in India as 20 per cent emulsifiable concentrate and 10 per cent water dispersible powder. The concentration in which this insecticide is generally recommended range from 0.02 to 0.08 per cent. It is less toxic to mammals as compared to parathion. It is comparatively safer to handle than parathion.

(c) *Carbamates:* Carbamates are derivative of carbonic acid. In 1951 the carbamate insecticides were introduced in to the market by the chemical company in Switzerland.

General structural formula:   R-O-C(O)-N(CH³) - R¹      R is alcohol, oxime or phenol.

R1 is hydrogen or a methyl group.

The carbamates are inhibitors of cholinesterase. Some of the carbamates are

(i) *Carbaryl (Sevin):* In 1956, carbaryl was the first successful carbamate insecticide which was introduced in to the market. It has two distinct characters. It has very low mammalian oral and dermal toxicity and a rather broad spectrum of insect control.

Structural formula:

$$O - C - N \begin{matrix} H \\ CH_3 \end{matrix}$$

*(ii)* **Baygon (propoxur):** It is also a carbamate insecticide, used to control cockroaches and other household pests in restaurants, kitchens and home. For home use it is formulated in bottled sprays.

*iii.* **Aldicarb(Temik):** It is used as insecticides and as well as nematicide.

Structural formula : $CH_3 - S - \underset{\underset{CH_3}{|}}{\overset{\overset{O}{|}}{C}} - C = N - C - N \begin{matrix} H \\ CH_3 \end{matrix}$

*(d)* *Synthetic pyrethroids:* In recent years synthetic pyrethroids have emerged as a potentially very useful class of insecticides with a high insect/mammal toxicity ratio, rapid detoxication in mammals and lack of cumulative toxicity.

The selective toxicity of pyrethroids to insects as compared to mammals appears to be largely due to their rapid biotransforamtion in mammals by way of ester hydrolysis and for aromatic and methyl hydroxylation. Several pyrethroids were intermediate between parathion and DDT with respect to their persistence in soil. The pyrethroids are extremely toxic to aquatic organisms, unlike the case for mammals. These are called 1V[th] generation pesticides.

*(e)* *Dinitro phenols:* Dinitrophenols are insecticides and as herbicides. Their mode of action as fungicides is the same uncoupling of oxidative phosphorylation in cell with an attendant upset of the energy system with in cell.

Dinocap(karathane) have been in use since the late 1930 both as an acaricides and for powdery mildew on a number of fruit and vegetable crops. It undoubtedly acts in the vapour phase, since it is quite effective against powdery mildews whose spores germinate in the absence of water. This is popular home fungicide.

(dinocap -2,4,dinitro-6-(2-otyl)phenyl crotonate).

*(f)* *Botanicals:* Botanical insecticides are of great interest to many, because, they are "natural", insecticide toxicants derived from plants. Tobacco, pyrehrum, derris, hellobore, quasia, and turpentine were some of the more important plant products in use before the organized search for insecticides began.

There are 5 natural or plant derived insecticides that are of interest to gardeners in general, but especially to the organic gardeners, pyrethrum, rotenone, sabadilla, ryania and nicotine. All except nicotine are exempt from the requirement of a tolerance when applied to growing fruit and vegetables. This is, they can be eaten anytime after application, but these botanical insecticides must be used according to label directions. Botanical insecticides use reached its maximum in the United states in 1966 and has declined steadily. Botanical insecticides are really safer than most of the currently available synthetic insecticides. Botanicals are expensive to extract from plant tissue.

**(i) Nicotine:** Smoking tobacco was introduced in England in 1585 by Sir Walter Releigh. As early as 1690, water extracts of tobacco were reported as being used to kill sucking insects on garden plants. The active principle in tobacco extracts was known to be nicotine and extracts were sold as commercial insecticides, for home, farm and gardens.

Nicotine sulfur, as it is commonly marketed, is highly toxic to all warm-blooded animals, as well as insects, for example $LD_{50}$ for rats is 50-60 mg/kg. Nicotine sulfate used primarily for piercing-sucking insects such as leafhoppers, aphids, scaley trips and white flies, but it can kill all insects and spider and mites on which it is sprayed directly. Its use for most greenhouse pests is also acceptable. There are several ornamental plants that are sensitive to nicotine, such as roses. Nicotine is also registered for out-of-door use as a dog and cat repellent as well as for furniture in the home.

(ii) **Rotenone:** Rotenoids, the rotenone related materials, have been used as crop insecticides since 1848, when they were applied to plants to control leaf-eating caterpillars. However, they have been used for centuries in South America to paralyze fish, causing them to come to surface and get caught.

Rotenoids are produced in the roots of two genera of the legume family, Derris, grown in Malaya and East Indies and Lonchcarpus, grown in South America. Rotenone is harmless to plants, highly toxic to fishes, insects, especially caterpillars. Its life in the sun is short, two to three days. It is useful against caterpillars, aphids, beetles, spider, mites, ants, rose slugs and other pests.

Rotenone is the most useful piscicide available, for reclaiming lakes for game fishing. Poisoning by rotenone in man is rare and it has been used by direct application for head lice, scabies and other ectoparasites. Local effects include conjuctivities, pharyngitis and dermatitis. Orally, rotenone preparations produce gastrointestinal irritation, nausea, and vomiting. Inhalation of the dust is more hazardous and it can cause respiratory stimulation followed by depression with fits and convulsions.

(iii) **Pyrethrum:** It is extracted from the flowers of Chrysanthemum grown in Kenya, Africa and South America. It has an oral $LD_{50}$ of 1500 mg/kg and is one of the oldest household insecticides available. In the early 19th century during the Napoleonic wars, ground dried flower heads were used to control body lice. Pyrethrum acts on insects with phenomenal speed causing immediate paralysis, thus its popularity in fast knockdown household aerosol spray. Pyrethrum has been approved by EPA, and has more uses than any other insecticide, pyrethrum is a mixture of four compounds. pyrethrum I, II, cinerin I and II.

## Properties of Pesticides

Some properties of pesticides are important and determine their mode of action, potential as pollutant and short or long term presence in the environment. They are as follows.

1. *Stability and persistence:* The stability and persistence of a pesticide in aquatic system is a function of its chemical structure. Pesticides range in stability from those that are very unstable and breakdown in a few hours (*e.g.* Malathion) or few days *e.g.* Diazinon; Methoxychlor) to extremely stable compounds able to persist as residues for months (*e.g.* comphechlor) or year (*e.g.* DDT.). Persistence in the total aquatic system is greatest for organochlorine insecticides, intermediate for organophosphate and carbamate insecticides and least for herbicides. Pesticides that are highly persistent, present a potential hazard to the productivity of aquatic systems, because the aquatic biota will be exposed to residues for considerable periods even after only a single contamination, and if such contamination is repeated or occurs continuously, there is potential for bioaccumulation of the more persistent pesticide in some components of an aquatic system.

2. *Toxicity:* High toxicity to the aquatic fauna or flora is an important criterion for a pesticide to be considered as a pollutant of aquatic systems. If a persistent pesticide does not cause any serious harm, it means that it cannot be considered as an important pollutant.

Pesticides differ in toxicity to different aquatic organisms. Some pesticides are extremely toxic to fish at very low concentrations and to aquatic invertebrates at even lower levels. For, example $LC_{50}$ (96) value of DDT to rainbow trout is 0.018 ppm, $LC_{50}$ (24 hr) of malathion is 0.1 ppm, and of carbaryl is 3.5 ppm; and $LC_{50}$(48 hr) of herbicide Diquat is 20. ppm. Toxicity may be confined to a small group of organisms and thus be highly specific, or at the opposite extreme, affects almost all forms of biota in water toxicity may be acute or chronic. Acute effect can be easily detected but chronic effect is difficult to detect.

3. *Solubility:* High water solubility is a characteristic which can increase or decrease the potential of pesticide as a pollutant of aquatic systems. Pesticides differ greatly in solubility. For example, solubility of DDT in water is 0.0012 ppm, Endrin 0.23 ppm, parathion 24 ppm, carbaryl 40 ppm, and herbicides, Monuron and 2,4-D is 280 and 890 ppm respectively. Herbicide like Diquat and Dalapon are about 70 to 80 per cent soluble in water.

If a pesticide is easily soluble, it can drain into aquatic systems more readily from agricultural land and permeate rapidly through the whole of the system. However, more soluble pesticides tend to be less persistent in water and more easily diluted. But relatively insoluble pesticides are not readily leached into aquatic systems and once in a system are rapidly bound to living or dead organic matter or bottom sediment. Therefore, they affect the biota only if the chemical is very toxic, accumulate in the tissue of organisms or is bound to organic matter that provides food for other organisms.

4. *Adsorption:* Most pesticides tend to carry an electric charge that enables them to be adsorbed into soil particles. The rate of adsorption (and, conversely, of movement through the soil) differs from pesticide to pesticide, but all behave in the same basic way. Herbicides are much more strongly adsorbed into soils with a high exchange capacity.

5. *Degradation:* In addition to soil adsorption, pesticides undergo major structural changes that completely alter their toxic properties. Some of these changes are biochemical, others are photochemical and still others are inorganic chemical reactions with water or other inorganic substances in the soil.

Biochemical degradation represents the quasinormal activities of the detritus food chain, pesticides serving as a source of energy for bacteria involved in their breakdown. This process commonly detoxifies the chemical. But it may reduce or alter its toxicity spectra. In some cases it may even amplify them. Photochemical decomposition has similar result. In photochemical breakdown the chemical reaction is carried out through the adsorption of solar energy rather than by bacterial metabolism. Inorganic decomposition occurs by hydrolysis or reaction with acids or base in the interstitial waters. Organic pesticides may be degraded, some very slowly and some rapidly. Aldrin is transformed by bacteria into its epoxide, dieldrin, which is even more toxic than the parent molecule. The breakdown rate of a pesticide is strongly affected by soil temperature, moisture texture, etc.,

6. *Bioconcentration and Biomagnification:* Process of bioconcentration is quite complex and depends upon several factors such as the time of exposure, metabolism, rate of uptake, within the organism, rate of excretion, potential storage and physiological condition of the organism etc. Bioconcentration is important for determining the effect of pesticide.

The process of uptake and bioconcentration from the medium in which organism lives is some time confused with that of biological magnification. The latter may be defined as the accumulation of a pesticide in an animal at any particular tropic level at a concentration greater than in its food or the preceding tropic level so that animals at the top of the food chain accumulate the maximum residues.

7. *Amount used:* Heavy use of pesticide, especially in or close to the aquatic system is also an important factor in the degree of contamination of any system by a particular pesticide. Applications of pesticide by spraying leads to drift and atmospheric pollution and causes considerable fallout on to system with a large surface area.

## Mode of Entry of Pesticide in the Non Target Organism

Most pesticides are intended to kill specific pests or groups of pests, while having minimal toxic effects on human and other non target species. However both wild life and humans can also be at risk. Worker exposed to pesticides are at higher risk. There is more chance of entry of pesticide through skin that is through dermal exposure. Pesticide may enter the non target organism through respiratory tract. Non human species often have much higher pesticide exposure than do humans, birds, other animals and beneficial insects may suffer adverse effect or die as a result of pesticide exposure. Birds are killed not only by pesticide spraying, but through eating of pesticide treated seeds. Even in the 1990s fish and aquatic species die or suffer adverse effect caused by pesticide run off from land or pesticide spills. So pesticide enter the non target organism through food, water, dermal routs or respiratory routes etc.

Recent studies have emphasized the skin as a prime route of absorption for certain occupational and environmental chemicals. The main barrier to the penetration of pesticide and other substances is the stratum corneum of the epidermis, it has been proposed that this layer functions as a two compartment system. The lypophilic compartment, is composed mostly of lipids and is the pathway through which non polar molecules diffuse. The intracellular material, namely proteins, is the compartment through which water and polar molecules diffuse. The flux of water through the horny layer is a function of its water content the higher its water content the more easily molecule can move through the horny layer. For strongly lipid soluble molecules that enter the horny layer easily is evident that the rate limiting barrier is not the horny layer but the lipid/aqueous fluid interface at the base of the horny layer. Vehicles influences skin penetrations by altering the partition coefficient. In addition a vehicle can enter the stratum corneum and alter its barrier characteristics. Direct and indirect factors may affect absorption, indirect factors include race, age, sex, skin condition and injuries, personal hygiene and allergy, temperature and humidity at work place. For example infant skin is more permeable than the adult skin which explains some facilities among children treated for lice with malathion or lindane.

Either polar and non polar pesticides can diffuse through the horny layer by different molecular mechanism but generally lipid soluble pesticide are more readily absorbed.

## Impacts of Pesticides on Human Population

Person engaged in the manufacturing of pesticides are subject to pesticidal exposure. This result in chronic poisoning. Laws *et al.*, 1967 revealed that workers exposed to DDT for an average of 15 years (11-19 years) at an estimated daily dose of about 5 to 18 mg per man (0.04 mg / man / day) resulted in the storage of DDT in fat tissues ranging from 38 to 64.7 ppm as compared to 4 to 8 ppm in general population. Despite such a high level of exposure no ill effect was noticed in these workers in clinical laboratory tests.

A slow accumulation of Aldrin and Dieldrin occurs in workers who handle these insecticides in factories. The symptoms developed are headache, fatigue, loss of appetite, loss of weight and memory. In non fatal poisoning with Aldrin, Dieldrin and Endrin, the patients recover-in due course of time. The recovery time is generally 0 to 5 months for Endrin and 1 to 4 months for Aldrin and Dieldrin.

Organophosphates ranks first in causing occupational poisoning. A number of cases of accidental poisoning through these pesticides have been reported. There were about 1,400 cases in California alone (Metcalf 1957) and about 6,000 cases of parathion poisoning in Japan has been reported. As these pesticides inhibit the cholinesterase, the measurement of cholinesterase level in blood gives an estimate of the degree of poisoning. In chronically or mildly poisoned workers the degree of poisoning can be detected by measuring the cholinesterase level before the external symptoms begin to appear.

Recently Ramachandran et al.,(1973) have recorded higher concentration of DDT in body parts and blood of human beings causing anxiety, tension, cancer, mutation, stress reactions, congenital uterine malformation and impotency. Insecticides like BHC, aldrin,dieldrin, chlorodane and endosulfan are extremely toxic to living beings. These are considered to affect the vital organs heart, brain, kidneys and lever producing chronic disturbances.

Pesticide poisoning in Kerala (1951) resulted in the death of 112 people while in Indore (1968) 35 cases of malathion poisoning were reported. Recently (Dec 3, 1984) Bhopal industrial disaster was the worst ever pesticidal (MIC) accident in the history of man, taking an unpredentual and still unaccounted death toll leaving no fewer than 50,000 Effected, quickly dwarfed by the tidal wave of man's suffering that spread across the central city like the poison cloud. This carbaryl leakage caused an increased risk of sleeping, digestive problem, vision problems, sterility, kidney and liver infections as well as the brain damage.

## Transport of Pesticide in the Environment

Herbicide and insecticides are applied over large areas of agricultural fields and forests, and farmers may apply them a dozen times or more during a sowing season for each applications, less than half of the pesticide actually reaches to the environment.

The insect, weed or other pest, most become a pollutant. Sometimes foggy weather prevents pesticides from being airborne away from the point of application, posing a problem to those exposed to the trapped pesticides. Most pesticides are applied to crops by spraying. They then drift in the air currents from the point source and the largest amount settle on land and water close to the point of application, but smaller amounts, swept higher into the atmosphere with the winds, can be carried thousands of miles away. Certain polychlorinated pesticides detected in wilderness lakes in the northern United States or Canada are not used in those countries and are assumed to have been blown from Mexico or other Latin American countries. Once soil and water become contaminated with these persistent pesticides, they may remain so for many years, especially in northern locations, where cold weather and lack of intense sunlight prevent them from degrading.

Agricultural lands are major non point source of pesticides, fertilizers, eroded soil, and manure. Runoff from lands to which pesticides have been applied is responsible for most surface water contamination with pesticides. A comprehensive study of the Mississippi river basin, for example, detected more than 40 pesticides. One, the herbicide atrazine was present in 95 per cent of the samples. Pesticides are also found in runoff from municipal streets and grounds, areas sprayed by utilities, golf play grounds, course greens, and gardens of home owners. Water soluble pesticides not only can be found in runoff, but can move down through soil to reach ground water. Chlorinated pesticides are much less water soluble and cling to soil particles, so they are less likely to contaminate ground water. Ground water contamination is a greater concern than surface water contamination because even pesticides that have only short lives in surface water may degrade very slowly in ground water. Ground water is also much harder to cleanup.

## Impact of Pesticides on Environment

The use of pesticides is a necessary evil of the modern agro-technology and perhaps their demand would never like to cease. Actually they are directed against economic pests but they also affect non-target organisms and the environment. Many pesticides such as DDT and other Chlorinated hydrocarbons are highly persistent and they can more rapidly and easily through a single ecosystem or from one ecosystem (river) to another (ocean). For example DDT may be washed away from a sprayed cotton field by runoff waters and eventually be carried to a river and finally to the ocean. Pesticides like DDT, endrin, dieldrin, etc, may gradually seep downward into ground water and eventually contaminate public drinking water supplies.

When water evaporates from an irrigated field or from a river or lake, the pesticide molecules may co-distill, *i.e.*, may be carried into the atmosphere along with the evaporating molecules of water. In a sprayed field DDT and other pesticides adhered to soil particles may be carried away by dust erosion and then eventually return to land, lake, river or ocean, many thousands of miles away from the site application. As the different components of the biosphere are functionally interrelated, pesticide pollution has spread into all of them. Trace amounts of pesticides have been found in the fatty tissues of seals and penguins in the Antarctic (Moran *et. al.*, 1973).

*(i) Toxicity Doses:* Different investigations have adopted different methods to assess the lethality of pesticides. Toxicity of a pesticide is evaluated by determining various parameters like Lethal Concentration (LC), Sub Lethal Concentration (SLC), Medium Lethal Concentration, Medium Tolerance Limit (TLM), Medium Effective Dose (MED) and Safe Concentration (SC). Lethal Concentration is the one which kills a definite population of an animal species employed for the test in a fixed period of time, whereas, $LC_{50}$ is the concentration that would theoretically kill 50 per cent of the population, which in turn represents median tolerance limit (TLM) and Median Lethal Concentration (Finney, 1971; Buikema et al., 1982). It is customary to represent lethality of a pesticide to a particular animal species in terms of mortality and time. Toxicity of pesticides is assessed by most investigators by determining the concentration which kills 50 per cent of the test species for different periods of exposure like 24, 48, 72 and 96 hours. This is usually done by plotting dosage mortality curves after exposing the animals to different concentrations of a test substance for a predefined period of time. As there is a direct relationship between the weight of the animal and dose of the pesticide, lethal dose (LD) is always expressed in terms of micro/milli grams/kg body weight of the animal. If the pesticide is solvent (water) as with aquatic organisms, its concentration is expressed as parts per million (ppm) or parts per billion (ppb) or mg/litre. The lethality of pesticide is also dependent on its concentration and period of exposure time. Thus it is customary to express the concentration of a pesticide that kills certain percentage of test species, say 50 per cent as $LC_{50}$ (x gms/y hrs).

For aquatic animals, $LC_{50}$ values of a toxicant are determined by exposing the animals in a static medium to different concentrations of a toxicant for a period of time, and noting down the concentration where 50 per cent mortality is observed. To determine $LC_{50}$ there are many methods in practice such as graphical method following dose response curve, statistical method following probit analysis (Finny, 1971) and Dragstedt-Behrens method using cumulative mortality (Carpenter, 1975). $LC_{50}$ values are essential to establish tolerance limits and safe level of the toxic agents for the biota and also for observing various symptoms of poisoning. A survey of literature shows that different pesticides have been tested for their toxicity to crustaceans by following different methods. These pesticides include synthetic organic compound like organochlorines, organophosphates, Carbonate and Synthetic pyrethroids.

*(ii) Impact of Pesticides on Crustaceans:* It is a fact that several non-target organisms such as crabs, fishes etc., are sensitive to a wide variety of pesticides, in addition to the target species. It has now become a normal practice to test all new pesticides for their toxicity. This assessment of toxicity would help in knowing the potentiality of a chemical so that new and more powerful formulations may be speeded

up in the manufacture of pesticides. The non-target organisms respond differently to different dosages of these compounds. These may be doses so low where no mortality is obtained and a dose which is fatal to all test species. Dose response studies occupy a primary position and are helpful in evaluating the toxicity of a test chemical, since it is from dose response studies that may be in a position to arrive at an arbitrary lethal concentration.

Toxicity evaluation of pesticides has been done for a few crustaceans with reference to the organochlorines such as Kelthane (Surendranath *et al.*, 1987 a,b), dieldrine (Parrish *et al.*, 1973), BHC (Mary, 1984; Geethanjali 1985), DDT (Hansan *et al.*, 1973; Mary, 1984), lindane (Srinivasalu Reddy and Ramana Rao 1986), aldrine (Mary, 1984), endosulfan (Mcleese and Metcalf, 1980; Renuka Devi and Venkatachari, 1984, Renuka Devi, 1986; Rajashri, 1986; Rajendra Prasad Naidu and Padmanabha Naidu, 1989; Nagendra Reddy, 1989), Organophosphates such as elsaan (Surendra Babu *et al.*, 1983 a) malathion (Bhagyalakshmi and Ramamurthi, 1981; Nagabhushanam *et al.*, 1983), methyl parathion (Srinivasalu Reddy and Ramana Rao, 1986), methyl parathion (Venkatachari and Renukadevi 1984), Monocrotophos (Nagabhushanam *et al.*, 1983; Venkatachari *et al.*, 1987), Carbamates such as Sevin (Chandrashekharan Natarajan, 1982), furadon (Renuka Devi and Venkatachari, 1984; Renuka Devi, 1986), and Synthetic pyrenthroids such as fenvalerate (Neeraja Kumari, 1986; Neeraja Kumari, *et al.*, 1987 a).

The above studies showed that the toxicity of a pesticide varies depending upon the species studies and the type of pesticide used. For the freshwater crab, *Oziotelphusa sensex sensex* the toxicity of the pesticide is in the order OP > OC> carbamates. Also in the same species the toxicity of different pesticides belonging to one class varies. In view of the extensive use of the organophosphate, Monocrotophos in the pest control operations an extensive study was undertaken by the author to evaluate to its toxicity to the freshwater crab, Barytelphusa guerini (Miline Edwards)\using different methods of toxicity evaluation and its relation to size and sex (Table 10.1, Fig 10.1).

**Table 10.1 : LC$_{50}$ Values of monocrotophos measured at dirrerent exposure periods for the crab Barytelphusa guerini of different sizes and sexes. The value expressed in ppm are mean ± S.D. of six observations**

| Period of Exposure | Different Methods | SMALL | | LARGE | |
|---|---|---|---|---|---|
| | | Male | Female | Male | Female |
| 24 Hours | Graphical method | 11.00 | 11.00 | 12.50 | 13.00 |
| | Probit Method | 9.80 | 10.00 | 12.0 | 12.50 |
| | Dragstedt-Behrens | 10.37 | 10.95 | 11.84 | 13.41 |
| | Average | 10.39± | 10.65± | 12.11± | 12.97± |
| | | 0.67 | 0.86 | 0.63 | 0.54 |
| 48 Hours | Graphical method | 5.00 | 5.00 | 5.00 | 6.50 |
| | Probit Method | 4.60 | 5.10 | 4.80 | 5.80 |
| | Dragstedt-Behrens | 5.19 | 5.50 | 5.19 | 6.40 |
| | Average | 4.93± | 5.20± | 4.99± | 6.23± |
| | | 0.40 | 0.31 | 0.24 | 0.36 |
| 72 Hours | Graphical method | 3.20 | 2.90 | 4.20 | 4.10 |
| | Probit Method | 3.20 | 3.00 | 3.80 | 3.90 |
| | Dragstedt-Behrens | 3.00 | 3.20 | 4.28 | 4.60 |
| | Average | 3.10± | 3.03± | 4.10± | 4.20± |
| | | 0.12 | 0.15 | 0.23 | 0.32 |
| 96 Hours | Graphical method | 1.40 | 2.20 | 2.20 | 2.40 |
| | Probit Method | 1.70 | 2.30 | 2.10 | 2.40 |
| | Dragstedt-Behrens | 1.87 | 2.23 | 2.20 | 2.50 |
| | Average | 1.66± | 2.24± | 2.16± | 2.43± |
| | | 0.21 | 0.06 | 0.07 | 0.07 |

## Metabolism of Pesticides

A consideration of the role of metabolism of complex organic pesticide molecules in relation to their selective toxicity involves the broad principles of xenobiotic metabolism in general.

e.g.:

### Organophosphate metabolism:

eg: Methyl parathion.

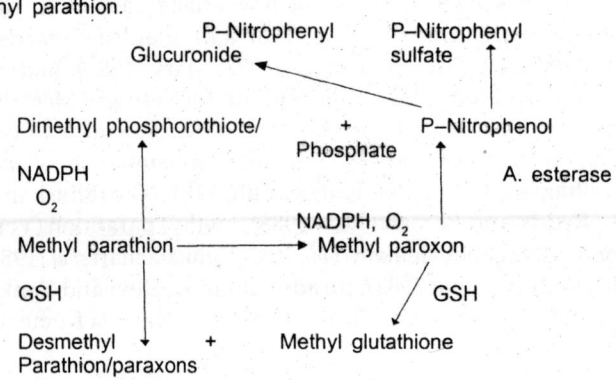

**Fig. 10.1**

All of metabolic reaction shown here for Methyl parathion are catalyzed by enzymes present in mammalian liver cells. Thus an oxidative reaction leads to the formation of oxygen analogue, methyl paraoxon, the active metabolite that inhibits acetyl cholinesterase, Oxidative cleavage to Dimethyl phasphorothioate and P-Nitrophenol, hydrolysis of Methyl paradxon and Glutathione linked Dimethylation of the parent compound or its oxygen analogue are enzyme catalyzed reactions that yield relatively nontoxic derivatives. Thus, for methyl parathion both activation and a detoxication reaction can be classified as phase-I. This includes oxidative desulfuration and oxidative cleavage and hydrolysis of Methyl paraoxon into its relatively nontoxic derivatives, Dimethyl phosphate and P-Nitrophenol. There is also the possibility for a variety of conjugation reactions. For eg: The derivative P-Nitrphenol can be conjugated either as the sulphate or the Glucuronide. This may be an important consideration in biological monitoring of exposure. It is important to recognize that this may also exists as conjugates. Removal of methyl group, catalyzed by Glutathione alkyl transferase, might be viewed as a type of conjugation reaction, since the methyl group of methyl parathion becomes attached to Glutathione. However the effect is more like a phase-I reaction to yield the more polar, less toxic Desmethyl parathion or Desmethyl paraoxon.

### Table 10.2 : Toxicity of different pesticides to crustaceans

| Sl. No. | Name of the Pesticide | Species Name | Duration | Value | Authors | |
|---------|----------------------|--------------|----------|-------|---------|---|
| I. | **Organochlorines** | | | | | |
| 1. | Kelthane | *Crangon franciscorum* | $LC_{50}$/24 hrs | 777-2138 ppb | Khorram & Knight | (1977) |
| | | | $LC_{50}$/48 hrs | 437-832 ppb | " | |
| | | *Metapenaeus Monoceros* | $LC_{50}$/48 hrs | 0.259 ppm | Surendranath *et al.,* | (1987a) |
| | | | $LC_{50}$/96 hrs | 0.156 ppm | " | |
| 2. | Dieldrin | *Penaeus duorarum* | $LC_{50}$/96 hrs | 00.9 µgm/ltr. | Parrish *et al.,* | (1973) |
| | | *Palaemonetes pugio* (Grass Shrimp) | $LC_{50}$/96 hrs | 11.4 µgm/ltr. | " | |

*Contd....*

| Sl. No. | Name of the Pesticide | Species Name | Duration | Value | Authors | |
|---|---|---|---|---|---|---|
| 3. | BHC | Oziotelphusa senex senex | $LC_{50}$/24 hrs | 39 ppm | Geethanjali | (1985) |
| | | | $LC_{50}$/48 hrs | 28 ppm | " | |
| | | | $LC_{50}$/72 hrs | 15 ppm | " | |
| | | | $LC_{50}$/96 hrs | 12 ppm | " | |
| | | Macrobrachium Kistnensis | $LC_{50}$/96 hrs | 8.622 µgm/ltr | Pawar & Katdare | (1983) |
| | | Cardina Rajdhari | $LC_{50}$/96 hrs | 31.34 µgm/ltr | " | |
| | | Macrobrachium lamerrii | $LC_{50}$/96 hrs | 0.0029 ppm | Mary | (1984) |
| 4. | DDT | Macrobrachium lamerrii | $LC_{50}$/96 hrs | 0.0043 ppm | Mary | (1984) |
| | | Palaemonetes pugio | $LC_{50}$/24 hrs | 0.0007 ppm | Hansen et al., | (1973) |
| 5. | Endrin | Palaemonetes pugio | $LC_{50}$/24 hrs | 0.0015 ppm | Hansen et al., | (1973) |
| 6. | Lindane | Metapenaeus dobsoni | $LC_{50}$/96 hrs | 0.00643 ppm | Srinivasulu Reddy & | (1986) |
| | | Panaeus indicus | $LC_{50}$/96 hrs | 0.00038 ppm | Ramana Rao | |
| | | Penaeus monodon | $LC_{50}$/96 hrs | 0.0012 ppm | " | |
| 7. | Aldrin | Macrobrachium lamerrii | $LC_{50}$/96 hrs | 0.0061 ppm | Mary | (1984) |
| 8. | Endosulfan | Crangon septumspinosa | $LC_{50}$/96 hrs | 0.2 ppb | McLeese & Metcalf | (1980) |
| | | Oziotephusa senex senex | $LC_{50}$/96 hrs | 15.14 ppm | Rajendra Prasad Naidu | (1985) |
| | | | | | Rajendra Prasad Naidu & Padmanabhanaidu | (1989) |
| | | Oziotelphusa senex senex | $LC_{50}$/96 hrs | 18.62 ppm | Rajeswari | (1986) |
| | | Barytelphusa guerini | $LC_{50}$/96 hrs | 17.78 ppm | Nagender Reddy | (1989) |
| | | Oziotelphusa senex senex | Small Males | | | |
| | | | $LC_{50}$/24 hrs | 7.32 ppm | Renuka Devi & Venkatachari | (1984) |
| | | | $LC_{50}$/48 hrs | 6.21 ppm | Venkatachari & Renuka Devi | (1984) |
| | | | $LC_{50}$/72 hrs | 5.83 ppm | & Renuka Devi | (1986) |
| | | | $LC_{50}$/96 hrs | 4.44 ppm | " | |
| | | | Small Females | | | |
| | | | $LC_{50}$/24 hrs | 10.09 ppm | " | |
| | | | $LC_{50}$/48 hrs | 9.23 ppm | " | |
| | | | $LC_{50}$/72 hrs | 7.96 ppm | " | |
| | | | $LC_{50}$/96 hrs | 6.86 ppm | " | |
| | | | Large Males | | | |
| | | | $LC_{50}$/24 hrs | 9.79 ppm | " | |
| | | | $LC_{50}$/48 hrs | 8.38 ppm | " | |
| | | | $LC_{50}$/72 hrs | 6.32 ppm | " | |
| | | | $LC_{50}$/96 hrs | 5.26 ppm | " | |
| | | | Large Females | | | |
| | | | $LC_{50}$/24 hrs | 11.28 ppm | " | |
| | | | $LC_{50}$/48 hrs | 9.44 ppm | " | |
| | | | $LC_{50}$/72 hrs | 8.42 ppm | " | |
| | | | $LC_{50}$/96 hrs | 7.23 ppm | " | |

**II. Organophosphates**

| Sl. No. | Name of the Pesticide | Species Name | Duration | Value | Authors | |
|---|---|---|---|---|---|---|
| 1. | Elsan | Metapenaeus Monoceros | $LC_{50}$/48 hrs | 0.013 ppm | Surendra Babu et al., | (1983a) |
| 2. | Malathion | Macrobrachium lamerrii | $LC_{50}$/24 hrs | 0.63 ppm | Nagabhushanam et al., | (1983) |
| | | | $LC_{50}$/48 hrs | 0.35 ppm | " | |
| | | | $LC_{50}$/72 hrs | 0.22 ppm | " | |
| | | | $LC_{50}$/96 hrs | 0.13 ppm | " | |
| | | Oziotelphusa senex senx | $LC_{50}$/24 hrs | 15.00 ppm | Sreenivasulu Reddy et al. | (1986a) |
| | | Oziotelphusa senex senex | $LC_{50}$/48 hrs | 23.00 ppm | Bhagyalakshmi & Ramamurthy | (1981) |
| | | Palaemonetes pugio | $LC_{50}$/24 hrs | 0.032 ppm | Hansen et al., | (1973) |
| 3. | Methyl parathion | Oziotelphusa senex senex | $LC_{50}$/24 hrs | 3.00 ppm | Nagarathnamma & Ramamurthy | (1981) |
| | | | $LC_{50}$/48 hrs | 1.00 ppm | " | |
| | | Penaeus monodon | $LC_{50}$/96 hrs | 0.148 ppm | Srinivasalur Reddy & Ramana Rao | (1986) |

*Contd....*

| Sl. No. | Name of the Pesticide | Species Name | Duration | Value | Authors | |
|---|---|---|---|---|---|---|
| | | Penaeus indicus | LC$_{50}$/96 hrs | 0.098 ppm | " | |
| | | Metapenaeus dobsoni | LC$_{50}$/96 hrs | 0.115 ppm | " | |
| | | Palaemonetes vulgaris | LC$_{50}$/96 hrs | 3.0 µgm/ltr | Eisler | (1969) |
| 4. | Sumithion | Oziotelphusa senex senex | LC$_{50}$/24 hrs | 0.6 ppm | Bhagyalakshmi & Ramamurthy | (1981) |
| | | | LC$_{50}$/48 hrs | 0.4 ppm | Bhagyalakshmi & Ramamurthy | (1981) |
| | | | | | & Balavenkatasubbaiah et al. | (1983) |
| | | | LC$_{50}$/72 hrs | 0.3 ppm | Bhagyalakshmi & Ramamurthi | (1981) |
| | | Macrobrachium kistnensis | LC$_{50}$/96 hrs | 0.9197 µgm/ltr | Pawar & Katdare | (1983) |
| | | Caridina rajdhari | LC$_{50}$/96 hrs | 0.021 µgm/ltr | " | |
| | | Macrobrachium lamerrii | LC$_{50}$/96 hrs | 0.0012 ppm | Mary | (1984) |
| 5. | Dimecron | Macrobrachium kistnensis | LC$_{50}$/24 hrs | 6.43 ppm | Mirajkar & Sarojini & Sarojini & Mirajkar | (1982) (1982) |
| | | | LC$_{50}$/48 hrs | 3.32 ppm | " | |
| | | | LC$_{50}$/72 hrs | 2.180 ppm | " | |
| | | | LC$_{50}$/96 hrs | 1.165 ppm | Mirajkar & Sarojini | (1982) |
| | | | | | Sarojini & Mirajkar | (1982) |
| | | | | | Mirajkar et al., | (1982) |
| | | Macrpbracjoi, lamerrii | LC$_{50}$/24 hrs | 1.75 ppm | Nagabhushanam et al., | 1983 |
| | | | LC$_{50}$/48 hrs | 1.63 ppm | " | |
| | | | LC$_{50}$/72 hrs | 1.50 ppm | " | |
| | | | LC$_{50}$/96 hrs | 1.38 ppm | " | |
| 6. | Monocrotophos | Macrobrachium lamerrii | LC$_{50}$/24 hrs | 5.37 ppm | Nagabhusanam et al., | 1983 |
| | | | LC$_{50}$/48 hrs | 4.46 ppm | " | |
| | | | LC$_{50}$/72 hrs | 3.11 ppm | " | |
| | | | LC$_{50}$/96 hrs | 1.91 ppm | " | |
| 7. | Dursban | Palaemonetes pugio | LC$_{50}$/24 hrs | 0.0032 ppm | Hansen et al., | 1973 |
| 8. | Phosphamidon | Macrobrachium malcomsoni | LC$_{50}$/96 hrs | 1.505 ppm | Srinivasulu Reddy et al., | 1985 |
| | | Penaeus monodon | LC$_{50}$/96 hrs | 1.434 ppm | Srinivasulu Reddy & Ramana Rao | 1986 |
| | | Penaeus indicus | LC$_{50}$/96 hrs | 0.828 ppm | " | |
| | | Metapenaeus dobsoni | LC$_{50}$/96 hrs | 1.095 ppm | " | |
| 9. | Dichlorovos | Macrobrachium lamarrii | LC$_{50}$/96 hrs | 0.0036 ppm | Mary | 1984 |
| 10. | Matasystox | Macrobrachium lamerrii | LC$_{50}$/96 hrs | 1.291 ppm | " | |
| 11. | Dimethoate | Macrobrachium lamerrii | LC$_{50}$/96 hrs | 0.0029 ppm | " | |
| 12. | Phenthoate | Penaeus indicus | LC$_{50}$/24 hrs | 0.0146 ppm | Surendra Babu et al., | 1983b |
| | | | LC$_{50}$/48 hrs | 0.0127 ppm | " | |
| | | Metapenaeus monoceros | LC$_{50}$/24 hrs | 0.0222 ppm | " | |
| | | | LC$_{50}$/48 hrs | 0.0129 ppm | " | |
| 13. | Ekalux | Barytelphusa cunicularis | LC$_{50}$/24 hrs | 0.4677 ppm | Jaiswal et al., | 1989 |
| | | | LC$_{50}$/48 hrs | 0.3236 ppm | " | |
| | | | LC$_{50}$/72 hrs | 0.1648 ppm | " | |
| | | | LC$_{50}$/96 hrs | 0.1474 ppm | " | |
| 14. | Chlorpyrifos | Oziotelphusa senex senex | | | | |
| | | | Small Male : | | | |
| | | | LC$_{50}$/24 hrs | 0.70 ppm | Renuka Devi & Venkatachari | 1984 |
| | | | LC$_{50}$/48 hrs | 0.57 ppm | Venkatachari & Renuka Devi | 1984 |
| | | | LC$_{50}$/72 hrs | 0.32 ppm | & Renuka Devi | 1986 |
| | | | LC$_{50}$/96 hrs | 0.22 ppm | " | |
| | | | Small Female : | | | |
| | | | LC$_{50}$/24 hrs | 0.94 ppm | " | |
| | | | LC$_{50}$/48 hrs | 0.60 ppm | " | |
| | | | LC$_{50}$/72 hrs | 0.45 ppm | " | |
| | | | LC$_{50}$/96 hrs | 0.30 ppm | " | |

Contd....

| Sl. No. | Name of the Pesticide | Species Name | Duration | Value | Authors | |
|---|---|---|---|---|---|---|
| | | | Large Male : | | | |
| | | | $LC_{50}/24$ hrs | 1.06 ppm | " | |
| | | | $LC_{50}/48$ hrs | 0.61 ppm | " | |
| | | | $LC_{50}/72$ hrs | 0.43 ppm | " | |
| | | | $LC_{50}/96$ hrs | 0.32 ppm | " | |
| | | | Large Female : | | | |
| | | | $LC_{50}/24$ hrs | 1.21 ppm | " | |
| | | | $LC_{50}/48$ hrs | 0.91 ppm | " | |
| | | | $LC_{50}/72$ hrs | 0.73 ppm | " | |
| | | | $LC_{50}/96$ hrs | 0.58 ppm | " | |
| **III.** | **Carbamates** | | | | | |
| 1. | Sevin | Penaeus monodon | $LC_{50}/96$ hrs | 43 ppb | Chadrasekaran & Natarajan | 1982 |
| | | | $LC_{50}/24$ hrs | 0.038 ppm | Hansen et al. | 1973 |
| 2. | Furadan | Macrobrachium kistnensis | $LC_{50}/96$ hrs | 157.3 µgm/ltr. | Pawar & katdare | 1983 |
| | | Cardidina rajdhari | $LC_{50}/96$ hrs | 0.3324 µgm/ltr | " | |
| | | Oziotephusa senex senex | | | | |
| | | | Small Male : | | | |
| | | | $LC_{50}/24$ hrs | 59.03 ppm | Renuka Devi & Venkatachari | 1984 |
| | | | $LC_{50}/48$ hrs | 48.34 ppm | Venkatachari & Renuka Devi | 1984 |
| | | | $LC_{50}/72$ hrs | 38.43 ppm | & Renuka Devi | 1986 |
| | | | $LC_{50}/96$ hrs | 31.07 ppm | " | |
| | | | Small Female : | | | |
| | | | $LC_{50}/24$ hrs | 68.02 ppm | " | |
| | | | $LC_{50}/48$ hrs | 58.70 ppm | " | |
| | | | $LC_{50}/72$ hrs | 44.96 ppm | " | |
| | | | $LC_{50}/96$ hrs | 32.95 ppm | " | |
| | | | Large Male : | | | |
| | | | $LC_{50}/24$ hrs | 89.36 ppm | " | |
| | | | $LC_{50}/48$ hrs | 68.04 ppm | " | |
| | | | $LC_{50}/72$ hrs | 54.27 ppm | " | |
| | | | $LC_{50}/96$ hrs | 44.45 ppm | " | |
| | | | Large Female : | | | |
| | | | $LC_{50}/24$ hrs | 70.96 ppm | " | |
| | | | $LC_{50}/48$ hrs | 60.37 ppm | " | |
| | | | $LC_{50}/72$ hrs | 48.15 ppm | " | |
| | | | $LC_{50}/96$ hrs | 38.43 ppm | " | |
| **IV.** | **Synthetic Pyrithroids** | | | | | |
| 1. | Fenvalerate | Mysiodopsis batia (Mysid shrimp) | $LC_{50}/96$ hrs | 0.008 µgm/ltr | McLeese et al., | 1980 |
| | | Pink shrimp | $LC_{50}/96$ hrs | 0.84 µgm/ltr | McLeese et al., | 1980 |
| | | Homarus americanus (Lobster) | $LC_{50}/96$ hrs | 0.14 µgm/ltr | " | |
| | | Crangon septumspinosa (Sand shrimp) | $LC_{50}/96$ hrs | 0.04 µgm/ltr | | |
| | | Oziotephusa senex senex | $LC_{50}/24$ hrs | 10 mg/ltr | Neeraja Kumari et al., | 1987a |
| | | | $LC_{50}/48$ hrs | 6 mg/ltr | " | |
| | | | $LC_{50}/72$ hrs | 5 mg/ltr | " | |
| | | | $LC_{50}/96$ hrs | 4 mg/ltr | " | |
| | | | $LD_{50}/24$ hrs | 7.6 mg/Kg. | " | |
| | | | $LD_{50}/48$ hrs | 5.8 mg/Kg. | " | |
| | | | $LD_{50}/24$ hrs | 7.6 mg/Kg. | " | |
| | | | $LD_{50}/48$ hrs | 5.7 mg/Kg. | " | |
| | | | **$KD_{50}$** | **380 µg/Kg.** | | |
| | | | 10 gm body weight : | | | |
| | | | $LD_{50}/24$ hrs | 3.0 mg/Kg. | " | |
| | | | $LD_{50}/48$ hrs | 1.6 mg/Kg. | " | |
| | | | 15 gm body weight : | | | |

*Contd....*

| Sl. No. | Name of the Pesticide | Species Name | Duration | Value | | Authors | |
|---------|----------------------|--------------|----------|-------|---|---------|---|
| | | | $LD_{50}$/24 hrs | 5.0 | mg/Kg. | " | |
| | | | $LD_{50}$/48 hrs | 2.7 | mg/Kg. | " | |
| | | | 20-30 gm body weight : | | | | |
| | | | $LD_{50}$/24 hrs | 8.0 | mg/Kg. | " | |
| | | | $LD_{50}$/48 hrs | 6.0 | mg/Kg. | " | |
| V. | Pesticide mixture | | | | | | |
| 1. | Mixutre of Furadan, | *Oziotelphusa senex senex* | | | | Small Male : | |
| | | | $LC_{50}$/24 hrs | 28.18 | ppm | Renuka Devi | 1986 |
| | | | $LC_{50}$/48 hrs | 22.79 | ppm | " | |
| | | | $LC_{50}$/72 hrs | 14.85 | ppm | " | |
| | | | $LC_{50}$/96 hrs | 12.08 | ppm | " | |
| | | | Small Female : | | | | |
| | | | $LC_{50}$/24 hrs | 28.59 | ppm | Renuka Devi | 1986 |
| | | | $LC_{50}$/48 hrs | 24.81 | ppm | " | |
| | | | $LC_{50}$/72 hrs | 19.45 | ppm | " | |
| | | | $LC_{50}$/96 hrs | 12.00 | ppm | " | |
| | | | Large Male : | | | | |
| | | | $LC_{50}$/24 hrs | 35.15 | ppm | " | |
| | | | $LC_{50}$/48 hrs | 24.20 | ppm | " | |
| | | | $LC_{50}$/72 hrs | 18.46 | ppm | " | |
| | | | $LC_{50}$/96 hrs | 12.64 | ppm | " | |
| | | | Large Female : | | | | |
| | | | $LC_{50}$/24 hrs | 31.50 | ppm | " | |
| | | | $LC_{50}$/48 hrs | 24.30 | ppm | " | |
| | | | $LC_{50}$/72 hrs | 17.58 | ppm | " | |
| | | | $LC_{50}$/96 hrs | 12.41 | ppm | " | |

## Precautionary Measures

Before applying pesticides-general instructions

1. Know the pest, and how much damage is really being done.

2. Use pesticides only when really needed.

3. Seek advice on the proper method of control.

4. Use only the recommended pesticide for the problem. Choose the least toxic to mammals and if possible the least persistent.

5. Read the label, including the small print.

6. Make sure the appropriate protective clothing is available and is used and that all concerned with the application also understand the recommendation, and are fully trained in how to apply pesticides.

7. Commercial operators using large quantities of organophosphate pesticides should visit their doctor and have a blood cholinesterase test, and have repeat checks during the season.

8. Check application equipment for leaks, calibrate with water and ensure it is in proper working order.

9. Check that pesticides on the form are in a dry, locked store, avoid inhaling pesticide mists or dusts, especially in confined spaces such as the pesticide store.

10. Take only sufficient pesticide for the day's application from the store to the site of application. Do not transfer pesticides into other containers, especially beer and soft drink bottles.

## While mixing pesticides and during application

1. Wear appropriate protective clothing. If it is contaminated, remove and replace with clean clothing.

2. Never work alone when handling the most toxic pesticides.

3. Recheck the instructions on the label.

4. Never eat, drink or smoke when mixing or applying pesticides.

5. Always have plenty of water available for washing.

6. Make sure pesticides are mixed in the correct quantities.

## After application

1. **RETURN** unused pesticide to the store.

2. **NEVER** leave pesticides in application equipment. Clean equipment and return to store.

3. Remove and clean protective clothing.

4. Wash well and put on clean clothing.

5. Keep a record of the use of pesticides.

6. Do not allow other persons to enter the treated area for the required period if restrictions apply to the pesticide used.

## SUMMARY

Pesticides are very important to control pests when used in a proper way. But indiscriminate use of pesticide brings number of problems to the non target organisms. So pesticides must be used not indiscriminately as at present, but only on a prescription by designated agricultural authorities. More important, we must ensure strong extension, information and training services for the teachers to taught media, farmers and the general public. Both the late prime minister Rajiv Gandhi, and the planning commission have pleaded for a policy on pesticides. It is time that the scientists themselves press the government on evolving a pragmatic policy. Use of plant origin pesticide is also one of the method to minimise the effects. Biological control is also a one of the methods. Finally we can conclude that pesticides are boon to the agriculture when used in proper manner.

## REFERENCES

● Agarwal, S.K. 1996. *"Industrial Environment Assessment and Strategy"*, 2nd Ed, A.P.H. Publishing Corporation, Ansari Road, Daryaganj, New Delhi-110002.

● Buikema, A.L., Niederlchner, B.R. & Cairns. J. 1982. *Biological Monitoring* Part IV. Toxicity testing Water Res. 16:239-262.

● Curtis, D. Klasen, Mary. O. Amdur, John Doull, *"Casarett and Doull's Toxicology"* 3rd Ed, Macmillan publishing Company, New York.

● Carpenter, P.L. 1975. *Immunology and Serology*, W.B. Saunders Company, Philadelphia 254.

● Chandrashekaran, V.S. & Natarajan. R. 1982. Acute toxicity of pesticide Sevin (Crabamate) and its effects on the oxygen consumption of Juveniles of the tiger prawn *Peneaus monodon* (Fabricius) In: Physiological responses of animals to pollutants proc. All India Symp., Aurangabad, 9-11 Dec. PP 48-52

- Dhingra, K.C. 1985. *"Handbook of pesticides"* Published by small industry research institute, 4\43, Roop Nagar, Delhi-110007.

- Dinesh Mani and Mishra S.G. 1994. *"Agricultural Pollution"* Vol II, Ashish publishing house, 8\81, Punjabi Bagh, New Delhi.

- Finney, D.J. 1971. *Probit Analysis,* Cambridge Unversity, Press, London.

- Geethanjali. K. 1985. *Effects of Organochlorine Pesticide BHC on the Physiology of edible freshwater crab., Oziotelphusa sensex sensex (Fabricius).* M.Phil. dissertation, S.V. University, Tirupati.

- Hansen. D.J. Schimmel. S.C. & Keltner. Jr. J.M. 1973. Avoidance of Pesticide of grass Shrimp (*Palaemonetes pugio*), *Bull. Environ. Contam. Toxicol* 9:129-133

- Lucio G.Costa, Corrado L.Galli Sheldon D.Murphy. 1987. *"Toxicology of pesticides; Experimental, Clinical & Regulatory Perspectives"* Springer-Verlag, Berlin Heidelberg New York.

- Marquita.K.Hill. 1997. *"Understanding Environmental Pollution* "1ˢᵗEd, published by the press syndicate of the University of Cambridge,Pittu Building, Trumpington street,Cambridge.

- Mary Avelin 1984. Effect of Pesticides on some aspects of Physiology of the freshwater prawn, *macrobrachium lamerrii.* Ph.D. thesis Marathawada University, Aurangabad.

- Mc.Leese, D.W Metcalfe. C.D. 1980. Toxicities of eight organochlorine compounds in sediment and sea water to *Crangon septemspinosa. Bull Environ. Contam. Toxicol* **25**: 921-926

- Nagender Reddy, A. 1989. Endosulfan induced metabolic alterations in the freshwater field crab, *Barytelphusa guerini* Ph.D. thesis, Osmania University, Hyderabad.

- Nagabhushanam, R. & Sambasiva Rao. K. 1983. Effect of monocrotophos on oxygen consumption of freshwater prawn *Caridina rajadhari;* VI All India Symp. Comp. Anim. Physiol, Jaipura, 10-12, March.

- Nagabhushanam, R., Gyananath. G. & Sarojini. R. 1983. Toxicity of three orgamophosphate compounds and their effect on the Gonad of freshwater Prawn. *Macrobrachium lamerrii.* And *J. Comp. Anim. Physiol.,* **1**: 71-75

- Neeraja Kumari, B. 1986. Studies on pyrethroid neutrotoxicity in the Freshwater Field crab, *Oziotelphusa sensex sensex,* (Fabricius) with special reference to neuroendocrine influence. Ph.D. Thesis. S.V. University, Tirupati.

- Neeraja Kumari, B. Yellamma. K. & Murali Mohan. P., 1987. Toxicological evaluation of fenvalerate as the freshwater field crab. *Oziotepphusa sensex* sensex. *Environment and Ecology,* **5**: 451-455

- Rajendra Prasad Naidu, K. & Padmanabha Naidu.B. 1989. Glucose Metabolism in the gill of *Oziotelphusa sensex sensex* (Fabricius) during endosulfan stress XI. All India Symp. Camp, Anim. Physiol. Nagpur 29-31 Janruary.

- Rajeswari, K. 1986. Effect of endosulfan toxicity on ion regulation in the freshwater crab. M.Phil. dissertation, S.V. University, Tirupati

- Ramachandran *et al.,* 1973. DDT and its Metabolites in Human body Fat in India; *Bull World Health Organ.;* **49**: 637.

- Renuka Devi, B. 1986. A comparative study of the toxicity of pesticide in an edible freshwater field crab, *Oziotelphusa sensex,* sensex Ph.D. Thesis, S.K.University, Ananthapur

- Renuka Devi, B. & Venkatachari, S.A.T. 1984. Comparative study of the toxicity of pesticides in an edible freshwate field crab. *Oziotelphusa senex* senex Ph.D. Thesis, S.K. University, Anantapur.

- Sharma, B.K. & Kaur. H. 1995. *"Environmental Chemistry"* 2ⁿᵈ Ed, Goel Publishing House, Meerut.

- Shepard, H.H., 1939. The Chemistry and toxicology of insecticides, Burgen Publication Co., Minneapolis, 383

- Sehrader, G. 1959. Unpublished speech given to the agricultural faculty, University of Bonn, Dec. 2, 1959. reported in holmstedt and liljestrand *op. Cit.,* (1963)

- Srinivasulu Reddy, M. & Ramana Rao., K.V. 1986. Acute toxicity of insecticides to penaeid prawns Environment and Ecology 4:221-223

- Surendra Babu, K., Siva Prasad Rao. K., Sreenivasa Babu.K., Ramana Rao. K.V. & Sasira Babu. K., 1983a. Correlation between the toxicity of elsan and AChE inhibition in selected tisues of the marine prawn *Metapenaeus monoceros*. VI All India Symp. Comp. Anim, Physiol, Jaipur. 10-12 March.

- Venkatachari, S.A.T. & Renuka Devi. B. 1984. Differential toxicity of three organophosphate pesticides to the freshwater crab, *Oziotelphusa senex senex* and its relation to size and sex. Nat. Symp. Ass. Environ. Pollut. Due to industrilization and urbanisation, Aurangabad, 20-22 December.

- Venkatachari, S.A.T., Gangotri. M.S. & Vasantha. N. 1987. Neuroendocine involvement in the regulation of lactate and succinate denydrogenase activities in the freshwater crab, *Barytelphusa guerini* (Milne Edwards) (Decapoda; Potamidea) *Curr. Sci.,* **56**: 1081-1083).

- Venkatachari, S.A.T., Venkteshwarlu. M. and Hussain. M.G. 1987. Toxicity of Monocrotophos Pesticide to the Freshwater Crab, *Berytelphusa guerini* (M. Edwards), Proc. of the Nat. Symp. on Environ. Pollut. and Pest. Toxicol. of Acad. of. Env. Biol held at Uni. of Jammu. Jammu. Dec. 10-12.

- Venkateshwarlu, M. 1999. Studies on Freshwater crab *Barytelphusa guerini* with special reference to the pesticidal impact. Ph.D. Thesis. Gulbarga Uni. Gulbarga.

- Wyland J.Hayes, Jr.Edward R.Laws, Jr *"Hand book of pesticide Toxicology"* Vol.1&3, Harcourt Brace Jovanovich Publication SanDiego, New York.

# 11

# Biochemical Effects of Pollutants on Fish

*G. Tripathi and Priyanka Verma*

## Introduction

The contamination of environment is called pollution in scientific language. It may also be defined as an addition or excessive addition of certain materials to the physical environment (water, air and land) which makes it harmful for the living organisms. However, pollutants are the materials which cause pollution of environment. Smokes from vehicles and industries, sewage from houses and hotels, radioactive substances from nuclear plants, discarded household articles and industrial wastes are the common pollutants. Not always the waste materials pollute the environment. Sometimes useful materials may also contaminate the environment. For instance nitrogen and phosphorus are used to enrich the soil for increased crop yields, but pollute the water if present in excess. Now environmental pollution has become a global problem and challenge to the scientists in particular.

Since the green revolution, enormous amount of pesticides have been used to save the crops from pests to meet the demands of growing population. In India, 125 pesticides are registered in agriculture and in public health programmes. Today most of the fresh waterbodies are being polluted by the increased production and utilization of pesticides and herbicides used in agricultural practices for pest control. Increased mining activities and industrial uses of the metals (Chandravarthy and Reddy, 1994) and disposals of waste from taxtile and dyeing industries, paper mills, petroleum refineries, dairy farms etc. are also polluting the aquatic environment. These pollutants contaminate rivers, lakes and ponds. The toxicants not only accumulate in fish but also in other organisms which contribute food for fishes (Butler *et al.*, 1970). Aquatic environments are effected not only by a single but also many pesticides, metals and organic wastes at a time. Such xenobiotics affect metabolic activities and alter, physiological state of organisms by changing important biochemical constituents of fishes. Certain metabolic disorders may sometimes cause death. Heavy mortality in aquatic organisms has been occasionally and sadly experienced in the past.

It is well known that agents responsible for pollution cause several biochemical alteration by affecting the enzyme system. For instance, the waste materials are commonly disposed or drained into the homes of fishes. These toxic waste materials in various ways are taken into the body of fishes and in turn may go in to the human body by eating them.

Therefore, it seems essential to review the toxic effects of pollutants on fish metabolism as they form an important part of human food because of being one of richest source of protein and also as a valuable link in the food chain of aquatic ecosystem. In this chapter we describe effects of various pollutants specially pesticides and heavy metals on biochemical make up of fishes (Fig. 11.1).

## Pollutants–Induced Metabolic Changes

In fishes, most of the toxic effects are due to poisoning of metabolism. Alterations in the biochemical values in fish due to environmental pollution provide an indication to understand the mode of action and type of pollutants. Accumulation of toxic substance in the body leads to physio-pathological and biochemical disorders. The variation in toxicity depends upon a number of factors. These factors are – species peculiarities (size, age, sex, physiological state, mode of breathing, starvation, parasitic infection), ecological peculiarities (temperature, pH, dissolve oxygen, $CO_2$, hardness of water) and pesticide specialties (rate of absorption, technical grade or commercial grade, rate of degeneration) (Dutta *et al.*, 1992). Generally poisoining occurs through pollutants–induced alteration in enzyme

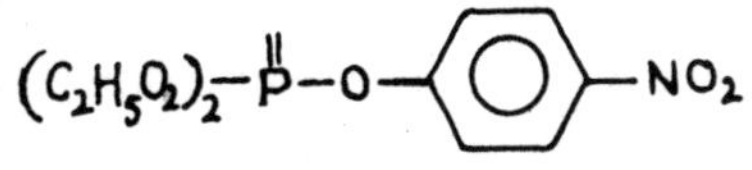

$(C_2H_5O)_2-\overset{O}{\overset{\|}{P}}-O-\langle\ \rangle-NO_2$

**Parathion**

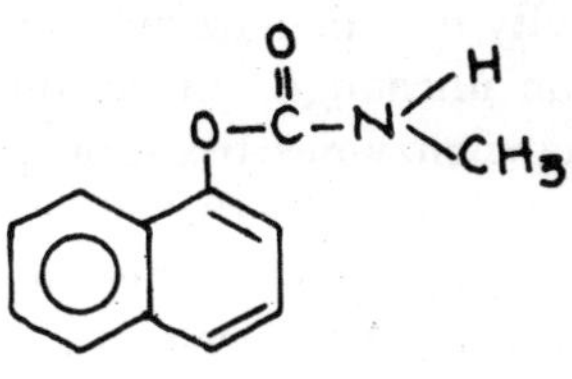

**Carbaryl**

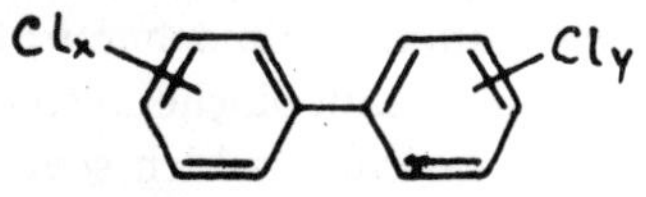

**Polychlorinated biphenyls**

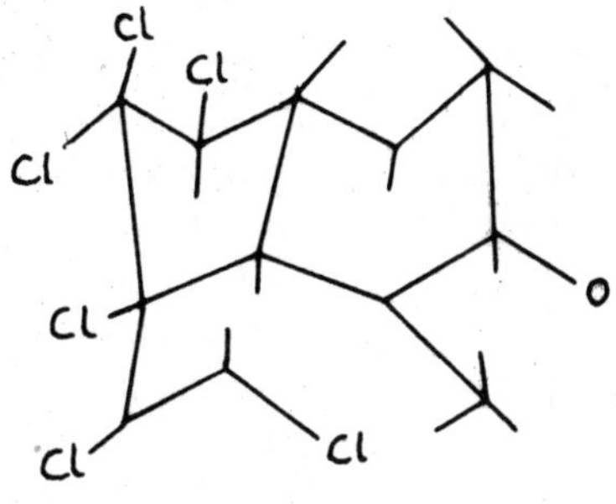

**Dieldrin**

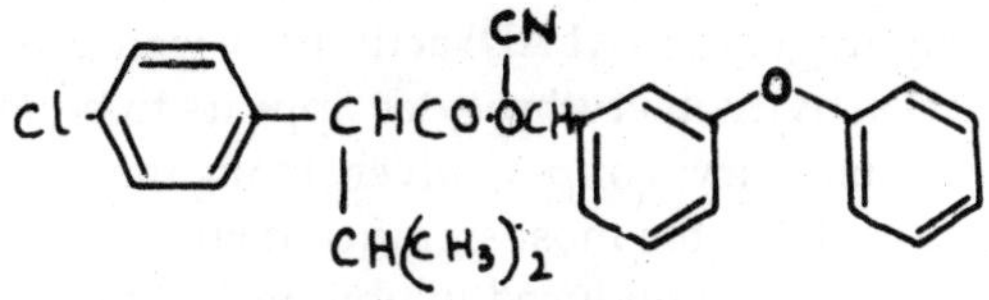

**Fenvalerate**

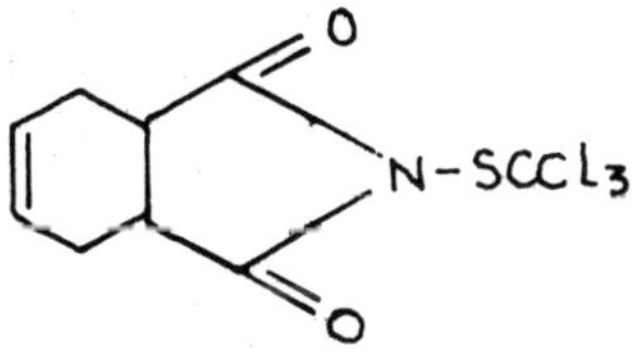

**Captan**

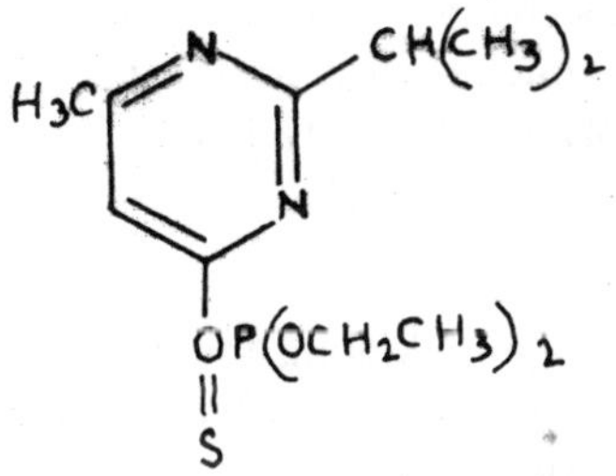

**Diazinon**

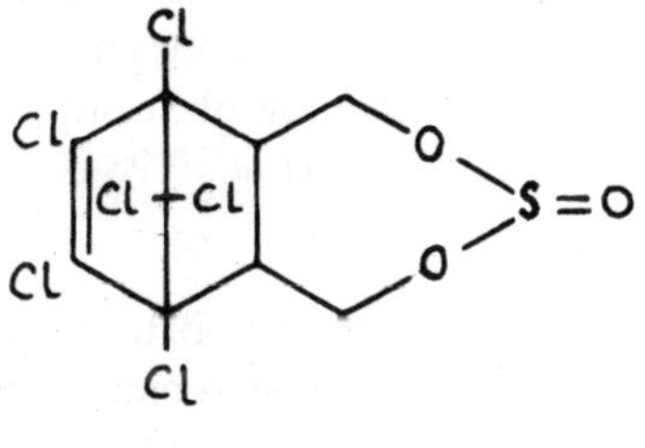

**Endosulfan**

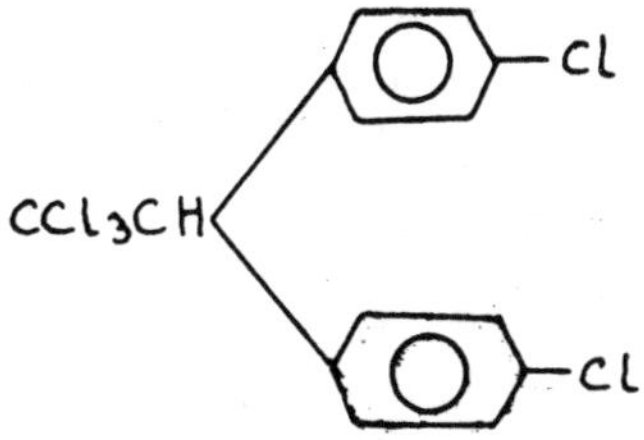

$CCl_3CH$

**DDT**

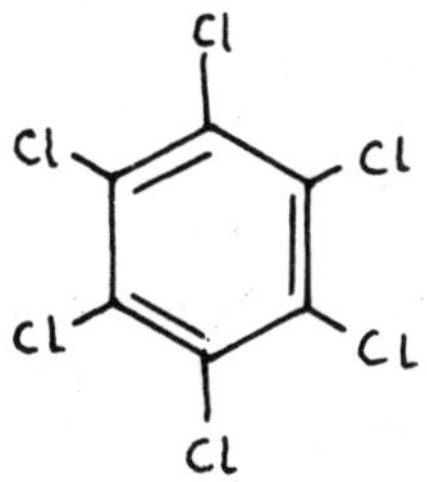

**BHC**

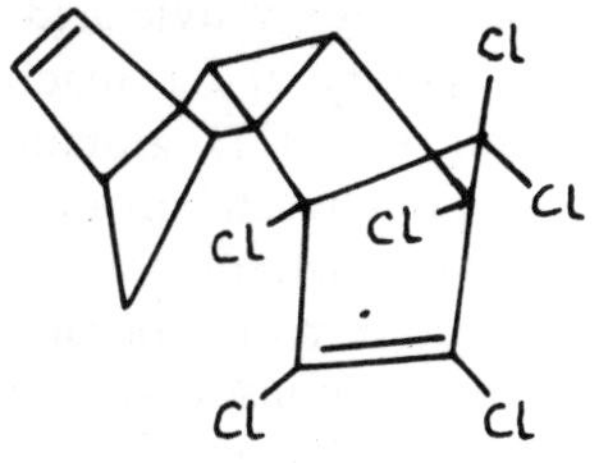

**Aldrin**

**Fig. 11.1.** Structural formulae of some pesicides.

systems. Pollutants increase the activity of some enzymes and decrease the activity of others, while the activities of few enzymes remain unchanged in various tissues of fishes. Enzymes mediated toxicological responses may be pollutant, enzymes, tissue or species–specific. It is inferred from several investigation that biochemical parameters could be effectively used to detect the effect of pollutants. Some important biochemical effects of pollutants in fishes have been reviewed in the present chapter. Certain toxicants which severely effect metabolic system have been described as follows:

## Lead

It is one of the heavy metal pollutants of the environment and a neurotoxic substance that cause behavioural dysfunction in fishes. The toxic effects of lead poisoning in fishes have been reviewed from time to time with reference to both haematological and biochemical variables. It is well known that high concentration of lead acts as cumulative general metabolic poison (WHO, 1977). It inhibits neural (Weber et al., 1983) and reproductive (Weber, 1993) activities in fishes. The reduction in D-aminolevulinic acid dehydrogenase. (ALAD) activity by lead is an example of a toxicant – induced response. Inhibition of ALAD activity in erythrocytes appears to be relatively specific for lead (Mehrle and Mayer, 1985). Although mercury, copper, silver, manganease, cadmium and zinc change the activity of ALAD in fish, but lead has the most significant effect (Hernberg and Nikkanen, 1972; Jackin, 1973; Hodson et al., 1977). The lead–induced inhibition of ALAD activity has been proposed as a short term indicator of long term toxicity in fish (Hodson 1976; Hodson et al., 1979). The protein and free amino acid were found to be decreased in gill and brain of Anabas scanden exposed to lead nitrate (Chandravarthy and Reddy, 1994). Exposure of fish to toxicants can cause change in rate of break down of erythrocytes, haemolysis and impairement of oxygen–carrying of haemoglobin, caused by oxidation of the molecule to methaemoglabin. The toxicants such as lead, cadmium, mercury, chloramine and pulpmill effluent can cause anaemia in fish. The exact mechanism is not known in every case. However, it is known that lead inhibits the enzyme delta–aminolevulinic acid dehydrogenase (ALAD) which is involved in synthesis of haemoglobin. Suppression of ALAD activity is used as a specific indicator of lead intoxication in fish (Hodson et al., 1984).

## Copper

Copper is another important aquatic pollutants. Among aquatic founa, fishes are one of the major group of vertebrates most sensitive to water pollution. Increase in lactate dehydrogenase (LDH) activity indicates that the rate of anaerobic glycolysis increases in copper exposed fish. Exposure to copper induces degeneration of gills causing reduction in oxygen availability which would necessitate shifting of energy metabolism towards anaerobic pathway. It also appears that aerobic oxidation of pyruvate through krebs cycle is adversely affected as revealed by inhibition in the activity of pyruvate dehydrogenase (PDH) and succinate dehydrogenase (SDH) in liver. Reduction in level of lactic acid in blood and liver and increase in pyruvic acid stand in support of this assumption. Increase in malate dehydrogenase (MDH) activity under anaerobic condition and elevation in the activities of glutamate oxalacetate transaminase (GOT), glutamate pyruvate transaminase (GPT) and decrease in protein level clearly indicate protein catabolism as a source of energy to the fish under copper stress. Decrease in xanthine oxidase (XO) activity shows retardation of purine metabolism and increase in GDH activity reflects increase in formation of ammonia (Sastry et al., 1997). The decrease in gill $ATP_{ase}$ activity has been reported in response to sublethal concentration of copper exposed to coho salmon (Lorz and McPherson, 1976). Asztalos and Nemcsok (1985) have found that the treatment of copper sulphate paraquat causes manifold increase in level of LDH in blood sera.

Metallothioneins are the important stress protein known throughout the living world. They are low molecular mass protein rich in cysteine and have ability to bind with IB and II B group metals

(Cu, Zn, Cd, Mg). They are primarily thought to function as regulators of the intracellular metabolism of copper and zinc. In fish, the elevation of metallothionein level is proportional to the degree of metal exposure (Hogstrand *et al.,* 1991)

## Cadmium

Cadmium is regarded as one of the most toxic metal pollutants having high toxicity at low concentration. It is found in small quantities in natural water and in the effluents of electroplating and paint industries. It has various routes of entry into the environment. Among other majer sources some agricultural practices such as phosphatic fertilizers, town–refuse composts application, sewage sludge disposal and mining, metal refining waste incineration and automobiles add cadmium into the environment. Most information available on cadmium toxicity is related to short term survival (Pickering and Gast, 1972; McCarthy *et al.*, 1978) apart from that dealing with the long term effect of exposure of fish to sublethal concentration (Spehor, 1976; Maza *et al.*, 1995). Liver and kidney are recognized as the major target tissues of cadmium toxicity (Friberg *et al.*, 1985). Sastry and Shukla (1990) reported decrease in the activity of glucose – 6 phosphatase and increase in the activities of hexokinase, lactate dehydrogenase and succinate dehydrogenase in liver and muscles of *Channa punctatus* chronically exposed to cadmium for 15 to 30 days. The enzyme activity decreases after 60 days of exposure of cadmium.

Cadmium produces marked alteration in the activity of different enzymes which varies with the period of exposure and the types of tissues. On chronic exposure to cadmium for 15 days an increase in the activity of lactate dehydrogenase in liver, gills, muscle and kidney indicates enhancement in rate of glycolysis. This increase may be correlated to cadmium–induced damage of the gill epithelium which can reduce the oxygen uptake capacity and bring about hypoxia in organs of vital importance (Gill *et al.*, 1988; Sastry and Shukla, 1993). Decrease in activity of pyruvate dehydrogenase (PDH) and succinate dehydrogenase (SDH) in liver and gills indicates oxygen stress, energy crisis and mitochondrial distrurbance. It also indicates that pyruvate is not metabolised aerobically. The level of lactate decrease and pyruvate increases in blood and liver. However, muscle lactate becomes elevated and the level of pyruvate is reduced.

Increase in muscle lactic acid may be due to inadequacy of oxygen supply to cells. Decrease in the level of lactic acid in blood and liver suggests that gluconeogenesis has been impaired (Sastry and Subhadra, 1982). Inhibition of the activity of succinate dehydrogenase (SDH) indicates that the aerobic metabolism has been impaired in liver and gill and the metal has a pronounced effects on oxidative metabolism of fish (Sastry and Shukla, 1994). Increase in malate dehydrogenase (MDH) activity indicates formation of malate from alternative sources, probably protien which may be increasingly metabolised to fullfill energy requirement of the fish under stressful environment. Increase in activity of transaminases (GPT and GOT) and decrease in protein level lend support to the above view. Such an increase in activity of transaminase is due to tissue damage. Increase in the activity of glutamate dehydrogenase (GDH) in all the tissues except gills shows that formation and excretion of ammonia is increased in cadmium exposed fish. Similarly, enhanced activity of xanthine oxidase (XO) in all the tissues show that metabolism of purines and formation of uric acid are increased in experimental fish. Inhibition of insuline secretion in cadmium treated striped mullet (*Mugil cephalus*) has also been reported (Thomas and Neff, 1985).

Wofford and Thomas (1988) reported that the exposure of striped mullet and Atlantic Croaket (*Micropogonias undulatus*) to either cadmium or the PCB mixture Aroclor 1254 increases the *in vitro* production of malondialdehyde in hepatic microsomal preparations. Malondialdehyde is a breakdown product which is used as an index of lipid peroxidation. In fact, exposure of fish to certain pollutants can cause lipid peroxidation, a chemical process resulting in the oxidative deterioration of polyunsaturated lipids in biological membrane and ultimately, cellular damage (Thomas, 1990).

The response of different enzymes to cadmium exposure is not similar. The activities of some enzymes are elevated while others are inhibited. Thus it can be said that the long term exposure to cadmium results increase in glycolysis and impairment of oxidative metabolism.

## Chromium

Chromium from industrial wastes can pollute water bodies including sea, coasts river mouth, ponds, ditches and so on. Chromium compounds have been reported to be toxic and carcinogenic (Forstner and Wittman, 1979; Venko, 1985). Studies on the toxicity of Cr (III) on some parameter in few freshwater teleosts have been reported by Patel and Sexena (1983). Sublethal effects of chromium in fish are directly related to the inhibition of various metabolic processes (Nath and Kumar, 1987). Chromium compound also cause renal failure leading to the loss of osmoregulatory ability and respiration in fish. It appears that this heavy metal ion depresses ion transport in several important osmoregulatory systems of teleosts (Olson et al., 1973), leading to structural damage to various organs, like gill, brain and kidney (Renfro et al., 1973). It also alters the membrane permeability of the intestinal epithelial cells and other layers of cells by altering the activity of $ATP_{ase}$, resulting in a breakdown of the active transport mechanism needed for the absorption of nutrient, ions and metabolites. It is possible that inhibition of $ATP_{ase}$ by Cr (VI) blocked the active transport system of the gill epithelial as well as chloride cells, glomerular and epithelial cells of the tubules and thus altered the osmoregulatory mechanism.

Gills of the fish are one of the first tissues which comes into direct contact to the external media and thus, Cr (VI) ion probably causes tremendous damage to this tissue. A fraction of the Cr (VI) is absorbed or crossed through gills into the circulation and reaches to various organs and tissues.

## Mercury

It is a very rare element found in the earth's crust and one of the most hazardous pollutants. It is the most potential biocide to aquatic fauna even at fairly low concentration. The concentration of mercury in freshwater world wide is increasing rapidly, almost doubling every decade with the discharge of effluents from the industries involved in the production of chlorine, caustic soda, paints, pesticides, fertilizers and electrical equipments (Shaw and Panigrahi, 1990). Mercury can readily accumulate in the soft tissues of aquatic fauna resulting increase in biotransport, distribution and toxicity (Patel et al., 1990). It may bind to high and low affinity sites of the DNA molecules and produces confirmational changes (Lavie and Eviater, 1988). It also effects nitrogen metabolism causing a progressive decrease in protein level on days 1 to 15 but the level regresses and attains almost normal value on days 30. Mercury increases the level of free amino acids and protease, hence, high activity of protease (a lysosomal enzyme) in the organs of fish might be due to the damage caused by mercury to lysosomes. The increase in free amino acids would also serve as a precursors for energy production under stress and for the synthesis of required proteins to face the metal challenge (Sreedevi et al., 1992). The impact of mercury on nitrogen metabolism is orgen dependent viz., more on liver, less on brain and intermediate on muscles (Sivaramakrishna and Radhakrishnaiah, 1998). The liver exhibited greater degree of changes as it is the centre for operation of various metabolic functions including the synthesis of metallothioneins, less degree of changes observed in the brain could partly be due to lower proteolytic activity in it and depressed de novo protein syntheis as reported by Sharma and Davis (1980).

Exposure to heavy metals including mercury promotes transcription of metallothionein gene. This property serves as a protective function during exposure to heavy metals by sequestering most of the free metal ions within the cell, thereby preventing them from binding to the sulphydryl groups of other functionally important proteins. Metallothionein levels in fish have been proposed as specific biochemical indicators of heavy metal contamination (Klavelr Kamp et al., 1989; Roesijadi et al., 1992).

## Ammonia

Ammonia is the major nitrogenous excretory product of teleost fish, that is lost from the body across the gills to the aqueous environment. Increase in deamination produces a significant elevation in the level of ammonia in liver and blood of the fish. Excess accumulation of ammonia in the blood could lead to ammonia toxicity. Part of excess ammonia is converted to less toxic urea (Rao et al., 1983) in liver because liver is the main organ where detoxification of the toxic substances takes place, thereby the urea level also increases significantly in the liver and blood. Increase in the urea level may serve as an ion regulator and prevent the flux of toxic metal ions from exterior to interior. Arillo et al., (1981) have reported elevated renin activity in rainbow trout after exposure to ammonia. Mock and Peters (1990) reported a decline in plasma lysozymes activity in rainbow trout after exposure to a high ammonia level.

## Organochlorine

Organochlorine compounds having carbon, hydrogen and chlorine as base molecular constituents. They are well known for their toxicological properties. Endosulfan, aldrine, dieldrin, DDT, BHC, lindane, heptachlor, etc. are commonly used to control various types of pests and pathogens. They produce toxic effects in non-target species including fishes. Among these endosulfan is a potential environmental pollutant due to its wide spread use in the control of over 100 agricultural insects, pests attacking 60 food and non-food crops (EPA, 1980). This insecticide belongs to cyclodiene group and is a central nervous system (CNS) poison, (Naqvi and Vaishnavi, 1993). Fishes are extremely sensitive to this compound and their toxicity generally increases with increasing temperature. It may cause massive mortalities in fishes. It produces marked changes in $Na^+$ and $K^+$ concentration, decrease the blood $Ca^{2+}$ and inhibits $Na^+$, $K^+$ and $Mg^{2+}$ dependent $ATP_{ase}$ in brain. Swarup et al., (1981) reported that freshwater fish, *Cirrhinus mrigala* exhibits a marked change in the sodium and potassium concentration of various tissues. Sodium concentration is also elevated in all the tissues of fish exposed to technical endosulfan. Endosulfan and its isomets have been shown to decrease the protein, glycogen and lipid contents of the liver and glycogen of the muscle in the freshwater fish *Channa punctatus* (Murty and Devi, 1982).

The activities of liver succinate dehydrogenase and cytochrome oxidase of black bullhead (*Ictalurus melas*) are inhibited by aldrin (Calvin and Phillips, 1968). It may cause various adverse effects on reproduction including decreased fertility and viability of the young ones (Vettorazzi, 1975). It is also known that long term feeding of aldrin may increase tumour formation at lower dosage. Dieldrin inhibits the activity of liver succinate dehydrogenase in rainbow trout (Mayer, 1971). The $ATP_{ase}$ system in fish is adversely affected by some environmental pollutants such as aroclors and polychlorinated terphenyl (Yap et al., 1971; Cutkomp et al., 1972; Koch et al., 1972). These compounds have greatest effects on $Mg^{2+} ATP_{ase}$ and lesser effects on $Na^+$ and $K^+ ATP_{ase}$. The $Na^+$, $K^+$ - $ATP_{ase}$ of rainbow trout is inhibited by DDT, dicofol, dieldrin, heptachlor, lindane, methoxychlor, perthane, strobane, thiodon, toxaphene and PCBs (aroclors 1242 and 1254) but not by endrin, mirex and 2,4-D (Davis and Wedemayer 1971; Davis et al., 1972).

Endosulfan insecticide is a polychlorinated compound used for controlling a variety of insect. It is practically water insoluble but readily adheres to clay particles. Endosulfan has been shown to increase the activity of alkaline phosphataes in the liver, muscles, kidney and brain of many species of freshwater teleost (Shafi, 1980). It has also been shown to inhibit the activity of $ATP_{ase}$ in several tissues of the freshwater teleosts. $ATP_{ase}$ in variation–dependent forms is a membrane–bound enzymes and responsible for the transport of ions through the membrane and thus regulates osmatic pressure, cellular volume and membrane permeability (Kundu et al., 1992) The activities of cytoplasmic malate dehydrogenase, mitochondrial malate dehydrogenase and lactate dehydrogenase are decreased in liver and muscle tissues of the freshwater catfish *Clarias batrachus* exposed to endosulfan (Tripathi and Shukla, 1990). Mishra and Shukla (1997) finding that endosulfan indicates a decline in the catalytic activity of LDH in the liver and the skeleton muscle, and but has no effect on total protein content. The enzyme LDH catalyzes the reversible reduction of pyruvate to lactate. LDH is used to detect tissue damage in fish for a long time (Kristofferson *et al.*, 1974; Nemcsok and Boross, 1982). The reduction in the activity of this enzyme may be due to nonproductive binding of endosulfan or its metabolite (S) with the enzyme moleculas and / or by blocking the enzyme synthesis. Endosulfa-induced reduction in the activities of ATP$_{ase}$, succinate dehydrogenase and mixed function oxidase has also been reported in vertebrates including fishes (Dalela *et al.*, 1978; Davis and Wedemeyer, 1971; Davis *et al.*, 1972).

It can be said that endosulfan interfers with fish protein metabolism or decrease the activity of fish (Day, 1984). A change in the rate of oxygen consumption indicates that the neurotoxicity of this compound is similar to other chlorinated hydrocarbon compounds.

The enzyme peroxidase plays an important role in the biosynthesis of the hormone, thyroxine. In this process it catalyzes the oxidation of inorganic iodide to active iodine in the first step and the oxidised iodine is subsequently incorporated into tyrosine moiety. Teleost lack a definite thyroid gland instead thyroid follicles are located in the kidney (Ahuja, 1962). The peroxidase activity primarily originates in these follicles to regulate the thyroid hormone synthesis. Thyroid hypofunction due to environmental toxicants such as carbon disulphide, organochlorines etc. may be mediated through inhibition of peroxidase. As thyroxine promotes growth, reproduction, osmoregulation and other important processes of life and is associated with iodinating peroxidase, an attempt has been made to study the effect of water pollution on the enzyme. In general the activity of the enzyme will be more in kidney than in other tissues like heart, gills, liver, spleen and ovary/testis, due to the presence of many thyroid follicles in it, thus, kidney in toleost plays an important role in the iodine metabolism of fish (Chitra and Kumar, 1997). The inhibition of peroxidase enzyme activity in fish by various industrial pollutants was reported by Mukherjee and Bhattacharya (1975). De and Bhattacharya (1976) showed that cytochrome-C could effectively reverse the inhibitory effect of industrial pollutants on fish thyroid peroxidase activity. The enzyme activity remains lower in the fish from polluted water as compared to those in the non-polluted water. In fact, fish from polluted or abnormal environments suffer from retarded growth and other physiological dysfunction due to thyroid deficiency. Environmental pollutants considerably depreas thyroid function in fish.

## Organophosphates

The use of organophosphorous pesticides has increased at a faster rate than organochlorine because of their high efficiency and biodegradebility. They are highly toxic and relatively unstable compound. The common organophosphates are malathion, parathion, carbophenothion, diazinen, chlorphyrifos, monocrotophos etc. They effect the synaptic points of nervous system of animals by intrfering with the action of the enzyme cholinesterase.

Methyl parathion is one of the most toxic insecticides belongs to the organophosphorus group. This compound has relatively short half–life in the environment and in the tissues of homeothermic animals. It causes dose dependent inhibition of brain and plasma cholinesterase activity, hyperglycemia and elevates plasma carticosterone concentration. The exposure of methyl parathion to the freshwater fish, *Tilapia mossambia* for 48 hours. decrease the level of succinate and lactate dehydrogenase, glycogen and total carbohydrate content in gills, liver and muscle tissues (Rao and Rao, 1979). The treatment of organophosphates of fishes inhibits the activities of several enzymes such as glucose – 6 phosphates, acid phosphatese, pyruvate dehydrogenase, succinate dehydrogenase and cholinesterase in the brain and acetylcholinesterase as well as cytochrome oxidase in the brain, kidney, gill, liver and muscle (Sastry and Sharma, 1980; Natarajan , 1984). Sastry and Sharma (1980) shows that the activity of alkaline phosphates, $ATP_{ase}$ and lactate dehydrogenase remain unaltered in brain of *Ophiocephalus punctatus* after 15 days of the exposure of an organophosphate pesticide. The sublethal concenteation of methyl parathion inhibits 30-55 per cent activity of cytoplasmic MDH, mitochondrial MDH and LDH of the liver and skeletal muscle after 7 days of the exposure of this pesticide to a freshwater cat fish *Clarias batrachus* (Tripathi and Shukla, 1990). The activities of these enzymes recovers after 7 days and reach the control level on the 28th days. The inhibition caused by the pesticides may be due to binding of methyl parathion (or their metabolities) with enzyme molecules and/or by blocking the enzyme synthesis. The recovery in the enzyme activity after 7 days in methyl parathion exposed individuals may be a kind of metabolic adaptation involving synthesis of the enzymes and/or degradation of the pesticides. The withdrawal of this pesticide from the medium after one week of exposure restores the activities of the enzymes to control level. The recovery may be due to dissociation of parathion (or their metabolites) from the enzyme molecules and / or by fresh synthesis of the enzymes. The treatment of actinomycin D and cycloheximide inhibits completely or partially the withdrawal–dependent increase in the activity of all the three metabolic enzymes. It has been suggested that the treatment of methyl parathion reduces the efficiency of energy production and protein synthesis.

Acetylcholinesterase is an enzyme which modulates the quantity of neurotransmitter acetylcholine in the nervous system. It is sensitive to particular forms of pollution stress. Malathion, parathion and other organophosphate insecticides inhibit the activity of acetylcholinesterase. Measurement of this enzyme is used to detect organophosphate poisoning of fish in field (Coppage et al., 1975). It has been reported that collagen deposition in skeletal tissues of fish is markedly reduced if exposed to a variety of pollutants such as organochlorine and organophosphate pesticides, producing changes in the mechanical properties of the skeleton (Pavlov et al., 1990). Such a biochemical change result in the "broken back" syndrome in which muscular contraction causes fractures in the weakened skeletal system (Mehrle and Mayer, 1975). Barron and Adelman (1984,1985) showed supperession of the RNA/DNA ratio in fathead minnows (*Pimephales promelas*) in response to exposure of a variety of toxicants.

Oraganophosphorus insecticides are highly toxic to birds and small mammals for a brief period after application, occasionally affecting local wildlife populations.

## Carbamates

The carbamate pesticides are relatively lesser toxic to organochlorines and commonly used in argicultural practices. They are known to inhibit the activity of acetylcholinesterase in fish. In most salmonids inhibition of acetylcholinesterase alters respiration, swimming, feeding and social interaction (Klaverkamp et al., 1977; Post and Leisure, 1974; Bull and McInery, 1974). Inhibition of brain acetylcholinesterase in fish has been used to detect the pollution of pesticides in natural water (Williams and Sova, 1966; Holland et al., 1967) but the explanantion between the relation of inhibition to exposure and death is controversial (Cox 1968; Gibson et al., 1969). The pesticide induced death of fish in laboratory occurs due to loss of activity of acetylcholinesterase from 54 per cent to 92 per cent to that of its activity normal in brain tissue (Weiss, 1961). However, the fishes have been survived at activities as low as 10-20°C of normal (Weiss, 1961; Gibson et al., 1969).

Impact of various xenobiotics on fish has been throughly described (Kennedy, 1995). Similarly, biochemical effects of stress including toxicant induced responses have been well documented (Pickering and Pottinger, 1995). Environmental impacts of agricultural pesticides have also been assessed (Levitan *et al.*, 1995). Nemcsok and Benedeczky (1995) have nicely reviewed the pesticide metabolism and the adverse effects of metatoblites of fishes. There is sufficient experimental exigence for transport of pesticides through field soild (Flury, 1996) and such transport has serious effects on aquatic ecosystem.

Cytochrome P-450 isoenyzmes (Phase II enzymes) are ethoxyresorufin O-deethylase (EROD), aryl hydrocarbon hydroxylase (AHH), testosterone 6B – hydroxylase (T6H), fatty acid hydroxylase (FAH) etc. They are a multigene family whose isoforms exhibit differing but often overlapping, substrate specificities for compounds of both endogenous and exogenous origin. These enzymes in liver of fish can also be selectively induced by exposure of various pollutants (Leaver *et al.*, 1992).

## Synthetic Pyrethroids

Discoveries of new synthetic insecticides have sparked exciting advancement in the control of insect enemies. Modern insecticides are effective, reliable and cheap but their frequent usage have reduced their effectiveness against different domestic and agricultural pests due to increasing resistance problem. The use of pesticides to control agricultural pests is now increasing every day. Synthetic pyrethroids are presently used as alternative to organochlorine, organophosphate and carbamate insecticides because of their improved potential stability as well as their low mammalian toxicity (Sogorb *et al.*, 1988). These compounds have relatively short half-lives in the environment and in the tissues of homeothermic animals. They are highly effective at lower temperature in controlling unwanted animal life such as mosquitoes, flies, midges and agricultural pests. Toxic effects of cypermethrin (a synthetic pyrethroid) on the activity of GOT, GPT and LDH in liver, kidney and heart in response to sublethal concentration exposed to fish show marginal changes over that of their control values. The alteration in transaminase and dehydrogenase activity in cypermethrin treated fish may be due to server cellular damage leading to the release of these enzymes and impaired carbohydrate and protein metabolism. Changes in transaminase are stress mediated (Knox and Greengard, 1965). The increase in GOT activity over their control in heart, liver and kidney upto 12th day represents necrosis in tissues leading to increase in the activity of transaminase. The increase in GOT and GPT activity indicates preponderance of anaerobic nature of carbohydrate *metabained* in fish, possibly to meet the increased energy demands under sustained and prolonged toxic stress. Increased LDH activity, indicating cell nerosis as pointed by Nemcsok *et al.*,(1985), may be also due to the injuries of gill epithellium resulting in oxygen depletion in fish, and to the fact that the decomposition process of energy supplying glucose changed in to lactate production (Sivakumari *et al.*, 1997).

The use of highly potent and photable pyrethroid pesticides have been on the increase during the last decade (Elliott, 1977). Pyrethroids are being promoted for a variety of large scale pest control programmes in agriculture, forestry and public health because of their high potency and photostability (Khan, 1983). Among the pyrethroids the neurotoxic organic insecticides fenvalerate (Cyano–3 phenoxy phenye) methyl 4 chloro (1 methythyl benzene acetate) is used extensively for the control of infection of boll weevil, *Anthonomon grandis* and boll worm, *Heliothis* zea on cotton, tabacco plants and vegetables (Sarthwick *et al.*, 1983). Fenvalerate intoxication indicates effects on nervous system, respiratory structure and renal ion regulation. It has been suggested that fenvalerate may have adverse effects on gill structure and could cause disruption in oxygen uptake and ion balance and may contribute to the increase in ventilation volume and decrease in oxygen uptake efficieny. Radaiah *et al.*, (1989) studied the toxic effect of fenvalerate on aldolase activity in fish and observed that the activity of aldolase increases with the duration of exposure in various tissues such as liver, kidney, gill and brain. It shows maximum increase in liver.

# Stress Responses

Pollutant-induces various stress responses in fish. The stress response deals with an integrated pattern of adjustment to the physiology and behaviour of animal which promotes the best chance of survival in the face of a noxious or threatering situation. According to Pickering (1993) the stress response is characterized by a switch from an anabolic to a catabolic state, there by providing the fish with the necessary resources to avoid or overcome the immediate threat, and has evolved as an adaptive response to short–term, or acute stress. If the fish is faced with a continuous, or chronic, stress from which there is no escape such as sublethal pollution etc., the adaptive value of the response is compromised. It is important to recognize that the stress response in the individual fish involves adjustments at all levels of organizations including molecular, biochemical, physiological, structural and behavioural. These result in effects at the population and ecosystem level (Bartell, 1990; Shuter, 1990).

The precise form of the stress response, both in quantitative and qualitative terms, varies according to the nature of the stress. But it is generally accepted that there is a core component of endocrinological and physiological changes which is a common feature of the response to most, if not all, forms of environmental stress (Pickering and Pottinger, 1995). Traditionally, changes in growth, mortality rate and reproductive success have been used as indicators of environmental stress. However, this approach is not advantageous because irreversible damage to fish population may have occurred before any remedial action can be taken. Therefore, attention has recently been given to some of the biochemical changes associated with stressed fish, because of their potential value in providing a sensitive, early indication of environmental problems. Pickering and Pottinger (1995) have suggested that most forms of stress activate a primary, neuroendocrine, response involving stimulation of the sympathetico–chromaffin system and hypothalamic–pituitary–interrenal (HPI) axis in particular, but also many other components of the endocrine system. This response has far reaching secondary consequences for all aspects of the fish biology as it switches from predominantly anabolic to catabolic pathways. In the short–term such changes are of adaptive value by virtue of mobilizing reserves and providing the fish with sufficient energy to avoid or overcome the immediate threat. In addition to stimulating the neuroendocrine components of the stress response, certain forms of stress such as due to exposure of pollutants etc. may also induce detoxification systems or cause direct cellular demage.

Overall it can be said that pollutants remarkably changes the biochemical constituents in the body of fish (Table 11.1). It must be remembered that a biochemical approach to detect and measure pollutant induced stress responses is a very important window to view the wider issues of stress biology for future perspectives and accomplishments.

Pollution has become a major global problem. Everyday tons of pollutants are released into aquatic environment. Heavy metals and pesticides are not present as a natural pollutant in the atmosphere but are introduced in te air as a result of industrialization and undesirable human activities. They are disturbing the delicate ecological balance and fish metabolism is greatly affected. Pollution of environment by heavy metals and pesticides is of prime importance. Unrestrained release of heavy metals and pesticides in environment *via* discharges of industrial effluents, sewage and agrochemicals into water resources has not only rendered it unusable but at the same time has produced great harm to fish. Direct binding of the heavy metal to enzyme protein leads to formation of protein metal complex. Heavy metals are also capable of displacing metal situated at the active site of enzymes, thus normal functioning of cell is distrubed and this in turn decrease the enzyme activity. Extensive use of pesticides has resulted into agricultural development and maximum crop production. But on the other hand, during rainy season these pesticides drain into water bodies thus causing pollution hazards to aquatic life. These pesticides accumulate in fishes and in turn hamper human health too via ecological cycling and biological

## Table 11.1 : Effect of pollutants on biochemical constituents in fish

| Pollutant | Tissue | Biochemical Constituent | Reference |
|---|---|---|---|
| 1. Lead | Brain and Gill<br>RBC | ⇓ Protein and free amino acid<br>⇓ δ- aminolevulinic acid dehydrogenase (ALAD) | Chandravarthy and Reddy,<br>(1994.) Hodson et al., (1984) |
| 2. Copper | Liver | ⇓ SDH and PDH<br>⇓ Protein level and X O<br>⇑ MDH, LDH, GOT and GPT | Sastry et al., (1997) |
| 3. Cadmium | Liver and muscle<br><br>Liver and Gill<br>All the tissue<br>except gill | ⇓ G-6-PDH<br>⇑ Hexokinase, LDH and SDH<br>⇓ PDH and SDH<br>⇑ MDH, GDH, GOT, XO and GPT<br>⇓ Protein level · | Sastry and Shukla (1990)<br><br>Sastry and Shukla (1994)<br>Thomas and Neff (1985). |
| 4. Chramium | Kidney Brain<br><br>Gill and Instestine | Loss of osmoregulatory ability,<br><br>Depress ion transpotation, Alter membrane permeability and Altering activity of ATP$_{ase}$ | Renfro et al., (1973) |
| 5. Mercury | | ⇓ Total Protein level<br>⇑ Level of amino acid and protease | Sreedevi et al., (1992) |
| 6. Ammonia | Plasma<br>Liver and Blood | ⇓ Plasma lysozymes activity<br>⇑ Urea level serve as an ion regulator | Mock and Peters (1990)<br>Rao et al., (1983). |
| 7. Organochlorine<br>a. Endosuflan | Liver<br>Muscles<br>Blood<br>Brain | Protein, glycogen and lipid content.<br>⇓ Glycogen<br>⇓ Blood Ca+2 level<br>⇓ Na+, K+ and Mg2+ dependent ATP$_{ase}$ | Murty and Devi (1982)<br>Naqvi and Vaishnavi (1993) |
| Endosulfan | Liver and Muscles | Cytoplasmic MDH, Mitochondrial MDH and LDH | Tripathi and Shukla (1990) |
| Endosulfan | Liver and Muscle | ⇓ LDH<br>⟺ Total protein | Mishra and Shukla (1997). |
| b. Aldrin | Liver | ⇓ SDH and Cytochrome oxidase | Calvin and Phillips (1968) |
| c. Dieldrin<br>8. Organophosphates | Liver | ⇓ SDH | Mayer (1971) |
| a. Methyl Parathion | Gill, Liver and Muscle<br><br>Liver and Muscles<br>Brain | ⇓ SDH, LDH, Glycogen and total carbohydrate<br><br>⇓ 30-55% activity of c- MDH, m–MDH and LDH<br>⟺ Alkaline Phosphates, ATP$_{ase}$ and LDH | Rao and Rao (1979)<br>Tripathi and Shukla (1990).<br><br>Sastry and Sharma (1980) |
| 9. Carbamates | Brain | ⇓ Acetylcholinesterase | William and Sava (1966)<br>Holland et al., (1967) |
| 10. Synthetic Pyrethroids<br>a. Cypermethrin | Liver, Kidney<br>and heart | Marginal change on activity of GOT, GPT and LDH | Knox and Greengard (1965). |
| b. Fenvalerate | Liver, Kidney,<br>Brain and Gill | ⇑ Aldolase Activity | Radaiah et al., (1989). |

maginification. The toxicity of pollutants depends on a number of factor including species peculiarities, ecological peculiarities and pesticide specialties. Exposure of fish to toxicants may induce detoxification system or cause direct cellular damage. Use of biochemical approach may provide an early warning of potentially damaging changes in stressed fish.

Almost all pollutants either interact directly with the enzyme system or effect their synthesis and degradation in cells. They cause some serious abnormalities in biological system leading to ill health and sometimes death. So studies regarding the effects of pollutants on metabolism is important to prevent fish mortality. As a precautionary measure all types of waste discharge should be properly treated. Any spillage or unused product should not be allowed to spread to vegetation or waterways and should be properly disposed of. Let us hope in the near future we will be able to control this serious worldwide problem with scientific approach and public awareness.

## SUMMARY

Rapid growth of human population and industrialization is directly or indirectly affecting the aquatic ecosystems. Thousands of tons of hazards toxicants are released everyday in the environment. Most of them are highly toxic and non-biodegradable. They have a longer persistence and affect non-target species and also causes ecological imbalance. Among aquatic founa fishes are most sensitive group for pollutants. Such biocides find their way with runoff water and adversely affect homes of fishes. Toxicants greatly affect fish metabolism and poison the biochemical machinery. Pesticides and heavy metals decrease the concentration of some biomolecules and increase the concentration of others. However, the concentration of some biochemical constituents remain unchanged. Alterations in biochemical make up of an organism hamper metabolic activity leading to serious abnormalities and some times death. At this crucial juncture knowledge about biochemical effects of pollutants provides an opportunity to save the life of fishes and in turn human health too.

## GLOSSARY

*Acetylcholinesterase* – The enzyme present in synaptic cleft that hydrolyzes acetylcholine to choline and acetic acid.

*Acid Phosphatases* – Enzyme that catalyze hydrolysis of an orthophorphoric monoester to an alcohol and orthophosphate and have acidic pH optima.

*Acute Toxicity* – A relatively short term lethal or other effect, usually defined as occuring with 4 days for fish and macroinvertebrates and shorter times for smaller organisms.

*Adenosine Triphosphate (ATP)* – An energy rich nucleotide conenzyme that takes part in many biological reactions. It contains a base adenine, a pentose sugar ribose and 3 inorganic phosphates. ATP reacts with water in the presence of phorphorylase to form ADP, phosphate and release energy which is utilized for various body function.

*Alkaline Phosphatase* – A hydrolytic enzyme which catalyzes the removal of 5' – phosphate residue from nucleic acid.

*Anabolism* – Chemical upbuilding of complex sustances by protoplasm.

*Catabolism* – Part of metabolism dealing with decomposition of complex substances into simple ones with release of energy.

*Chronic Toxicity* – Long term effects that may be related to changes in appetite, growth, metabolism, repoduction and even death or mutations.

*Cycloheximide* – It is a glutarimide antibiotic from *Streptomyces griseus* and effective inhibitor of cytoplosmic (not mitochondrial) protein synthesis in eukaryotes. It binds to a 60 S subunit of ribosome and primarily blocks the translocation step of translation which is dependent an elongation factor (EF2).

*Cytochrome* – A hemoprotein acting as an electron carrier.

*Cytochrome P 450* – It is one of the family of heme monoxygenases catalyzing oxidation of a wide variety of structurally diverse compound.

*Dehydrogenase* – Catalyses reaction involving electron transfer to or from an external electron carrier (NAD or NADP).

*Enzyme*–Organic substance that brings about acceleration of chemical reaction without itself undergoing any change.

*Exposure Time* – Time of exposure of test organism to test solution.

*Fish* - Fishes are essentially aquatic and jaw bearing vertebrates. They are characterized by the presence of gills for respiration and paired fins for swimming.

*Glucokinase (Hexokinase)* – An enzyme that catalyses the conversion of glucose-6-phosphate utilizing a molecule of ATP.

*Haemolysis* – Escape of haemoglobin from red blood corpuscles owing to damage to surface membrane.

*Heavy Metal* – Those element in which d-orbit is half filled or unfilled. It is also called as transition element, e.g., Zn, Cu, Ni, Pd, Cd, Fe, Cr.

*Lactate Dehydrogenase* – The enzymes which reversibly catalyzes conversion of lactate to pyruvate in presence of a coenzyme (NAD / NADH).

*Lethal Concentration (LC)* – Toxicant concentration producing death of test ogranism. Usually defined as median (50 per cent) lethal concentration, LC 50, *i.e.*, concentration killing 50 per cent of exposed organisms at a specific time of observation, for example, 96-h LC50.

*Metabolism* – Sum total of chemical reactions, both anabolic and catabolic that occur in living cells.

*Metallothionein* – It refers to a collective name for a group of cysteine rich, low molecular mass (Mr 6600) proteins that bind heavy metals (specially zinc ions) and have a role in homeostasis and detoxification.

*Peroxidase* – Catalyze the oxidation of an organic or inorganic substance by $H_2O_2$.

*Pesticides* – A chemical used to kill pest organism.

*Pollutants* – Any substance chemical, physical, biological etc. which produces harmful effects in the environment is called a pollutant.

*Pollution* – An undesirable change in the chemical and biological characteristics of our air, land and water, that will harmfully affect human life.

*Toxicant* – Poison, chemical exhibiting toxicity.

*Toxicity* – Adverse effect to a test organism caused by pollutants, generally a poison or mixture of poisons. Toxicity are classified according to duration – short term, intermediate/or long term. It is a resultant of concentration and time, modified by variables such as temperature, chemical form and availability.

*Xenobiotics* – Compound foreign to an organism.

# REFERENCES

- Ahuja, S.K. (1962). Thyroid follicles in the kidney of carps. *Curr. Sci.* **31**: 466.
- Arillo, A., Biancamaria U., and Vallarino, M. (1981). Renin activity in rainbow trout (*Salmo gairdneri*) and effect of environmental ammonia. *Comp. Biochem. Physiol.* **68**:307-311.
- Asztalos, B., and Nemcsok, J. (1985). Effect of pesticides on the LDH activity and isoenzyme pattern of carp (*Cyprinus carpio*) sera. *Comp. Biochem. Physiol.* **82**:217-219.
- Barron, M.G., and Adelman I.R. (1984). Nucleic acid, protein content and growth of larval fish sublethally exposed to various toxicant *Can. J. Fish. Aquatic Sci* **41**: 141-150.
- Barron, M.G., and Adelman I.R. (1985). Temporal characterization of growth of fathead minnow (*Pimephales promelas*) larvae during sublethal hydrogen cyanide exposure. *Comp Biochem. Physiol.* **81** C: 314-344.

● Bartell, S.M. (1990). Ecosystem context for estimating stress. Induced reductions in fish population. *Am Fish. Sec. Symp.* **8**: 167-182.

● Bull, C.J., and MC Inerny, J.E. (1974). Behaviour of juvenile coho salmon exposed to sumithion, an organophosphate insecticide. *J. Fish. Res. Board. Can.* **31**: 1867-1872.

● Butler, P.A., Childress R. and Jr. Wilson A.J., (1970). In FAO Tech. Conference on marine pollution and its effects on living resources and fishing. Rome. Italy, Dec. 9-18, 13.

● Calvin, H.J. and Phillips, A.T. (1968). Inhibition of electron transport enzymes and cholinesterase by endrin. *Bull Environ. Contam. Toxicol.* **3**: 106-113.

● Chandravthy V.M. and Reddy S.L.N. (1994). *In vivo* recovery of protein metabolism in gill and brain of a freshwater fish, Anabas scandens after exposure to lead nitrate. *J Environ Biol.* **15**: 75-82.

● Chitra, K.V. and Kumar N.S.R. (1997). Effect of water pollution on peroxidase activity in fish, Channa gachua, *J. Environ Biol.* **18**: 191-194.

● Coppage, D.L., Matthews, E., Cook, G.H., and Knight, J. (1975). Brain acetylecholinestarase inhibition in fish as a diagnosis of environmental poisoning by malathion, O,O-dimethyl S (1,2-dicarboxyethyl) phosphorodithinate. *Pestic. Biochem. Physiol.* **5**: 536-542.

● Cox, W.S. (1968). Enforcing insecticide content water quality standards. *Science.* **159**: 1123-1124.

● Cutkomp, L.K., Yap, H.H., Desaiah, D. and Koch, R.B. (1972). The sensitivity of fish ATP$_{are}$ to polychlorinated biphenyls. *Environ. Health Perspect.* **1**: 165-168.

● Dalela, R.C., Bhatnagar, M.C., Tyagi, A.K. and Verma, S.R., (1978). Adenosine triphosphatase activity in few tissues of a freshwater teleost, Channa gochua, following *in-vivo* exposure to endosulfan. *Toxicology* **11**: 361.

● Davis P.W. and Wedemeyer G.A. (1971). Na+, K+ activated ATP$_{ase}$ inhibition in rainbow trout : A site for organochlorine pesticide toxicity; *Comp. Biochem. Physiol.* **40**: 823-827.

● Davis P.W., Friedhaff J.M. and Wedemeyer G.A. (1972). Organochlorine insecticides, herbicide and polychlorinated biphenyl (PCB) inhibition of Na+, K+, ATP$_{ase}$ in rainbow trout, *Bull. Environ. Contam. Toxicol.* **8**: 69-72.

● Day, A.C.(1984). Distribution of malate dehydrogenase in different tissues of rainbow trout. Salmo gairdneri of different ages. *Comp. Biochem. Physiol.* **77** B: 675-678.

● De, S.N. and Bhattacharya, S. (1976). Effect of some industrial pollutants on fish thyroid peroxidase activity and role of cytochrome C there on. *Ind. J. Exp. Biol.* **14**:561-563.

● Dutta H.M., Munshi. J.S., Roy P.K., Singh W.K. and Richmonds C.R. (1992). Variation in toxicity of malathion to air and water breathing teleost. *Bull Environ Contam. Toxicol.* **49**: 279 284.

● Elliott, M. (1977). Synthetic pyrethroids. In M. Elliott, ed. Synthetic pyrethroids. American chemical society symposium series 42. Washington, D.C. 1-28.

● EPA, Environmental Protection Agency (1980). Ambient water quality criteria for endosulfan. *Env. Res. Lab.* Gulf Breeze, FLA, Rept. No. 4405-80-046, 108.

● Flury, M. (1996). Experimental evidence of transport of pesticides through field soils – A review. *J. Environ. Quality.* **25**: 25-45.

● Forstner, U., and Wittman, G.T.U. (1979). Metal pollution in the aquatic environment, Springer Verlag, New York, 486-532.

● Friberg, L., Kjellstorm, T., Elinder, C.G., and Norberg, G.F. (1985). Cadmium and health : A toxicological and epidemiological appraisal, Vol. I (CRC press. Boca Raton, FL) 248.

● Gibson, R.F., Ludke, J.L., and Ferguson, D.E. (1969). Sources of error in the use of fish-brain acetylcholinesterase as a monitor for pollution. *Bull. Environ. Contam. Toxicol.* **4**: 17-23.

● Gill, T.S., Pant, J.C., and Tewari, H. (1988). Bronchial pathogenesis in a freshwater fish Puntius conchonius, chronically exposed to sublethal concentration of cadmium. *Ecotoxicol. Environ. Safety.* **15** : 153-161.

● Hernberg, S. and Nikkanen, J. (1972). The effect of lead on 6 – animolevulinic acid dehydrogenase *Prac. Lek.* **24**: 77-83.

● Hodson, P.V. (1976). A -Aminolevulinic acid dehydrotase activity in fish blood as an indicator of a harmful exposure to lead. *J. Fish. Res. Board Can.* **33**: 268-271.

- Hodson, P.V., Blunt, B.R. Spray, D.J and Austen, K (1977). Evaluation of erythrocyte deltaaminolevulinic acid dehydratase activity as a short-term indicator in fish of a harmful exposure to lead. *J. Fish. Res. Board.Can.* **34**: 501 – 508.

- Hodson, P.V., Blunt, B.R., Jensen, D., and Morgan, S. (1979). Effect of fish age on predicted and observed chronic toxicity of lead to·rainbow trout in lake ontario water. *J. Great Lakes Res.* **5**: 84-89.

- Hodson, P.V., Blunt, B.R., and Whittle, D.M. (1984). Monitoring lead exposure of fish. In : contaminant Effects on fisheries, edited by V.W. Cairns, P.V. Hodson and J.O. Nriagu, New York, NY, John Wiley and Sons. 87-98.

- Hogstrand, C., Litner G. and Haux C. (1991). The importance of metallothionein for the accumulation of copper, zinc and cadmium in environmentally exposed perch, *Perca fulviatils, Pharmacol. Toxicol.* **68**: 492-501.

- Holland, H.T., Coppage, D.L. and Butler, P.A. (1967). Use of fish brain acetylcholinesterase to monitor pollution by organophosphorus pesticides. *Bull. Environ. Contam. Toxicol.* **2**: 156-162.

- Jackin. E. (1973). Influence of lead and other metals on fish A-aminolevulinate dehydrase activity. *J. Fish. Res. Board* Can. **30**: 560-562.

- Kennedy, C.J. (1995). Xenobiolics – Bioche. *Mole. Biol. Fishes* (Ed. P.W. Hochachka and T.P. Mommsen) **5**: 281-312.

- Khan, N. Y. (1983). An assessment of the hazard of synthetic pyrethroid insecticides to fish and fish habitat. In pesticide chemistry – Hyman welfare and environment (Eds : J. Miyamoto and P.C. Kearney) 1$^{st}$ Ed., vol. 3 : 437-450.

- Kalverkamp, J.F., Duangsawadsi, M., McDonald, W.A., and Majewski, H.S. (1977). An evaluation of fenitrothion toxicity in four life stages of rainbow trout, *Salmo gairdneri*. In Aquatic Toxicology and Hazard Evaluation (F.L. Mayer,and J.L. Hamelink, Eds.) ASTM STP **634**: 231-240.

- Klaverkamp, J.E., Macdonald W.A., Duncan D.A. and Wageman R. (1984). Metallothionein and acclimation to heavy metals in fish; a review. In : Contaminant Effects on fisheries, edited by V.W. Cairns, P.V. Hodson and J.O. Nriagu, NewYork, NY, John Wiley and Sons, 99-113.

- Knox, W.L. and Greengard, O. (1965). In an introduction to Enzyme Physiology. Pergamon Press, New York, Vol. **3**: 247.

- Koch, R.B., Desaiah, D., Yap H.H. and Cutkamp. L.K. (1972). Polychlorinated biphenyls. Effect of long term exposure of ATP$_{ase}$ activity in fish, *Pimephales promelas. Bull. Environ. Contain Toxicol.* **2**: 87-92.

- Kristafferson, R., Broberg, S., Oikari, A., and Pekkainen, M.(1974). Effect of sublethal concentration of phenol on some plasma enzyme activities in the pike (*Esox lucius* L.) in brackish water. *Ann. Zool. Fennici.* **11**: 220-223.

- Kundu, R. Lakshmi, R. and Mansuri, A.P. (1992). The entry of mercury through the membrane: an enzymological study using a tolerant fish Boleophthalmus dentatus. *Proc. Acad. Environ. Biol.* **1**: 1-6.

- Lavie, B., and Eviater, N. (1988). Multilocus genetic resistance and susceptability to mercury and cadmium pollution in the marine gastropode Cerithium scabridum. *Aquatic. Toxicol.* **13**: 291-296.

- Leaver, M.J., Clarke D.J. and George S.G. (1992). Molecular studies of the phase II xenobiotic conjugative enzymes of marine pleuronectid flatfish. *Aquatic Toxicol,* **22**: 465-278.

- Levitan, L., Merwin, I., and Kovach, J. (1995). Assessing the relative environmental impacts of agricultural pesticides : The quest for a holistic method. *Agricul. Eco. Environ.* 153-168.

- Lorz, H.W. and Mc Pherson, B.P. (1976). Effects of copper or zinc in fish on the adaptation to sea water and ATP$_{ase}$ activity and the effects of copper on migratory disposition of coho salmon (*Oncorhinchus kisutch*) *J. Fish. Res. Board. Can.* **33**: 2023 – 2030.

- Mayer, F.L. JR. (1971). Dynamics of dieldrin in rainbow trout and effect's on oxygen consumption. Ph.D. Thesis, Utah State University. Logan, Utah, U.S.A.

- Maza Usha, De Silva, S. and Mitchell, B.M. (1995). Effect of Sublethal concentrations of cadmium of food intake, growth and digestibility in the gold fish *Carassius auratus. J. Environ. Biol.* **16**: 253-264.

- McCarthy, L.S., Henery, J.A.C. and Houston, A.H. (1978). Toxicity of cadmium to gold fish, *Carassius auratus* in hard and soft water. *J. Fish. Res. Bd. Can* **35**: 35-42.

- Mehrle, P.M. and Mayer, F.L.(1975). Toxaphene effects on growth and bone composition of fathead minnows (*Pimphales promelas*) *J. Fish. Res. Board Can.* **32**: 593-598.
- Mehrle, P.M. and Mayer,. F.L. (1985) Biochemistry / Physiology. In fundamentals of Aquatic Toxicology. Methods and Applications (G.M. Rand, and S.R. Petrocelli, Eds.) 262-282 Hemisphere Publishing Corp., New York.
- Mishra, R. and Shukla, S.P. (1997). Impact of endosulfan on lactate dehydrogenase from the freshwater catfish Clarias batrachus, *Pesti. Biochem Physicol.* **57**: 220-234.
- Mock, A., and Peters, G. (1990) Lysozyme activity in rainbow trout, Oncorhynchus mykiss stressed by handling, transport and water pollution, *J. Fish. Biol.* **37**: 873-885.
- Mukherjee, S., and Bhattacharya, S. (1975). Changes in the kidney peroxidase activity in fish exposed to some industrial pollutants. Environ. *Physiol. Biochem.* **5**: 300-307.
- Murty, A.S. and Devi. A.P.(1982). The effect of endosulfan and its isomers on tissue protein, glycogen and lipids in the fish, *Channa punctatus. Pesti. Biochem. Physicol.* **17**: 280.
- Naqvi, S.M. and Vaishnavi, C (1993). Bioaccumulative potential and toxicity of endosulfan insecticide to non-target animals. A mini review. *Comp. Biochem. Physiol.* **105**: 347-361.
- Natarajan, G.M. (1984). Effect of lethal (LC50/ 48hr) concentration of metasystox on some selected enzyme systems in the air-breating fish, *Channa striatus* (Bleeker). *Comp. Physiol. Ecol.* **9**: 29-32.
- Nath, K. and Kumar, N. (1987). Effects of hexavalent chromium on the carbohydrate metabolism of a freshwater tropical teleost *Colisa fasciatus. Bull. Inst. Zool. Acad. Sin.* **26**: 245-248.
- Nemcsok, J. and Boross, L. (1982). Comparative studies on the sensitivity of different fish species to metal pollution. *Acta Biol. Hung.* **33**: 23-27.
- Nemcsok, J., Orban. L., Asztaloz B., Buzas Z, Nemeth A., and Boross L. (1985). Investigations on paraquat toxicity in fishes. *Water Intnat.* **10**: 79-81.
- Nemcsok, J., and Benedeczky, I. (1995). Pesticide metabolism and the adverse effects of metabolities on fishes. *Biochem. Mole. Biol. Fish.* **5**: 313-349.
- Olson, K.R., Bergman, H. L. and Fromn, P.O. (1973). Uptake of methylmercuric chloride and mercuric chloride by trout : a study of uptake pothways into the whole animal and uptake by erythrocytes *in vitro. J. Fish Res. Board. Can.* 30 : 1293-1299.
- Patel, R., and Saxena, A.B. (1983). Effects of potassium chromate on freshwater fishes, *Puntius ticto and Channa striatus. Indian J. Zool.* **11**: 43-49.
- Patel, B., Chandy, J.P. and Patel, S. (1990). Effect of mercury, selinium and glutathione are sulfhydryl levels and glutathione educatase in blood clam *Anodonta granosa (L). Ind. J. Mar. Sci.* **19**: 187-190.
- Pavlov, D.F., Kozlovskaya V.I. and Flerov, B.A.(1990). The use of collegen for assessing the toxicity of pollutant to fish *Trudy Inst. Biol. Vnutr. Vod.* **57**: 85-94.
- Pickering, Q.H. and Gost, M.H. (1972). Acute and chronic toxicity of cadmium to the fatehead minnow, *Pimephales promelas. J. Fish. Res. Bd. Can.* **29**: 1099-1106.
- Pickering, A.D. (1993). Endocrine induced pathology in stressed salmonid fish. *Fish Res.* **17**: 35-50.
- Pickering, A.D. and Pottinger, T.G.(1995). Biochemical Effects of Stress. *Biochem. Mole, Biol. Fish.* **5**: 349-376.
- Post, G., and Leisure, R.A. (1974). Sublethal effect of malathion to three salmonid species. *Bull. Environ. Contam. Toxicol.* **12**: 312-319.
- Radaiah, V., Joseph, K.V., and Rao, K.J. (1989). Toxic effect of fenvalerate on fructose−1,6, diphosphate aldolase activity of liver, gill, kidney and brain of the freshwater teleost, *Tilapia mossambica. Bull. Environ. Contam. Toxicol.* **42**: 150-153.
- Rao, K.S.P. and Rao, K.V.R.(1979). Effect of sublethal concentration of methyl parathion on selective oxidative enzymes and organic constituents in the tissues of the freshwater fish, *Tilapia mossambica. Current Sci.* **48**: 526 − 528.
- Rao, R, Rao, M.R.S. and Rao, K.V.R. (1983). Toxic impact of phenthoate on protein and ammonia .netabolism in tissues of the snail. *Pila globosa* (Swainson) *Proc. Indian Natn. Sci. Acad.* **49**: 416-420.

- Renfro, J.L., Schmidt – Nielson, B., Miller, D., Benos, D. and Allen, J. (1973). Methylmercury and inorganic mercury : uptake distribution and effect on osmoregulatory mechanisms in fishes. In : F.J. Vernberg and W.B. Vernberg (Eds.), pollution and physiology of marine organisms, Academic press, New York, 101-122.
- Roesijadi, G. (1992). Metallothioneins in metal regulation and toxicity in aquatic animals. *Aquatic Toxicol.* 81-114.
- Sarthwick, L.J., Smith, S. and Willis, G.H. (1983). Compartmentalization of permethrin on cotton leaves in field during spray application season. *Environ Toxicol Chem.* **2**: 29-34.
- Sastry, K.V., and Sharma, K. (1980). Diazinon effect on activities of brain enzymes from *Channa punctatus. Bull. Environ. Contam. Toxicol.* **24**: 326-332.
- Sastry, K.V., and Subhadra (1982). Effect of cadmium on some aspects of carbohydrate metabolism in the freshwater catfish *Heteropneustes fossillis. Toxicol. Lett.* **14**: 32-45.
- Sastry, K.V., and Shukla, V. (1990). Toxic effect of cadmium on some biochemical and physiological parameters in the teleost fish *Channa punctatus.* Biojournal. **2**: 325-332.
- Sastry, K.V., and Shukla, V. (1993) Acute and chronic effects of cadmium on the rate of oxygen uptake and metabolism of fish. *J. Ecobiol.* **5**: 295-298.
- Sastry, K.V. and Shukla, V. (1994). Actue and chronic toxic effects of cadmium on some haemotological, biochemical and enzymological parameters in the freshwater teleost fish *Channa punctatus. Acta. Hydrichin. Hydrabiol.* **22**: 171-176.
- Sastry, K.V., Sachdeva, S. and Rathee, P. (1997). Chronic toxic effects of cadmium and copper, and their combination of some enzymological and biochemical parameters in *Channa punctatus. J. Environ. Biol.* **18**: 291-303.
- Shafi, S.A.(1980) Thiodone toxicity. Non- specific phosphomonoesterase in nine freshwater teleosts. *Toxicol. Lett.* **6**: 339.
- Sharma, K.C. and Davis, P.S. (1980). Effect of methyl mercury on protein synthesis in the liver of the Eurpoean carp, *Cyprinus carpio. Ind. J. Exp. Biol.* **18**: 1054-1055.
- Shaw, B.P. and Panigrahi, A.K. (1990). Geographical distribution of mercury around chloralkali factry. *J. Environ. Biology.* **8**: 277-281.
- Shuter, B.J. (1990). Population level indicators of stress. *Am.* Fish. *Soc. Symp.* **8**: 145-166.
- Sivakumari, K., Manavalaramanujam R., Ramesh, M. and Lakshmi R. (1997). Cypermethrin toxicity Sublethal effects on enzyme activities in a freshwater fish, *Cyprinus carpio. J. Environ. Biol.* **18**: 121-125.
- Sogorb, A., Andrew Moliner, E.S., Almar, M.M., Ramo, J. Del. and Nunez, A. (1988). Temperature toxicity relationships of fluvinalate (Synthetic Pyrethroid) on Procambarus Clarkii (Girard) under laboratory conditions. Bull. *Environ. Contain. Toxicol.* **40**: 13-17.
- Spehar, R.C. (1976). Cadmum and zinc toxicity to flag fish. Jordanella floridae IBID 33: 1939-1945.
- Sreedevi, P.B., Sivaramakrishna, Suresh A. and Radhakrishnaiah, K.(1992). Effect of nickel on some aspects of protein metabolism in the gill and kidney of the freshwater fish *Cyprinus carpio* (L). *Environ Polut.* **76**: 355-361.
- Thomas, P. and Neff, J.M.(1995) Plasma corticosteroid and glucose responses to pollutants in striped mullet. Different effects of naphthalene, benzo (a) pyrene and cadmium exposure. In Marine Pollution and Physiology : Recent Advance Belle W. Baruch Libr. Mar. Sci. 13, edited by F.J. Vernberg, F.P. Thurberg, A. Calabrese and W.B. Vernberg, South Carolina, University of South Carolina Press, pp. 63-82.
- Thomas, P. (1990). Molecular and Biochemical responses of fish to stressors and their potential use in environmental monitoring. *Am. Fish. Soc. Symp.* **8**: 9-28.
- Tripathi, G. and Shukla S.O.(1990) Malate and lactate dehydragenase of a freshwater catfish. Impact of endosulfan. *Biomed. Environ. Sci.* **3**: 52.
- Venko, V. (1985). Chromium : a review of environmental and occupational toxicology. *J. Hug. Epidemiol. Microbiol. Immunol.* **29**: 26-37.

- Vettorazzi, G.(1975). State of the art of the toxicological evaluation carried out by the joint FAO/WHO expert committee on pesticide residues. I organohologenated pesticides used in public health and agriculture. *Residue review,* **56**: 107-134.
- Weber, D.N., Russo, A.C., Seale, D.B., and Spieler, R.E. (1983). Water brone affects feeding abilities and neurotransmitter levels of juvenile fathead minnows (*Pimephales promelas*) *Aquat. Toxicol.* **21**: 71-80.
- Weber, D.N. (1993). Exposure to sub-lethal levels of water borne lead alters reproductive behaviour patterns in fathead minnows *(Pimephales promelas). Neurotoxicol.* **14**: 347-358.
- Weiss, C.M., (1961). Physiological effect of organic phosphorus insecticides on several species of fish. *Trans. Am. Fish. Soc.* **90**: 143-152.
- WHO. (1977). Environmental Health Criteria. 3. Lead. World Health Organisation, Geneva.
- Williams, A.K., and Sava, R.C. (1966). Acetylcholisterase levels in brain of fishes from polluted water. *Bull. Environ Contam. Toxicol.* **1**: 198-204.
- Wofford, H.W. and Thomas, P. (1988). Effect of xenobiotics on peroxidation of hepatic microsomal lipids from striped mullet (*Mugil cephalus*) and Atlantic Croaker (*Micropogonias undulatus*) *Mar. Environ Res.* **24**: 285-289.
- Yap. H.H., Desaiah, D., Cutkomp, L.K and Koch, R.B.(1971). Sensitivity of fish. $ATP_{ase}$ to polychlorinated biplhenyls. *Nature* **233**: 61.

# 12

# Studies on Fluoride, Aluminium and Arsenic Toxicity in Mammals and Amelioration by Some Antidotes

*N. J. Chinoy*

Human eagerness to perform better and better with respect to production of food, energy and convenience products in order to improve the living standards are the causes of chemical pollution. This eagerness led to tremendous growth in production of chemicals. A large number of populations are occupationally exposed to a variety of chemicals in their daily life. Many of these chemicals are hazardous and have also been involved in numerous industrial disasters. The extensive use of pesticides in the present decade are also major culprits of environmental pollution. The smelting of metals and burning of coal in industries as well as volcanic eruptions are also adding more harmful chemicals in the environment. Their levels which are far beyond the permissible quantity for human beings become toxic and affect their health status. Hence it is essential to evaluate the effects of environmental toxicants on animals and human beings.

Although different toxicants are known, emphasis has been laid on fluoride, aluminium and arsenic toxicity in this article. In many countries, the most critical environmental issues today is groundwater contamination. About 70 per cent of all the water available in our country is polluted. We face a paradoxical situation. On one hand, we suffer from acute water scarcity with even our major cities having 40-50 per cent shortfall in their needs. But on the other hand, we are mismanaging our water resources so appallingly that if we go by WHO standards, almost all our surface water is polluted. Therefore, the preservation, protection and management of the quality of life is dependent on the environmental components apart from the industrial, agricultural and other economic parameters.

Trace elements are a group of chemicals which play a dual role in many systems. They are essential and beneficial for human health at minute concentrations, but exert toxic effects if their required levels are exceeded. Few such trace elements are fluorine, arsenic and aluminium. Their occurrence, distribution, properties, biological role and effects have been reviewed. Studies on the combined effects of aluminium and fluoride in biological systems have come up in recent years and are very controversial. Aluminium is known to decrease the intestinal absorption of fluoride and thus help in its increased excretion in human beings thereby reducing its toxicity. However, reports by Dai *et al.* (1994) have shown that the combined effects of aluminium and fluoride aggravated toxicity in blood and femur bone of male chicks.

There is a paucity of data on combined effects of sodium fluoride and arsenic both in humans and animals. Recently, at a meeting in Shenyang in China, in August 1999, many effects of their toxicity on animal and human health were elucidated.

## SOURCES

### Fluoride

Fluoride is found in our natural environment and under normal conditions is present in our food, water, soil, air, vegetation and body and it may be significantly increased by industrial sources (WHO, 1984). Water is invariably considered as the major carrier of fluoride. Fluoride also finds its way into the body through fluoridated tooth pastes. In India, around 10 of the population are known to use toothpastes.

## Arsenic

Arsenic is a natural part of the environment and it is present in low levels in soil, water, food and air. According to WHO, maximum permission level is 0.05 mg/L (Caussy, 1999). It has been estimated that in India and Bangladesh over 20 million people have ingested water containing arsenic concentration exceeding this limit. Soil usually contains the most with average levels of about 5000 parts of arsenic per billion parts of soil (ppb). Arsenic is also known to be widely distributed in a large number of minerals. The highest mineral concentrations generally occur as arsenides of copper, lead, silver or gold as the sulfide. In addition to the normal levels of arsenic in air, water, soil and food, some regions contain unusually high natural levels of arsenic in rock and this can lead to very high levels in soil or water. In addition to this, pollution through use of pesticides, non ferrous smelters, coal fires and geothermal power plants also contribute to arsenic in the environment.

## Aluminium

Human beings are exposed to aluminium through food, water and air-borne dust particles. Aluminium is added to drinking water as aluminium sulfate at the treatment plants, to flocculate the organic matter and to clear the water. Soil contamination is one of the factors responsible for the elevated concentration of aluminium found in vegetables. Certain plants like tea are known aluminium accumulators. One of the potential sources of additional dietary aluminium is aluminium cookware like skillets, pressure cookers, roasting pans, sauce pans, frozen dinner trays, foils and wrappers. The use of aluminium in over the counter drugs such as antacids, analgesics and anti-diarrhoeals has increased substantially in recent times. Another source of aluminium is through aluminium containing food additives which are generally used as buffers, neutralizing agents, dough strengtheners, emulsifying agents for processed cheese, stabilizers, thickners, texturizers etc.

## Chemistry

Fluoride belongs to the sub group VII-A of the periodic system. The outermost orbital contains 7 electrons and its valency is 1 (Underwood, 1977).

Arsenic can exist in -3, +3 or +5 oxidation states. It is the 20th most abundant element in the earth's crust but 12th most common in the human body. Its atomic number is 33 and atomic mass is 74.9216 and belongs to the sub-group Va of the periodic system. Arsenic has both cationic and anionic forms.

Aluminium is a silvery white, ductile and malleable metal. It belongs to group III A of the periodic table and in compounds it is usually found as Al III. It forms about 8 per cent of the earth's crust and is one of the most reactive of the common metals. Aluminium possesses high electrical and thermal conductivity, low density and great resistance to corrosion. It is often alloyed with other metals.

## DISTRIBUTION IN AIR, WATER AND SOIL

### Fluoride

Minute traces of fluoride are found in air. Sources of fluoride in air include effluents from volcanoes, and a variety of industrial processes, outcropping of fluoride containing minerals, ocean spray, smoke from the burning of coal, and fluoride containing soil. Fluorides account for about 0.032 per cent of the earth's crust. Its content in the soil usually increases with depth. Air borne fluoride is returned by the way of snow and rainfall when occurring over land, it eventually reaches the oceans *via* rivers.

### Arsenic

Arsenic is mobile within the environment and may circulate many times in various forms through the atmopshere, water, soil, food and fly ash (Zheng *et al.*, 1999). Air borne arsenic is mainly inorganic and is present mainly in particulate form as arsenic trioxide, with background levels of 1 to 10 ng/

$m^3$ in rural areas and 20 ng/$m^3$ in urban areas. Fresh water normally contains 0.15-0.45 µg/L arsenic mainly in inorganic forms. Mineral waters may contain upto 50 times, hot springs upto 300 times more arsenic than normal background levels. High levels of arsenic have been found in waters from areas of thermal activity. Cases of arsenic in drinking water have been reported from Argentina, Bangladesh, Bosnia, China, Chile, Ghana, Hungary, India, Mexico, Thailand, United States of America, Canada and New Zealand. Arsenic contamination is regarded as a world wide problem (Yamamura, 1999; Hoque, 1999).

The levels of arsenic in soil is about 7 mg/kg, but could be as high as 1000 mg/kg in the vicinity of metal smelters and in agricultural soils where pesticides, herbicides and defoliants are extensively used (Merian, 1991).

## Aluminium

Aluminium does not occur naturally in the metallic, element state, but is widely distributed in the earth's crust in combination with oxygen, fluorine, silicon and other constituents. The most important raw material for the production of aluminium is bauxite, which contains 40-60 per cent alumina (aluminium oxide). Other raw materials sometimes used in the production of aluminium include cryolite, aluminium fluoride, fluorspar, corundam, and kaolin minerals (U.S. Department of Health and Human Services, 1997).

## IMPORTANCE

### Fluoride

Fluoride ion could play a significant role in the prevention of human dental caries. Fluoride is also beneficial for the maintenance of a normal skeleton in the adults. Fluoride may be necessary for normal hematocrit levels, fertility and growth. It acts as a pharmacological agent in correcting some dietary imbalance or deficiency. However, higher levels cause endemic fluorosis which is a public health problem in several parts of the world. Skeletal fluorosis is characterised clinically by restricted movements of joints, stiffness and deformities of the spine. Chronic fluoride toxicity causes dental fluorosis. In some endemic areas of India *"genu valgum"* was described as the manifestation of fluoride toxicity among population groups in whom dietary calcium was low (Krishnamachari and Krishnaswamy, 1973). Genu valgum is a crippling form of fluoride toxicity which occurs in relatively younger children around 8-10 years. It has certain distinctive epidemiological and clinical characteristics such as predominantly male involvement, its occurrence in adolescence, evidence of secondary hypothyroidism (Krishnamachari and Krishnaswamy, 1974) and elevated levels of circulating immunoreactive parathyroid hormone·(Sivakumar and Krishnamachari, 1976).

### Arsenic

Arsenic compounds have been used in medicine for centuries. Fowler's solution, which is 1 per cent aqueous solution of arsenic trioxide was widely prescribed for the treatment of a wide variety of ailments, including skin conditions such as psoriasis and eczema, as well as epilepsy and asthma.

### Aluminium

Studies of interactions of aluminium with other materials that may be found at hazardous waste sites show that aluminium has a protective role against the toxic effects of some other chemicals. For example, aluminium hydroxide, commonly found in antacids, can decrease the intestinal absorption of fluoride in humans (Spencer *et al.*, 1980).

Aluminium exposure is a risk factor for the development or acceleration of the onset of Alzheimer's disease (AD) in humans (Crapper McLachlan *et al.*, 1989). Aluminium exposure as a single risk factor began to be examined in the early 1980s, when reports of the increased level of aluminium in brains of AD patients suggested that this might also be a factor. Several studies examined the water borne aluminium and AD relationship (Frecker, 1991). In addition exposure from aluminium containing antiperspirants (Graves *et al.*, 1990) and antacids (Flaten *et al.*, 1991) have also been explored as risk for dementia and/or AD.

## HALF LIFE AND LD$_{50}$

### Fluoride

The half life of fluoride in blood and soft tissues has been reported to be few hours, while in skeleton, it has a longer half life of about 8 years (WHO, 1970; Grandjean, 1985). The LD$_{50}$ values for male and female nice are 54.41 and 51.6µg/kg body weight respectively.

### Arsenic

The 96 hour LD$_{50}$ of arsenic trioxide in Swiss mice is 39.4 mg/kg (NAS, 1977; USEPA, 1981). In humans acute symptoms may occur within minutes or hours of ingestion depending upon the vehicle, solubility and particle size.

### Aluminium

LD$_{50}$ value of aluminium chloride was found to be 4 g/kg body weight in male mice (Chinoy and Bhattacharya, 1997).

## EFFECT ON PROTEIN METABOLISM

### Fluoride

Fluoride is known to reduce protein synthesis (Hongslo and Holland, 1979) by impairment of the polypeptide chain initiation (Hoertz and McCarty, 1971). Holland (1979) found that fluoride inhibits growth of cell cultures as well as protein and DNA synthesis which are the main targets of its cytotoxic action. Morphological alteration of chromosome (Tsutsui *et al.*, 1984) and decreased nuclear DNA levels (Holland, 1980) observed as a result of fluoride treatment would affect the protein synthesis. The protein levels in stomach, duodenum and ileum of fluoride treated rabbits was also decreased (Shashi *et al.*, 1987) as well as in various tissues of fluoride treated male and female rats, mice, guinea pigs and rabbits (Chinoy and Sequeira, 1989a; Chinoy, 1991a,b; 1992, 1995, 1996; Chinoy et al., 1991a; 1993a,b; Chinoy and Patel, 1996; Chinoy and Sharma, 1998).

### Arsenic

The high retention of arsenic in the skin seen in the animals receiving arsenic (III) may be explained by reaction of trivalent arsenic with sulfhydryl groups of proteins which are abundant in the skin (Vahter and Norin, 1980). As (III) and As (V) inhibit DNA, RNA and protein synthesis and replace phosphate in the nucleotides during DNA synthesis (WHO, 1981; Merian, 1991).

### Aluminium

Aluminium salt when ingested at toxic levels caused profound disorders in phosphate metabolism. Considerable experimental evidence indicates that aluminium alters second messenger systems of C-AMP and G-Proteins (Steinweis and Gilman, 1982; Johnson et al., 1990; 1992). Studies from our laboratory have shown that aluminium toxicity caused decrease in protein and some enzymes in tissues of mice (Chinoy and Bhattacharya, 1997).

# CARBOHYDRATE METABOLISM

## Fluoride

Fluoride has been reported to induce dramatic changes in carbohydrate metabolism (Dousset *et al.,* 1987) mainly by causing allosteric inhibition of some key enzymes in glycolysis and tricarboxylic acid cycle (TCA).

Accumulation of glycogen has been reported in gastrocnemius muscle, liver, vas deferens and uterus of different animal models treated with NaF (Chinoy and Sequeira, 1989a, Chinoy *et al.,* 1993b; 1994a,b; Chinoy and Patel, 1996; Chinoy and Sharma, 1998) which was correlated with the decrease in the activity of phosphorylase. A diminished activity of glucose-6-$PO_4$ dehydrogenase depressing glycogen turnover has been reported (Carlson and Suttie, 1966). The concentrations of serum catecholamines in fluorotic mice were significantly elevated in comparison to control after 45 and 60 days treatments (Chinoy and Patel, 1996), whereas, blood glucose declined (Patel *et al.,* 1994) which also indicates an alteration in carbohydrate metabolism.

## Arsenic

Carbohydrate depletion, resulting mainly from inhibition of gluconeogenesis is proposed to be a major problem in poisoning with trivalent arsenicalz (Szinics and Forth, 1988). All animals which died after arsenic intoxication showed a significant decrease in the levels of glycogen in liver (Reichl *et al.,* 1990). Arsenicals cause inhibition of pyruvate dehydrogenase, the subsequent depletion of acetyl CoA and inhibition of gluconeogenesis.

## Aluminium

De Bruin (1976) reviewed the effects of aluminium on carbohydrate metabolism. The treatment is known to produce hyperglycaemia.

The treatment with $AlCl_3$ (30 and 60 days) to mice caused a significant enhancement in the levels of glycogen in vas deferens, muscle, liver of male mice. The elevated glycogen levels in these tissues was accompanied by a significant decrease in the activity of phosphorylase. As a result of decreased glycogen utilization significant decline was obtained in the blood glucose levels of aluminium chloride treated mice. Hence it is evident that the effects of fluoride, arsenic and aluminium on glycogen and phosphorylase in liver, muscle, vas deferens and uterus were similar in causing an accumulation of glycogen but an inhibition of phosphorylase (Chinoy and Sharma, 1998; Chinoy and Bhattacharya, 1996; Chinoy *et al.,* 2000).

## Lipid Metabolism

Fluoride has been implicated in arteriosclerosis, hence the interaction of fluoride and lipid metabolism assumes considerable significance (Exner and Waldbott, 1957). Rats supplemented with 100 ppm of fluoride resulted in marked reduction in plasma free fatty acids.

Chinoy and associates reported an accumulation of cholesterol in testis and ovary concomitant with the decrease in the activities of 3ß and 17ß HSD and circulating testosterone and estradiol levels in fluoride treated rats and mice (Chinoy, 1992; 1996; Narayana and Chinoy, 1994a).

Recent work has revealed that fluoride administration inhibited the activities of superoxide dismutase, glutathione peroxidase and catalase in the ovary and testis of treated mice which increased ovarian lipid peroxidation, thus rendering the tissue susceptible to injury (Chinoy and Patel, 1998; Chinoy and Sharma, 1998). The most important consequences are the denaturation of proteins and the peroxidation of membrane lipids with an increase in the permeability of the cell membrane (Subramaniam *et al.,* 1994).

## Arsenic

There is very little information regarding the effect of arsenic on lipid metabolism.

## Aluminium

Recent work from our laboratory (Chinoy and Bhattacharya, 1996) has revealed that aluminium treatment to mice caused an accumulation of testicular cholesterol and a reduction in activity of 3ß and 17ß HSD which might have resulted in reduced steroidogenesis in the testis and thus decrease in serum testosterone levels as found after fluoride ingestion.

## Genotoxicity

Fluoride has been reported to cause decrease in DNA and RNA synthesis in cultured cells (Strochkova et al., 1984), in rabbit ovary (Shashi, 1994) and in the ovary and uterus of fluorotic mice which could affect their metabolism (Patel and Chinoy, 1998).

Conflicting reports are available in the literature regarding the genotoxic effects of fluoride. Jachimczak and Skotarczak (1978) have reported that sodium fluoride induces chromosome aberrations in cultured human leucocytes whereas, Obe and Slacik-Erben (1973) found negative results. Thompson et al. (1985) found no fluoride induced increase in the frequencies of chromosomal aberrations or SCEs in human lymphocyte cultures. However, studies carried out by Sheth et al. (1994) revealed an increase in the frequency of SCE in fluorotic individuals of North Gujarat, India, as compared to the control ones indicating that fluoride might have a genotoxic effect. The frequency of micronuclei in peripheral blood lymphocytes of 40 workers chronically exposed to fluoride at a phosphate fertilizer factory in North China was significantly higher than that of controls (Zhang and Meng, 1999).

Several assays performed in vitro on mammalian cells have shown that arsenicals display evident clastogenic properties and can induce a slight increase of SCEs (Lee et al., 1999; Xie et al., 1999a; Zhang et al., 1999). Induction of cancer appears to be the most striking long-term effect of chronic exposure to inorganic arsenic (Lee et al., 1999; Ng et al., 1999).

## Aluminium

Manna and Das (1972) reported that a significant incease of chromatid type of aberrations (including gaps, breaks, translocation and ring formations), with non random distribution over the chromosome complement occurred in the bone marrow cells of mice dosed intraperitoneally with $AlCl_3$. Prolonged treatment of rats with $Al_2(SO_4)_3$ or $KAl(SO_4)_2$ resulted in a dose dependent inhibition of dividing bone marrow cells and an increase in chromosomal aberrations (Bhamra and Costa, 1992). Aluminium caused a concentration dependent change in number of sister chromatid exchange (SCE) in cultured human lymphocytes and increased the unscheduled DNA synthesis in cultured human astrocytes (De Boni et al., 1980). There have been no reports concerning genetic effects of aluminium in humans following oral exposure. The combined sodium fluoride and aluminium chloride coadministration to female mice for 30 days caused a significant decline in the levels of DNA, RNA, DNA/RNA ratio and RNA/protein ratio in liver and muscle, which indicates disturbances in the process of transcription and translation by the toxicants (Patel and Chinoy, 2000).

## Human Intake

Historically, recognition of fluoride as a preventive agent for dental caries resulted in the addition of small amounts of fluoride (about 1 ppm F) to drinking water in the U.S.A. in 1945. This measure was generally accepted and recommended by health authorities and dentists (Horowitz, 1973; WHO, 1970; 1984). However, recently there have been serious reservations on this aspect in countries like USA, New Zealand etc.

Due to the ubiquitous presence of fluoride in our environment, significant and variable quantities of fluoride are found in our diet. The amount of fluoride present in foods is variable, and there are no foods totally devoid of it.

## Aluminium

The actual concentration of aluminium in food and beverages from various countries will vary widely depending upon the food product, the type of processing used, in particular the levels of aluminium containing food additives permitted and the geographical area in which food crops are grown. In general, the foods highest in aluminium are those that contain aluminium additives (*e.g.* grain products (flour), processed dairy products, infant formulae etc.). The cooking and storage of food in aluminium containers, particularly in the case of foods that are acidic, salty or alkaline such as tomatoes in aluminium pans causes a significant increase in the level of aluminium in the food. Aluminium levels in drinking water, distributed through household plumbing or as bottled water, vary according to the natural levels found in the source and whether aluminium flocculants were used during purification process (WHO, 1997). The use of antacids and buffered analgesics may result in large intakes of aluminium far in excess of that normally consumed in food. Aluminium compounds are widely used in the preparation of cosmetics, particularly in antiperspirants (WHO, 1997).

## Arsenic

The natural concentration of total arsenic in drinking water varies in different parts of the world and could be severely contaminated through industrial operations. Leaching of arsenic from coal preparation wastes and fly ash from coal-fired power plants may also result in the contamination of water (Williams, *et al.*, 1977; Chu *et al.*, 1978).

Most of the arsenic in marine organisms occurs in the form of either fat soluble or water soluble organo arsenic compounds (Lunde, 1975). Wine may contain appreciable amounts of arsenic due to use of the arsenic containing insecticides. Elevated arsenic levels have been found in some bottled mineral waters.

## ORGANS AND ORGAN SYSTEM

### Digestive System

### Fluoride

The major route of fluoride entry into the body is through the digestive tract. Human beings are usually found to absorb a minimum of 45 per cent of the fluoride normally present in the diet (Ham and Smith, 1954). Stomach and bowel disorders are major features of intolerance to fluoride intake. Formation of hydrofluoric acid in the gut appears to account for the symptoms of nausea, vomiting, abdominal pain, and diarrhea associated with fluoride poisoning as well as widespread damage to the stomach mucosa (Susheela *et al.*, 1992; Waldbott *et al.*, 1978).

### Stomach

Shashi *et al.* (1987) reported a significant inhibition of protein synthesis in stomach of fluoride intoxicated rabbits. As a consequence of fluoride intoxication, erosion and necrosis of mucosal and submucosal layer, diffuse punctate hemorrhages and disintegration of gastric glands occur which produce severe systemic effects such as depilation and spastic paralysis (Shashi *et al.*, 1987).

### Intestine

Fluoride not only affects cellular protein synthesis in gastrointestinal organs but also causes alterations in the permeability of membrane and membrane bound enzymes especially in the intestinal cell lining. According to Rastogi *et al.* (1987), ATP ase activities of brush border preparations in male albino rats declined significantly indicating fluoride induced damage to the intestinal brush border membrane.

# Aluminium

The gastrointestinal tract is the most important port of entry for aluminium. The mechanism of gastrointestinal absorption of aluminium is fairly complex and has not yet been fully elucidated (Vander Voet, 1992). Variable quantities of $Al(OH)_3$ or $Al_2(CO_3)_3$ given to volunteers or patients for different periods of time resulted in significant increase in plasma and/or urinary aluminium concentrations (WHO, 1997). In the Down syndrome patients uptake was apparently 5 times higher than in controls.

After absorption, aluminium is bound in the plasma primarily to transferrin and to a lesser extent, to albumin (Martin, 1986). The distribution of aluminium depends on the animal species used, route of administration and the aluminium compound administered (WHO, 1997).

# Arsenic

Absorption of inorganic arsenic from the gastrointestinal tract can occur following the ingestion of food, water, beverages or drugs, containing arsenic or as a result of inhalation and subsequent mucociliary clearance. The absorption of ingested arsenic will depend on the solubility of the compound given in solution or as undissolved particles.

Nausea, vomiting and diarrhea are very common symptoms in humans following oral exposure to inorganic arsenicals, after both acute and high dose exposure (Armstrong *et al.*, 1984; Levin-Scherz *et al.*, 1987).

# EFFECTS ON LIVER

## By Fluoride

Liver being the principal organ for detoxification encounters most of the toxicants that gain entry into the body. Hence the hepatic tissue bears the major brunt of structural insults meted out by toxic substances. In many of the hepatocytes, the nuclei were pushed to one side while in some nuclear material was extruded out suggesting apoptosis. The hepatic lobules were hyalinized with loss of cells and the cytoplasm was vacuolized. The arrangement of hepatic cord was also disturbed (Chinoy *et al.*, 1991a). Zonal necrosis and nuclear degeneration was the most common feature observed in fluoride treated rats and guinea pigs (Chinoy et al., 1993b; Kour *et al.*, 1981). Sodium fluoride (10 mg/kg body weight) for 30 days caused ultrastructural changes in the liver which included hepatic cell cytoplasmic vacouolisation and fatty deposition. The nuclei were pyknotic, irregular nuclear membrane and disorganisation of chromatin was observed. The mitochondria were enlarged with damaged cristae. The hepatocytes showed accumulation of glycogen granules (Sharma and Chinoy, 2000). Fluoride induced changes in various biochemical parameters of liver were reported (Bogin et al., 1976; Chinoy *et al.*, 1991a,b, 1994c) in different animal models.

## By Aluminium

Stein *et al.* (1987) using laser microprobe analysis observed concomitant storage of Al and Fe in hepatocyte and Kupffer cell lysosomes, respectively and within lysosomes of macrophages in liver, spleen and other tissues. Thus lysosomes seems to be a target for storage and perhaps the damage. Apart from the damage to the lysosomes, the repeated application of Al also exerts a selective influence on the synthesis of enzymes. However, biochemical studies have failed to show an effect of aluminium in rat liver mitochondria and microsomes as well as guinea pig liver mitochondria (Biggs, 1963).

Berlyne *et al.* (1972) found that aluminium was specifically taken up by the nuclei of the hepatocytes and that the DNA of the nucleus had a specific affinity for aluminium and hence enzymes were altered in the liver.

## By Arsenic

Exposure to inorganic arsenic compounds has been associated with the development of chronic pathological liver changes. Several authors have reported cases of liver damage following treatment with arsenic in the trivalent inorganic forms (Huet *et al.*, 1975; Szuler *et al.*, 1979). Oral exposure of humans to inorganic arsenicals often produce a swollen and tender liver (Chakraborty and Saha, 1987; Mazumdar *et al.*, 1988). However, there is usually only marginal evidence of hepatic cell injury i.e. elevated serum enzyme levels (USDHHS, 1998) and histological examination suggests that the principal lesion is a portal tract fibrosis and cirrhosis that result in portal hypertension (Mazumdar *et al.*, 1988). Thus, the hepatic effects may be largely vascular in origin. Studies from our laboratory on fluoride, arsenic combined treatment (Chinoy, 1999a) revealed zonal necrosis, structural alteration, disorganization of hepatocytes with pyknotic nuclei, cytoplasmic vacuolization and fatty deposition. The histocytometry of liver cells also supported the above results. The same study also showed changes in biochemical parameters like decline in protein levels, inhibition of phosphorylase and accumulation of glycogen.

## RESPIRATORY SYSTEM

### Fluoride

Next to gastrointestinal tract, respiratory system is a potential route of entry of fluoride into the human body especially in the vicinity of industries. Airborne fluoride is readily absorbed through the respiratory tract and immediately ionizes in contact with blood and is carried to different parts of the body.

Inhalation of fluoride affects the respiratory process. Elkins (1959) described nose bleeds and sinus trouble from high hydrogen fluoride exposures. Impaired nasal respiration (Rybicki, 1970) wheezing and discomfort in the nose and throat in workers in a cryolite plant were reported by Johnson et al. (1973).

In mouse, rat and guinea pigs exposed to different concentrations of hydrogen fluoride, irritation of the mucous membrane of the nose and eyes, acute inflammation, focal necrosis of the nasal mucosa and tracheobronchitis were observed (Wohlschlage *et al.*, 1976).

In acute toxicity, respiratory depression and coagulation, necrosis and congestion in lung were observed. Kaltreider *et al.* (1972) reported pneumonia, carcinoma and lung abscess besides the common respiratory obstacles in inhabitants of industrial vicinity. Thus exposure to fluoride compounds are harmful and damage respiratory tract.

### Arsenic

Human exposure to inorganic arsenic through inhalation usually occurs occupationally or during cigarette smoking. Inhaled arsenic is mainly in the form of an aerosol. In many work places, the particles containing arsenic are of relatively large size (Pinto and McGill, 1953) resulting in deposition primarily in the upper respiratory passages (nasal cavity, nasopharynx, larynx, trachea and bronchus). Effects on the lung may actually be more pronounced following high dose (*i.e.* near lethal) oral exposure, where edema and hemorrhagic lesions have been noted (Campbell and Alvarez, 1989; Fincher and Koerker, 1987).

### Aluminium

Historically, pulmonary fibrosis have been associated with various types of occupations within the aluminium industry. Occupational aluminium exposure is reported to cause pathological lung functions, abnormal chest X-rays, development of intestinal fibrosis and other problems (Nutrition News, 1998). The lungs are constantly exposed to aluminium primarily as particulates of aluminium silicate and other poorly soluble compounds. Some of these particulate matter is probably phagocytosed by alveolar macrophages. The remainder are probably taken up by macrophages in the pulmonary tissues and held indefinitely in the lungs. Although the concentration of aluminium in the lungs increases with age (Alfrey, 1983), under normal environmental conditions this accumulation appears to be of little pathological significance. In contrast, pulmonary disease has been well documented in workers exposed to very large quantities of aluminium containing dusts and fumes (Van de Vyver and De Broe, 1985).

## CARDIOVASCULAR SYSTEM

### Fluoride

There is scant information available on the role of fluoride on cardiovascular functions. Vascular changes characterized by microvascular injury, perivascular disintegration of tissue cells and vascular proliferation were predominated by fluoride ingestion (Branemark, 1967). High doses of fluoride have been reported to cause severe heart damage leading to cardiac irregularities, low blood pressure and irregular electrocardiogram in humans (Zhiliang et al. 1987). Aortic calcification and degeneration of smooth muscle fibers in the tunica media of the aorta were reported in fluoride intoxicated rabbits (Susheela and Kharb, 1990). The aorta is known to accumulate the highest amount of fluoride as compared to other soft tissues. In male albino mice the protein levels, DNA and RNA in the ventricle were significantly decreased (Chinoy and Biringwala, unpublished observations). The decrease in RNA levels in ventricle of fluorotic mice might be due to fluoride interaction with DNA to inhibit RNA synthesis. On the other hand, the cholesterol level in ventricle was significantly increased.

### Aluminium

Very little work has been done concerning aluminium and its role in the metabolism of cardiac tissue. Biochemical studies have demonstrated that aluminium has a specific activating effect on the myocardial succinate oxidase system (Bradley, 1990). It was observed that the aluminium concentration increased in aorta with age (Popov et al., 1966). Hypertrophy of the ventricles and increased capillary permeability in the workers of aluminium plant have been reported (WHO, 1970).

### Arsenic

An increased mortality from cardiovascular disease has been observed in two epidemiological investigations on smelter workers exposed to high levels of airborne arsenic (Lee and Fraumeni, 1969; Axelson et al., 1978).

A high prevalence of a peripheral vascular disease called "black foot disease" was found in a population living in China (Province of Taiwan), where the arsenic levels in well water used for drinking purposes ranged from 0.01-1.82 mg/litre (Tseng et al., 1968; Tseng, 1977). The severity of the disease was related to duration of water intake. Further supporting evidence that arsenic in drinking water was causative factor in "black foot" disease is that no new cases of the disease have appeared in children in the area, since the installation of tap water systems with low levels of arsenic in the water. Butzengeiger (1949) described peripheral vascular lesions in 23% of 180 vintners with chronic intoxication. In six cases the inadequate peripheral circulation caused gangerene. Chronic nephritis, cardiac failure has also been reported.

## BLOOD

### Fluoride

The blood acts as a transport medium for fluoride and about 75% of the blood fluoride is present in the plasma, the rest is mainly in or on the red blood cells (Hosking and Chamberlain, 1977). Macuch et al. (1963) have found low haemoglobin, increased erythrocyte and abnormal lymphocyte counts in children exposed to fluoride residues. The studies in fluoride afflicted human population of endemic district of Mehsana in North Gujarat, India, revealed a significant decrease in haemoglobin concentration suggesting an anaemic condition (Chinoy et al., 1994d).

Erythrocyte membrane abnormality and echinocyte formation were also reported in rabbits and human beings exposed to fluoride (Susheela and Jain, 1986).

## Aluminium

There have been numerous publications since 1957 dealing with the changes in the aluminium content in human blood. The content in the blood of female newborns was somewhat high than that of males. Blood aluminium has also been observed to increase in pregnant women throughout normal pregnancy (Bibileishvili, 1965; Laptieva, 1967).

The concentration of aluminium was elevated in leukemia and in Hodgkins disease (Bradley, 1990). The concentration of aluminium in blood and tissue of patients with a variety of neoplasms has been demonstrated to be different from control subjects (Mulay *et al.*, 1971). Some neoplastic tissues had elevated aluminium levels while others had depressed levels.

## Arsenic

Data indicating any quantitative relationship relevant to man between arsenic exposure and its concentrations in the blood are not available. Cheng and Zhu (1999) have reported inhibitory effect of arsenic trioxide on the immune system in mice.

The cholinesterase activity in blood was found to decrease in fluorotic rats (Wang et al., 1999).

# URINARY SYSTEM

## Fluoride

The principle route of excretion of absorbed fluoride is through urine. Urinary fluoride concentration is one of the indices of fluoride intake. In adults exposed to high fluoride concentrations or for a longer period, kidney gets damaged and therefore the excretion of fluoride is significantly diminished which reflects in an increase in fluoride content of bone (Kono *et al.*, 1984). The changes in kidney include necrosis of convoluted tubules (Kour and Singh, 1980a) and inflammation of glomeruli which led to impaired kidney function such as polyuria (Jankauskas, 1974). Nephropathy, is a major manifestation of fluoride toxicity in the initial stages of exposure. Fluoride is implicated in the etiology of kidney stones.

Bhatnagar and Susheela (1998) studied chronic fluoride toxicity in glomerulus of the rabbit kidney. The authors reported major abnormalities in visceral epithelial cells including loss of foot processes, distortion and fusion of foot process and detachment of the epithelial cell layer in some parts causing denudation of glomerular basement membrane. Similar observations have been made in fluorotic mice kidney (Chinoy and Sharma, 2000).

## Aluminium

Aluminium is now widely recognised to be a toxic element and has been implicated in a number of pathological conditions, including dialysis dementia (Kerr and Ward, 1986).

In rats given Al intravenously (in the form of aluminium chloride), excretion of Al by the kidney is inefficient due partly to protein binding, but at high Al concentrations, mainly due to the formation of insoluble colloids (Lote *et al.*, 1992).

Significant aluminium levels were found in cytoplasm and mitochondria of proximal tubule cells of kidney after acute aluminium citrate administration (Spencer et al., 1995). Similarly significant increase in kidney aluminium concentrations in two types of human kidney diseases, lipid nephrosis and tuberculoma have been reported (Bradley, 1990).

## Arsenic

In dogs an *in vivo* oxidation of trivalent to pentavalent arsenic occurred (Ginsburg, 1965). Braman and Foreback (1973) reported the presence of methylated forms of arsenic in the urine of four subjects. Dimethyl arsenic acid was also the major form of arsenic found in the urine of smelter workers occupationally exposed to arsenic, chiefly in the form of arsenic (III) oxide (Smith *et al.*, 1977). The elimination of arsenic in rats is very slow because of the accumulation in red blood cells. In animals other than the rat, absorbed arsenic is excreted from the body at a much higher rate, mainly *via* the kidneys.

## CENTRAL NERVOUS SYSTEM

Lu *et al.* (1961) found stimulation of CNS by intraperitoneal injection of NaF to rats which is attributed to the inhibition of cholinesterase activity. The cholinesterase activity in mice brain (cerebral hemisphere) was significantly decreased by NaF treatment for 30 days (Chinoy and Biringwala, unpublished observation). This might be due to the alteration in $Ca^{2+}$ ion concentration in brain, which is essential for the release of acetylcholine from synaptic vesicles.

In humans, the partial and complete paralysis of arms and legs in advanced fluorosis is usually considered to be related to pressure upon the spinal cord by newly formed bone protruding into it and upon nerves at the point of their exit from the spine. However, it has been suggested that the spinal cord lesions and muscular damage in patients suffering from occupational fluorosis are also the result of a direct action of the fluoride ion on the ganglion and muscle cells (Franke *et al.*, 1975). A neuropathological analysis by Chlubek *et al.* (1998) revealed marked shrinkage of cerebellar granular and Purkinje cells, perivascular myelin swelling and astroglia reaction, especially in the white matter of brain in NaF treated (60 ppm) rats.

## Aluminium

Considerable evidence indicates that aluminium is neurotoxic to experimental animals. The toxicity is characterized by neurological impairment, neurofibrillary pathology in large and medium size neurons predominantly in the spinal cord, brain stem and selected areas of cortex (WHO, 1997). Crapper *et al.* (1973) have reported very high levels of aluminium, (9 to 11 µg/g dry weight) in brain tissue from patients who had Alzheimer's disease.

Considerable experimental evidence implicates aluminium in alterations of the second messenger systems of C-AMP and G-proteins (Steinweis and Gilman, 1982; Johnson *et al.*, 1990, 1992).

## Arsenic

A large number of epidemiological studies and case reports indicate that digestion of inorganic arsenic can cause injury to the nervous system. Acute high dose exposures (1 mg As/kg/day or above) often lead to encephalopathy, with signs and symptoms such as headache, lethargy, mental confusion, hallucination, seizures and coma (USDHHS, 1998). Intermediate and chronic duration exposures to lower levels (0.05-0.5 mg As/kg/day) are typically characterized by a symmetrical peripheral neuropathy (Franzblau and Lilis, 1989; Huang *et al.*, 1985). This neuropathy usually begins as a numbness in the hands and feet, but later may develop into a painful "pins and needles" sensation. The sensory and motor nerves are both affected, and muscle weakness often develops, sometimes leading to wrist drop or ankle drop (Chhuttani *et al.*, 1967). Histological examination of nerves from affected individuals reveals a dying back axonopathy with demyelination (Goebel *et al.*, 1990). Disturbance in the functional state of the central nervous system were reflected as changes in conditional reflexes. Histopathological changes in the brain included pericellular oedema, plasmatic impregnation of the vascular walls, plasmolysis and karyolysis of the neurons (Rozenshtein, 1970). Inhibition of cholinesterase activity was observed in rats exposed for 3 months to arsenic (III) oxide (Rozenshtein, 1970).

## MUSCLE

### Fluoride

Fluoride is known to affect the structure and functions of muscle. The fluoride treated rabbits revealed degeneration of muscle fibres, defects of plasma membrane as evident from the enhanced levels of serum creatinine phosphokinase (Kaul and Susheela, 1974). Fluoride also affects the biochemical parameters of muscle. Bogin et al. (1976) found a significant decline in alkaline phosphatase and isocitrate dehydrogenase in the skeletal muscle of mice maintained on water containing 100 ppm NaF.

The effects of fluoride, arsenic and aluminium administration on muscle are almost similar. Studies from our laboratory have revealed that administration of fluoride, arsenic or aluminium alone or in combination resulted in a significant decrease in the activities of SDH and ATP ase in gastrocnemius muscle of mice. The muscle SDH is an oxidative enzyme involved in the contractile mechanism of the muscle (George and Berger, 1966). Hence the decline in SDH activity would affect the conversion of succinate to fumarate and may cause a block in the Krebs cycle. The treatment also resulted in significant decline in the protein levels, whereas, glycogen accumulated due to decrease in phosphorylase activity. The activity of cholinesterase was decreased affecting muscle contraction (Chinoy, 1999a; Chinoy et al., 1991a; 1993b; 1994a,b; Chinoy et al., 2000).

### Endocrine Glands

Extensive investigations carried out during the past one and a half decade have revealed that fluoride toxicity is not confined to the bone and dental tissues alone but involves more than one endocrine organ in adults as well as children. Alteration in hormonal profile are now believed to be related to chronic exposure to environmental fluoride.

### Thyroid

High concentration of fluoride interferes with the thyroid function. In fluoride fed animals, swelling of mitochondria with disintegrated cristae in follicular epithelial cells of thyroid gland was observed (Chongwan and Daijei, 1988). Fluoride may inhibit the proteinases responsible for splitting thyroglobulin molecule into thyroxine and triodothyroxine (Willems et al., 1972). Fluoride may affect the feedback mechanism mediated through the hypothalamus and adenohypophysis which regulates thyroid secretion through TSH.

Recent studies in human population affected by fluorosis revealed low serum thyroid hormones namely T3, T4 and TSH (Chinoy, 1996; Chinoy and Narayana, 1992; Mathews et al., 1996). Desai et al. (1993) also observed a significant positive correlation between overall prevalence of goiter and dental fluorosis among endemic population of Gujarat. Experimental studies in animals revealed thyroid hyperplasia, colloid goiter, degeneration of follicular epithelium and true glandular hypertrophy (Wadhwani and Ramaswamy, 1953).

### Parathyroid Gland

The parathyroid gland plays an essential role in endemic fluorosis since its function is to mainly regulate calcium metabolism. Fluoride is known to stimulate parathyroid and thereby enhance circulating parahormone levels. Teotia and Teotia (1973) reported an increase in parathyroid hormone (PTH) levels manifesting secondary hyperparathyroidism in patients with skeletal fluorosis including children living in endemic areas.

Observations on increased hormonal levels were substantiated by Makhni et al. (1980) at autopsy in two fluorosis patients whose parathyroid glands weighed atleast four times the normal weight due to the increased size and number of the parenchmal cells which led to hyperactivity of the gland.

## Thymus
Fluoride is known to injure thymic epithelial cells and thymocytes and affect the growth in mice (Chen *et al.*, 1999). The mitochondria were swollen and their cristae were lost.

## Adrenal
Several authors reported an increase in weight of adrenal gland after fluoride intoxication. A significant increase in plasma epinephrine and hyperglycemia was induced by fluoride (McGown and Suttie, 1977). It is likely that these changes represent a general stress response, secondary to metabolic poisoning by fluoride and mediated through sympathetic nervous system. The histology of adrenal gland revealed pycnosis in some regions of the cortical cells and the medulla showed extensive vacuolization as well as hypertrophy of chromaffin cells, suggesting alterations in adrenal function (Chinoy, unpublished observations). The adrenal ascorbic acid concentration was increased by 10 mg NaF treatment to mice in response to the imposed stress which is overcome by increased utilization and storage of ascorbic acid (Chinoy, 1978; Chinoy, 1991a,b).

There is paucity of data concerning changes in adrenal activity and aluminium concentrations. Soroka (1964) analysed the content of several metals including aluminium in the adrenal of dogs following excitation of the central nervous system (CNS) with caffeine and depression with ether anaesthesia. The results showed that both CNS excitation and depression resulted in decrease of about 50 to 65 per cent of the normal aluminium concentration of the adrenal gland within 1 hour after administration of the drugs, with a gradual return to normal during the second hour.

## Pancreas
NaF treatment brought about no alteration in the histology of pancreas of mice as compared to control except that the Islet cells appeared more pyknotic as compared to normal (Patel *et al.*, 1994).

Clinical study on the effect of high fluoride intake revealed that the B-cells of pancreatic islets were damaged (Xie *et al.*, 1999b). Hence insulin production may be affected.

Nechaev and Soroka (1967) found that patients with increased pancreatic activity associated with chronic pancreatitis and cholangiohepatitis had higher levels of aluminium.

## Pituitary
Investigation of a cluster of pituitary adenomas in workers in the aluminium industry by Cullen *et al.* (1996) revealed no association with any work activity or location in the industry to suggest a work related or exposure-related cause for disease.

## Arsenic
There is paucity of data on effects of arsenic on endocrine glands of animals and humans. However, studies from our laboratory have elucidated its effects on ovary and uterus which are discussed in a later part.

# REPRODUCTIVE TOXICITY

## Fluoride
The interrelationship of fluoride and reproductive functions were unknown until 1970. Messer *et al.* (1972; 1973; 1974) found that fluoride plays an important role in reproduction and its deficiency causes fertility impairment in mice. Degenerative changes including atrophy and necrosis of seminiferous tubules as well as lack of differentiation and maturation of spermatocytes were reported in fluoride treated mice (Kour and Singh, 1980b). Chinoy and Sequeira (1989a,b) studied the effects of fluoride treatment on the structure and functions of reproductive organs of male mice. After sodium fluoride

treatment seminiferous tubules were found to be necrotic, decreased in their diameter (Chinoy and Sequeira, 1989b) with vacuolization of germinal cells. The accumulation of cholesterol, concomitant with decline in 3β and 17β hydroxysteroid dehydrogenase activities and serum testosterone levels suggested that fluoride interferes with cholesterol metabolism and steroidogenesis in 45 and 60 days NaF treated mice and rats (Chinoy, 1991a,b; Patel and Chinoy, 1997; Chinoy and Mehta, 1999; a, b; Chinoy and Sharma, 1998).

Next to testis, cauda epididymis was the most affected organ by fluoride. Following different doses of fluoride ingestion in mice, rats, rabbits and guinea pigs, the cauda epididymis revealed reduced epithelial cell height, disorganization of secretory epithelium, degeneration and confluence of tubules, pyknotic nuclei of the epithelium and hyalinization of the interstitium. These changes in the histology affected the secretions of cauda epididymis and rendered its internal milieu hostile for maturation of spermatozoa leading to their low sperm count, motility and finally fertility rate was decreased in mice, rats and rabbits by fluoride treatment (Chinoy and Sequeira, 1989a,b; 1992; Chinoy et al., 1991b; Chinoy et al., 1994b; Chinoy, 1995).

Sodium fluoride treatment brought about structural alterations in the vas deferens of mice and rat wherein pyknosis of epithelium, clumping of stereocilia, cell debris in lumen, increase in lamina propria and a decrease in thickness of muscle coat was observed by Chinoy and Sequeira (1989b).

According to Narayana and Chinoy (1994b) after 50 days of NaF treatment to rats, the sperm showed loss of acrosome, deflagellation and reduction in the sperm acrosomal acrosin activity, which is important for gamete fusion. Observations in NaF treated rabbit sperm also revealed disappearance of acrosome, head to head agglutination and deflagellation (Chinoy et al., 1991b). Human spermatozoa lost their motility in vitro in the presence of 250 mM NaF within 20 minutes incubation (Chinoy and Narayana, 1994).

## Uterus and Ovary

Fluoride treatment caused a significant decrease in total protein levels in uterus of NaF treated mice (Chinoy and Patel, 1996). This decline in protein levels in the uterus would affect the activities of its various enzymes. There was an increase in glycogen in uterus which might also be related to the decrease in the activity of phosphorylase in NaF treated mice (Patel et al., 1994). This might be the main causative factor for the accumulation of glycogen in the uterus.

Sodium fluoride (5mg/kg body weight) was effective from the 45th day of treatment in causing a significant decline in DNA and RNA levels of mice ovary, indicating alterations in its nucleic acids and protein metabolism (Patel and Chinoy, 1998).

## Aluminium

Aluminium chloride was found to be embryotoxic and teratogenic when given parenterally to rats (Benett et al., 1975) and mice (Wide, 1984; Cranmer et al., 1986).

A single intratesticular injection of 27.4 mg/kg of aluminium sulphate given to rats caused focal necrosis in testis within 2 days after injection, while this dose also destroyed all the spermatozoa within 7 days after aluminium injection (Kamboj and Kar, 1964). The same authors also found that daily injection of the above dose of aluminium sulphide to mice for 30 days reduced the weight of testis and caused shrinkage of the tubules and spermatogenic arrest at the primary spermatocyte or spermatogonial stages without affecting the interstitium (Kamboj and Kar, 1964).

Aluminium has been found in the prostate, seminal fluid, testicle and seminal vesicle of normal males. According to Llobet et al. (1995), four weeks aluminium nitrate treatment (50, 100 and 200 mg/kg/day) intraperitoneal to male mice showed significantly decreased testicular and epididymal weights, decreased spermatid counts, epididymal sperm counts and a decline in the rate of pregnancy. However, the sperm motility was unaffected and the percentage of morphologically normal spermatozoa in all mice exposed to aluminium were comparable to the values in control mice. Histological changes including necrosis of spermatocytes/spermatids were observed in the testis of male mice treated with 100 and 200 mg/kg/day of aluminium nitrate, whereas tubular diameters were unaffected by aluminium administration.

Reports from our laboratory by Chinoy and Bhattacharya (1997) revealed that aluminium treatment caused alterations in the metabolisms of the testis and cauda epididymis whose homeostasis was disturbed. This has serious repercussions on the sperm motility and fertility rate since normal internal milieu of epididymis is necessary for proper maturation for sperm. Aluminium treatment caused disturbances in oxidative, energy and carbohydrate metabolisms in testis and cauda epididymis as there was decrease in SDH, ATPase and phosphorylase with concomitant increase in glycogen levels. Protein and sialic acid levels were declined after aluminium administration. Steroidogenesis was also affected as 3ß and 17ß HSD activities were decreased, whereas, testicular cholesterol levels were increased (Chinoy and Bhattacharya, 1996). Thus, it is evident that the aluminium treatment altered carbohydrate, protein, oxidative metabolisms, steroidogenesis, sperm motility and caused a reduction in fertility in mice.

## Arsenic

Only limited information exists on the reproductive effects of inorganic arsenic. The histological studies on ovary of mice administered combined treatment of sodium fluoride and arsenic trioxide for a duration of 30 days revealed structural alterations (Chinoy, 1999b). The treatment brought about disintegration, necrosis and dense vacuolization in the stromal tissue, follicular atresia, pyknosis in the follicular cell nuclei and hemorrhage. Further, the corpus luteum diameter and number of primary and secondary follicles were decreased. The above data clearly elucidates alterations in ovarian structure and folliculogenesis, which would influence its functions. The combined treatment also resulted in changes in histology of uterus. Vacuolization in the myometrium and endometrium occurred in treated group of animals as compared to control. Atrophy and confluence of the endometrial gland with pyknosis of their cell nuclei was also observed. These changes would influence the growth of the organ as well as its enzymes, secretions and metabolism.

The protein levels were significantly reduced by sodium fluoride and arsenic trioxide combined treatment in both ovary and uterus of mice (Chinoy, 1999b). This study also elucidated that combined sodium fluoride and arsenic trioxide treatments brought about alterations in uterine carbohydrate metabolism. An accumulation of glycogen was obtained in the present study which might be related to the decrease in the activity of phosphorylase in the uterus as obtained for fluoride and aluminium treatment. The results also elucidated accumulation of cholesterol with a corresponding decline in activities of 3ß and 17ß hydroxysteroid dehydrogenases which would adversely affect steroidogenesis in ovary. These results imply that circulating hormonal levels *i.e.* estradiol and progesterone might also be affected.

Thus, combined, fluoride and arsenic treatment affected protein metabolism in ovary, and uterus, carbohydrate metabolism in uterus and steroidogenesis in ovary of mice.

## Influence of Fluoride, Aluminium and Arsenic on Biological Free Radicals

Free radicals and lipid peroxidation play an important role in fluorosis (Sun *et al.*, 1994). Fluoride is known to stimulate the so-called respiratory burst and the production of superoxide radicals in neutrophils of humans, rabbits and guinea'pigs. The high reactivity of superoxide radicals may lead to chemical modification and impairment of proteins, lipids, carbohydrates and nucleotides in living cells (Rzeuski *et al.*, 1998). High fluoride concentrations are likely to inhibit superoxide dismutase (SOD) and glutathione peroxidase (GSH-PX) activities, resulting in the accumulation of large amounts of free radicals and peroxides causing cell damage in people living in areas endemic to fluorosis (Li and Cao, 1994). Studies from our laboratory (Chinoy and Patel, 1998) revealed that fluoride administration at a dose of 5 mg/kg body weight for 45-60 days to mice inhibited the activities of SOD, GSH-PX and catalase in the ovary and increased ovarian lipid peroxidation, thus rendering the tissue susceptible to injury. The production of superoxide radicals is caused by incomplete oxygen oxidation. These radicals are liable to react with several molecules, provoking their destabilization. The most important consequences are the denaturation of proteins and the peroxidation of membrane lipids, with an increase in the permeability of the cell membrane (Subramaniam *et al.*, 1994). Epidemiological studies of patients with dental and skeletal fluorosis from endemic regions in China also revealed an inhibition of GSH-PX and SOD activities in blood with increased lipid peroxide levels in serum (Bian *et al.*, 1994). The depleted GSH by NaF treatment strongly suggests that, like several compounds, fluoride might also be largely dependent on GSH for detoxification (Li *et at.* 1999). Similar studies from our laboratory (Chinoy *et al.*, 1995; 1997a,b) have also revealed depleted GSH levels in reproductive organs and in sperm suspensions of rats and guinea pigs treated with fluoride. Studies by Dai *et al.* (1999) on endemic fluorotic patients has indicated that drinking water containing high fluoride concentration for a long time caused reduced levels of GSH and GSH-Px. Fluoride induced lipid peroxidation could be reduced by oral intake of glutathione and selenium in rats (Liang *et al.*, 1999; Li *et al.*, 1999). Similarly some herbal antioxidants have also been used in reducing free radical damage in case of chronic fluorosis in China (Liu, 1999).

## Aluminium

Lipid peroxidation has been proposed as a mechanism of cellular membrane damage during heavy metal induced toxicity (Stacey and Kappus, 1982). Brain being rich in polyunsaturated fatty acids is highly susceptible to lipid peroxidation (Sun and Sun, 1974).

Aluminium has some influence on membrane lipids or other organic molecules of the cell and thus facilitates lipid peroxidation which is believed to be an indicator of membrane damage resulting from the degradation of polyunsaturated fatty acids (Tam and McCay, 1970). Aluminium is also known to alter physical properties of the membrane (Vierstra and Haug, 1978). A selective binding of aluminium to phosphatidylserine, a major phospholipid of the brain has been also reported (Blaustein, 1967). It has been shown that free radical damage to polyunsaturated fatty acids, carbohydrates, amino acids and nucleic acids have resulted in elevation of Thiobarbituric acid - reactive substance (TBA-RS) mainly because of generation of malonaldehyde (Gutteridge, 1982).

## Arsenic

There is very limited information regarding arsenic and free radical toxicity. Glutathione (GSH: *viz.* reduced glutathione) is the most abundant naturally occurring non-protein thiol in the body and is involved in numerous biochemical reactions within cells. The fundamental role of GSH may be the protection of thiol groups present in tissue from oxidative stress by xenobiotics (Larsson *et al.*, 1983).

Arsenic has a high affinity for thiol groups, especially dithiol groups of proteins (Aposhin *et al.*, 1984). Studies on Syrian golden hamsters (Hirata *et al.*, 1988) have suggested that GSH is needed to protect cells from damage by arsenite. Low levels of GSH prevent the efficient methylation of arsenite and cause it to accumulate in the cells. The high arsenite concentrations lead to cell damage particularly in the proximal tubules of kidney. Agents that reduce GSH levels may increase the toxic effects of arsenite.

## Reversal of Toxicity

Chinoy and co-workers (Chinoy *et al.*, 1991b; 1994a; 1995; Chinoy and Sequeira, 1992; Narayana and

Chinoy, 1994b; Patel and Chinoy, 1997; Chinoy and Sharma, 1998; Chinoy and Patel, 1998; Chinoy and Mehta, 1999a) have reported partial or incomplete recovery in several biochemical parameters in various organs of mice and rats, after the withdrawal of NaF treatment for one or two months. But after two months, Chinoy and Sequeira (1989a) found marked recovery in the histoarchitecture of reproductive organs of male mouse. Therefore toxic effects induced by fluoride were found to be partially reversible after cessation of fluoride treatment.

## Aluminium

In view of the observed aluminium induced toxic effects, withdrawal studies were carried out in our laboratory. During this study $AlCl_3$ was fed for 30 days and the treatment withdrawn afterwards for 30 days (Chinoy *et al.*, 2000). The results revealed that in many of the parameters, recovery was only partial from aluminium induced toxicity, as compared to control. This may be due to delayed sequestration of aluminium from the body as evident by high serum aluminium levels in the study (Chinoy *et al.*, 2000).

## Arsenic

There is hardly any data regarding withdrawal studies on arsenic toxicity alone.

Reversible studies were carried out in our laboratory (Chinoy, 1999a,b) with combination treatment of NaF and $As_2O_3$ for 30 days in mice and the treatment withdrawn for 30 days afterwards. These studies elucidated that toxic affects were partially recovered and a longer period of withdrawal would be needed for a better recovery.

## Beneficial Effects of Ascorbic Acid (AA), Calcium (CA) and Vitamins on Fluoride, Aluminium and Arsenic Induced Effects

In view of millions of people afflicted with fluoride, aluminium and a variety of pathological manifestations in soft tissues of both animals and human beings, necessitates the investigation of therapeutic agents which are easily available, cheap and have promising results in mitigation of fluoride, aluminium and arsenic induced health hazards in endemic populations.

## Mechanism of Action

The participation of AA in cellular oxido-reduction reactions occurs *via* the formation of its free radical, monodehydro ascorbic acid (MDHA) which is a more powerful reducing agent than AA by virtue of possessing an unpaired electron, which subsequently gets oxidized to dehydroascorbic acid (DHA). DHA could be converted back to AA by glutathione (Chinoy, 1978). Hence AA functions as a powerful anti-oxidant. Ascorbic acid is also known to bind with macro molecules like nucleic acid and protein (Chinoy, 1978) by charge transfer complex formation, which appears to be a very active source of energy for biological processes.

## Ascorbic Acid

A number of studies have demonstrated mitigation of fluorosis in experimental animals and fluorotic human population by the ingestion of ascorbic acid (Wadhwani, 1954; Yu and Hwang, 1985; Chinoy *et al.*, 1991b; 1994b; 1995; 1997a,b; Narayana and Chinoy, 1994b; Patel and Chinoy, 1997; Chinoy and Patel, 1998; Chinoy and Sharma, 1998).

Ascorbic acid is known to inhibit phosphodiesterase (PDE) (Pasternak, 1979) and thereby increase C-AMP levels. The increase in C-AMP, a "second messenger" might have resulted in the recovery in the activities of several enzymes in different tissues. Ascorbic acid itself is known to activate several hydroxylating enzymes and those involved in the oxido-reduction reactions in various tissues (Chinoy, 1978). Antioxidative preparations containing glutathione, ß carotene and superoxide dismutase has been used for the cure of endemic, fluorosis and arsenism (Qiu and Sun, 1999). Similarly preventive antifluorosis preparations containing zinc salt, boron or selenium compounds have also been used by Sun *et al.* (1999) in China.

The therapeutic role of ascorbic acid in alleviation of aluminium and arsenic induced toxicity was also evident in treated mice (Chinoy 1999a,b; Patel and Chinoy, 2000; Memon and Chinoy, 2000).

## Vitamin E

Vitamin E is one of the most active and major lipid soluble antioxidant in tissues (Chinoy and Sharma, 1998) which reduces cell injury by preventing oxidation *in vivo* of polyunsaturated fatty acids (PUFAs) to hydroperoxides and thus protects structural integrity of membranes and prevents occurrence of atherosclerosis. Vitamin E has also been related to changes in calcium homeostasis in tissues (Meerson *et al.*, 1982). Vitamin E has come under much scrutiny for its possible therapeutic roles in numerous disease states especially those involving oxidation related events (Phelps, 1987). Chinoy and Sharma (1998) have reported that ingestion of vitamin E to fluorotic male mice brought about a significant recovery in NaF induced reproductive failure. Vitamin E administration to fluoride fed mice brought about significant recovery in the activity of SOD, levels of lipid peroxides in ovary, as well as serum calcium and potassium levels. Vitamin E also reduces cell injury and has a therapeutic role as a potent biological antioxidant (Chinoy and Sharma, 1998; Sharma and Chinoy, 2000).

A similar mitigation of aluminium toxicity in mice was found by vitamin E administration which caused recovery in steroidogenesis, protein metabolism, phosphorylase activity, sperm motility and fertility rate (Chinoy et al., 2000; Patel and Chinoy, 2000). Combined fluoride and aluminium induced free radical toxicity in cerebral hemisphere of mice was mitigated by use of ascorbic acid, calcium or vitamin E, administered alone or in combination during withdrawal period (Memon and Chinoy, 2000).

## Arsenic

There is hardly any data regarding beneficial role of vitamin E and D in arsenic related toxicity. However, Hsu *et al.* (1999) and Xia *et al.* (1999) have reported that selenium can alleviate the symptoms of arsenic poisoning in arsenic exposed persons. Treatment of arsenic related skin cancer with recombinant interferon Alfa-2b have been attempted by Liang *et al.* (1999).

## Calcium

It is well known that calcium (Ca) combines with fluoride to form an insoluble compound $CaF_2$ thereby reducing its absorption. Calcium activates several enzymes, whereas both calcium and ascorbate are known as inhibitors of phosphodiesterase (PDE) and enhance C-AMP levels (Rasmussen, 1989). Ameliorative role of Ca for mitigation of fluoride and aluminium induced toxicity in mice, rats, rabbits has already been reported (Patel and Chinoy, 2000; Memon and Chinoy, 2000; Mehta and Chinoy, 2000). But its action in mitigating arsenic toxicity is not yet known and needs further research.

## Vitamin D

The chief function of vitamin D is to promote the intestinal absorption of calcium and phosphorus and thus maintain an optimal blood concentration of these elements for calcification of bone. In addition to its role in promoting the intestinal absorption of calcium and phosphorus, vitamin D increases tissue citrate levels which acts as a chelator for aluminium. Thus incorporation of vitamin D might help to sequestrate aluminium from the body.

Vitamin D administration was also found to be beneficial to some extent in fluoride and aluminium toxicity.

Ingestion of vitamin D during the withdrawal period of NaF treated mice was found to be very beneficial in recovery of all NaF induced effects, thus elucidating its ameliorative role in recovery from toxic effects of NaF and aluminium on the reproductive functions and fertility of male mouse (Chinoy and Sharma, 1998; Sharma and Chinoy, 2000; Chinoy *et al.*, 2000). Similar results were also found in female mouse after vitamin D administration during the withdrawal period (Chinoy and Patel, 1998).

Thus fluoride and aluminium induced effects are transient and reversible by the use of vitamins. But the role of these therapeutic agents in mitigating arsenic toxicity need to be explored by detailed study.

## Supplementation of Amino Acids and Protein Supplemented Diet

Studies conducted in our laboratory (Chinoy and Mehta, 1999a) revealed that amino acids (glycine and/or glutamine) were beneficial in promoting the recovery from fluoride induced toxicity. The ameliorative effect of these amino acids was probably due to their roles in various physiological functions, including as biologically active antioxidants (Harper, 1965).

Feeding a protein supplemented diet to mice given alongwith sodium fluoride in different doses helped in suppressing the toxicity whereas a protein deficient diet aggravated it (Chinoy and Mehta, 1999b).

It is thus evident that AA, vitamin E, D, calcium, amino acids and protein supplementation induced a pronounced recovery. Therefore, their deficiency might cause aggravation of fluorosis in fluoride endemic areas. Their combined treatments manifested an additive/synergistic effect for recovery of all parameters almost to control levels (Chinoy and associates).

Thus fluoride, aluminium and arsenic induced effects are transient and reversible by the use of above mentioned therapeutic agents and could be recommended to prevent health hazards.

## SUMMARY

Studies on fluoride, aluminium and arsenic toxicity in mammals and amelioration by some antidotes was reviewed. The sources, distribution (in air, water and soil), importance, their half life and $LD_{50}$ details are presented together with the effects on the three toxicants on protein, carbohydrate, lipid, nucleic acid metabolisms, genotoxicity and free radical toxicity. Their effects on various organs and organ systems in humans and animals have also been presented. Data on the recovery from induced toxicity of several organs due to the beneficial and ameliorative effects of some antidotes vix. Vitamins C,E,D; Calcium, administered alone or in combination as well as other dietary factors i.e. a protein supplemented diet have been reviewed. The data has revealed that the effects of fluoride, aluminium and arsenic on various parameters of a number of organs are by and large, similar. Further more it is evident that the induced toxicity is transient and reversible by the antioxidant and ameliorative action of some antidotes, majority of them being dietary factors. The data has immense significance in view of millions of people affected by these toxicants the world over and especially those suffering from malnutrition.

## ACKNOWLEDGEMENTS

The author is thankful to Ms. Sreelata Nair, Shri Devendra Sinh Jhala, Ms. Arti Sharma, Ms. Trupti Patel and Ms. Sunita Chawla for their help rendered during the compilation of the review.

## REFERENCES

● Alfrey, A.C. (1983) Aluminium. *Advances in Clinical Chemistry.* **23**: 69-91.

● Aposhian, H.V., Carter, D.E., Hoover, T.D., Hus, C., Maiorino, R.M. and Stine, E. (1984). *Fundam. Appl. Toxicol.,* **4**: 558.

● Armstrong, C.W., Stroube, R.B., Rubio, T., *et al.* (1984). Outbreak of fatal arsenic poisoning caused by contaminated drinking water. *Arch Environ. Health.* **39**: 276-279.

- Axelson, O., Dahlgren, E., Jackson, C.D. and Rehnlund, S.O. (1978). Arsenic exposure and mortality: a case-referent study from a Swedish copper smelter. *Br. J. Ind. Med.,* **35**: 8-15.
- Benett, R.W., Persaud, T.V. and Moore, J.L. (1975). Experimental studies on the effects of aluminium on pregnancy and fetal development. *Anat. Anz.* **138**: 365-378.
- Berlyne, G.M. *et al.,* (1972) Hyperaluminanemia from aluminium resins in renal failure. *Lancet.* **1**, 564.
- Bhamra, R.K. and Costa, M. (1992). Trace elements aluminium, arsenic, cadmium, mercury, nickel. In: Environmental toxicants: Human exposures and their health effects. Lippmann, M. (Ed.). New York Van Nostrand Reinhold Company, 575-632.
- Bhatnagar M. and Susheela, A.K. (1998). Chronic fluoride toxicity: An ultrastructural study of glomerulus of the rabbit kidney. *Environmental Science,* **6**(1): 43-54.
- Bian, J.C., Xian, S.M., Ye, P. *et al.* (1994). Determination and analysis of trace elements anti-oxidant material of the Int. Soc. for Fluoride Research, ISFR, 1994, 5-9 Sept., Beijing, China.
- Bibileishvili, Z.V. (1965). Change in trace element concentration and activity of some enzymes in blood of females, Soobshah. Akad. Nauk Gruz. SSR, 39(3), 58. *Chem. Abstr.,* **64**: 7131, 1966.
- Biggs, M.H. (1963). Effect of calcium and aluminum ions on succinate oxidation by liver mitochondria, N.Z.J. Sci., 6, 14.
- Blaustein, M.P. (1967). Phospholipids as ion exchangers: Implications for a possible role in membrane excitability and anaesthesia. *Biochem. Biophys. Acta.* **135**: 653-668.
- Bogin, E., Abrams, M., Avidar, Y. and Israeli, B. (1976). Effect of fluoride on enzymes from serum, liver, kidney, skeletal and heart muscles of mice. *Fluoride,* **9**(1): 42-46.
- Bradley, A.C. (1990). Biological properties of Aluminium. In: Systemic aspects of Biocompatibility. Volume I. CRC series in biocompatibility. (Eds.) David, F. Williams. CRC Press, Beca Roton, Florida, U.S.A., pg. 187-210.
- Brauman, R.S. and Foreback, G.C. (1973). Methylated forms of arsenic in the environment. *Science,* **182**: 1247-1249.
- Braemark, P.I. (1967). Local tissue effects of sodium fluoride. Odont. Revy., 18: 273-294.
- Butzengeiger, K.H. (1949). Arsenism I. ECG changes and other cardiac and circulatory phenomena. II: Mucosal symptoms and pathogenesis. *Dtsch.Arch. Klin. Med.,* **1974**: 1-16.
- Campbell, J.P. and Alvarez, J.A. (1989). Acute arsenic intoxication. *Am. Fam. Physician,* **40**: 93-97.
- Carlson, J.R. and Suttie, J.W. (1966). Pentose phosphate pathway enzymes and glucose oxidation in fluoride fed rats. *Amer. J. Physiol.,* **210**(1): 79-83.
- Caussy, D. (1999). WHO Strategic Plan for Arsenic Mitigation in the South East Asia Region. PAN Asia Pacific Conference on Fluoride and Arsenic Research. Shenyang, China, August, 16-20, 1999, pp.4.
- Chakraborty, A.K. and Saha, K.C. (1987). Arsenical dermatosis from tubewell water in West Bengal. *Indian J. Med. Res.,* **85**: 326-334.
- Chen, P.Z., Sun, H.Y., Qin, Y.P. *et al.* (1999). Effect of maternal exposure to fluoride on the thymic ultrastructure and enzymohistochemistry for filial generation. PAN Asia Pacific Conference on Fluoride and Arsenic Research Shenyang, China, August 16-20, 1999, pp.108.
- Cheng, J. and Zhu, S.F. (1999). The immunological effect of $As_2O_3$ in mice. PAN Asia Conference on Fluoride and Arsenic Research. Shenyang, China, August 16-20, 1999, pp.41.
- Chinoy, N.J. (1978). Ascorbic acid turnover in animal and human tissues. *J. Anim. Morphol. Physiol.,* Silver Jubilee Volume, pp.68-85.
- Chinoy, N.J. 1991a. Effects of fluoride on physiology of some animals and human beings. *Ind. J. Environ. Toxicol.,* **1**(1): 17-32.
- Chinoy, N.J. 1991b. Effects of fluoride on some organs of rats and their reversal. *Proc. Zool. Soc.,* Calcutta, **44**(1): 11-15.

- Chinoy, N.J. 1992. Fluoride toxicity in female mice and its reversal. Recent Advance in Life Sciences. Eds. Saxena, A.K., Ramamurthy, R., Srirama Reddy, G. and Saxena, V.L. Indian Society of Life Sciences, Manu Publications, Kanpur, U.P., India, pp.39-50.
- Chinoy, N.J. 1995. Role of fluoride in animal systems: A review. Toxicity and monitoring of xenobiotics, 13-30.
- Chinoy, N.J. (1996). Fluorosis prone areas in India and affects of fluoride on human health. Latest Advances in Environmental Conservation. Ed. Mathur, R., Mathur, A. and Sharma, S. Scientific Publishers, Jodhpur, India, 79-93.
- Chinoy, N.J. (1999a). Effects of sodium fluoride and arsenic trioxide on liver, gastrocnemius muscle of mice and their reversal by vitamin C. PAN Asia Conference on Fluoride and Arsenic Research. Shenyang, China, August 16-20, 1999, pp.13.
- Chinoy, N.J. (1999b). Combined toxicity of fluoride and arsenic trioxide in ovary and uterus of mice and its amelioration by ascorbic acid. PAN Asia Pacific Conference on Fluoride and Arsenic Research, Shenyana, China, August 16-20, 1999, pp.57.
- Chinoy, N.J. and Sequeira, E. (1989a). Fluoride induced biochemical changes in reproductive organs of male mice. Fluoride, 22(2): 78-85.
- Chinoy, N.J. and Sequeira, E. (1989b). Effects of fluoride on the histoarchitecture of reproductive organs of male mouse. Reprod. Toxicol., 3(4): 261-267.
- Chinoy, N.J. and Sequeira, E. (1992). Reversible fluoride induced fertility impairment in male mice. Fluoride, 25(2): 71-76.
- Chinoy, N.J. and Bhattacharya, S. (1996). Effects of a single dose of aluminium chloride on some reproductive organs and fertility in male mice. Indian J. Environ. and Toxicol., 6(1): 10-13.
- Chinoy, N.J. and Bhattacharya, S. (1997). Effects of chronic administration of aluminium chloride on reproductive functions of testis and some accessory sex organs of male mice. Indian J. Environ. & Toxicol., 7(1): 12-15.
- Chinoy, N.J. and Mehta, D. (1999a). Beneficial effects of some amino acids on testis of mice treated with sodium fluoride. Fluoride, 3(3): 162-170.
- Chinoy, N.J. and Mehta, D. (1999b). Effects of protein supplementation and deficiency on fluoride induced toxicity in reproductive organs of male mice. Fluoride, 32(4) : 204-214
- Chinoy, N.J. and Narayana, M.V. (1992). Studies on Fluorosis in Mehsana District of North Gujarat. Proc Zool. Soc., Calcutta, 45(2): 157-161.
- Chinoy, N.J. and Narayana, M.V. (1994). In vitro fluoride toxicity in human spermatozoa. Reprod. Toxicol., 8(2): 155-159.
- Chinoy, N.J. and Patel, D. (1996). Ameliorative role of amino acids on fluoride induced alterations in uterine carbohydrate metabolism in mice. Fluoride, 29(4): 217-226.
- Chinoy, N.J. and Patel, D. (1998). Influence of fluoride on biological free radicals in ovary of mice and its reversal. Environmental Sciences, 6(3): 171-184.
- Chinoy, N.J. and Sharma, A. (1998). Amelioration of fluoride toxicity by vitamin E and D in reproductive functions of male mice. Fluoride, 31(4) : 203-216.
- Chinoy, N.J. and Sharma, A. (2000). Fluoride induced renal damage and its reversal by some antidotes. XXIIIrd World Conf. of the ISFR, June 11-14, Szczecin, Poland.
- Chinoy, N.J., Joseph, R., Sequeira, E. and Narayana, M.V. 1991a. Effects of sodium fluoride on the muscle and liver of albino rats. Ind.J. Environ. Toxicol., 1(2): 129-134.
- Chinoy, N.J., Sequeira, E. and Narayana, M.V. 1991b. Effect of vitamin C and calcium on the reversibility of fluoride induced alterations in spermatozoa of rabbit. Fluoride, 24(1): 29-39.
- Chinoy, N.J., Mathews Michael and Barot, V.V. (1993a). Toxic effects of sodium fluoride ingestion in mice. Ind. J. Environ. Toxicol., 3: 30-34.
- Chinoy, N.J., Sharma, M. and Mathews Michael (1993b). Beneficial effects of ascorbic acid and calcium on reversal of fluoride toxicity in male rats. Fluoride, 26(1) : 45-56.

- Chinoy, N.J., Walimbe, A.S., Vyas, H.A. and Mangla, P. (1994a). Transient and reversible fluoride toxicity in some soft tissues of female mice. *Fluoride*, 27(4) : 205-214.

- Chinoy, N.J., Reddy, V.V.P.C. and Mathews Michael (1994b). Beneficial effects of ascorbic acid and calcium on reproductive functions of fluoride treated prepubertal male rats. Fluoride, 27(2) : 67-75.

- Chinoy, N.J., Patel, S., Bhatt, N. and Mathews Michael (1994c). Effects of fluoride on some soft tissue functions of fresh water fish *Channa punctatus*. Proc. Acad. *Environ. Biol.*, 3(2) : 191-196.

- Chinoy, N.J., Barot, V.V., Mathews Michael, Barot, J.M., Purohit, R.M., Godasara, N.B. and Parikh, D.J. (1994d). Fluoride toxicity studies in Mehsana District, North Gujarat. *J.Environ.Biol.*, 15(3) : 163-170.

- Chinoy, N.J., Narayana, M.V., Dalal, V., Rawat, M. and Patel, D. (1995). Amelioration of fluoride toxicity in some accessory reproductive glands and spermatozoa of rat. *Fluoride.*, 28(2) : 75-86.

- Chinoy, N.J., Patel, B.C., Patel, D. and Sharma, A.K. (1997a). Fluoride toxicity in the testis and cauda epididymis of guinea pig and reversal by ascorbate. *Med. Science Res.* 25(2) : 97-100.

- Chinoy, N.J., Shukla, S., Walimbe, A.S. and Bhattacharya, S. (1997b). Fluoride toxicity on rat testis and cauda epididymal tissue components and its reversal. *Fluoride.*, 30(1) : 41-50.

- Chinoy, N.J., Bhattacharya, S. and Chawla, S. (2000). Effects of aluminium on some soft tissues of male mice and its reversal. International Conference on Probing in Biological Systems. Feb. 7-11, 2000, Institute of Science, Mumbai.

- Chinoy, N.J. (unpublished observation).

- Chinoy, N.J. and Biringwala, K. (unpublished observation).

- Chongwan, Z. and Daijei, H. (1988). Ultrastructural findings in liver, kidneys, thyroid gland and cardiac muscle of rabbits following sodium fluoride administration. *Fluoride*, 21(1) : 32-38.

- Chhuttani, P.N., Chawla, L.S. and Sharma, T.D. (1967). *Arsenical Neurology*, 17: 269-274.

- Chlubek, D., Nowacki, P., Mikolajek, W., Lagocka, R., Jakubowska, K. and Rzeuski, R. (1998). Neurotoxicity of fluoride in rats - Neuropathological studies. *Fluoride*, 31(3) : S24 (Abstract).

- Chu, T.-Y.J., Ruane, R.J. and Krenkel, P.A. (1978). Characterization and reuse of ash pond effluents in coal-fired power plants. *J. Water Pollut. Control. Fed.*, 50: 2494-2508.

- Cranmer, J.M., Wilkins, J.D., Cannon, D.J. and Smith, L. (1986). Fetal placental-maternal uptake of aluminium in mice following gestational exposure. *Neurotoxicology*, 7: 601-608.

- Crapper McLachlan, D.R., Lukiw, W.J. and Kruck, T.P.A. (1989). New evidence for an active role of aluminium in Alzheimer's disease. *Can. J. Neurol. Sci.*, 16: 490-497.

- Crapper, D.R., Krishnan, S.S. and Dalton, A.J. (1973). Brain aluminum distribution in Alzheimer's Disease and experimental neurofibrillary degeneration, *Science*, 180, 511.

- Cullen, M.R., Checkoway, H. and Alexander, B.H. (1996). Investigation of a cluster of pituitary adenomas in workers in the aluminium industry. *Occupational and Environment Medicine.* 53: 782-786.

- Dai, G.J., Zhang, Z.Y., Shai, C. et al. (1999). The levels of lipid peroxidation and antioxidation of patients with endemic fluorosis and the influence of interference. PAN Asia Pacific Conference on Fluoride and Arsenic Research, Shenyang, China, August 16-20, 1999, pp.9.

- Dai, G.Y., Cai, O.H., Zhou, L.Y., Wei, Z.D. and Zhang, H. (1994). Experimental study of combined effect with fluoride and aluminium. Proceedings of the XXth Conference of the International Society for Fluoride Research, Beijing, China, Abs. No.0-12:42.

- De Boni, U., Serger, M. and Crapper McLachlan, D.R. (1980). Functional sequences of chromatin bound aluminium in cultured human cells. In: Aluminium Neurotoxicity, Liss, L. (Ed.). Park Forest South Illinois, Pathotox Publishers, Inc., pp.6581.

- Agents. Elsevier/North Holland, Biomedical Press, Amsterdam, pp.471-525.

- Desai, V.K., Solanki, D.M., Kantharia, S.L. and Bhavsar, B.S. (1993). Monitoring of neighbourhood fluorosis through a dental fluorosis survey in schools. *Fluoride*, 26(3) : 181-186.

- Dousset, J.C., Rioufol, C., Philibert, C. and Bourbon, P. (1987). Effects of inhaled HF on cholesterol, carbohydrate and tricarboxylic acid metabolism in guinea pigs. *Fluoride*, **20**(3): 137-141.
- York, p.71.
- Exner, F.B. and Waldbott, G.L. (1957). The American Fluoridation Experiment. New York, Devin Adair.
- Fincher, R.M. and Koerker, R.M. (1987). Long-term survival in acute arsenic encephalopathy. Follow-up using newer measures of electrophysiologic parameters. *Am. J. Med.*, **82**: 549-552.
- Flaten, T.P., Glattre, E., Viste, A. and Soreide, O. (1991). Mortality from dementia among gastroduodenal ulcer patients. *J. Epidemiol. Community Health*, **45**: 203-206.
- Franke, J., Rath, F., Runge, H. *et al.* (1975). Industrial Fluorosis. *Fluoride*, **8**: 61-85.
- Franzblau, A. and Lilis, R. (1989). Acute arsenic intoxication from environmental arsenic exposure. Arch. *Environ. Health*, **44**: 385-390.
- Frecker, M.F. (1991). Dementia in Newfoundlands: Identification of a geographical isolate? J. Epidemiol. *Community Health*, **45**: 307-311.
- George, J.C. and Berger, A.J. (1966). Avian Myology. Academic Press, New York.
- Ginsburg, J.M. (1965). Renal mechanism for excretion and transformation of arsenic in the dog. *Am. J. Physiol.*, **268**: 832-840.
- Goebel, H.H., Schmidt, P.F. and Bohl, J. *et al.* (1990). Polyneuropathy due to acute arsenic intoxication. Biopsy studies. *J. Neuropathol. Exp. Neurol.*, **49**: 137-149.
- Grandjean, P. 1985. Long term significance of industrial fluoride exposure: A study of Danish cryolite workers. November 13-17, 1983, New Delhi. ISFR Publication, 1985, p.5-16.
- Graves, A.B., White, E., Koepsell, T.D., Reifler, B.V., Van Belle, G. and Larson, E.B. (1990). The association between aluminium containing products for Alzheimer's disease. *J. Clin. Epidemiol.*, **43**: 35-44.
- Gutteridge, J.M.C. (1982). Free radical damage to lipids, amino acids, carbohydrates and nucleic acids determined by thiobarbituric acid reactivity. *Int. J. Biochem.*, **14**: 649-653.
- Ham, M.P. and Smith, M.D. (1954). Fluorine balance studies on three women. *J. Natr.*, **52**: 225-232.
- Harper, H.A. (1965). Review of Physiological Chemistry. Asian edition, Singapore, Maruzen.
- Hirata, M., Hisanaga, A., Tanaka, A. and Noburu, I. (1988). Glutathione and methylation of inorganic arsenic in hamsters. *Applied Organometallic Chemistry*, 2: 315-321.
- Hoerz, W. and McCarty, K.S. (1971). Inhibition of protein synthesis in rabbit reticulocyte lysate system. *Biochem. Biophys. Acta.*, **228**: 526-535.
- Holland, R.I. (1979). Fluoride inhibition of protein and DNA synthesis in cells *in vitro*. *Acta Pharmacol et Toxicol.*, **45**: 96-101.
- Holland, R.I. (1980). Cytotoxicity of fluoride. *Acta Odont. Scand.*, **58**: 69-89.
- Hongslo, J.H. and Holland, R.I. (1979). Effect of sodium fluoride on protein and DNA synthesis, ptrnithine decarboxylase activity and polyamine content in LH cells. Acta pharmacol. *Toxicol.*, **44**: 350-355.
- Horowitz, S.H. (1973). A review of systemic and topical fluorides for the prevention of dental caries, *Comm. Dent. Oral Epidemiol.*, **1**: 104-114.
- Hosking, D.J. and Chamberlain, M.J. (1977). Studies in man with fluoride. *Clin. Sci.*, **42**: 153-161.
- Hoque, B.A., Yamamura, H.A., Heijnen, G. *et al.* (1999). Arsenic problem in drinking water in Bangladesh context. PAN Asia Pacific Conference on Fluoride and Arsenic Research, Shenyang, China, August 16-20, 1999, pp.21.
- Hsu, K.H., Chiou, H.Y., Chen, C.J. (1999). Arsenic metabolism in humans and its modulation by selenium. PAN Asia Pacific Conference on Fluoride and Arsenic Research, Shenyang, China, August 16-20, 1999, pp.58.
- Huang, Y.Z., Qian, X.C., Wang, G.Q. et al. (1985). Endemic chronic arsenism in Xinjiang. *Clin. Med. J.* (Eng.), **98**: 219-222.
- Huet, P.M., Guillaume, E., Cote, J., Legare, A., Lavoie, P. and Viallet, A. (1975). Noncirrhotic presinusoidal portal hypertension associated with chronic arsenic intoxication. *Gastroenterology*, **68**: 1270-1277.

- Jachimczad and Skotarczak, B. (1978). The effect of fluoride and lead ions on the chromosomes of human leukocytes *in vitro. Genet. Pol.,* **19**: 353-357.

- Jankauskas, J. (1974). Effect of fluoride on the kidney (A review), *Fluoride,* **7**: 93-105.

- Johnson, W.M., Shuler, P.J., Curtis, R.A., Wallingford, K.M., Mangin, H.J., Parnes, W. and Donaldson, H.M. (1973). Industrial hygiene survey. Ormet Corporation Aluminium Facilities, Honnibal, Ohio, U.S. Department of Health, Education and Welfare. Public Health Service National Institute for Ocupational Safety and Health, Cincinnatti.

- Johnson, G.V.W., Codgill, K.W. and Jope, R.S. (1990). Oral aluminium alters *in vitro* protein phosphorylation and kinase activities in rat brain. *Neurobiol. Aging.,* **11**: 209-216.

- Johnson, G.V.W., Watson, A.L.Jr., Lartius, R., Vemura, E. and Jope, R.S. (1992). Dietary aluminium selectively decrease MAP-2 in brains of developing and adult rats. *Neurotoxicology,* **13**: 463-474.

- Kaltreider, N.L., Elder, M.J., Cralley, L.V. and Colwell, M.O. (1972). Health survey of aluminium workers with special reference to fluoride exposure. *J. Occup. Med.,* **14**: 531-541.

- Kamboj, V.P. and Kar, A.B. (1964). Antitesticular effect of metallic and rare earth salts. *J. Reprod. Fertil.,* **7**:21-28.

- Kaul, R.D. and Susheela, A.K. (1974). Evidence of muscle fibre degeneration in rabbits treated with sodium fluoride. *Fluoride,* **7**(4): 177-181.

- Kerr, D.N.S. and Ward, M.K. (1986). The history of aluminium related disease. In: Aluminium and Other Trace Elements in Renal Disease, Taylor, A. (Ed.), pp.1-14, Bailliere Tindall, London.

- Kono, K., Yoshida, Y., Watanabe, M. (1984). Urinary fluoride excretion in fluoride exposed workers with diminished renal function. *Industr. Health,* **22** : 33-40.

- Kour, K., Koul, M.L. and Koul, R.L. (1981). Histological changes in liver following sodium fluoride ingestion. *Fluoride,* **14**(3): 119-123.

- Kour, K. and Singh, J. (1980a). Histological findings in kidney of mice following sodium fluoride administration. *Fluoride,* : 163-167.

- Kour, K. and Singh, J. (1980b). Histological findings in mice testes folowing fluoride ingestion. *Fluoride,* **13**(4) : 160-162.

- Krishnamachari, K.A.V.R. and Krishnaswamy, K. (1973). Genuvalgum and osteoporosis in an area of endemic fluorosis. *Lancet,* : 887-889.

- Krishnamachari, K.A.V.R. and Krishnaswamy, K. (1974). An epidemiological study of the syndrome of genu valgum among residents of endemic areas for fluorosis in Andhra Pradesh. *Ind. J. Med. Res.,* **62** : 1415-1417.

- Laptieva, E.D. (1967). Trace elements in blood of donors and parturient women with physiological blood loss during delivery, *Zdravookhr. Tadzh.,* **3**: 578.

- Larsson, A., Orrenius, S., Homgreen, A. and Mannerwik, B. (eds.) (1983). Functions of Glutathione, Raven Press, New York.

- Lee, A.M. and Fraumeni, J.F. Jr. (1969). Arsenic and respiratory cancer in man: an occupational study. *J. Natl. Cancer Inst.,* **42**: 1045-1052.

- Lee, T.C., Yih, L.H., Huang, S.C. (1999). Cytogenetic alterations induced by inorganic arsenic in human cells. PAN Asia Pacific Conference on Fluoride and Arsenic Research, Shenyang, China, August 16-20, 1999, pp.33.

- Levin-Scherz, J.K., Patrick, J.D., Weber, F.H. *et al.* (1987). Acute arsenic ingestion. *Am. Emerg.Med.,* **16**: 702-704.

- Li, J. and Cao, S. (1994). Recent studies on endemic fluorosis in China. *Fluoride,* **27**(3) : 125-128.

- Li, Y.Y., Sun, G.F., Li, F.J. *et al.* (1999). Effect of Se and GSH on lipid peroxidation induced by fluoride: An experimental study. PAN Asia Pacific Conference on Fluoride and Arsenic Research, Shenyang, China, August 16-20, 1999, pp.111.

- Liang, G., Zhang, X.M., Zhao, H. *et al.* (1999). The effect of GSH taken orally on lipid peroxidation induced by fluoride. PAN Asia Pacific Conference on Fluoride and Arsenic Research, Shenyang, China, August 16-20, 1999, pp.55.

- Liu, J.L. (1999). Free radical damage and antagonizing effect of herbal antioxidant in case of chronic fluorosis. PAN Asia Pacific Conference on Fluoride and Arsenic Research, Shenyang, China, August 16-20, 1999, pp.112.

- Llobet, J.M., Colomina, M.T., Sirvent, J.J., Domingo, J.L. and Corbella, J. (1995). Reproductive toxicology of aluminium in male mice. *Fundamental and Applied Toxicology,* **25**: 45-51.

- Lote, C.J. *et al.* (1992). Effect of citrate on plasma aluminium concentration and aluminium excretion in the rat. *Clin. Sci.,* **83**: 431-435.

- Lu, F.C., Mazurkiewiez, I.M., Grewal, R.S, Allmark, M.G. and Boivin, P. 1961. The effects of sodium fluoride on responses to various control nervous system agents in rats. *Toxicol. Appl. Pharmacol.,* **3**: 31-38.

- Lunde, G. (1975). Isolation of an organoarsenic compound present in codliver. *J. Sci. Food Agric.,* **26**: 1247-1255.

- Macuch, P., Balazoa, G., Bartosova, L., Hiluchan, E., Ambrus, J., Janovicova, J. and Kirilculova, V. (1963). Hygienic analysis of the influence of noxious factor on the environment and state of health of the population in the vicinity of an aluminium plant. *J. Hyg. Epidem.,* **7** : 389-403.

- Manna, G.K. and Das, R.K. (1972). Chromosome aberration in mice induced by aluminium chloride. *Nucleus,* **15**: 180-186.

- Makhni, S.S., Sidhu, S.S., Singh, P. and Singh, G. (1980). The parathyroid in human fluorotic syndrome. *Fluoride,* **13** : 17-19.

- Martin, R.B. (1986). The chemistry of aluminium as related to biology and medicine. *Clin. Chem.,* **32**: 1797-1806.

- Mathews Michael, Barot, V.V. and Chinoy, N.J. (1996). Investigations of soft tissue functions in fluorotic individuals of North Gujarat. *Fluoride,* **29(2)** : 63-71.

- Mazumdar, D.N., Chakraborty, A.K., Ghose, A. *et al.* (1988). Chronic arsenic toxicity from drinking tube well water in rural. *West Bengal. Bull.,* WHO 66: 499-506.

- McGown, E.L. and Suttie, J.W. (1977). Mechanism of fluoride induced hyperglycemia in the rat. *Toxicol. Appl. Pharmacol.,* **40**: 83-90.

- Meerson, F.Z., Kagan, V.K., Kozlov, Yu, P., Belkina, L.M., Arckhipenko, Yu. V. (1982). The role of lipid peroxidation in pathogenesis of ischemic damage and the antioxidant protection of the heart. *Basic Res. Cardiol.,* **77**: 465-485.

- Mehta, D. and Chinoy, N.J. (2000). Reversibility of fluoride induced effects on some organs of male mice by vitamin C and calcium. International Conference on Probing in Biological Systems. February 7-11, 2000, Institute of Science, Mumbai.

- Memon, R. and Chinoy, N.J. (2000). Fluoride and/or aluminium induced free radical toxicity in cerebral hemisphere of male mice and mitigation by antidotes. International Conference on Probing in Biological Systems. February 7-11, 2000, Institute of Science, Mumbai.

- Merian, E. (Ed.) (1991). Metals and their Compounds in the Environment: Occurrence, Analysis and Biological Relevance. pp. 751-767, Weinheim, New York.

- Messer, H.H., Armstrong, W.D. and Singer, L. (1972). Fertility impairment in mice on a low fluoride intake. *Science,* **177**: 893-894.

- Messer, H.H., Armstrong, W.D. and Singer, L. (1973). Influence of fluoride intake on reproduction in mice. *J. Nutr.,* **103**: 1319-1326.

- Messer, H.H., Armstrong, W.D. and Singer, L. (1974). Essentiality and function of fluoride. In: Hoekstra, W.G., Suttie, J.W., Ganther, H.E. and Mertz, W. (Eds.) Trace Element Metabolism in Animal, Baltimore, University Park Press, 425-437.

- Mulay, I.L. *et al.* (1971). Trace-metal analysis of cancerous and non-cancerous human tissues, *J. Nat. Cancer Inst.,* **47**(1), 1.

- Narayana, M.V. and Chinoy, N.J. (1994a). Effects of fluoride on rat testicular steroidogenesis. *Fluoride,* 27(1): 7-12.

- Narayana, M.V., and Chinoy, N.J. (1994b). Reversible effects of sodium fluoride ingestion on spermatozoa of rat. *Int. J. Fertil.,* **39**(6): 337-346.

- National Academy of Sciences (NAS), 1977. Medical and biologic effects of environmental pollutants, Arsenic. Washington D.C., National Academy of Sciences.

- Nechaev, E.V. and Soroka, V.R. (1967). Correlation between trace elements and enzyme activity of pancreatic juice, *Chem. Abstr.*, **67**, 71909.

- Ng, J.C., Qi, L.X., Wang, J.P. *et al.* (1999). Study of arsenic carcinogenicity using the *in vitro* and *in vivo* systems. PAN Asia Pacific Conference on Fluoride and Arsenic Research, Shenyang, China, August 16-20, 1999, pp.35.

- Nutrition News (1998). Risk of aluminium toxicity in Indian context. National Institute of Nutrition, Hyderabad, Vol.19(3).

- Obe, G. and Slacik-Erben (1973). Suppressive activity by fluoride on the induction of chromosome aberrations in human cells with alkylating agents *in vitro*. *Muta. Res.*, **19**: 369-371.

- Pasternak, C.A. (1979). In: An Introduction to Human Biochemistry. Oxford University Press, New York, Toronto, pp.199-219.

- Patel, D. and Chinoy, N.J. (1997). Synergistic action of ascorbic acid and calcium in mitigation of fluoride induced toxicity in uterus of mice. *Ind. J. Environ. and Toxicol.*, **7(1)**: 16-19.

- Patel, D. and Chinoy, N.J. (1998). Ameliorative role of amino acids on fluoride induced alterations in mice (Part II) : Ovarian and uterine nucleic acid metabolism. *Fluoride*, **31(3)**: 143-148.

- Patel, T. N. and Chinoy, N.J. (2000). Combined fluoride and aluminium toxicity in liver and gastrocnemius muscle of female mice and its amelioration. International Conference on Probing in Biological Systems. February 7-11, 2000, Institute of Science, Mumbai.

- Patel, D., Milind, V.S., Narayana, M.V. and Chinoy, N.J. (1994). Effects of sodium fluoride on physiology of female mice and its reversal. *Proc. of Academy of Environ. Biol.*, **3(2)**: 197-205.

- Phelps, D.L. (1987). Current perspectives on vitamin E in infant nutrition. *Am. J. Clin. Nutr.*, **46**: 187-191.

- Pinto, S.S. and McGill, C.M. (1953). Arsenic trioxide exposure in industry. *Ind. Med. Surg.*, **22**: 281-287.

- Popov, K., Rusanov, E.and Balevska, P. (1966). Trace elements of the human aorta depending on age, hemodynamics and some diseases. *Int. Cong. Gerontol. Proc.* **2**, 393, Chem. Abstr., 71, 20269, 1969.

- Qiu, L.Y. and Sun, G.F. (1999). Effect of ß-carotene and SOD on lipid peroxidation induced by fluoride. PAN Asia Pacific Conference on Fluoride and Arsenic Research, Shenyang, China, August 16-20, pp.53.

- Rasmussen, H. (1989). The cycling of calcium as an intracellular messenger. Scientific American, October, pp.66-72.

- Rastogi, R., Upreti, R.K. and Kidwai, A.M. (1987). Effect of fluoride on the intestinal epithelial cell brush border membrane. *Bull Environ. Contam. Toxicol.*, **39**: 162-167.

- Reichl, F.X., Szinicz, L., Kreppel, H., Fichtl, B. and Forth, W. (1990). Effect of glucose in mice after acute experimental poisoning with arsenic trioxide ($As_2O_3$). *Arch. Toxicol.*, **64**: 336-338.

- Rozenshtein, I.S. (1970). Sanitary toxicological assessment of low concentrations of arsenic trioxide in the atmosphere. *Hyg. Sanit.*, **35(1-3)**: 16-22.

- Rybicki, J. (1970). Effect of fluorine on the upper respiratory tract and ears of workers in an aluminium factory. *Med. Pr.*, **21**: 192.

- Rzeuski, R., Chinbek, D. and Macho, Z. (1998). Interactions between fluoride and biological free radical reactions. *Fluoride*, **31(1)**: 43-45.

- Sharma, A. and Chinoy, N.J. (2000). Fluoride induced ultrastructural and histopathological changes in liver of mice and its reversal by antidotes. International Conference on Probing in Biological Systems. Feb. 7-11, 2000, Institute of Science, Mumbai.

- Shashi, A. (1994). Preliminary observation on alterations in rabbit ovary DNA and RNA content in experimental fluorosis. *Fluoride*, **27(2)**: 76-80.

- Shashi, A., Thapar, S.P. and Singh, J.P. (1987). Effects of fluoride administration on organs of gastrointestinal tract - an experimental study on rabbits - effect on tissue proteins. *Fluoride*, **20(3)**: 183-188.

- Sheth, F.J., Multani, A.S. and Chinoy, N.J. (1994). Sister chromatid exchanges: A study in fluorotic individuals of North Gujarat. *Fluoride*, **27(4)**: 215-219.

- Sivakumar, B. and Krishnamachari, K.A.V.R. (1976). Circulating levels of immunoreactive parathyroid hormone in endemic genu valgum. *Fluoride*, **9(4)**: 185-186.

- Smith, T.J., Crecelius E.A. and Reading, J.C. (1977). Airborne arsenic exposure and excretion of methylated arsenic compounds. Environ. *Health Perspect.*, **19**: 89-93.

- Soroka, V.R. (1964). Participation of adrenal glands in the metabolism of some trace elements during medicinal excitation and inhibition of the central nervous system. Chem. Abstr., 61, 13783.

- Spencer, H., Kramer, L., Norris, C., *et al.* (1980). Effect of aluminium on fluoride and calcium metabolism in man. Trace Subst. Environ. Health, **14**: 94-102.

- Spencer, A.J., Wood, J.A., Saunders, H.C., Freeman, M.S., and Lote, C.J. (1995). Aluminium deposition in liver and kidney following acute intravenous administration of aluminium chloride or citrate in conscious rats. *Human and Experimental toxicology*, **14**: 787-794.

- Stacey, N.H., Kappus, H. (1982). Cellular toxicity and lipid peroxidation in response to mercury. Toxicol. *Appl. Pharmacol.*, **63**: 29-35.

- Stein, G., Laske, V., Muller, A. et al. (1987). Aluminium induced damage of the lysosomes in the liver, spleen and kidneys of rats. *J. Appl. Toxicol.*, **7(4)**: 253-258.

- Steinweis, P.C. and Gilman, A.G. (1982). Aluminium A requirement for the activation of the regulatory component of adenylate cyclase by fluoride. *Proc. Natl. Acad. Sci.* (USA), **79**: 4888-4891.

- Strochkova, L.S., Zahvoronkov, A.A., Autsyn, A.P. (1984). Effects of fluoride on morphological modifications in Hela cell culture. *Tsitologiya*, **26**: 299-306.

- Subramaniam, S., Shyama, S. and Shyamaladevi, C.S. (1994). Protective effect of vitamin E against CMF-induced damages in small intestinal brush border membrane of rats. Ind. J. of Pharmacol., **26**: 213-217.

- Sun and Sun (1974). Synaptosomal plasma membranes: Ocyl group composition of phosphoglycerides and Na$^+$, K$^+$ ATPase activity during fatty acid deficiency. *J. Neurochem.*, **22**: 15-18.

- Sun, G.F., Shen, H.Y. and Ding, G.Y. (1994). Effects of extraneous GSH on toxicity and metabolism of fluoride. In : Proc. of XXth Conference of the Int. Soc. Fluoride Research, ISFR, 1994, 5-9 Sept., Beijing, China.

- Sun, S.Z., Chen, Y.Y., Chen, X.M. *et al.* (1999). Investigation of prevention and cure of endemic fluorosis and arsenism. PAN Asia Pacific Conference on Fluoride and Arsenic Research, Shenyang, China, August 16-20, pp.50.

- Susheela, A.K. and Jain, S.K. (1986). Fluoride toxicity: Erythrocyte membrane abnormality and echinocyte formation. In: Fluoride Research Studies in Environmental Science. (Eds. H. Tsunoda and M.H.Yu). Elsevier Science Publ., B.V. Amsterdam, 27, 231-239.

- Susheela, A.K. and Kharb, P. (1990). Aortic calcification in chronic fluoride poisoning: Biochemical and Electron microscopic evidence. *Experimental and Molecular Pathology*, **53**: 72-80.

- Susheela, A.K., Das, T.K. and Gupta, I.P., Tandon, R.K., Kaker, S.K., Ghosh, P. and Deka, R.C. (1992). Fluoride ingestion and its correlation with gastrointestinal discomfort. *Fluoride*, **25(1)**: 5-22.

- Szinicz, L. and Forth, W. (1988). Effect of As$_2$O$_3$ on gluconeogenesis. Arch. *Toxicol.*, **61**: 444-449.

- Szuler, I.M., Williams, C.N., Hindmarsh, J.T. and Park-Dincsoy, H. (1979). Massive variceal hemorrhage secondary to perisinusoidal portal hypertension due to arsenic poisoning. *Can. Med. Assoc. J.*, **120**: 168-171.

- Tam, B.K. and McCay, P.B. (1970). Reduced triphosphopyridine nucleotide oxidase-catalyzed alterations phospholipid peroxidase. *J. Biol. Chem.*, **245**: 2295-2300.

- Teotia, S.P.S. and Teotia, M. (1973). Secondary hyperparathyroidism in patients with endemic skeletal fluorosis. Br. *Med. J.*, **1**: 637-639.

- Thompson, E.J., Kilanowski, F.M. and Perry, P.E. (1985). The effect of fluoride on chromosome aberration and sister chromatid exchange frequencies in cultured human lymphocytes. *Muta. Res.*, **144**: 89-9.'.

- Tseng, W.P. (1977). Effects and dose response relationships of skin cancer and Blackfoot disease with arsenic. *Environ. Health Perspect.*, **19**: 109-119.

- Tseng, W.P., Chu, H.M., How, S.W., Fong, J.M., Lin, C.S. and Yeh, S. (1968). Prevalence of skin cancer in an endemic area of chronic arsenicism in Taiwan. *J. Natl. Cancer Inst.*, **40**: 453-463.

- Tsutsui, T., Suzuki, N. and Ohmori, M. (1984). Sodium fluoride induced morphological and neoplastic transformation, chromosome aberrations, sister chromatid exchanges and unscheduled DNA sythesis in cultured Syrian hamster embryo cells. *Cancer Res.*, **44**: 938-941.

- Underwood, E.J. (1977). Trace Elements in Human and Animal Nutrition. Academic Press, New York.

- US Environmental Protection Agency (US EPA) (1981). An exposure and Risk Assessment for Arsenic. EPA office for Water Regulations and Standards, Washington, D.C.

- US Department of Health and Human Service (1997). Toxicological Profile for Aluminium. U.S. Dept. of Health and Human Services, Public Health Service. Agency for Toxic Substances and Disease Registry. Atlanta, Georgia, pp.1-207.

- U.S. Department of Health and Human Services, Public Health Service (1998). Draft, Toxicological Profile for Arsenic, Atlanta, Georgia.

- Vahter, M. and Norin, H. (1980). Metabolism of $^{74}$As labelled trivalent and pentavalent inorganic arsenic in mice. *Environ. Res.*, **21**: 446-457.

- Van der Voet G.B. (1992). Intestinal absorption of aluminium. In: Aluminium in biology and medicine. New York, Chichester, Brisbane, Toronto, John Wiley and Sons, pp.109-122 (Ciba Foundation Symposium, No.169).

- Van de Vyver, F.L., De Broe, M.E. (1985). Aluminium in tissues. *Clinical Nephrology*, **24** (Suppl.1): 537-557.

- Vierstra, R. and Huag, A. (1978). The effect of Al$^{+3}$ on the physical properties of membrane lipids in *Thermoplasma acidophilium*. *Biochem. Biophys Res. Comn.*, **84**: 138-143.

- Wadhwani, T.K. (1954). Mitigation of fluorosis (Experimental). *Ind. J. Med. Gaz.*, **87**: 5-7.

- Wadhwani, T.K. and Ramaswamy, A.S. (1953). Pathological changes in tissues of rats and monkeys in fluorine toxicosis. *V. Indian. Inst. Sci.*, **35A**: 223-230.

- Waldbott, G.L., Burgstahler, A.W. and McKinney, H.L. (1978). Fluoridation. the Great Dilemma. Coronado Press Inc., Lawrence, Kansas, pp.148-174.

- Wang, S.X., Gao, J.G., Chen, Y.X. (1999). Effect of fluorine on ChE activity and Ach content in rats blood and the histochemical changes. PAN Asia Pacific Conference on Fluoride and Arsenic Research, Shenyang, China, August 16-20, 1999, pp.107.

- WHO (1970). Fluorides and Human Health. Geneva, World Health Organization, p.364 (Monograph Series No.59).

- WHO (1981). Environmental Health Criteria 18: Arsenic. International Programme on Chemical Safety Geneva. Printed in Finland. 81/5113 - Vammalan Kirjapaino OY, Vammala - 7000.

- WHO (1984). IPCS International Programme on Chemical Safety. Environmental Health Criteria. 36. Fluorine and Fluorides. Published by United Nations Environment Programme, the International Labour Organization, and the World Health Organization, Geneva, 1-136.

- WHO (1997). Geneva Environmental Health Criteria, 194: Aluminium-1-282. Printed in Finland 97/PLL/11539-Vammala-5000.

- Wide, M. (1984). Effect of short term exposure of five industrial metals on the embryonic and fetal development of the mouse. *Environ. Res.*, **33**: 47-53.

- Willems, C., Sande, B.J. and Dumont, J.E. (1972). Inhibition of thyroid secretion by sodium fluoride *in vitro*. *Biochem. Biophys. Acta*, **264**: 197-204.

- Williams, J.M., Hewerka, E.M., Vanderborgh, N.E. *et al.* (1977). Environmental pollution by trace elements in coal preparation wastes. In: Proceedings of the 7th Symposium on Mine Drainage Control, at NCA/BRC Coal Conference, Louisville, October 19, 1997, Los Alamos, new Mexico, Los Alamos Scientific Laboratory.

- Wohlschlage, J., Dipasquale, L.C. and Vernot, E.H. (1976). Toxicity of solid rocket motor exhaust - effects of HCl, HF and alumina on rodents. *J. Combust. Toxicol.*, **3**: 61-70.

- Xia, Y.J., Hou, S.F., Wu, K.G. *et al.* (1999). Effects of organ-selenium on cell membrane structure and function of endemic arsenism. PAN Asia Pacific Conference on Fluoride and Arsenic Research, Shenyang, China, August 16-20, 1999, pp.59.
- Xie, Y.X., Jiang, X.Y., Zhang, A.H. *et al.* (1999a). A study on the genetic damage to the peripheral lymphocytes of the patients with endemic arsenism caused by burning coal. PAN Asia Pacific Conference on Fluoride and Arsenic Research, Shenyang, China, August 16-20, 1999, pp.81.
- Xie, Y.P. and Ge, X.J., Jiang, M.Y. *et al.* (1999b). Clinical study on the effect of high fluoride on the function of the pancreatic islets ß cells. PAN Asia Pacific Conference on Fluoride and Arsenic Research, Shenyang, China, August 16-20, 1999, pp.139.
- Yamamura, S.T. (1999). Arsenic and Fluoride in Drinking Water, WHO's Recent endeavours. PAN Asia Pacific Conference on Fluoride and Arsenic Research, Shenyang, China, August 16-20, 1999, pp.3.
- Yu, M.H. and Hwang, H.L.S. (1985). Influence of protein and ascorbic acid on fluoride induced changes in blood composition and skeletal fluoride deposition in mice. In: Fluoride Research. Studies in Environmental Science. *Tsunoda, H. and Yu, M.H. (Eds.)*, **27**: 203-210.
- Zhang, B. and Meng, Z.Q. (1999). Observation of micronuclei in lymphocytes of workers exposed to fluoride. PAN Asia Pacific Conference on Fluoride and Arsenic Research, Shenyang, China, August 16-20, 1999, pp.137.
- Zhang, A.H., Huang, X.X., Sun, Y. *et al.* (1999). Detection by SCGE of DNA damage in blood cells of the patients with arsenism caused by burning coal. PAN Asia Pacific Conference on Fluoride and Arsenic Research, Shenyang, China, August 16-20, 1999, pp.83.
- Zheng, B.S., Ding, Z.H., Zhu, J. *et al.* (1999). The major ingestion pathways of arsenic in endemic arsenosis areas in Guizhou province, China. PAN Asia Pacific Conference on Fluoride and Arsenic Research, Shenyang, China, August 16-20, 1999, pp.44.
- Zhiliang, Y., Yihua, L., Linsheng, Z. and Zhengping, Z. (1987). Industrial fluoride pollution in the metallurgical industry in China. *Fluoride*, **20(3)**: 119-125.

# 13

# Involvement of Radicals in Atomospheric Reactions and Chemical Toxicity : An Overview

*Vrajesh Tripathi*

## Introduction

Life is being exposed to a number of pollutants and chemicals which have different physical state and chemical nature. A role for free radical has been proposed in the toxicity of numerous chemicals and pollutants. The radical is defined as any molecule that contains one or more unpaired electrons. Free nature of the electrons in free radicals makes them able to combine readily within a tissue in order to achieve a more stable paired eletron states. Radicals are involved in many atmospheric reactions and are also generated in metabolic pathways. In atmosphere mainly oxygen radicals are formed in photolytic and oxidation reaction (Hippeli & Elstner, 1991). In biological system mainly superoxide anions ($O_2^-$) hydroxy radical (OH·), hydroperoxy radical ($HO_2$·) are formed. Since singlet oxygen ($1O_2$), hydrogern peroxide ($H_2O_2$), hypochlorous acid (HOCl) and peroxide and hydroperoxide and epoxide metabolites of endogenous lipids and xenobiotics (foreign to life) contain chemically reactive oxygen-containing functional groups (Saltman, 1989), but are not radicals and do not necessarily interact with tissues through radical reactions, so reactive oxygen species (ROS) terms is more commonly used. However, carbon, nitrogen, and sulphur centered radicals may also occur in biological systems and are more important in initiating and /or propagating various types of injury.

In biological system, the known cellular sources of ROS are phagocyte activation, mitochondrial and microsomal electron transport systems, soluble oxidase enzymes, auto-oxidation of endogenous or exogenous substrates, and transition metals. The capacity of specific pathways to produce free radicals varies with the cell type, but all aerobic cells appear capable of producing free radicals and reaction with biomolecules including DNA, protein and lipids occur (review: Keherer, 1993 ref. therein). But cells have enzymatic and non-enzymatic defence mechanism (through antioxidants) for protection and repair of biomolecules against such oxidative changes. These include superoxide dismutases, catalase, glutathione system, vitamin E, ascorbate, urate, histidine, methionine, and several others (review: Chow, 1991; Kakkar & Vishwanathan, 1992; Edge *et al.*, 1997 ref, therein). Free radicals, however, are not always harmful rather needed for life. Hydrogen peroxide, oxidized halogens, and oxidant radicals contribute in the destruction of invasive pathogens, induce the release of cytokines and exert influence on some reproductive events (Mendoz & Ramos, 1997). However, the oxidative stress mechanism has been implicated in the pathogenesis of certain injury and disease states also. Therapeutic application of antioxidant in controlling diseases are encouraging but are not conclusive. (Book, Eds.: Blake & Winward, 1995). An important part of the cellular defence to oxidative stress is the specific induction of new gene expression in response to specific oxidative stressors. Some of the genes induced response to oxidative stress as superoxide dismutase and glutathione peroxidase are directly invloved in the neutralization of oxygen radicals and their precursors (Jansen *et al.*, 1993; Pahl and Baeurle, 1994). Others such as p 21, c-fos, and caspases are involved in the control of cell proliferation and apoptosis in response to oxidative stress (Simon *et al.*, 1997).Some of signal transducer and activator of transcription (STAT) factors are activated by $H_2O_2$ (Simon *et al.*, 1998) and ROS has been shown to participate in local immune repsonse in lung diseases *via* interleukin-6 release also, from bronchial epithelial cells (Yoshida, 1999).

Voluminous literature related to radical implication in biological or related processes is available.

The current chapter is designed to provide an overview of the basic mechanism involved in atmospheric processess and chemical toxicity only, that may be helpful in understanding the subject. The detail account can be seen in the references mentioned or from other sources.

## ATMOSPHERIC PROCESS

### Source of Atmospheric Pollutants

The worlds greatest problem is air pollution which may directly influence plants, animals and man or indirectly through global climate changes due to anthropogenic gas emissions and stratospheric ozone depletion as a result of the emissions of chlorofluorocarbons. The physico-chemical and biological processess, form and release many compounds in environment. The gaseous pollutants in the atmospheric environment emitted from various sources such as $CO_2$ from respiration, biological degradation and combustion; CO from mainly combustion; Hydrocarbons (without $CH_2$) from trees, industries, and motor vehicles; $CH_4$ from swamps, rice fields and ruminants; $SO_2$ from volcanoes, coal and combustion; NOx from combustion; $NH^+_4$ from soil, biological degradation and cattle. Volcanic ashes contain arsenic, mercuric and fluorine, $CO_2$, $SO_2$, HCl, HF, $CH_2$, aldehydes, ketones, benzene and toluene etc. Atmospheric aerosol particles are classified as primary or secondary. Primary particles are produced by sources such as combustion devices and are imported into the atmosphere in particulate form. Secondary particles are formed in the atmosphere by chemical reactions among primary and secondary gabeous species.

### The Oxyradical's Reactions in Atmosphere

After emissions, particulate forms are removed from atmosphere by sink processes such as wet and dry deposition or chemical processes leading to the formation of photochemical oxidants and strong acids. Photolysis or photodissociation results in molecule destruction caused by light absorption (review: Hippeli & Elstner, 1991). The photolysis of nitrogen dioxide, ozone, and formaldehyde has been shown by the following reactions.

$$NO_2 + hv\ (\leq 400nm) \longrightarrow NO^* + <O>$$
nitrogen dioxide
$$<O> + O_2 \longrightarrow O_3$$
$$O_3 + hv\ (\leq 300nm) \longrightarrow O^*_2 + O^*$$
Ozone
$$O^* + H_2O \longrightarrow 2^*OH$$
$$H_2CO + hv\ (\leq 330\ nm) \longrightarrow H^* + HCO^*$$
Formaldehyde
$$H^* + O_2 \longrightarrow HO^*_2$$
$$HCO^* + O_2 \longrightarrow HO^*_2 + CO$$
$$HO^*_2 + NO^* \longrightarrow {}^*OH + NO_2$$

The properly weighed, average tropospheric concentrations of the major oxidant, the *OH can be estimated by calculating the global rate of loss of methyl chloroform (Prinn et al, 1987). The CO, $CH_4$ $SO_2$ and $NO_2$ are oxidized by OH* radical, yielding their corresponding acids

(a) CO Oxidation

$$CO + {}^*OH \longrightarrow CO_2 + H^* \quad \text{Initiation}$$
$$H^* + O_2 \longrightarrow HO^*_2 \quad \text{Propagation}$$
$$HO^*_2 + NO^* \longrightarrow {}^*OH + NO_2$$

$$\overline{CO + O_2 + NO^* \longrightarrow CO_2 + NO_2}$$
$$\text{and } HO^*_2 + HO^*_2 \longrightarrow H_2O_2 + O_2 \quad \text{Termination}$$

## (b) $CH_4$ Oxidation

$$CH_4 + *OH \longrightarrow CH_3^* + H_2O$$
$$CH_3^* + O_2 \longrightarrow CH_3O_2^*$$
$$CH_3O_2 + NO^* \longrightarrow CH_3O^* + NO_2$$
$$CH_3O^* + O_2 \longrightarrow HCHO + HO_2^*$$
$$HCHO + *OH \longrightarrow CHO^* + H_2O$$
$$CHO^* + O_2 \longrightarrow CO + HO_3$$
$$CO + *OH \longrightarrow CO_2 + H^*$$
$$H^* + O_2 \longrightarrow HO_2^*$$
$$3HO_2^* + 3NO^* \longrightarrow 3*OH + 3NO_2$$
$$\overline{CH_4 + 4O_2 + 4NO^* \longrightarrow CO_2 + 2H_2O + 4NO_2}$$

and

$$CH_3O_2^* + HO_2^* \longrightarrow CH_3OOH + O_2$$

If there is fall in *OH or NO* concentration by any means, the methane degradation rate may slow down or terminate. The monthly average net yield of *OH, CO and $O_3$ can be calculated from the methane oxidation chain reactions (Tie et al., 1992: ref. therein). Increased methane concentrations may contribute to global warming, enhance formation of tropospheric ozone, suppress *OH and affect stratospheric ozone (Thompson el al., 1992)

## (c) $SO_2$ Oxidation

$$SO_2 + OH \longrightarrow SO_2OH$$
$$SO_2OH + O_2 \longrightarrow SO_3 + HO_2$$
$$SO_3 + N_2O \longrightarrow H_2SO$$
$$HO_2 + NO^* \longrightarrow *OH + NO_2$$
$$\overline{SO_2 + O2 + NO + H_2O \longrightarrow H_2SO_4 + NO_2}$$

Other than gas phase oxidation of sulphur dioxide, liquid phase oxidation may occur by hydrogen peroxide in an acid catalyed reaction (Fuhrer, 1985; Mohnen, 1988).

$$SO_2 + H_2O_2 \longrightarrow H_2SO_4$$

The aquocous phase oxidation significantly decrease ozone concentration in troposphere (Lelieveld and Crutzen, 1990).

## (d) $NO_2$ Oxidation

During daytime $NO_2$ react with *OH to form nitric acid while at night $NO_2$ can react with $O_3$ which also leads to the formation of nitric acid.

$$NO_2 + O_3 \longrightarrow NO_3 + O_2$$
$$NO_3 + NO_2 \longrightarrow N_2O_5$$
$$N_2O_5 + H_2O \longrightarrow 2HNO_3$$

The nitric acid and sulphuric acid, both can react with ammonia forming ammonium nitrate or ammonium sulphate respectively.

# Photosmog

Photosmog (smoke + fog, under light) can be formed by strong sunlight irradiation and high temperature exposure over smoke and fog concentration leading to an increased photooxidants. Oxyradicals are important for production of photochemical smog. It is believed that most of the hydrocarbon is removed by free radical chain reaction involving hydroxy1 radicals (Kerr et al., 1976).

The reactions involved are:

$$NO_2 + O_2 + h\upsilon \longrightarrow NO^* + O_3$$
$$O_3 + NO^* \longrightarrow NO_2 + O_2$$
$$RH + {}^*OH + O_2 \longrightarrow RO^*_2 + H_2O$$
$$RO^*_2 + NO^* \longrightarrow RO^* + NO_2$$
$$RCH_2O^* + O_2 \longrightarrow HO^*_2 + RCHO$$
$$HO^*_2 + NO^* \longrightarrow {}^*OH + NO_2$$
$$NO_2 + {}^*OH \longrightarrow HNO_3$$
$$RO^*_2 + NO_2 \longrightarrow RO_2NO_2$$

where $RO^*_2$ may represent the acetic acid radical

$$CH_3COO^* + NO_2 \longrightarrow CH_3COO^* \text{ peroxyacety1 nitrate}$$

and

$$RO^*_2 + HO_2 \longrightarrow RO_2H + O_2$$

The concentration of the reactants show diurnal variation. In the morning, $^*OH$ radicals is generate $RO^*_2$ by ozone photolysis and reaction proceeds. At midday ozone concentration is maximum since gemerated photolysis is faster than ozone photolysis.

## Impact on Organism

The photochemical oxidants and strong acid pollutants produced in atmospheric reactions can make their direct effect or indirectly they may become tool for endogenous production of ROS that subsequently leads to deleterious effects in an organism.

In direct action, oxidants from the atmosphere may react with naturally emitted unsaturated volatile organic compounds close to the surface of leaves, increasing the ozone formation (Oswald and Elstner, 1986). The reactions of the plant stress hormone ethylene with ozone or other components of air pollution may produce $H_2O_2$ and formaldehyde. These compounds, together with acid mist and aerosols may attack the outer surface of plants, damaging in particular the cuticular waxes (Elstner et al., 1985). Chronic injury of leaves through photooxidants and / or dry acidic depositions may result in a partial loss of resistance resulting infections of plants. The correlation of necrotic events and fungal infections has been demonstrated by Oswald and Elstner (1986). The physiological processes like photosynthesis, stomatal opening, carbon partitioning, respiration and antioxidant systems, are all affected by the individual pollutants or their combinations (review: Darrall, 1989). The plants have endogenous defence mechanism to deal with pollutants (review: Srivastava, 1999) but that becomes inadequate at higher doses of pollutants.

There is no single influence of just one component of air pollutants on aerobic cells. Moreover, it is almost impossible to differntiate between the individual influences under natural conditions. Most of the workers, however, have used higher doses than ambient level of pollutants like $SO_2$, NOx, Ozone, Peroxy1acety1 nitrate (PAN) and their derivatives etc. in their experimentations. The primary target in higher animals of airborne pollutants is the respiratory system. Ozone at high concentration causes lung injury (review : Lippman, 1989; Hatch et al., 1994), stimulate a late non-specific hyperreactive response in asthmatics with or without an early stimulus of an allergen (Konig et al., 1987), increase level of xenobiotic- metabolizing activity (Takahashi & Miura, 1989). Involvement of free radicals in lung injury is well documented (Cross et al., 1994; Pryor, 1994). $NO_2$ may damage the lung directly via its oxidant properties. At high level of exposure, $NO_2$ causes serious effects including broncospasm and pulmonary oedema (Kulle & Clements, 1987). Increased suceptibility of respiratory system to pathogens infection has been shown in mammals (Fenters et al., 1971; Morrow, 1984; Samet et al., 1987; Jakob, 1980). Cigarette smoking and enhance risk of cancer is well established and $NO_2$ & $H_2O_2$ are both components of cigarette smoke, $NO_2$ may exceed 300 ppm in smokestream (Forth et al., 1990).

NO$_2$-induced damage is believed to involve free radical mediated peroxidative destruction of unsaturated membrane compounds (Pryor, 1976; Mustafa, 1978). Oxyradicals, hydrogen peroxides, peroxynitrate, and peroxynitrite are major oxidants of cigarette smoke (Pryor and Stone, 1993). Cigarette smoke oxidizes biological molecules and increases free radical production by phagocytes (Church & Pryor, 1985; Hoshino *et al.*, 1990), glutathione has major antioxidant defence role in oxidant- induced lung injury and inflammation (review: Rahman & MacNee, 1999).

Soot particles which are less than 5 mm in size with carbon core, 5μm adsorbed organic compounds such as polycyclic aromatic compounds, nitromatics and quinones (Larersgoiti *et al.*, 1977) are hazardous. Organic extracts from diesel particles have been shown to be mutagenic (Mitchell, 1988), and carcinogenic (review : Mccdellan, 1987). In general, the carcinogenic activity of polycyclic hydrocarbons of diesel emissions has been correlated with their ability to form free radicals (Southorn & Powis, 1988). Several other particulate compounds of air such as diatomite, tremolite, talcum caoline minusile form *OH (Kennedy *et al*, 1989). The *OH is thought to be the most likely mediator for asbestos-induced carcinogenecity (Kamp *et al.*, 1992). Role of oxyradicals in mutagenecity and DNA damage induced by crocidolite asbestos is recognised (Xu *et al.*, 1999).

## Radiation Toxicity

Ionizing radiations, which begins free radical studies in biology, cause deleterious biological effects by involving ROS. Damage to critical cell targets caused by direct ionization is less frequent than indirect actions. Indirect effect of ionzing radiation proceed by ionizing water molecules present in cell. Ionization of water molecule is responsible for the generation of the primary radiolysis species, the hydrated electron (e$^-$ eq), the hydrogen atom (H*) and the hydroxyl free radical (*OH). In the presence of oxygen, H*. & e$^-$ eq are rapidly converted to superoxide radical anion (O$_2$). The hydrolytic species generated in aerated solutions and in cellular system are form of activated oxygen and are the major cause of radiation damage to biological system (Greenstock, 1983). Generation of oxygen radicals appear to be involved in cellular damage. Antioxidant functions of Vit E, Vit A, ascorbic acid, zinc selenium and beta-carotene have been shown to possess various degrees of radioprotective effects (Weis & Kumar, 1988; Weis & Simic (eds), 1987).

Exposure of ultraviolet (UV), non-ionizing radiation, occur from both natural and artificial sources. The sun is the principal source of exposure for life. Solar UV undergoes significant absorption by the atmosphere. The stratospheric ozone depletion will make higher intensities of UV influx. UV in the electromagnetic spectrum lies within the range of 100 nm (which corresponds to a photon energy of approximately 12 ev) to 400 nm. For biological purposes UV can be classified into UVA (315-400nm), UVB (220-315 nm) and UVC (100-280 nm) region. Only UVB is affected by changes in the atmospheric ozone column. UVC is almost completely absorbed by ozone and O$_2$ in the atmosphere. Even with severe ozone reduction UVC would still be effectively absorbed by the remaining O$_2$. Man made sources of UV include tungusten lamp, mercury lamp (low, medium, and high pressure), mercury lamp with metal halides, xenon lamps, hydrogen and deuterium lamps, flash tubes, welding arcs, carbon arcs, fluorescent lighting tubes, fluorescent sunlamp (UVB emitters), fluorescent UVA tubes, excimer laser, dye laser, and gas laser.

To produce any change, UV must be absorbed by the biomolecule. This invloves absorption of a single photon by the molecule and the production of an excited state in which one electron of the absorbing molecule is raised to a higher energy level. The primary products of UV exposure are genereally ROS or free radicals which can produce effects that can last for hours, days or even years (detail of UV radiation, see EHC 160, WHO 1994). In human UVR can affect skin immune system, eye and environment, and involved in mutagenesis, carcinogenesis and modulation of proliferative activity. The UVC and UVB are capable of inducing direct tissue sensitization reactions but UVA requires a

photosensitizer to induce its effect (Urbach, 1992). Apart from endogenous chromophores many drugs and chemicals produce photosensitization reactions (review:Epstein & Wintroub, 1985; Kochevar, 1987; Henegouwen, 1991). A correlation between UV radiation and oxidants are there (Tyrrel, 1991) but it has been difficult to demonstrate clearly the specific role of ROS in the manifestation of phototoxicity and oxidative stress. However, results derived from studies involving antioxidants in such process give considerable information (Muizzuddin *et al.*, 1999; review: Black & Roth.1991; Tyrrel, 1991; Edge *et al.*, 1997).

# CHEMICAL TOXICITY

Researches have shown that, apart from air-borne pollutants, many drugs, industrial chemicals, pesticides and other substances are not toxic as such but effects when metabolized to electrophilic internmediates or to radical species which can interact with cellular molecules. Such interactions can modify cellular components resulting in cellular structure damage. A number of chemicals such as alkanes, haloalkanes, aromatic carbon system, aryl halides, bipyridyl compounds, nitrogen and sulphur based systems are activated to toxic forms (review: Guengerich & Liebler, 1985).

The pollutants or chemicals may interact with macromolecules in several ways. The mechanism of action of each xenobiotic is not completely understood. Xenobiotics is thought to depend at least in part upon their bioactivation by cytochromes P450, lipoxygenases and prostaglandin H synthase to electrophilic and/or free radical reactive intermediate that covalently bind to or oxidize cellular macromolecules such as DNA, protein and lipids resulting in pathogenesis. Before discussing the possible mechanism of action of xenobiotics, it may be relevant to recapitulate, in short, the cytochrome P450 system and lipid peroxidation process.

## Cytochrome P450 System

The general reaction catalyzed by cytochrome P450 is as follows :

$$NADPH + H + O_2 + \text{S-H} \longrightarrow NADP + H_2O + \text{S-OH}$$

The substrate Ⓢ may be a steroid, fatty acid, drug, or any other chemical that has an alkane, alkene, aromatic ring, or heterocyclic ring substituent that can serve as a site for oxygenation involving oxygenases. In mammalian cells, cytochrome P450 serves as terminal electron acceptor in electron transport systems which are present either in endoplasmic reticulum or inner mitochondrial membrane. The cytochrome P450 catalyzed reactions require two electrons to accomplish the task of heme iron reduction, oxygen binding, and oxygen cleavage, but cytochrome P450 may only accept one electron at a time. In fact NADPH-dependent flavoprotein reductase, which accepts two electrons from NADPH simultaneously but transfers the electrons individualy either to an intermediate iron-sulfur protein (mitochondria) or directly to cytochrome P450 (endoplasmic reticulum.)

In the endoplasmic reticulum, NADPH donates electrons to a flavoprotein called NADPH-cytochrome P450 reductase which contain both FAD and FMN as prosthetic groups. FAD serves as the entry point for electrons from NADPH and FMN serves as the exit point, transferring electrons individvually to cytochrome P450. In certain reactions catalyzed by microsomal (suspension of endoplasmic reticulum) cytochrome P450, the transfer of the second electron may occur from cytochrome $b_5$. Cytochrome $b_5$ is reduced either by NADPH-cytochrome P450 reductase or NADH cytochrome $b_5$ reductase.

In mitochondria, a flavoprotein NADPH- adrenodoxin reductase acts as the electron acceptor from NADPH. One adrenodoxin molecule receives an electron from mitochondrial flavoprotein reductase and interacts with a second adrenodoxin, which then transfers its electron to the cytochrome P450.

The cytochrome P450 metabolizes a variety of lipophilic compounds of endogenous or exogenous origin. These enzymes may catalyze simple hydroxylation of the carbon atom of methyl group, insertion

of hydroxyl group into a methylene carbon of an alkane, hydroxylation of an aromatic ring to form a phenol, or addition of an oxygen atom across a double bond to form an epoxide. In dealkylation reactions, the oxygen inserted into the carbon-hydrogen bond amine, or sulfhydroxyl compounds. Oxidation of nitrogen, sulfur, and phosphorous atoms and dehalogen reactions are also catalyzed by cytochrome P450. Cytochrome P450 oxidizes a variety of xenobiotics particularly lipophilic compounds. The addition of a hydroxyl group makes the compound more polar and thus more soluble in aqueous environment of the cell (Okita & Masters, 1997 ref. therein).

## Lipid Peroxidation

The biological membranes contain polyunsaturated fatty acids which are susceptible to oxidation. In the presence of lipoxygenases or cyclo, oxygenases, oxygenated lipids are produced under controlled conditions. Oxygenated lipids can act as mediator of inflamation (Smith & Marnett, 1991; Yamamoto, 1992). The enzymatic reactions may involve the formation of potentially toxic free radicals which are stabilized within the enzyme active site and the non-radical product released is not usually pro-oxidants (Schewe et al., 1986). The lipid peroxidation reactions are complex involving many components and reaction products (review: Girotti, 1985; Gardner, 1989; Buetner, 1993). In general, lipid peroxidation reactions are as follows

$$X^* + LH^* \longrightarrow L^* + XH \qquad \text{Initiation}$$
$$L^* + O_2 \longrightarrow LO^*_2 \qquad \text{Propagation}$$
$$LO^*_2 + LH \longrightarrow L^* + LOOH$$
$$LO^*_2 + LO^*_2 \longrightarrow \text{Products} \qquad \text{Termination}$$

where

X is reactive oxidant, and L is lipid

The first step is abstraction of a hydrogen atom from an unsaturated fatty acid. The formation of lipid alkyl radical ($L^*$.) is followed by its rapid reaction with oxygen to form a lipid peroxyl radical ($LO^*_2$). The peroxyl radical is capable of abstracting a hydrogen atom from an unsaturated fatty acid with the concomitant formation of a lipid radical and lipid hydroperoxide (LOOH). The peroxyl and alkyl radicals are regenerated, the cycle of propagation may continue indefinitely or until one or other of the substrate is consumed or radical-radical reaction terminates the process.

## Mechanism of Chemical Toxicity

The chemicals and pollutants which are activated to toxic forms are numerous. Their interaction with biomolecule and ultimate effect, may involve different mode and mechanism of action. The possible mechanism of action of such chemicals have been categorised by Comporti (1989) as follows:

(a) Chemicals giving reactive free radicals that alkylate cellular macromolecules but do not induce glutathione (GSH) depletion (eg. Carbon tetrachloride, $CCI_4$; monobromotrichloromethane, $BrCI_3$).

(b) Chemicals that are converted to electrophilic intermediates giving extensive GSH conjugation and consequent GSH depletion (e.g. Bromobenzene, Acetaminophen).

(c) Chemicals giving intermediates that generate reactive oxygen species by redox cycling processess (e.g. Paraquat, menadione.)

## Process Involving Alkylation

The chemicals of this group are metabolized in the drug metabolizing system i.e. mixed function oxydase system invoing the NADPH cytochrome P450 electron transport chain at the level of endoplasmic reticulum. The formation of free radicals ($CCI^*_3$ and $CCI_3OO^*$) has been shown in the process (Poyer et al., 1978; McCay, 1984). The involvement of cytocrome P450 IIE1 in activating halogenated hydrocarbons, including $CCI_4$, has been reviewed by Raucy et el. (1993).

These free radicals can either act directly or by binding covalently to membrane lipids and proteins

(Gomez *et al.*, 1973) with resulting alkylation reactions and possible enzyme inactivations. The second indirect way that the free radical interact first to membrane unsaturated fatty acids that subsequently promote lipid peroxidtion.

**Covalent Binding:** The attack of trichloromethyl radicals to the double bonds of phospholipid unsaturated fatty acids lead to the formation of branched chain fatty acids (Gordis, 1969) and this may be followed by cross-linking with neighbouring fatty acid chains (Link *et al.*, 1984). Similar free radical reactions can ultimately lead to covalent binding of xenobiotics to various biomolecules. The relationship between covalent binding and toxicity is not very clear, some compounds bind but apparently do not damage cells (Roberts, 1990). Hence, depending on the specific molecules attacked, the irreversible binding of free radical metabolited to tissue macromolecules seems capable of disrupting function, such as alkylation of thiol groups or their oxidation to disulfides resulting in inactivation of such molecules or loss of their biological activity.

**Lipid Peroxidation:** Lipids have been extensively studied because of their critical structure and functional role in membranes. The unsaturated and polyunsaturated fatty acids in biological membranes causes membrane less compact and more fluid, which is important for the proper functioning of biological membrane and it has been shown that lipid peroxidation reduces the membrane fluidity (Bruch & Thyer, 1984). Also, the hydroperoxides and carbonyl group changes phospholipid's hydrophobic region to hydrophilic centres which alters the lipid-protein interaction compelety. The peroxidized fatty acid may enter into contact with external aqueous phase (Witting, 1965) and due to this membrane permeability may be increased. Because of increased permeability, swelling of mitochondria, the vesiculation of endoplasmic reticulum, the leakage of enzymes and co-enzymes, the hemolysis of RBC etc is possible. The abnormal bond developed between two adjacent fatty acids during lipid peroxidation, can influence those protein structures and functions which derive some of their structures from closely associated membrane lipid (Demopoulos, 1973). Lipid-protein and protein-protein cross linking is possible if lipid peroxy radicals abstract hydrogen atoms from neighbouring protein (Tappel, 1965). The significance of reactive products of lipid peroxidation such as 4- hydroxynoneol (4-HNE) is that they combine reactivity with diffusibility and are capable of spreading the damage away from the original locus of activation of the hepatotoxin, something of which the free-radical metabolites are not capable. 4HNE and other hydroxyalkenals react with thiol and amino groups of proteins, and inhibit a wide range of enzyme processess (Esterbauer *et al.*, 1990). The aldehyde binding to functional-SH groups of protein, during lipid peroxidation, influence the protein function. Thus, fatty acid hydroperoxides are detrimental to cells but mechanism exist to remove them from membrane phospholipid (Janero, 1990). When such processes are overwhelmed, it seems clear that cell injury will ensue.

## Process Involving Glutathione Depletion

Glutathione has several important functions. It is a reductant, conjugated to drugs to make them more water soluble (see redox cycling processes), involved in transport of amino acids across cell membrane, part of some leukotriene structure, a cofactor for some enzymatic reactions and an aid in rearrangement of protein disulfide bonds.

In other process, some chemicals are metabolized to form epoxide (addition of an oxygen atom across a double bond) which may react with GSH to give glutathionyl conjugate (Jollow, *et. al.*, 1974). The reaction involves nucleophilic- SH group association with electrophilic centre (epoxy group) of the active metabolites, catalyzed by gluathione-S-transferases (Jakoby, 1978). Such GSH-conjugates are ultimately excreted in urine (Boyland & Chasseaud, 1969). More active metabolites means more utilization of GSH for their removal which results in marked decrease in GSH cellular stores. It is known that GSH being hydrogen donor in both selenium dependent (Flohe *et al.*, 1976) and selenium independent

(Burk *et al.*, 1978) GSH peroxidases, GSH prevent formation of lipid peroxides. The possibility of cellular membrane lipid peroxidation will be more if GSH store is depleted because of GSH conjugate formation or by other means.

## Redox Cycling Process

Most eukaryotic life is dependent upon molecular oxygen for the provision of energy through the coupling of oxidation to energy transfer via the phosphorylation of ADP. The $O_2$ undergoes a concerted four electron reduction to water by the mitochondrial electron transport chain system. In the electron transport chain of mitochondria, most of electron transfer is tightly coupled, but a small amount of leakage occur, primarily from NADH-coenzyme-Q-reductase complex and from autooxidation of co-enzyme Q itself. In this process of concerted reduction, particulary reduced oxygen results and various oxyradicals are produced in biological system. The one, two, and three electron reduction produces, superoxide radicals, hydrogen peroxide, and hydroxyl radicals, respectively.

Superoxide anion radical ($O^-_2$) can dismutate to $H_2O_2$ as

$$2O^- + 2H^* \longrightarrow H_2O_2 + O_2$$

then

$$O^-_2 + H_2O_2 \longrightarrow O_2 + {}^*OH + OH^- \text{ (Haber Wesis reactions)}$$

This reaction is catalyzed in biological system by complexed iron (McCord & Day, 1978)

$$O^-_2 + Fe^{3+} \longrightarrow O_2 + Fe^{2+}$$

then

$$Fe^{2+} + H_2O_2 \longrightarrow Fe^{3+} + OH^- + OH^* \qquad \text{(Fenton reaction, Walling, 1975)}$$

$$\overline{O^-_2 + H_2O_2 \longrightarrow OH^- + OH^* + O_2}$$

The hydroxyl radical is the most potent oxidant known, capable of reacting indiscriminately with virtually all organic chemicals, including critical cellular macromolecules, possibly leading to protein degradation and enzyme inactivation, lipid peroxidation, DNA damage or cell death (Borg & Schaich, 1984).

Many chemicals and pollutant metabolites, possibly interact with oxygen by this pathway and generate ROS. The mechanism of chemical's cytotoxicity induced by oxyradicals either involve lipid peroxidation (e.g. paraquat) or independent of lipid peroxidation (e.g.menadione). It is believed that chemicals of the first group act as an uncoupler of the microsomal electron transport chain by receiving electrons from NADPH cytochrome P450 reductase. Bipyridylium compounds, for example paraquat, are easily reduced by cellular reductases. The first oxygen species produced in the aerobic reaction of paraquat with microsomes is the single electron reduction product superoxide anion which is dismutated by enzyme superoxide dismutase to hydrogen peroxide. Alternatively $H_2O_2$ can be produced by the direct reduction of $O_2$ by the paraquat radical (Masson & Hotzman, 1975).

The quinone is reduced to hydroquinone by two electron derived from NAD (P)H. The reaction is catalyzed by cytosolic DT-diphorase enzyme. The one electron reduction of menadione to semiquione-free radical is catalyzed by flavoezymes, mainly NADPH-cytochrome P450 reductase. Semiquinone free radical is reoxidized by $O_2$ giving superoxide anion (Thor *et al.*, 1982) which is dismutated to $H_2O_2$ in superoxide dismutase catalyzed reaction. The $H_2O_2$ is reduced by selenoprotein GSH-peroxidase and GSSG formed is reduced back to GSH by NADPH- linked GSH reductase. If GSSG is not reduced back, it is excreted out which may result in intracellular GSH depletion (Eklov *et al.*, 1984). In addition, oxidation and arylation of protein-thiol group inactivate protein function in the quinone metabolism and this may affect several cellular processes.

The quinoid compound, for example menadione, can undergo one or two electron - reduction reactions.

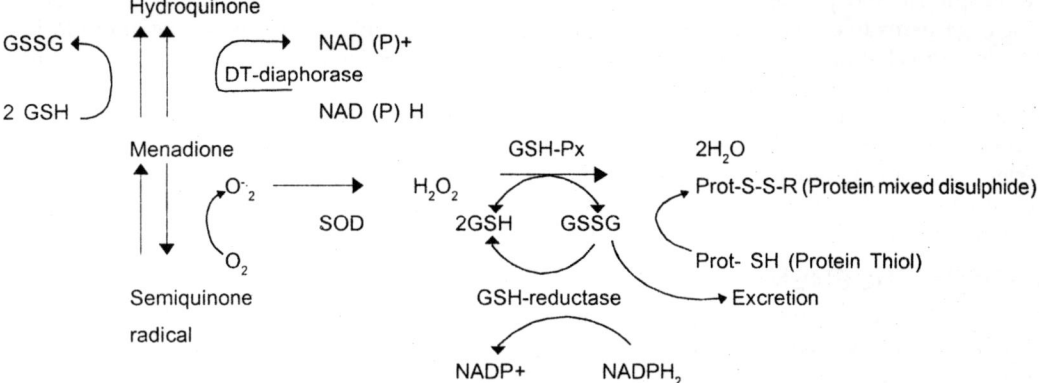

**Fig. 13.1** : Menadione and associated metabolities (Comporti, 1989)

Number of nitroheterocyclic compounds (nitroimidazoles, misonidazole, metronidazole, nitrofurantonin etc.) can be activated by flavoproteins. Oxygen is activated by the nitroradical anion formed during reduction step (Masson, 1979; Adam *et al.*, 1980). Although not occuring with all nitro compounds, this type of redox cycling appears to be responsible for much of the cytotoxicity of these agents (Kedderis & Miwa, 1988).

## Chemical Toxicity and Calcium Homeostasis

The intracellur content of calcium is normally 10,000 fold less than in the extracellular fluid and any perturbation that effects calcium transport is capable of seriosly affecting cell functions. The initial pathological events in the membrane (lipid peroxidation, covalent binding, loss of protein thiols etc.), probably lead to a disturbance of the mechanisms that regulate concentration of free cytosolic calcium. A variety of toxic agents (p-chloromercuribenzoate, diamide, t-butylhydroperoxide, menadione etc.) can inhibit the calcium sequestration activity of liver microsomes by affecting protein sulfhydroxyl group (Di Monte *et al.*, 1984; Moore *et al.*, 1985). Decrease in protein thiols essential for calcium transport result in perturbation of calcium homeostasis. The thiol group of calcium ATP ase enzymes can be inactivated by ROS (Scherer & Deamer, 1986). Reactive oxygen species mediator can decrease cellular energy which can affect calcium and other ions gradient (review : Pound, 1990; Farber, 1990; Reed, 1990; Orrenius *et al.*, 1992). It has also been proposed that oxidant induced cell death and its prevention by some oncoprotein, involves $Ca^{2+}$ mobilization (Ichimiya *et al.*, 1998)

## Perspectives

The atmospheric chemistry is dynamic involving interaction among different component gases. Their interactions are affected by factors such as radiation, temperature, humidity etc. In living system the environmental pollutants or chemicals induce toxicity through generation of ROS. The question that remains to be answered that what is the pathological significance of increase in radical formation. How does it contribute to the ensueing cell damage? These questions have been partly answered by studies where free radical scavengers/antioxidants were given to animals subejcted to several diseases. The sequence of events in ROS generation, their effect at molecular level and dose and mechanism of antioxidant action is not clearly known. It will be important to reconize the critical steps/ metabolites in prote'ctive action so that a suitable strategy for boosting metabolites through genetic manipulation may be adopted. For example, same of the transcription factors known to be involved in early gene expression are also regulated by ROS and in an elevated oxidants burden there is endogenous antioxidant up-regulation system. Hence, mechanistic studies of these aspect may be helpful in developing new thereapeutic strategy through genetic manipulations.

## SUMMARY

In atmosphere, free radicals are formed in photochemical primary reactions. This radicals initiate most of atmospheric and pollutants driven atmospheric conversions to various compounds. Exposure of living organisms to exogenous environmental agents is a potentially major source of oxidative stress. These include chemicals, *e.g.* drugs, pesticides and metals; particulate dusts, *e.g.* silica, asbestos, diesel particulates; gasses etc. ozone and NOx; and irradiations, *e.g.* UV and ionizing radiations. Much about the metabolism leading to cell death are not yet completely understood. It is clear that free radicals are involved as mediators in several biochemical reactions. The mechanism by which reactive oxygen species (ROS) mediated pathogenesis occur, seems likely to be multifactorial, such as alkylation of nucleic acids, calcium mobilization etc. This chapter includes the introduction of free radicals mediated reactions of atmosphere and an outline mechanism of the chemical toxicity to organisms.

## ACKNOWLEDGEMENT

The valuable suggestions and encouragement of Prof. H.S Srivastava, Head, Department of Plant Science, is gratefully acknowledged.

## REFERENCES

- Adams, G.E.; Strafored, I.J.; Wallace, R.G.; Wardman, P. and Watts, M.E. (1980). Toxicity of nitro compounds toward hypoxic mammalian cells *in vitro*: dependence or reduction potential. *J. Natl. Cancer Inst.* **64**: 555

- Black, S.H. and Roth, M.M.M. (1991). Protective role of butylated hydroxytoluene and certain carotenoids in photocarcinogenesis, *Photochem. and Phpobiol.* **53** (5):707-716

- Blake, D. and Winward, P.G. (1995) Eds: Immunopharmacology of free radicals species, Academic press.

- Borg, D.C. and Schaich, K.M. (1984). Cytotoxicity from coupled redox cycling of autooxidizing xenobiotics and metals. *Israel J. Chem.* **24**:38-53

- Boyland, E. and Chasseaud, L.F. (1969). The role of glutathione and glutathione-s- transferases in mercapturic acid biosynthesis, in: F.F. Nord (Ed.) Advances in enzymology. Vol.32. John Wiley and Sons, New York p.173

- Bruch, R.C. and Thayer, W.S. (1983). Different effect of lipid peroxidation on membrane fluidity as determined by electron spin resonance probes. Biochim. Biophys. Acta. 733:216

- Burk, R.F.: Nishiki, K.; Lawrence, R.A, and Chance, B. (1978). Peroxide removal by selenium dependent and selenium-independent glutathione peroxidase in hemoglobin- free perfused liver. *J. Biol. Chem.* **253**:43

- Buetner, G. (1993). The pecking order of free radicals and antioridants : lipid peronidation, L-tocopherol and abcorbate. Arch. Biochem. Biophysics 300, 535-543.

- Church, D.F. and Pryor, W.A. (1985). Free radical chemistry of cigarette smoke and its toxicological implications. *Environ. Health Perspect.* **64**: 111-126

- Chow, C.K. (1991). Vitamin E and oxidative stress. *Free Radical Biol. & Med.* **11**:215-232

- Comporti, M. (1989). Three models of free raidcal-induced cell injury. *Chem. Biol. Interactions.* **72**: 1-56

- Cross, EE; Van der Vliet, A.: O' Neill, C.A.; Louie S.; and Halliwell, B. (1994). Oxidants, antioxidants, and respiratory tract lining fluids. Environ. Health Perspect. 102, Suppl. 10:185-191

- Darrall, N.M. (1989). The effect of air pollutants on physiological processes in plants. Plant Cell Environ 12:1 30.

- Demopoulos, H.B. (1973). Lipid peroxidation *in vivo*. *J. Am Oil. Chem. Soc.* **42**:908

- Di Monte, D.; Bellomo, G.; Thor, H.; Niotera, P. and Orrenius, S. (1984). Menadione induced cytotoxity is associated with protein thiol oxidation and alteration in itracellular $Ca^{2+}$ homeostasis. Arch. Biochem. Biophys. 235:343

- Edge, R.; McGarvey, D.J.; Truscott, T.G. (1997). The carotenoids as anti-oxidants : A review. *J. Photochem, and Photobiol.* **41**(3) : 189-200

- Eklov, L.; Moldeus, P.; and Orrenius, S. (1984). Oxidation of glutathione during hydroperoxide metabolism. A study using isolated hepatocytes and the glutathione reductase inhibits (1, 3-bis (2 -chloroeth1). 1-nitrosurea, Eur. J. Biochem, 138:459

- Elstner, E.F; Oswald, W.F. and Youngman, R.J. (1985). Basic mechanisms of pigment bleaching and loss of structural resistance is spruce (*Picea abies*) needles: advances in phytomedical diagnostics. *Experientia.* 41:591-597

- Environmental Health Criteria 160: Ultraviolet Radiation, World Helath Organisation, Geneva (1994).

- Epstein, J.H. and wintroub, B.U. (1985). Photosensitivity due to drugs. Drugs 30: 42-57

- Esterbouer, H; Zollner, H; and Schour, R.J. (1990). Aldehydes formed by lipid peroxidation: mechanisms of formation, occurrence and determination. In 'Lipid' Oxidation' (ed. C.Vigo-Pelfrey) p. 239-283, CRC Press, Boca

- Fenters, J.D.; Erlich, R.; Findlay, J.; Soanglerand, J. and Tolkacz, V. (1971). Serologic respose in squirrel, monkeys exposed to nitrogen dioxide and influenza virus. *Am Rev. Respir. Dis.* **104** : 205-451

- Flohe, L; gunzler, W.A., and Landensterin, R. (1976). Glutathione peroxydase: a selanoenzyme, FEBS Lett., 32:132

- Forth, W.; Henschler, D. and Rummel, W. (eds) (1990). Allegemeine und spezille Pharmakilogie und Toxikologie, 5th edn, BI Wissen-schaftsverlag.

- Fuhrer, J. L. (1985). Formation of secondary air pollutants and their occurrence in Europe. *Experientia,* **41**:286-301

- Farber, J.L. (1990). The role of calcium in lethal cell injury. Chem. Res. Toxicol. 3: 503

- Gardner, H.W. (1989). Oxygen radical chemistry of polyunsaturated fatty acids. Free Rad. Biol. Med. 7,65-86.

- Giroti, A.W. (1985). Mechanisms of lipid peroxidation. J. Free Rad. Biol. Med. 1, 87-95

- Gomez, M.I.D.; Castro, J.A.; De Ferreyra, E.C.; D' Acosta, N. and De Castro, C.R. (1973). Irreversible binding of $_{14}CC_4$ to liver microsomal lipids and proteins from rat pretreated with compounds altering microsomal mixed-function oxygenase activity, *Toxicol. Appl. Pharmacol.* **25**: 534.

- Gordis, E. (1969). Liver metabolites of carbon tetrachloride. *J. Clin. Invest.,* **48**:203.

- Greenstock, C.L. (1983). Oxyradicals and radiobiological oxygen effect, *Israel J. Chem.* **24**: 1-10

- Guengerich, P.F. and Liebler, D.C. (1985). Enzymatic activation of chemicals to toxic metabolites. *Toxicology.* **14**: 259

- Hatch, G.E.; Slade, R., Harris, L.P.; Mc Donnel, W.F.; Devlin, R.B.; Koren, H.S.; Costa, D.L. and McKee, J. (1994). Ozone dose and effects in humans and rats. A comparison using oxygen-18 labeling and bronchoalveolar lavage. *Am. J. Respir. Crit. Care Med.* **150**: 676-683

- Henegouwen, GMJBV (1991). (Systemic) Phototoxicity of drugs and other xenobiotics. *J. Photochem. Photobiol.* **10**: 183: 210

- Hippeli, S. and Elstner, E.F. (1991). Oxygen radicals and air pollution. In: Oxidative Stress: Oxidants and antioxidants. Helmut Sies (Ed.), Academic Press Inc.

- Hosino, E.; Shariff, R.; Van Gossum, A.; Allard, J.P.; Pichard, C. Jeejeebhoy, K.N. (1990). Vit E suppresses increased lipid peroxidation in cigarette smokers. J. Parental Enternal Nutr. 4: 300-305.

- Inchimiya, M.; Chang, S.H.; Liu, H., Berezesky, I.K,; Trump, B.F. and Amstad, P.A. (1998). Effect of Bcl 2 on oxidant-induced cell death and intracellular $Ca^{2+}$ mobilization. *Am. J. Physiol.* 275:832-839

- Jakob, G.J. (1980). $NO_2$ induced susceptibility to acute respiratory illness : A perspective *Bull. N.Y. Acad Med.* 56:847-855 .

- Jakoby, W.B. (1978). The glutathione S- transferases: a group of multfunctional detoxification proteins, in: A Meister (Ed.), Advances in enzymology, Vol 46, John Wiley and Sons, New York p.383

- Janero, F.R. (1990). Malondialdehyde and thiobarbituric acid-reactivity as diagnostic indices of lipid peroxidation and peroxidative tissue injuri. *Free Rad. Biol. Med.* 9,515

- Jansen, Y. M.W.; Houten, B.V.; Born, P.J. A.; and Mossman, B.T (1993). Biology of disease: Cell and tissue repsonses to oxidative damage. *Lab. Invest.* 69:261-273.

- Jollow, D.J.; Mitchell, J.R.; Zampaglione, N. and Gillette, J.R. (1974). Bromobenzene induced liver necrosis Protective role of glutathione and evidence for 3, 4- bromobenzene oxide as the hepatotoxic metabolite. *Pharmacology.* 11:151

- Kakkar, P. and Viswananthan, P.N. (1992). Formation and scavanging of active oxygen species in immunological responses. *J. of Scientific & Industrial Res.* 51: 802-809.

- Kamp, D.W.; Graeeffa, P. Prylor, W.A. and Weitzman, S.A. (1992). The role of free radicals in asbestos induced diseases. *Free Radic. Biol. Med.* 12: 293-315

- Kedderis, G.L. and Miwa, G.T. (1988). The metabolic activation of nitroheterocyclic therapeutic agents. *Drug Metab. Rev.* 19:33

- Kehrer, J.P. (1993). Free radicals as , mediators of tissue injury and disease. *Critical Reviews in Toxicology.* 23 (1): 21-48

- Kennedy, T.P.; Dodson, R.; Rao N V (1989). Dust causing pneumoconiosis generate *OH and produce hemolysis by acting as Fenton catalysts. *Arch. Biochem. Biophys.* 269 (1): 359-364.

- Kerr, I.A.; Calvert, J.G. and Demerjian, K.L. (1976). Free radical in the production of photochemical smog. In Pryor W.A. (Ed.). Free radicals in biology, pp. 159-179. London and NY, Academic Press.

- Kochevar, E.I. (1987). Mechanisms of drug photosensitazation. *J. Photochem. and photobiol.* 10:183-210

- Konig, J.Q.; Pierson, W.E.; Marshal, S.G.; Covert, D.S.; Morgan, M.S. and Belle, G.V. (1987). The effects of ozone and nitrogen dioxide on lung funtion in health and asthmatics adolescents. Res. Rep. No. 14, Health Effects Inst., 215 First Street. Cambridge. MA 02142

- Kulle, T.J. and Clement, M.L. (1987). Susceptibility to virus infection with exposure to nitrogen dioxide. Res. Rep. No. 15., Health Effects Inst., 215 First Street. Cambridge. MA 02142

- Laresgoiti, A.; Loos, A.C and Springer, G.S. (1977). Particulate and smoke emission from light duty diesel engine, *Current Res.* 11(10): 973-978

- Lelieveld, J. and Crutzen, P.J. (1990). Influences of cloud photochemical processes on tropospheric ozone. *Nature.* 343 (6255): 227-233

- Link, B.; Durk, H.; Thiel, D. and Frank, H. (1984). Binding of trichloromethyl radicals to lipids of the hepatic endoplasmic reticulum during tetrachloromethane metabolism. *Biochem. J.* 223:577

- Lippmann, M. (1989) Health effects of ozone: A critical review. MPCA. 39: 672-695

- Masson, R.P., Holtzman, J.L. (1975). The role of catalytic superoxide formation in the $O_2$ in hibition of nitroreductase, Biochem. Biophys. Res. Commun. 67, 1267.

- Masson, R.P. (1979). Free radical metabolites of foreign compounds and their toxicological significance. In: E. Hodgson, J.R. Benal and R.M. Philpot (Eds.), Reviews in biochemical toxicology, Vol.1, Elsevier North Holland, New York. P. 151.

- McCord, J.M.; and Day, E.D.J. (1978). Superoxide dependent production of hydroxyl radical catalyzed by iron-EDTA complex. FEBS Lett. 86:139.

- McCay, P.B.; Lai, E.K.; Poyer, J.L., Dubose, C.M. and Janzen, E.G. (1984). Oxygen and carbon centered free radical formation during carbon tetrachloride metabolism. *J. Biol. Chem.* 259:2135

- McClellan, R.O. (1987). Health effects of exposure of diesel exhaust particles. *Annu. Rev. Pharmacol. Toxicol.* 27:279-300

- Mendoz, J.D. and Ramos, R.H.G. (1997). About utility of free radicals. *Rev. Med. Inst. Mex. Seg. Social.* 35(4): 309-313

- Mitchell, C.E. (1988). Damage and repair of mouse lung DNA induced by 1-nitropyrene. *Toxicol. Lett.* 42: 159-166

- Mohnen, V.A. (1988). The mountain cloud chemistry program. In proceedings of the USFRG research symposium. Effect of atmospheric pollutants on the spruce-forest of the eastern United States and the Federal Republic of Germany: Oct. 19-23. pp23. pp27-60. Burlington. Vermont. Broomall. P.A. Northeastern Forest Experiment station.

- Moore, M.; Thor, H. Moor, G.; Nelson, S.; Moldeus, P. and Orrenius, S. (1985). The toxicity of acetaminophen and N-acetyl-p- benzoquinone imine in isolated hepatocytes is associated with thiol depletion and increased cytosolic $Ca^{2+}$. *J. Biol. Chem.* 260:13035.

- Morrow, P.E. (1984). Toxicological data on NOx: An overview. *Toxicolol. Environ. Health* **13**: 205-227.

- Muizzuddin, N.; Shakoori, A.R. and Marenus, K.D. (1999). Effect of antioxidants and free radical scavengers on protection of human skin against UVB, UBA, and IR irradiation. *Skin Res. Technol.* 5/4: 260-265.

- Mustafa, M.G. and Tierney, D. (1978). Biochemical and metabolic changes in the lungs with oxygen, ozone and nitrogen dioxide toxicity. *Am Rev. resp. Dis.* **118**:1061-1090

- Okita, R.T. and Masters, B.S.S. (1997). Biotransformations: The cytochrome P450. In: Textbook of Biochemistry with clinical correlation 4th ed. Ed. T.M. Develin, Wiley-Liss, Inc. USA.

- Orrenius, S.; Burkitt, M.J.; Kass, G.E.N.; Dypbakt, J.M.; and Nicotera, P. (1992). Calcium ions and oxidative cell injury. *Ann. Neurol.* **32**: 533.

- Oswald, W.F. and Elstner, E.F. (1986). Fichtener krankungen in den Hochalgen den Bayerischen mittelyebinge. *Ber Deutsch. Bot. Ges.* **99**:313-339

- Pahl, H.L. and Baeuerle, P.A. (1994). Oxygen and the control of gene expression. Bioassay 16:497-502.

- Pounds, J.G. (1990). The role of cell calcium in current approaches to toxicology. *Environ. Health Perspect.* **84**: 7

- Poyer, J.L,; Floyd, R.A.; McCay, P.B.; Janzen, E.G and Davis, E.R (1978) Spin trapping of the trichloromethyl radicals produced during enzymic NADPH oxidation in the presence of carbon tetrachloride or bormotrichloromethane. *Biochim. Biophys. Acta.* **539**:402

- Prinn, R.; Cunnold, D.; Ramussen, R. *et al.* (1987). Atmospheric trends in methychloroform and the global average for the hydroxyl radical. *Science* **238**:945-950

- Pryor, W.A. (1976). Free radical reactions in biology: initiation of lipid autoxidation by ozone and nitrogen dioxide. *Environ. Health Persp.* **16**: 180-181.

- Pryor, W.A and Stone, K. (1993). Oxidants in cigarette smoke: radicals, hydrogen peroxides, peroxynitrate, and peroxynitrite. *Ann. NY Acad. Sci.* **686**:12-28.

- Pryor, W.A. (1994). Mechanisms of radical formation from reaction of ozone with target molecules in the lung. *Free Radic. Biol. Med.* **17**: 451-465.

- Rahman, I. and MacNee, W. (1999). Lung glutathione and oxidative stress: implications in cigarette smoke induced airway disease *Am. J. Physiol* **277**: L1067-1088

- Raucy, J.L.; Kraner, J.C. and Lasker, J.M (1993). Bioactivation of halogenated hydrocarbons by cytochrome P450 IIE1. *Crit. Review Toxicol,* **23**:1-20.

- Reed, D.W. (1990). Review of the current status of calcium and thiols in cellular injury. *Chem. Res. Toxicol.* **3**:495

- Roberts, S.A.; Price V.F. and Jollow, D.J. (1990) Acetaminophen structure-toxicity studies: *in vivo* covalent binding of a nonhepatotoxic analog, 3-hydroxy acetamide. *Toxicol. Appl. Pharmacol.* **105**: 195.

- Saltman, B. (1989). Oxidative stress: a radical view. Seminar *Hematol.* **26**: 249-286

- Samet, J.M.; Marbury, M.C. and Spengler, J.D. (1987). Health effect and sources of indoor air pollution. Part 1. *Am. Rev. Respir. Dis.* **136**: 486-508

- Scherer, N.M. and Deamer, D.W. (1986). Oxidative stress impairs the function of sarcoplasmic reticulum by oxidation of sulfhydryl group in $Ca^{2+}$ ATPase. *Arch. Biochem. Biophys.* 246:589

- Schewe, T., Rapoport, S.M., and kuhn, H. (1986). Enzymology and physiology of reticuloiyte lipoxygenase : Comparision with other lipoxygenase. 191-272.

- Simon, A. R. Fanburg, B.L., and Cochran, B.H. (1997). Oxidative stress and cell proliferation. In : Oxygen, gene expression, and cellular proliferation. Eds. L.B. clerch and D.J. Massaro. New York : Dekkar, p 123-138

- Simon, A.R.; Rai U,; Fanbury B.L.; and Cochran, B.H. (1998). Activation of the JAK-STAT pathway by reactive oxygen species. *Am. J. Physiol.* **275 (44):** CI640-1652.

- Smith, W.L. and Marnett, L.J. (1991). Prostaglandin endoperoxide synthase : structure and Catalysis. Biochem. Biophys. Acta. 1083, 1-17.

- Southorn, P.A. and Powis, G. (1988). Free radicals in medicine. II Involvement in human disease. Mayo. *Clin. Proc.* **63:** 390-408.

- Srivastava, H.S. (1999). Biochemical defence mechanisms of plants to increased levels of ozone and other atmospheric pollutants. *Current Science.* **76(4)** : 525-533.

- Takahashi, Y. and Miura, T. (1989). Effects of nitrogen dioxide and ozone in combination on xenobiotic metabolizing activities of rat lungs. *Toxicology* **59:** 253-262.

- Tappell, A.L. (1965). Free radical lipid peroxidation damage and its inhibition by Vit. E. and selenium, Fed. Proc. 24:73

- Thor, H.; Smith, M.T.; Hartzell, P.; Bellomo, G.; Jewell, A. and Orrenius, S. (1982). The meatabolism of menadione (2-methy1-1, 4-naphtoquinone) by isolated hepatocyte. *J. Biol. Chem.* **257:**12419.

- Thompson, A.M.; Hogan, K.B.; and Hoffman, J.S. (1992). Methane reductions: Implications for global warming and atmospheric chemical change. *Atm. Environ.* **26 (14):** 2665-2668.

- Tie, X.X.; Kao, C.Y.J.; and Mroz, E.J. (1992). Net yield of OH, CO, and $O_3$ from the oxidation of atmospheric methane. *Atmospheric Environ.* **26(1)** 125-136.

- Tyrrel, R.M. (1991). UVA (320-380) radiation as an oxidative stress. In: Oxidative stress: Oxidants and antioxidants, ED. Helmut Sies, Academic Press Inc.

- Urbach, F. (1992). Biological response to ultraviolet radiation. Valdenmar Pub. Co., Kensas, USA.

- Walling, C. (1975). Fenton's reagent revisited. Accounts. *Chem. Res.* **8:** 139-142.

- Weis, J.F. and Simic, M.G. (Eds.) (1987). Perspectives in radioprotection. New York : Pergamon, 1-407.

- Weiss. J.F. and Kumar, K.S. (1988). Antioxidant mechanisms in radiation injury and radioprotection. In: chow, C.K., Ed Cellular antioxidant defence mechanisms, Voll. ll. Boca Raton FL; CRC Press. 163-189.

- Witting, L.A. (1965). Lipid peroxidation *in vivo. J. Am. Oil Chem. Soc.* **42:**908

- Xu, A.; Wu, L.J.; Santella, R.M. and Hei, T.K. (1999). Role of oxyradicals in mutagenecity and DNA damage induced by crocidolite asbestos in mammalian cells. *Caner Res.* **59:**5922-5926.

- Yamamotto, S. (1992). Mammalian lipoxygenases : Molecular stnectures and functions. Biochim. Biophys. Acta 1128, 117-131.

- Yoshida, Y.; Maruyama, M.; Fujita, J. Arai, N.; Hayashi, R.; Araya, J.; Matsui, s.; Yamashita, N.; Sugiyama, E.; and Kobayashi, M. (1999) Reactive oxygen intermediates stimulate interleukin-6 production in human bronchial epithelial cells. *Am. J. Physiol.* **276(20):** L900-908.

# 14

# Chelating Agents and Their Use in Metal Poisoning

*Swaran J. S. Flora, Shashi N. Dube and Sushil K. Tandon*

Chelation is one of the most important chemical functions taking place in the bodies of living organism. It is also one of the important processes by which plants and animals utilise inorganic metals. Chlorophyll, the green matter of plant, is a chelate of magnesium. Haemoglobin, cytochrome C, catalase and peroxidase are chelators of iron. A host of other metalloenzymes could be used as examples involving chemical processes. Many of the successful drugs used in the treatment of disease are dependent upon chelation processes for their effective therapeutic properties. This chapter focuses on some metal chelating agents, their biological and therapeutic properties. The pharmacology and toxicology of chelating drugs in humans are briefly reviewed to introduce the problems associated with the present conventional chelating agents and challenges facing for an effective chelation of toxic metal. The beneficial and adverse effects including their limitations are briefly mentioned along with the recent developments to ameliorate most of the problems.

Chelation therapy has been the basis for the medical treatment of metal poisoning. Chelating agents have been used clinically as antidotes for acute and chronic metal poisoning. Chelators not only enhance excretion but in at least some cases they also decrease the metal's toxicity by preventing it from binding to cellular target molecules (Catsch et al. 1979). Calcium disodium EDTA and 2,3- dimercaprol (BAL) have been the mainstay of chelation therapy for toxic metal poisoning. A recent development in this field has been the identification and recognition of meso 2,3- dimercaptosuccinic acid (DMSA) as a promising and efficient oral agent for the treatment of lead poisoning. The better performance of DMSA over D- penicillamine has been attributed to two SH group having stronger binding sites. The relative safety of DMSA in childhood lead intoxication treated on outpatient basis is not associated with risk for increased lead absorption. DMSA and DMPS have been evaluated in human lead poisoning with promising results. Comparative studies have shown that thiol chelating agents are more effective than polyaminocarboxylic acids for the treatment of metal toxicity. Finally, recommendations for choice of chelating agents and dosing are offered as guidelines and are not rigid protocol.

## Chelating Agents and Chelation Therapy

Chelating agents are organic compounds capable of linking together metal ions to form complex ring-like structure called chelates. 'Chelate' is derived from the Greek word meaning the claws of a lobster and somehow the chelators act in this way. Chelators act according to a general principle: the chelator forms a complex with the respective (toxic) ion, and these complexes reveal a lower toxicity and are more easily eliminated from the body. It is essential that the chemical affinity of the complexing agent for the metal ion is higher than the affinity of the metal for the sensitive biological molecules. Thus chemical measurement of the stability constants of the metal-complexes formed may give a first indication of the effectiveness of a particular chelating agent. Chelation thus can be defined as the *incorporation of a metal ion into a heterocyclic ring structure.* An ideal chelating agent should possess the following characteristic:

- Greater affinity for the toxic metal that has to be chelated
- Ability to chelate with natural chelating groups found in biological system
- Low toxicity
- Ability to penetrate cell membrane to reach site of toxic metal deposit
- Minimal metabolism
- Rapid elimination of metal
- Highly water solubility

## Chemical Properties of Metal and their Complexes

The design of chelating agents for a toxic metal ion must take into consideration the co-ordination number of that metal ion. The use of a chelating agent which will occupy more of the co-ordination position of a metal ion will generally give a complex of greater stability than is found for those complexes with chelating agents which occupy fewer positions. These metal chelate complexes will also have a reduced tendency to undergo exchange reactions once they are formed. However, it is frequently advantageous to use a preferred donor atom in a chelating agent of lower density. Another important property of a metal complex in governing its property is its ionic charge. There is an hypothesis that large complexes ions with a positive charge will pass out of a cell very slowly because of their inability to pass through either the lipid portion of the cellular membrane or the cation transport system designed to move ions with +1 or a +2 charge across this membrane. Another important property of metal complexes is the stereochemistry of the toxic metal ion. Chelating agents tie up all the co-ordination position of a metal ion. It should be noted that metal chelating agents usually contain more than one functional group, in order to provide a chemical 'claw' to chelate the toxic metal. The link formed between the metal and chelating agent is of co-ordinate type which is generally similar to covalent type but the major difference is that both electron forming the link are supplied by the binding atom (the resulting compound is called 'metal complex' or 'co-ordinate compound'. A simplest example in this case can be a link formed by proton (hydrogen atom with a positive charge). Beside hydrogen atom there are number of other atoms which can take part to co-ordinate complex formation like sodium, magnesium, copper, zinc and various transition elements such as manganese, iron and cobalt. Chelation treatment can be now more completely defined as *an equilibrium reaction between a metal ion and a complexing agent, characterised by the formation of more than one bond between the metal and a molecule of the complexing agent resulting in the formation of a heterocyclic ring structure incorporating the metal ion (Aaseth 1983).*

Chemical formula of some of the chelating agents is given in Table 14.1 and Figure 14.1. One of the most important chelating agent from a pharmacological point of view is EDTA which has four linking sites on the molecule, 2 N plus 2 O. Thus it can absorb the chelated metal into upto three heterocyclic rings.

**Table 14.1 : Some Common Chelating agents their Physico-chemical and pharmacological properties**

| Chelating agent | Empirical Formula | LD50 species/ route (m mol/kg) | Side effects | Use |
|---|---|---|---|---|
| BAL | $C_3H_8OS_2$ | 0.73 mouse, i.p. | Blood Pressure, headache, nausea, vomiting | Arsenic, Lead |
| CaNa$_2$EDTA | $C_{10}H_{12}CaN_2Na_2O_8$ | 16.4 mouse, i.p. | Nephrotoxic, malaise, zinc Loss, Redistribution, | Lead |
| DMSA | $C_4H_6O_4S_2$ | 13.73 mouse, s.c. | none, mild allergic, skin reaction | Lead, Arsenic |
| DMPS | $C_3H_7O_3S_3.Na$ | 5.22 mouse, i.p. | As in DMSA | Mercury Lead |
| D-PA | $C_5H_{11}NO_2S$ | 2.53 mouse, i.p. | Anaphylactic reaction in allergic patient | Lead, Copper |

Abbreviation: BAL– British Anti Lewisite; CaNa$_2$EDTA – calcium disodium ethylenediamine tetraacetic acid; DMSA– meso 2,3–dimercaptosuccinic acid; DMPS – sodium 2,3–dimercaptopropane 1– sulfonate; D–PA – D–penicillamine.

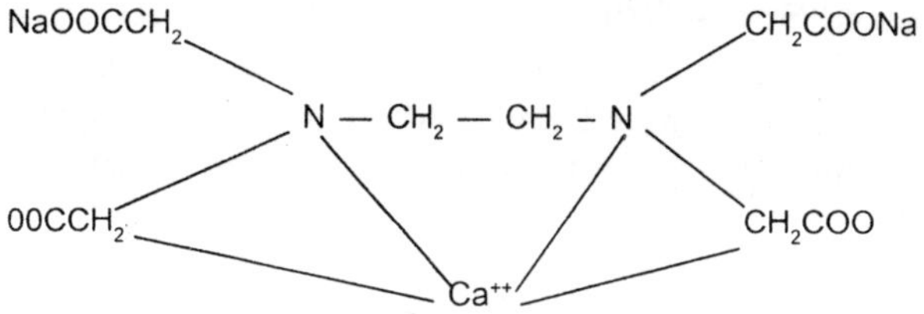

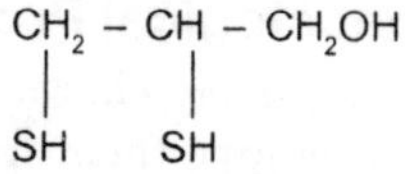

NaOOCCH$_2$

CH$_2$COONa

CH$_2$ – CH – CH$_2$OH

| | | | |
SH     SH

N — CH$_2$ — CH$_2$ – N

00CCH$_2$

CH$_2$COO

British Anti Lewisite

Ca$^{++}$

**Calcium disodium ethylenediaminetetraacetic acid**

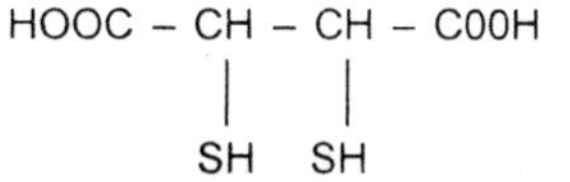

HOOC – CH – CH – COOH

| | | |
SH   SH

**Meso 2,3-dimercaptosuccinic acid**

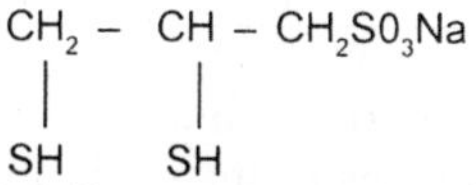

CH$_2$ – CH – CH$_2$SO$_3$Na

| | | |
SH     SH

**Sodium 2,3-dimercaptopropane 1-sulfonate**

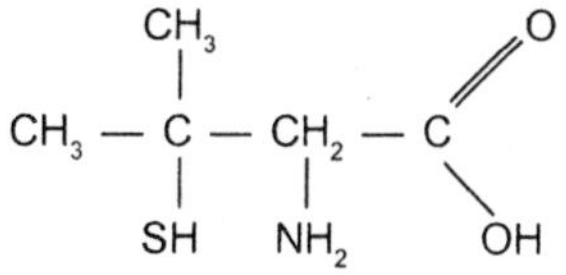

CH$_3$

O

CH$_3$ — C — CH$_2$ — C

| | |
SH   NH$_2$   OH

**D-Penicillamine**

$$H_2N(CH_2)_5NC(CH_2)_2CNH(CH_2)_5NC(CH_2)_2 CNH(CH_2)_5NCCH_3 . CH_3SO_3H$$

with O double bonds and OH groups below

OH       OH       OH

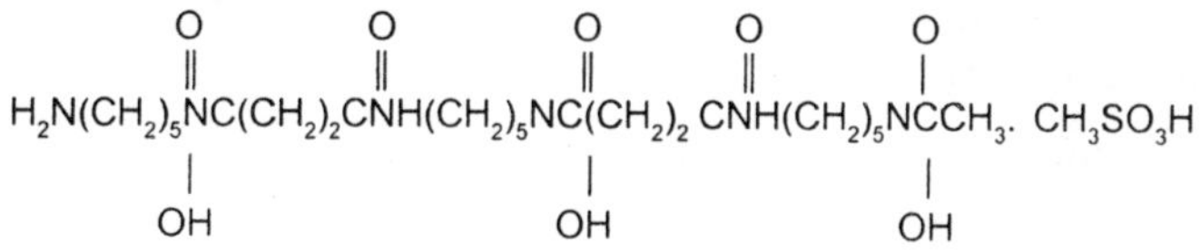

**Deferrioxamine Mesylate**

**Fig. 14.1 :** Chemical Structures of Some Common Chelating Agents

Determining factors for complex formation are the hardness/ softness characteristics of electron donor and acceptor. This characteristic not only determines the stability of the formed complex but also the chelating agent's degree of metal selectivity in relation to competing essential metals present in the biological fluid. Softness character can be explained as the ability of the empty frontier orbital of metal ions for accepting electrons and to the deformability of the outmost occupied electron orbital of donor groups. So called soft metal cations have large atomic radius and a high number of electron pair in the outer shell in contrast to the hard ions. Formation of a metal complex ML, involves that the metal cation, M, co-ordinates or accept free electron pairs that are furnished by electron-donor groups from the ligands, L. The interaction between a chelating agent and a toxic metal can be expressed in term of stability constants. Assuming the formation of the simple mononuclear complex only, the equilibrium concentration can be calculated from the law of mass action: (Aaseth 1983)

$$\text{Stability Constant, } K = \frac{[ML]}{[M] [L]}$$

Values within the [] denotes concentration in mol/litre

A metal with a higher stability constant competes for the chelating agent with a lower stability value and sooner or later removes the metal with a lower constant from the complex, even if this has already been formed. Relative concentration also influences this release and this is the major reason that is why calcium which is readily available in the body, binds to EDTA in large quantities if disodium EDTA is administered, even though it has a stability constant lower than that of lead.

## Chemical and Pharmacological Properties of Some Conventional Chelating Agents

There are a variety of incompletely characterised processes, which operate to limit the access of toxic metals to the body and to remove them from the body. The limited absorption of some toxic metals from the gastro-intestinal tract is the first barrier. Further, of the fraction of metal ions, which are absorbed, some will be rapidly excreted in the urine or faeces. The ones, which will be absorbed and incorporated into cells or other structures, will be turned over and excreted in part during the normal metabolic processes. For the number of toxic metals there are few normal processes within the system involving endogenous chelating agents like glutathione operating for the excretion and removal of the toxic metals. However, the half-lives of some metals vary enormously and in most of these cases direct action of chelating agents in accelerating the removal of toxic metals will be required. The extent of the increase in toxic metal excretion is determined by both the degree of exposure to the toxic metal and to the regimen used to administer the chelating agent (Ellenhorn 1988). Selected chelating agents and their various chemical and pharmacological properties are given below.

## Calcium Disodium Ethylenediaminetetraacetic acid (EDTA)

Calcium disodium ethylenediaminetetraacetic acid (CaNa$_2$EDTA) is a derivative of ethylenediaminetetraacetic acid (EDTA), a synthetic polyaminocarboxylic acid. It is a white crystalline solid with a molecular weight of 374.28 and empirical formula is $C_{10}H_{12}CaN_2Na_2O_8$. It is a weak tetrabasic acid. This chelating agent (chemical structure given in Figure 1) has been widely used as a chelator because of its ability to form complexes with several bivalent and trivalent metals. which has been used successfully for treating cases of lead poisonings.

*Metabolism and Kinetics:* A small amount of calcium disodium EDTA is absorbed in the gastro intestinal tract following oral administration in humans and laboratory animals. It is reported that more than 80 percent is eliminated in the faeces within 24 hours of administration and remaining amount is absorbed (Foreman and Trujillio 1954). It has been confirmed that EDTA does not penetrate cell membranes and has a biological half-life of 50-60 minutes; 90 percent is excreted within 6-8 hours after administration. Renal clearance is mainly through active tubular secretion without any significant re-absorption.

*Toxicity:* CaNa$_2$EDTA has the LD$_{50}$ value of 16.4 mmol/kg in mouse (Cantilena and Klaassen 1981). Intravenous administration of this drug results in good absorption but very painful at the injection site. Hence intravenous injection could be given either by diluting in 5 percent dextrose or saline (Klaassen 1990). Hypocalcemia is reported with the administration of Na$_2$EDTA. CaEDTA has the major toxic effects on the renal system causing the necrosis of tubular cells. Total destruction of the tubules has also been reported. These lesions along-with some alterations in the urine like hematuria, proteinuria and elevated BUN are generally reversible when the treatment ceases. Another side effect of EDTA is its ability to chelate various essential metals endogenous to the body, zinc in particular (Flora and Tandon 1990, Powell *et al.* 1999). Zinc administration during EDTA administration is generally recommended to reduce toxicity (Flora and Tandon 1990).

Other possible side effects related to EDTA include teratogenic effects (Kimmel 1977). Apgar (1977) found that the use of EDTA to remove endogenous zinc appeared to offer a mechanism for studying the effects of short-term zinc supplementation at critical periods in pregnant zinc deficient rats. Brownie et al. (1986) also reported teratogenic effects. They further concluded that incorporation of zinc as ZnEDTA or ZnCaEDTA afforded a considerable degree of protection against the production of teratogenic effects. Another reported disadvantage of CaNa$_2$EDTA is that it redistribute lead to the brain (Cory Slechta *et al.* 1987, Flora *et al.* 1995). They presented evidence that rats given lead as lead acetate in their drinking water and then treated with CaNa$_2$EDTA mobilised lead from their tissues and redistributed to brain and liver on the first day of treatment.

## 2.3: Dimercaprol; British Anti Lewisite (BAL)

BAL was developed primarily as antidote to lewisite during World War II and has become rapidly outmoded. The empirical formula of BAL is $C_3H_8OS_2$ and its molecular weight is 124.21. It is an oily, colourless liquid with a pungent, unpleasant smell typical of mercaptans.

*Metabolism and Kinetics:* BAL is highly liposoluble and thus permeates all the body tissue including brain. Its distribution is therefore both extracellular and intracellular. Highest concentration has been reported in the liver and kidney. The half-life is very short; after 4 hours only a small amount remains in blood. Studies using $^{36}S$ have shown that the major part of BAL derived S is excreted as dithiols and glucuronides.

It's reported $LD_{50}$ value is 0.73 mmol/kg (Zvirblis and Ellin 1976) and 1.48 mmol/kg (Aposhian and Aposhian 1990, Aposhian *et al.* 1982). BAL is unstable and susceptible to oxidation and therefore difficult to store as a ready for use preparation. It has a low therapeutic efficacy and due to its high toxicity, BAL is suited only for short treatment of acute toxicity.

*Toxicity:* BAL has number of serious disadvantages. It is not very stable. BAL has reported to cause increased arsenic and mercury burden along-with mobilisation of this metal from the various tissues of the exposed animals (Hoover and Aposhian 1983, Berlin *et al.* 1965). The injections are very painful, as because of its oily nature it requires deep intra-muscular administration. Numbers of other adverse effects too have been reported. BAL forms chelate complex between its sulfhydryl groups and lead. BAL has been found to be effective in treating lead (Flora *et al.* 1985). It is much more effective when given soon after exposure. BAL can be administered intramuscularly as a 10 per cent solution in oil. Peak concentration in blood reaches in 30 to 60 minutes. In lead poisoning, BAL is given intramuscularly at a dose of 4 mg/kg every 4 hours for 48 hours, then every 6 hours for an additional 7 days. On the whole BAL reduces essential metals less than EDTA. Effects reported in man are also alarming. The most frequent effect is a rise in both systolic and diastolic blood pressure accompanied by tachycardia. Other symptoms include vomiting, headache, lachrymation, rhinorrhea and salivation, profuse sweating, intense pain in the chest and abdomen and anxiety. Children too react to the drug in a similar way as adults, the doses are almost similar. The appearance of fever accompanied by neutropenia is a reaction peculiar to children. Even the most severe symptoms are however, reversible.

## D-Penicillamine

Penicillamine is D-β, β-dimethylcysteine and in clinical practice only D- isomer is used although can exist in two optical forms with dextro- and levo- configuration as well as in the racemic mixture DL-,. Its empirical formula is $C_5H_{11}NO_2S$ and molecular weight is 149.21. It is available as a hydrochloride salt in capsule, which is slightly hygroscopic crystalline powder, soluble in water and ethanol.

*Metabolism and Kinetics:* D-pencillamine (DPA) can penetrate cell membranes and then get metabolised. It can be absorbed through the gastro-intestinal tract and thus can be administered orally. Its absorption from the gastrointestinal tract is between 40 to 70 per cent. It is fairly stable as its SH group is very resistant to oxidation *in vivo*, attack from enzymes such as cysteine desulfhydrase and L-amino acid oxidase, compared to other monothiols. Excretion of DPA through urine is very fast. Small amount is also reported to cross hepatocyte membrane and excreted through bile.

*Toxicity:* It's reported $LD_{50}$ value in mouse by intraperitoneal route is 2.53 mmol/kg and through oral is 17 mmol/kg. The major toxic effect of DPA is antagonising pyridoxine and inhibiting pyridoxine dependent enzyme such as transaminases. It is thus advisable to supply a dietary supplement of pyridoxine in prolonged administration and also an additional supply of essential metals like iron. Other toxic effects include hypersensitive allergic reactions like fever, skin rashes, leukopenia and thrombocytopenia (Shannon et al. 1988). In few reports nephrotoxic effects too have been observed alongwith penicillin allergic reaction in sensitive individual due to cross reactivity. Prolonged treatment may also lead to anorexia, nausea and vomiting in human.

## Meso 2,3-dimercaptosuccinic Acid (DMSA)

The one chemical derivative of dimercaprol, which has gained more and more attention these days, is DMSA. DMSA is an orally active chelating agent, much less toxic than BAL and its therapeutic index is about 30 times higher (Kuntzelman *et al.* 1990). US FDA has approved this compound in 1991 for the treatment of children whose blood lead concentration was above 45 mg/dL (FDA 1991). The empirical formula of DMSA is $C_4H_6O_4S_2$ and its molecular weight is 182.21 it's a weak acid soluble in water.

*Metabolism and Kinetics:* DMSA distribution is predominantly extracellular since it is unable to cross hepatic cell membrane. Over 95 per cent of blood DMSA is protein bound mainly to albumin (Maiorino et al. 1990). DMSA appears to be transported by plasma albumin. It has been reported that 2-4 hours after DMSA administration only 12 per cent of meso DMSA excreted in urine was unaltered whereas about 88 per cent oxidized to form disulfates. The absorption of DMSA after oral administration is about 60 per cent. It is distributed predominantly in the extracellular fluid and excreted by the kidney with a half-life of about two days (Aaseth 1989). Aposhian group developed an assay for the determination of DMSA in biological fluid (Maiorino *et al.* 1986, 1987).

*Toxicity:* Using a percutaneous route the acute $LD_{50}$ for rats and mice is about 2 g/kg. The acute oral $LD_{50}$ is more than 5 g/kg while through intraperitoneal route the value is 3 g/kg in rats and mice. No intraperitoneal preparation of this compound is available. Graziano *et al.* (1978) reported that i.p. administration of 200 mg/kg DMSA could produce only a marginal change in growth but did not elicit any appreciable change in histopathological alterations in tissue nor cause haematological or biochemical change in blood. No significant loss of essential metals like zinc, iron, calcium or magnesium was observed. A slight increase in transaminase activities in serum, of human and animals has been reported after DMSA treatment (Graziano *et al.* 1985, Flora and Kumar 1993). Adverse reaction to DMSA includes gastrointestinal discomfort, skin reaction, mild neutropenia and elevated liver enzymes. Some evidence of embryotoxicity/fetal toxicity due to DMSA administration was also reported (Domingo 1998) which was attributed to the result of direct contact of the chelator and/or metabolites with the embryonic or fetal tissues more than the indirect result of maternal toxicity. No redistribution of lead also occurred on DMSA administration in rats (Cory Slechta 1987).

## Sodium 2,3-dimercaptopropane 1-sulfonate (DMPS)

DMPS was first introduced in Soviet Union in the 1950s as 'Unithiol'. Its empirical formula is $C_3H_7O_3S_3$.Na and molecular weight is 210.3. Its chemical structure is Show in Figure 14.1

*Metabolism and Kinetics:* DMPS is mainly distributed in the extracellular space, it may enter cells by specific transport mechanism. By the parenteral route acute $LD_{50}$ for various species is about 1 g/kg to 2 g/kg. After i.p. injection of lethal doses the animals were highly irritable for some minutes before they became apathetic and breathing ceased (Planas Bohme *et al.*, 1980). DMPS is rapidly eliminated from the body through the kidneys. The serum half-life is about 20 to 60 minutes. Following oral administration, about 60percent of the administered dose are absorbed in dogs (Wiedelmann *et al.* 1982) and 30 percent in rats (Gabard 1980), and plasma peak levels are reached after 30 to 45 minutes (Wieldenauer *et al.* 1982).

DMPS is not involved in important metabolic pathway and parts of administered substance are excreted in an unchanged form; Maiorino *et al.* (1988) showed several acyclic and cyclic oxidised metabolites in the urine of rabbits. Both urinary and biliary excretion of DMPS occurs (Zheng *et al.* 1990). DMPS administration through i.v. route should be given over a period of 5 min since hypotensive effects are possible.

*Toxicity:* No major adverse effects following DMPS administration in humans or animals have been reported (Hruby and Donner 1987). However, a dose dependent increase in the copper contents was found in the serum, liver, kidneys and spleen. The macroscopic and microscopic examination of several organs revealed no pathological changes. A significant report published by Szincicz *et al* (1983) described that after 10 weeks of DMPS administration there was a decrease in copper concentration in serum and in various organs, an increase in iron contents of liver and spleen and a decrease in haemoglobin, hematocrit, red blood cells, activity of alkaline phosphatase and zinc contents in the blood. Information regarding the developmental toxicity of DMPS is rather scarce. No abnormalities in the offsprings of chronically DMPS treated (orally) pregnant rats (125 mg/kg/day) were reported. Oral administration of DMPS also did not adversely affect late gestation, parturition, or lactation in mature mice and fetal and neonatal development does not appear to be adversely affected. No observed effect level (NOEL) for health hazards to the developing foetuses or pups, 630 mg/kg/day is much higher than the doses of DMPS usually given in the treatment of human metal poisoning.

## Deferroxamine (DFO)

Deferroxamine is a chelating agent that is synthesised by the actinomycete; *Streptomyces pilosus* to extract needed iron from its environment. It has a very high stability constant for iron (III) and forms a water soluble complex with iron (III) which is readily excreted in the urine. It undergoes extensive degradation in the gastro intestinal tract and for this reason is usually administered i.v. or s.c. Its principal use is the control of iron overload in individuals suffering from thalassemia and must receive blood transfusion during their lifetime. It is very expensive. Its empirical formula is $C_{25}H_{48}N_6O_8$ and the molecular weight as a mesylate salt is 656.8.

*Metabolism and Kinetics:* Deferroxamine is poorly absorbed in the gastrointestinal tract and thus must be administered by intravenous route (injection or infusion). Its distribution volume is extracellular and the protein - binding in plasma is low (<10 per cent). Its renal excretion is biphasic with the slow half-life being about 6 h. The acute toxicity ($LD_{50}$) in rat through iv route is 520 mg/kg.

*Toxicity:* Intravenous infusion is safe if care is taken not to administer the dose rapidly, which can result in hypotension. Numbers of side effects have been reported after continued and prolonged use of this compound in iron loaded patients. Major side effects include auditory, ophthalmic toxicity, bacterial and fungal infections, changes in blood histology, allergic and skin reactions and pulmonary, renal and neurological effects (Andersen 1999, Kontoghioghes 1995). Other complications associated with the use have been reported. DFO suppressed water intake; an effect, which persisted beyond sub-chronic DFO infusion in aluminium, loaded rabbits. The side effects of DFO therapy during iron chelation have included hypotension, anaphylactic reaction, abdominal pain, and gastrointestinal disturbances. Ocular toxicity of DFO came to light when four patients with thalassaemia major were treated with a high iv dose to counter the effects of iron overload.

## Miscellaneous Chelating Agents

In addition to the above, there are number of other chelating agents which are in use or recently been developed for treating cases of metal poisoning. Some of them are listed below describing briefly their chemical and pharmacological properties:

*Diethylenetriaminepentaacetic Acid (DTPA):* DTPA can bind atoms of plutonium and other actinides thus forming a complex that is quickly excreted from the body. Both zinc and calcium salt of DTPA are generally administered however, Ca-DTPA is more effective than zinc-DTPA. Its empirical formula is $C_{14}H_{23}N_2O_{10}$ and the molecular weight 497.4. The enteral absorption of DTPA is less than 10 per cent. The kidneys eliminate 24 hours after parenteral application 90-100 per cent of the administered dose. While this chelating agent was administered in the past to a number of subjects to increase the elimination of these metals, it is also an effective chelator in mobilising cobalt and zinc from exposed animals. Like EDTA, this chelating agent is also compromised with number of side effects. These include nephrotoxicity, loss of endogenous metals (zinc and calcium in particular). In recent years DTPA was also found not very toxic/lethal to the pregnant animals but still increased fetal mortality and the frequency of gross malformation with the highest susceptibility in early and midgestation. These effects were mainly attributed to the zinc and magnesium loss following administration. As described earlier both the zinc and calcium salts have characteristic, which made their use appropriate for therapy. Ca salts is more effective than zinc for early treatment, however after 24 hours both are equally effective. This compared efficiency coupled with lesser toxicity makes zinc-DTPA the preferred agent for protracted therapy (Seidel 1973, Lushbaugh and Washburn 1979).

*Triethylene Tetraamine (Trien):* This is an orally active chelating agent, is used primarily in the treatment of Wilson's disease when patients show immunological intolerance to DPA, the first drug of choice. Like DPA, this chelating agent also interacts with divalent cations by increasing the excretion of trace elements in the urine, presumably in the chelate form. The absorption of Trien through oral route is poor as less than 20 per cent of an oral dose was recovered in carcass and urine. After iv administration one half of the administered dose is rapidly excreted in the urine and the cumulative fecal excretion was approximately 20 per cent. The acute toxicity (LDS$_{50}$)of Trien is low *i.e.* 1.6-2.5 g/kg in mouse and rat. This chelator is generally free of side effects compared to DPA.

*Monoisoamyl DMSA (MiADMSA):* Recently some mono and diesters of DMSA especially the higher analogues have been developed and tried against cases of experimental metal poisoning (Flora *et al.* 1998, Tripathi and Flora 1998, Tripathi *et al.* 1997, Walker et al. 1992, Jones *et al.* 1992). Among these new chelators, monoesters are found to be more effective than DMSA in reducing cadmium and mercury burden. Maximum metal mobilisation occurred after treatment with MiADMSA; a C$_5$ branched chain alkyl monoester of DMSA. It is reported that the toxicity of DMSA with LD$_{50}$ of 16 mmol/kg is much lower than the toxicity of MiADMSA with LD$_{50}$ of 3 mmol/kg. It may be recalled that reported LD$_{50}$ of BAL is 1.1 mmole/kg. However, the interaction of MiADMSA and DMSA with essential metals is same. The no observed adverse effect levels (NOAELs) for maternal and developmental toxicity of MiADMSA were 47.5 mg/kg and 95 mg/kg/day respectively indicating that MiADMSA would not produce developmental toxicity in mice in the absence of maternal toxicity (Blanuska *et al.* 1997).

## Treatment of Some Toxic Metals Poisoning by Chelating Agents

*Arsenic:* Arsenic compounds have many medical and industrial applications. Though most of the arsenic based drugs have been phased out its industrial use like, in dyes, alloys, semiconductors and pesticides is still widespread. High levels of arsenic may also be found in drinking water. The world's recent and perhaps the worst arsenic contamination of drinking water is in the Indo-Bangladesh region. According to an estimate around 38 millions run the risk of arsenic poisoning. Inorganic trivalent form of arsenic is regarded as most toxic than pentavalent. Arsenic is also a known carcinogen. Arsenic exposure may lead to many adverse effects in the system. Arsenic was the first xenobiotic to which human liver disease was attributed. It also affects cardiovascular and nervous system. Blackfoot disease is characterised by a progressive loss of circulation in hand and feet.

Chelation therapy has been the basis for the medical treatment of arsenic poisoning. They have been used clinically as antidotes for acute and chronic poisoning. 2,3-dimercaprol (BAL) has long been the mainstay of chelation therapy of arsenic poisoning due to chemical warfare with arsine gas (AsH$_3$). After almost 50 years of research we still do not have an effective antidote for arsine which is almost 10 times more toxic than inorganic arsenic (Muckter *et al* 1997). All the three thiol chelators BAL, DMSA, and DMPS (at a dose of 160 mmol/kg) afforded protection against arsine at 2LD$_{50}$ dose in experimental animals. BAL was however toxic at a dose of 40 mmol/kg (Inns *et al.* 1993). It has generally been assumed that poisoning by arsine (Inns *et al.* 1993) and inorganic arsenic (III) in rats (Flora *et al.* 1995), mice (Kreppel *et al.* 1993), and guinea pigs (Reichi *et al.* 1991) all favour treatment with DMSA and DMPS.

The recommended dose of BAL for moderate arsenic poisoning is 2.5 mg/kg, 4 doses/day for first two days followed by 2 per day for third day and finally 1 dose per day for next 10 days. This compound however has limited use now because of number of serious side effects like increase in brain arsenic level.

DMSA has been tried successfully in animals as well as in few cases of human arsenic poisoning (Flora and Tripathi 1998). DMSA has been shown to protect mice due to lethal effects of arsenic. A subcutaneous injection of DMSA provided 80-100 per cent survival of mice injected with sc sodium arsenite (Ding and Liang 1991). We also reported a significant depletion of arsenic and a significant recovery in the altered biochemical variables of chronically arsenic exposed rats. This drug can be effective if given either oral or i.p. route. Patients treated with 30 mg/kg DMSA per day for 5 days showed significant increase in arsenic excretion and a marked clinical improvement. In a case of attempted suicide by ingesting 2 g of arsenic the patient was given a course of 300 mg DMSA orally every 6 hours for 3 days with good results (Aposhian 1983). It has been recommended that for treating mild arsenic poisoning an oral dose of 10 mg/kg DMSA thrice a day for 5-7 days may be given followed by two daily doses of 10 mg/kg for another 10-14 days. While for severe arsenic poisoning an oral dose of 18 mg/kg thrice a day for first 5-7 days followed by 2 doses of same strength for next 10-14 days are recommended. Number of other studies appeared in the recent past have recommended that DMSA could be safe and effective for treating arsenic poisoning. However, in an interesting prospective, double blind, randomised controlled trial study conducted on few selected patients from arsenic affected West Bengal (India) regions with oral administration of DMSA suggested that DMSA was not effective in producing any clinical or biochemical benefits or any histopathological improvements of skin lesions (Guha Mazumder et al. 1998). In an experimental study conducted by us recently provided an *in vivo* evidence of arsenic induced oxidative stress in number of major organs of arsenic exposed rats and that these effects can be mitigated by pharmacological intervention that encompasses combined treatment with N-acetylcystein and DMSA (Flora 1999). DMPS although known for its antidotal efficacy against mercury, too has been reported to be an effective drug for treating arsenic poisoning. This drug too can be administered both orally and intravenously. An oral dose of 100 mg/kg thrice a day for 10-12 days is effective against mild arsenic poisoning while no recommendation for treating chronic arsenic poisoning is available (Angle 1996). A maximal intravenous dose of 15 mg/kg DMPS in humans for the treatment of arsenic cardiomyopathy is recommended. In experimental animals i.p. administration of DMPS increased the lethal dose of sodium arsenite in mice by four folds. A quantitative evaluation of three drugs reveals that DMPS is 28 times more effective than BAL in arsenic therapy in mice (Hauser and Weger 1989), while DMSA and DMPS are equally effective.

*Aluminium:* Aluminium is no longer considered a non-toxic element since it is clear that aluminium overload causes major disturbances in subjects with severe renal insufficiency. Aluminium intoxication has become one of the most preoccupying problem in chronic hemodialysis patients. Brain aluminium accumulation has also been reported in victims of Alzheimer disease suggesting that aluminium may play a role in the pathology of this syndrome (Candy et al. 1986, Peri and Brady 1980).

The chelator desferrioxamine (or deferoxamine; DFO) is a well-known chelating agent for the removal of iron overload during dialysis. DFO is also known to remove aluminium. The effects of DFO are due to an increase in the ultrafilterable fraction of plasma aluminium and to an increase in the total plasma by mobilisation of tissue aluminium stores. The optimum dose of DFO and the mode of administration have yet to be determined. Commonly between 40 and 80 mg/kg is given parenterally once weekly although long term DFO is well tolerated in doses of 20-60 mg/kg, 1 to 3 times per week (Swartz 1985, Ackrill and Day 1985).

*Cadmium:* Cadmium is a widely studied toxic metal and has widespread industrial use. Cigarette smoke is the most significant source of exposure to cadmium among the general population. Cadmium effluent has been linked to the outbreak of Itai-Itai disease in Japan, Cadmium has been shown to be toxic to numerous organs in rats: liver, kidney, testis and spleen. Among these kidney is the critical organ on long term exposure and the proximal tubuli are primarily affected. At a later stage irreversible glomerular effects occur. Cadmium was also recently designated a human carcinogen. Cadmium is also known for its ability to produce low molecular weight metal binding protein known as *"Metallothionein (MT)"* which is cystein rich protein composed of 60 amino acid units.

Treatment of cadmium intoxication still remains a challenge to the toxicologists. The problem in cadmium chelation is special toxicokinetics which makes its entry into the intracellular sites and then binding itself to MT. Cadmium bound to MT slowly released into the blood and then gets deposited in proximal tubular cells of kidneys. In chronic exposure conditions, cadmium is mainly present in intracellular MT and there is very little extracellular cadmium in the body (Shaikh and Lucis 1972). Therefore an ideal chelating agent for treating cadmium should be able to reach inside the cells easily, chelate cadmium from MT and increase its excretion without causing tissue damage or increase in the cadmium levels of any organ. Large numbers of chelating agents have been tried in experimental animals (Jones and Cherian 1990). Initially BAL was tried but was shown to potentiate the toxicity. DMSA too has few beneficial effects, but among all these chelating agents, DTPA was an efficient antidote under certain experimental condition like injecting chelator and metal together. Oral administration of disodium salt of DTPA reduced intestinal absorption of cadmium and enhanced survival after oral exposure. Jones and his group have developed number of new chelators capable of mobilising cadmium (Jones eval 1994 a,b). Number of diethyldithiocarbamates were synthesised and evaluated for their ability to mobilise cadmium. Among the effective compounds are monoalkylesters or monoalkylamides of DMSA (Singh *et al.* 1996, Jones *et al.*, 1994 (a,b), amphpathic carbodithioates and N- (4-methoxybenzyl)-4-O- (-D-galactopyranosyl)-D-glucamine acrbodothioates (Jones *et al.* 1991-1994 a,b). Although most of these new compounds including the most promising one, monoisoamyl DMSA (MiADMSA) are effective but invariably they suffer from number of side effects. Recently, Flora *et al.* (1998) reported a beneficial role of zinc supplementation during chelation of cadmium by DTPA in rats. Thus search is still on to find a suitable, effective, and safe chelating agent for treating cases of cadmium intoxication. The implications for chelation therapy are important and require careful examination.

*Lead:* Exposure to lead *via* inhalation may occur in certain occupational environments. The addition of alkyl lead compounds to gasoline is also a source of lead exposure *via* inhalation. The general population is mainly exposed to lead from food (either the food items themselves or through contamination of food stored in containers partly made of lead such as soldered cans) or pottery glazed or painted with lead. Lead released from water pipes containing lead may contaminate drinking water. Lead and its compounds primarily affect the central and peripheral nervous system. Developing nervous system is the most sensitive target organ system. Severe inorganic lead intoxication may lead to encephalopathy with symptoms such as ataxia, coma and convulsion. Children are at particular risk to the neurotoxic properties of lead owing to their greater absorption of ingested lead, an immature blood-brain barrier and a nervous system under development. Lead also inhibits the biosynthesis of haem at several points through interaction with key enzymes, particularly δ-aminolevulinic acid dehydratase (ALAD). Lead has shown to impair renal mitochondrial function and haem biosynthesis (Woods 1995). In addition, renal gene expression modulated by lead (Mistry *et al.* 1985).

Historically, the drug of choice in treatment of lead toxicity is EDTA. The common practice of treating children with high lead exposure (blood lead levels of 70-100 mg/dl) with a combination of EDTA and BAL is believed to reduce mortality from about 30 per cent to 1 or 2 per cent and is more effective than the treatment with EDTA alone. Treatment with $CaNa_2EDTA$ requires hospitalisation with the resultant increased costs. This chelating agent is usually given by slow, intravenous infusion.

Treatment is given for 5 days and after a rest period of 5-7 days another 5 days treatment course may begin. For children the maximal daily dose is 75 mg/kg divided into two or three doses. The total dose of CaNa$_2$EDTA per 5-day course should not exceed 500 mg/kg for treating lead poisoning.

US Food and Drug Administration, has recently licensed the drug DMSA for reduction of blood lead levels. The recommended initial dose for treating lead poisoning in children is 30 mg/kg/day or 1050 mg/kg for 5 days, in three divided doses (Angle 1993). After the initial five days the dose is reduced by 1/3 to 20 mg/kg/day or 700 mg/m$^2$ in two divided doses for an additional two weeks (Ding and Liang 1991, Aposhian 1983, Aposhian and Aposhian 1990). Bentur et al. (1987) tried a gradually increasing dose for 5 days in a lead-poisoned patient. On first day the patient was given 3 gelatin capsules of DMSA each containing 270 mg of DMSA. On the second and third day the patient received 5 capsules, on fourth day 8 capsules while on fifth day the patient received 10 capsules. The patient was given lot of fluid. The author concluded that the oral use of DMSA is effective, safe and convenient both as provocative test in establishing diagnostic and as therapeutic test. Grandjean et al. (1991) treated a 54-year-old male with lead poisoning. A daily dosage of 30-mg/kg-body weight for three days and 20 mg/kg of DMSA for 4 days resulted in a decrease of blood lead content. For the treatment of lead poisoning the recommended dose is 500 mg to 1.5 g per day in four divided doses. The drug may be given for 5 days on an empty stomach. Experimental studies in rats demonstrated that DMSA given orally was more effective than D-penicillamine. It was reported that EDTA increases the lead content in the brain due to redistribution (Cory-Slechta 1987). DMSA when administered either alone or in combination with EDTA decreases the lead concentration in the brain (Cory-Slechta 1987, Flora et al 1995). Besunder et al. (1997) too recently confirmed our findings in rats (Flora et al. 1995, 1997) and recommended the administration of DMSA and EDTA to children hospitalised for chelation therapy instead of monotherapy with either agent.

DMPS appeared to be effective at least in reducing the body lead burden (Gabard 1980, Twarog and Cherian 1984). By the parenteral route, treatment of adults may be started with 250 mg DMPS (DMPS must not be mixed with other infusion or administered through intravenous route) and continued with 250 mg every 4 hours on the first day. On the second day 250 mg may be given every 6 hours. On the following days dosages should be adjusted to the clinical status and the results of the toxicological analysis. In children, 5 mg/kg per single dose should be given (Kemper et al. 1990). Oral DMPS treatment in adults may be given with an initial dose of 100-300 mg and continued with 100 mg every 6 or 8 hours. In case of chronic intoxication 100 mg given 3 times a day may be sufficient. In children, the oral dosage is 5 mg/kg/day.

*Mercury:* Mercury and its salts have widespread industrial applications like mercury vapour lamps and electronic apparatus, in pesticides, mercury cells for caustic soda and chlorine production in dental amalgam, antifouling paints, batteries and catalysts. The main form of mercury of environmental concern is methyl mercury. It is formed through methylation of inorganic mercury by microorganism in aqueous environment. The high concentration of mercury in certain species of fish is a public health concern among fish eating communities. Large-scale cases of mercury poisoning have been reported due to consumption of seed grain treated with methyl mercury compounds (Bakir et al. 1976). Primarily risk groups are pregnant and nursing women, owing to the susceptibility of the developing nervous system of foetus and infant to methyl mercury toxicity.

Human cases of mercury poisoning have been treated with the chelating agents like BAL, DPA, DMSA and DMPS. Due to low toxicity and high efficacy, DMSA and DMPS are currently favoured compared to the traditional treatment with BAL followed by DPA administration. Several studies explored antidotes against acute mercury (inorganic or organic) reducing mercury deposits in various organs and increasing its excretion. The high efficacy of DMSA in acute methyl mercury intoxication was observed (Aaseth and Friedhem 1976, Magos 1976). The monoalkyl esters of DMSA have also been proved very effective in mobilising mercury. Several such esters have been found to be more effective than DMSA and DMPS in reducing whole body mercury retention and increasing the urinary mercury excretion. Among these chelators, monoisoamyl DMSA ester has proved the most effective (Gale *et al.* 1993). However, human uses of these compounds have not yet been undertaken and await vigorous clinical and experimental trials including safety testing. Possibility of DMSA and DMPS chelation for extended time periods with a low rate of adverse side effects thus can be considered as the current recommended treatment. Recommended doses for DMSA has already been discussed above. In case of DMPS, it can be administered parenterally in adults with 250 mg (slow iv injection is recommended) and continued with 250 mg every four hours on the first day. On the second day 250 mg may be given every 6 hours. On the following days the doses may be adjusted to the clinical status. In children 5 mg/kg per single dose should be applied. Oral treatment in adults may be started with an initial dose of 100-300 mg and continued with 100 mg every 6 or 8 hours. 100 mg every 4 or 2 hours may be applied for oral continuation of therapy in severe cases. In case of chronic intoxication 100 mg given 3 times a day may be sufficient. In children the oral dosage is 5 mg/kg/day.

## Problems and Possible Remedies Concerning the Use of Chelating Agents in Metal Poisoning

Most of the currently used chelating agents have serious adverse effects. $CaNa_2EDTA$ is a general chelating agent that complexes a wide variety of metal ions and is used clinically. $CaNa_2EDTA$ cannot pass through cellular membranes and therefore restricted to removing metal ions from their complexes in the extracellular fluid. The principal toxic effect of $CaNa_2EDTA$ is on the kidneys (Flora and Kumar 1993, Tandon *et al.* 1985, Doolan *et al.* 1967). Renal toxicity may be related to the large amount of chelated metals that pass through the renal tubules in a relatively short period during therapy. Monitoring of zinc status is also recommended during therapy because of massive diuresis of endogenous zinc (Cantilena and Klaassen 1981). Addition of zinc during chelation with $CaNa_2EDTA$ has recently been proved beneficial in experimental animals (Flora and Tandon 1990, Flora 1991, Flora et al. 1994). Other minor problems with the treatment of $CaNa_2EDTA$ include malaise, fatigue, myalgia, anorexia, nausea and vomiting, sneezing, glycosuria, anemia, hypotension. Intramuscular $CaNa_2EDTA$ is painful also. BAL is the first chelating agent to be successfully introduced into clinical practice as an antagonist for cases of acute and chronic metal intoxication. It is also the most toxic of the agents approved for clinical use. One of the most consistent responses to dimercaprol is a rise in systolic and diastolic arterial pressure accompanied by tachycardia. Other serious side effects include headache, nausea, vomiting, lacrimation, rhinorrhea, abdominal pain, anxiety and unrest. Dimercaprol is contraindicated in patients with hepatic insufficiency.

The main disadvantage of treatment with the penicillamine as a chelating agent is that it might cause anaphylactic reaction in patient allergic to penicillin (Bell and Grandjean 1983). Prolonged use of penicillamine may induce several cutaneous lesions, dermatomyosites, adverse effects on collagen, dryness etc. The haematological effects include leukopenia, aplastic anemia and agranulocytosis. Renal toxicity is usually as reversible proteinuria while, elevation in liver enzymes indicate hepatotoxicity. Children undergoing D-penicillamine therapy should be monitored with blood counts, urinalysis and serum creatinine every 2-4 weeks.

In comparison to other chelating drugs, treatment with DMSA and DMPS has got less adverse effects. Few adverse effects include mild and transient elevation of SGPT and SGOT, mild abdominal disturbances and skin reaction possibly of allergic origin.

As evident from the above, the most important problem concerning the medical use of chelating agent is their low therapeutic range which is mainly due to the inherent toxicity of the chelator itself. Chelation is not specific to toxic ions and is causing disturbances of all biological processes depending on a physiological equilibrium of ions (Mehta and Flora 2001). In general, chelators with the intracellular activity are more toxic and have a lower therapeutic range than those distributed only in the extracellular spaces.

Recently, a number of strategies have been suggested to minimise the numerous problems. One of the important solution could be the use of an 'adjuvant' *viz.* essential metals, vitamins and amino acids, etc (Flora and Tandon 1995). In the first, the effects of p.o. zinc and copper supplementation on the safety and efficacy of $CaNa_2EDTA$ in the treatment of lead and cadmium poisoning in experimental animals have been examined (Flora and Tandon 1990, Flora *et al.* 1990, 1994, Flora 1991, Flora *et al.* 1998). However, it was also suggested that higher dose and prolonged administration of zinc should be avoided (Flora *et al.* 1994). In the second approach, efficacy of some naturally occurring compounds like vitamins and amino acids were tried both as potential chelating agents and/as an adjuvant to conventional chelating agents during experimental lead intoxication. Concomitant administration of thiamine, ascorbic acid or methionine during experimental lead intoxication have been proved beneficial (Flora *et al.* 1986, Tandon *et al.* 1987, Kim *et al.* 1990, Dhawan *et al.* 1988, Tandon *et al.* 1994). A somewhat different class of compounds the esters of dimercaptosuccinic acid has also been investigated as agents to mobilise lead from aged intracellular deposits (Jones 1991). The efficacy of S-adenosyl L-methionine in the prophylaxis of lead poisoning has been demonstrated in both human and animals (Battle *et al.* 1986, Paredes *et al.* 1985a,b). Methionine being a ready source of sulfhydryl group would increase the bioavailability of glutathione, which would provide additional complexing, sites for lead poisoning. It appears that dietary nutrients and antioxixdant when given during chelation therapy may have a beneficial role in controlling lead poisoning (Pande eval 2001). Although, most of the available information is on lead poisoning, similar work is required against other metals as well.

## Current Concern and Conclusions

Much of the current interest in chelating agents stems from concerns about the possible beneficial effects of removal of toxic metals in people with low level exposure without overt symptoms of toxicity. It is now well established that low level exposure to lead in early childhood may impair cognitive and behavioural development while lifetime accumulation of cadmium in liver and kidneys are associated with renal tubular dysfunction and hypercalciuria in later life. More recently there have been assertions that mercury vapours released from dental amalgams might be responsible for a spectrum of chronic health problems. Chelation therapy has long been the only method for reducing body burden of metals resulting from genetic disorders of metal metabolism such as copper accumulation in Wilson's disease, cystine crystal formation in cystinuria and removal of tissue iron in hemochromatosis. There is still a need for increased research efforts to provide a better understanding of what chelation therapy does and does not do and to identify its risks. In most cases it is not difficult to demonstrate increased excretion of the metal, but in few instances the clinical efficacy of the treatment has been demonstrated without any scientific rigor (Kosnett 1992). Although, there may be evidence for the ability of a particular agent to enhance excretion of a metal in question, there is a paucity of evidence that any of the uses of chelation therapy reverses toxicity at the cellular level or prevent progression of the pathology produced by the accumulated metal. Further, there has not been sufficient basic research to elucidate the cellular effects and mechanisms of action and effects of chelating agents on the biokinetics of toxic metals.

# GLOSSARY

**Ataxia** : failure of muscular coordination
**BAL** : a metal chelating agent
**BUN-Blood urea nitrogen** : British Anti Lewisite; 2, 3-dimereaprol thiol
**Carcinogen** : a cancer producing substance
**Chelate** : a compound in which the metal becomes incorporated into a ring structure
**Detoxication** : a reduction to toxicity
**DMSA** : Meso 2,3-dimercaptosuccinic acid; a thiol chelator for treating lead poisoning
**DMPS** : Sodium 2,3-dimercaptosuccinic acid; a chelator for treating mercury toxicity
**CaNa$_2$EDTA** : Calcium disodium ethylenediamine terraacetic acid; a general chelating agent
**DFO** : Deferroxamine
**DPA** : D-penicillamine; a chelate for treating Wilson disease
**DTPA** : Diethylenetriaminepenta acetic acid; a metal chealting compound
**Embroyotoxic** : Toxic to embryo
**Erythrocyte** : red blood cells
**Extracellular** : Outside the cells
**Glomerular** :
**Filteration** : the filteration of liquid in the kidney uriniferous tubules
**Interstitial fluid** : The plasma like fluid which bathes cells
**Intercellular** : Between the cells
**Intracellular** : Within the cell
**Lachrymation** : Tear formation
**Leukopenia** : Decrease in white blood cells
**Thrombocytopenia** : Decrease in thrombocytes
**LD$_{50}$** : Lethal Dose for 50% of the subject to which the agent was administered
**Ligands** : an organic molecule which donates electron to form coordinate covalent
**Nephrotoxic** : harmful to the kidney
**Neutropenia** : Decrease in neutrophylls
**Neonatal** : A newly born
**Parturition** : Giving birth to child
**Sulfhdryl group** : SH as in R-SH
**Rhinorrhea** : Running nose
**Salivation** : Excess saliva formation
**BUN-Toxicity** : Poisonousness

*Acute:* Clinical symptom develop quickly
*Chronic:* Action from small quantities for a long time

# ACKNOWLEDGEMENT

Authors thank Dr. R.V. Swamy, Director of the establishment for his suggestions and encouragement.

# REFERENCES

- Aaseth, J. (1983). Recent advances in the therapy of metal poisoning with chelating agent. *Human Toxicol.* 2, 257-272.

- Aaseth, J.O. (1989). Presentation of preliminary review on DMSA for heavy metal poisoning. Annual Metal European Associ. of Poison Control.

- Aaseth, J. and Friedheim, E.A.H. (1978). Treatment of methyl mercury poisoning in mice with 2,3-dimercaptosuccinic acid and other complexing thiols. *Acta Pharmacol. Toxicol.*, 42, 248-252.

- Ackrill, P. and Day, J.P. (1985). Desferrioxamine in the treatment of aluminum overload. *Clin. Nephrol.*, 24, S94-S97.

- Andersen, O. (1999). Principle and recent development in chelation treatment of metal intoxication. *Chem. Rev.*, **99**, 2683-2710.
- Angle, C.L. (1993). Childhood Lead Poisoning and Treatment. *Ann. Rev. Pharmacol. Toxicol.* 32: 4009-434.
- Angle, C.R. (1996). Chelation therapies for metal intoxication. In Toxicology of Metals, CRC Press, pp 487-503.
- Apgar, J. (1977). Use of EDTA to produce zinc deficiency in the pregnant rat. *J. Nutr.*, **107**, 539-545.
- Aposhian, H.V., Merhson, M.M., Brinkley, F.B., Hsu, C.A. and Hackley, B.E. (1982). Anti Lewisite activity and stability of mesodimercapto succinic acid. *Life Sci.*, **31**: 2149-2156.
- Aposhian, H.V. (1983). DMSA and DMPS- water soluble antidotes for heavy metal poisoning, *Ann. Rev. Pharmacol. Toxicol* 23: 193-215.
- Aposhian, H.V. and Aposhian, M.M. (1990). Meso-2,3-dimercapto-succinic acid: chemical, pharmacological and toxicological properties of an orally effective metal chelating agent. *Ann. Rev. Pharmacol. Toxicol.* **30**: 279-306.
- Bakir, F., Al-Kalidi, A., Clarkson, T.W. and Greenwood, M.R. (1976). Clinical observations on treatment of alkylmercury poisoning in hospital patients. *Bull. WHO*, **53**, 87-92.
- Battle, A.M., Del C, Paredes, S.R., Fukuda, I., Kozicki, P.A. and Rossetti, M.V. (1986). S-Adenosyl-L-methionine-a mechanism for its action on lead mobilization and disposal in lead poisoning, *Biochem. Arch.* 2: 293-303.
- Bell, C.L. and Grandjean, F.M. (1983). The safety of administration of penicillamine to penicilin-sensitive individuals. *Arthritis Rhem.* 26: 801-803.
- Bentur, Y., Brook, J.G., Behar, R., Taitelman, U. (1987). Meso 2,3 - dimercaptosuccinic acid in the diognosis and treatment of lead poisoning. *Clin. Toxicol.* 25, 39 - 51.
- Berlin, M., Jerksell, L.G., and Nordberg, G. (1965). Accelerated uptake of mercury by brain caused by 2,3- dimercaptopropanol (BAL) after injection into the mouse of methylmercuric compound. *Acta Pharmacol. Toxicol.*, **23**, 312-320.
- Besunder, J.B., Super, D.M., Anderson, R.L. (1997). Comparison of dimercaptosuccinic acid and calcium disodium ethylenediaminetetraacetic acid versus dimercaptopropanol and ethylenediaminetetraacetic acid in children with lead poisoning. *J. Pediatr.*, **130**, 966-971.
- Blanuska, M., Prester, L., Piasek, M., Kostial, K., Jones, M.M., Singh, P.K. (1997). Monoisoamyl ester of DMSA reduces Hg(NO3)2 retention in rats: 1. Chelation therapy during pregnancy. *J. Trace Elem. Exp. Med.*, **10**, 173-181.
- Brownie, C.F., Brownie, C., Noden, D., Krook, L., Haluska, M. and Aronson, A.L. (1986). Teratogrnic effect of calcium edetate (CaEDTA) in rats and the protective effect of zinc. *Toxicol. Appl. Pharmacol.*, **82**, 426-443.
- Candy, J.M., Klinowsky, J., Perry, R.H., Perry, E.K., Fairbairn, A., Oakley, A.E., Carpenter, T.A., Atack, J.R., Blessed, G. and Edwardson, J.A. (1986). Aluminosilicates and semile plaque formation in Alzheimer's disease. *Lancet* 1, 354-357.
- Cantilena, Jr L.R. and Klaassen, C.D. (1981). The effects of chelating agents on the excertion of endogenous metals, *Toxicol. Appl. Pharmacol.* 63: 344-50.
- Catsch, A., Harmuth-Hoene, A.E. and Mellar, D.P. (1979). The chelation of heavy metals, Pergamon Press, USA.
- Cory-Slechta, D.A., Weiss, B. and Cox, C. (1987). Mobilization and redistribution of lead over the course of calcium disodium ethylenediamine tetraacetate chelation therapy, *J. Pharmacol. Exp. Ther.* 243: 804-813.
- Cory-Slechta, D.A. (1987). Mobilization of lead over the course of DMSA Chelation therapy and long-term efficacy, *J. Pharmacol. Exp. Ther.* 246: 84-91.
- Dhawan, M., Kachru, D.N. and Tandon, S.K. (1988). Influence of thiamin and ascorbic acid supplementation on antidotal efficacy of thiol chelators in lead intoxication, *Arch. Toxicol.* 62: 301-304.

- Ding, G.S. and Liang, Y.Y. (1991). Antidotal effects of dimercaptosuccinic acid, *J. Appl. Toxicol.* **11**: 7-14.
- Doolan, P.P., Schwarz S.L., Hayes J. R.. Mullen J.L., Cummings N.B. (1967). An evaluation of nephrotoxicity of ethylenediaminetetracetic acid and diethylenetriamine penta acetate in rats. *Toxicol. Appl. Pharmacol.* **10**: 481-491.
- Domingo, J.L. (1998). Developmental toxicity of metal chelating agents. *Reproductive Toxicology* **12**, 499-510.
- Ellenhorn, M.J. and Barceloux DG. (1988). Medical Toxicology. New York, Elsevier.
- Fischbein A. (1992). Occupational and environmental lead exposure. In: Rom WN, ed. Environmental and Occupational Medicine. 2nd Edition. Boston: Little Brown
- Flora, S.J.S., Singh, S. and Tandon, S.K. (1985). BAL therapy in human lead poisoning. *Ind. J. Med. Sci.,* **39**, 187-191.
- Flora, S.J.S., Singh, S. and Tandon, S.K. (1986). Chelation in Metal Intoxication XVIII: Combined effects of thiamin and calcium disodium versenate on lead toxicity, *Life Sci.* **38**: 67-71.
- Flora, S.J.S. and Tandon, S.K. (1990). Beneficial effects of zinc supplementation during chelation treatment of lead intoxication in rats, *Toxicology* **64**: 129-39.
- Flora, S.J.S. and Kumar, P. (1993). Biochemical and Immunological evaluation of metal chelating drugs in rats. **Drug Invest. 5:** 269-273.
- Flora, S.J.S., Bhattacharya, R. and Vijayaraghavan, R. (1995). Combined therapeutic potential of meso 2,3- dimercaptosuccinic acid and calcium disodium edetate in the mobilization and distribution of lead in experimental lead intoxication in rats. *Fundamental & Applied Toxicology,* **25**: 233-240.
- Flora, S.J.S., Bhattacharya, R. and Sachan, S.R.S. (1994). Dose dependent effects of zinc supplementation during chelation treatment of lead intoxication in rats. *Pharmacol. Toxicol.* **74**, 330-33.
- Flora, S.J.S. and Tandon, S.K. (1995). Adjuvants for therapeutic chelating agents for lead intoxication. *Trace Elem. Electrolytes* **12**, 131-140.
- Flora, S.J.S., Dhawan, M. and Tandon, S.K. (1990). Influence of copper supplementation during chelation of lead, *Clin. Chem. Enzy. Comm.* **3**: 97-105.
- Flora, S.J.S. (1991). Influence of simultaneous supplementation of zinc and copper during chelation of lead in rats, *Human & Exper. Toxicol.* **10**: 331-336.
- Flora, S.J.S., Dube, S.N., Arora, U., Kannan, G.M., Shukla, M.K., and Malhotra, P.R. (1995). Therapeutic potential of meso 2,3- dimercaptosuccinic acid or 2,3- dimercaptopropane 1-sulfonate in rats. *Biometals* **8**, 111-116.
- Flora, G.J.S., Seth, P.K. and Flora, S.J.S. (1997). Recoveries in lead induced alterations in rat brain biogenic amines levels following combined chelation therapy weith meso 2,3- dimercaptosuccinic acid and calcium disodium versenate. *Biogenic Amines* **13**, 79-90.
- Flora, S.J.S., Pant, B.P., Tripathi, N., Kannan, G.M. and Jaiswal, D.K. (1997). Therapeutic efficacy of a few diesters of meso 2,3- dimercaposuccinic acid during sub-chronic arsenic intoxication in rats. *J. Occup. Health* **39**, 119-123.
- Flora, S.J.S. and Tripathi, N. (1998). Treatment of arsenic poisoning: an update. *Ind. J. Pharmacol.,* **30**, 209-217.
- Flora, S.J.S., Gubrelay, U., Kannan, G.M. and Mathur, R. (1998). Effects of zinc supplementation during chelating agent administration in cadmium intoxication in rats. *J. Appl. Toxicol.* **18**, 357-362.
- Flora, S.J.S. (1999). Arsenic induced oxidative stress and its reversibility following combined administration of N-acetylcysteine and meso 2,3-dimercaptosuccinic acid. *Clin. Exp. Pharmacol. Physiol.,* **26**, 865-869.
- FDA (Food and Drug Administration) (1991): Succimer (DMSA) approved for severe lead poisoning. JAMA **265**, 1802.
- Foreman, H. and Trujillo, T.T. (1954). The metabolism of $C^{14}$ labelled ethylenediaminetetraacetic acid in human being. *J. Lab. Clin. Med.,* **43**, 566-572.

- Gabard, B. (1980). Removal of internally deposited gold by 2,3 - dimercaptopropane sodium sulfonate (dimaval) Brit. *J Pharmacol*. **68**, 607-610.

- Gale, G.R., Smith, A.B., Jones, M.M. and Singh, P.K. (1993). Meso 2,3- dimercaptosuccinic acid monoalkyl esters: effects on mercury levels in mice. *Toxicology* **81**, 49-56.

- Grandjean, P., Jacobsen, IA and Jorgensen, P.J. (1991). Chronic lead poisoning treated with dimercaptosuccinic acid. *Pharmacol. Toxicol.*, **68**, 266-269.

- Grazinao , J.H., Cuccia, D., and Friedheim, E. (1978). The pharmacology of 2,3- diemercaptosuccinic acid and its potential use in arsenic poisoning. *J. Pharmacol. Exp. Ther.*, **207**, 1051-1055.

- Graziano, J.H., Siris, E.S., LoIacono, N., Silveberg, S.J. and Turgeon, L. (1985). 2,3- dimercaptosuccinic acid as an antidote for lead intoxication. *Clin. Pharmacol. Ther.*, **37**, 431-438.

- Guha Mazumder, D.N., Ghoshal, U.C., Saha, J., Santra, A., De, B.K., Chatterjee, A., Dutta, S., Ansle, C.R. and Centeno, J.A. (1998). Randomized placebo-controlled trial of 2,3-dimercapto succinic acid in therapy of chronic arsenicosis due to drinking arsenic contaminated subsoil water. *Clin. Toxicol.*, **36**, 683-690.

- Hauser, W. and Weger, N. (1989). Treatment of arsenic poisoning in mice with sodium dimercaptopropane 1-sulfonate. In Proc. Inter. Cong. Pharmacol., Paris, (abst).

- Hoover, T.D. and Aposhian, H.V. (1983). BAL increases the arsenic-74 content of rabbit brain. *Toxicol. Appl. Pharmacol.*, **70**, 160-162.

- Hruby, K. and Donner, A. (1987). 2,3-dimercapto 1-propane sulfonate in heavy metal poisoning. *Med. Toxicol* **2**, 317-323.

- Inns, R.H., Rice, P., Bright, J.E., and Marrs, T.C. (1993). Evaluation of the efficacy of dimercapto chelating agents for the treatment of systemic organic arsenic poisoning in rabbits. *Human Exp. Toxicol.*, **9**, 215-220.

- Jones, M.M. and Cherian, M.G. (1990). The search for chelate antagonists for chronic cadmium intoxication. *Toxicology* **62**, 1-25.

- Jones, M.M. (1991). New developments in therapeutic chelating agents as antidotes for metal poisoning. *Crit. Rev. Toxicol.* **21**: 209-33.

- Jones, M.M., Cherian, M.G., Singh, P.K., Basinger, M.A. and Jones, S.G. (1991a). A comparative study of the influence of vicinal dithiols and a dithiocarbamate on the biliary excretion of cadmium in rat. *Toxicol. Appl. Pharmacol.*, **110**, 241-250.

- Jones, M.M., Singh, P.K., Jones, S.G. and Holscher, M.A. (1991b). Dithiocarbamates of improved efficacy for the mobilization of retained cadmium from renal and hepatic deposits. *Pharmacol. Toxicol.*, **68**, 115-120.

- Jones, M.M., Singh, P.K., Gale, G.R., Smith, A.B., and Atkins, L.M. (1992). Cadmium mobilization *in vivo* by intraperitoneal or oral administration of monoalkyl esters of meso 2,3- dimercaptosuccinic acid. *Pharmacol. Toxicol.*, **70**, 336-340.

- Jones, M.M., Singh, P.K., Basinger, M.B. Gale, G.R., Smith, A.B. and Harris, W.R. (1994a). Design of in vivo cadmium mobilizing agents: synthesis and properties of monobenzyl meso 2,3- dimercaptosuccinate. *Chem. Res. Toxicol.*, **7**, 367-373.

- Jones, M.M., Singh, P.K., Basinger, M.A., Gale, G.R. and Smith, A.B. (1994b). Cadmium mobilization by monoaralkyl- and monoalkyl esters of meso 2,3- dimercaptosuccinic acid and a dithiocarbamate. *Pharmacol. Toxicol.* **74**, 76-83.

- Kemper, F.H., Jekat, F.W., Bertram, H.P. and Eckard, R. (1990). New Chelating Agents.In Basic Science in Toxicology. Volnasis GN, Srinis J, Sullivan FW, Turner P. Taylor & Francis Brighton, England, pp 523-546

- Kim, J.S., Blakley, B.R. and Rousseaux, C.C. (1990). The effects of thiamin on the tissue distribution of lead, J. *Appl. Toxicol.* **10**: 93-97.

- Kimmel, C.A. (1977). Effect of route of administration on the toxicity of EDTA in the rat. *Toxicol. Appl. Pharmacol.*, **40**, 299-306.

- Klaassen, C.D. (1990). Heavy metals and heavy metal antagonist in Goodman and Gilman's. The Pharmacological Basis of Therapeutics, pp1592-1614. Pergamon Press. USA.

- Kontoghiorghes, G.J. (1995). Comparative efficacy and toxicity of desferrioxamine and other iron and aluminium chelating drugs. *Toxicol. Letters* **80**, 1-18.

- Kosnett, M.J. (1992). Unanswered question in metal chelation, *Clin. Toxicol.*, **30**, 529-547.

- Kreppel, H., Paepcke, U., Thiermann, H., Szinicz, L., Reichl, F.X., Singh, P.K., and Jones, M.M. (1993). Therapeutic efficacy of new dimercaptosuccinic acid (DMSA) analogues in acute arsenic trioxide poisoning in mice. *Arch. Toxicol.*, **67**, 580-585.

- Kuntzelman, D.R., England, K.E., Angle, C.R. (1990). Urine lead (UPb) in outpatient treatment of lead poisoning with dimercaptosuccinic acid (DMSA). *Vet. Human Toxicol* **4**, 364-371.

- Lushbaugh, C.C. and Washburn, L.C. (1979). FDA IND approval for Zn-DTPA, new clinical agent for the decorporation therapy for actinides. *Health Phys.*, **36**, 472.

- Magos, L (1976). The effects of dimercaptosuccinic acid on the excretion and distribution of mercury in rats and mice treated with mercuric chloride and methylmercuric chloride. *Br. J. Pharmacol.*, **56**, 478-484.

- Maiorino R.M., Akins, J.M., Blaha, K., Carter, D.E., and Aposhian, H.V. (1990). Determination and metabolism of dithiol chelating agents. X. In humans, meso 2,3-dimercaptosuccinic acid is bound to plasma proteins via mixed disulfide formation. *J. Pharmacol. Exper. Ther.*, **254**, 570-577.

- Maiorino, R.M., Weber, G.L. and Aposhian, H.V. (1988). Determination and metabolism of dithiol chelating agents. III. Formation of oxidized metabolites o 2,3- dimercaptopropane 1-sulfonic acid in rabbit. *Drug Metabol. Disposit.*, **16**, 455-463.

- Maiorino, R.M., Weber, G.L., and Aposhian, H.V. (1986). Fluorimetric determination of 2,3-dimercaptopropane 1-sulfonic acid and other dithiols by precolumn derivatization with bromobimane and column liquid chromatography. *J. Chromatograph* **374**, 297-310.

- Maiorino, R.M., Barry, T.J. and Aposhian, H.V. (1987). Determination and metabolism of dithiol chelating agents: electrolytic and chemical reduction of oxidized dithiols in urine. *Anal. Biochem.*, **160**, 217-226.

- Mehta A., and Flora, S.J.S. (2001). Possible role of meral redistribution, hepatotoxicety and oxidative siress is chelating agent induced hepatic and reval merallothionein is rats. Food and Chemical Toxicology, in press.

- Mistry, P., Lucier, G.W. and Fowler, B.A. (1985). High affinity lead binding proteins in rat kidney cytosol mediate cell free nuclear translocation of lead. *J. Pharmacol. Exp. Ther.*, **232**, 462-469.

- Muckter, H., Liebl, B., Reichl, FX, Hunder, G., Walther, U., Fichtl, B. (1997). Are we ready to replace dimercaprol (BAL) as an arsenic antidote? Human Exp. *Toxicol* **16**, 460-465.

- Paredes, S.R., Juknat De Geralink, A.A., Battle, A.M., Del. C. and Conti, H.A. (1985a). Beneficial effect of S-adenosyl-L-methionine in lead intoxication : Another approach to clinical therapy, Inter. *J. Biochem* **17**: 625-629.

- Pande M., Mehta A., Pant B.P., and Flora, S.J.S. (2001). Combined administration of a chelating agent and an autioxidant in the prevention and treatment of acute lead intoxication in rats. *Environ. Toxicol. Pharmacol.* 173-184.

- Paredes, S.R., Hozicki, P.A. and Battle, A.M. and Del. C. (1985b). S-Adenosyl-L-methionine: A counter to lead intoxication, *Comp. Biochem. Physiol.* **B82**: 751-757.

- Perl, D.P. and Brody, A.R. (1980). Alzheimer's disease: X-ray spectrometric evidence of aluminum accumulation in neurofibrillary tangle-bearing neurons. *Science* **208**, 297-299.

- Planas Bohne F, Gabard, B., and Schaffer, E.H. (1980). Toxicological studies on sodium 2,3-dimercaptopropane 1-sulfonate in the rat. *Arzneim Forch/ Drug Res.* **30**, 1291-1294.

- Powell, J.J., Burden, T.J., Greenfield, S.M., Taylor, P.D. and Thompson, R.P.H. (1999). Urinary excretion of essential metal following intravenous calcium disodium edetate: an estimate of free zinc and zic status in man. *J. Inorgan. Biochem.,* **75**, 159-165.

- Reichi, F.X., Kreppel, H., and Szinicz, L. (1991). Effects of chelating agents on biliary excretion of arsenic in perfused liver of guinea pigs pretreated with As2O3. *Vet. Human Toxicol.,* **32**, 223-226.

- Seidel, A. (1973). Comparison of the effectiveness of CaEDTA and ZnDTPA in removing [241]Am from the rat. *Radiation Research* **54**, 304-315.

- Shaikh, Z.A. and Lucis, O.J. (1972). Biliary mobilization of cadmium by 2,3- dimercaptopropanol and some related compounds. *J. Toxicol. Environ. Health* **6**, 75-80.

- Shannon, M., Graef, J. and Lovejoy F.H. (1988). Efficacy and toxicity of D-penicillamine in low level lead poisoning. *J. Pediatr.,* **112**, 799-804.

- Singh, P.K., Jones, M.M., Kostial, K., Blanusa, M., Piasek, M. and Restek-Samarzija, N. (1996). Meso 2,3-dimercaptosuccinic acid mono-N-alkylamides: syntheses and biological activity as novel *in vivo* cadmium mobilizing agents. *Chem. Res. Toxicol.,* **9**, 965-969.

- Swartz, R.D. (1985). Deferoxamine and aluminum removal. *Am. J. Kidney Dis.* **6**, 358-364,

- Szincicz, L., Wiedeman, P., Haring, H. and Weger, N. (1983). Effects of repeated treatment with sodium 2,3-dimercaptopropane-1-sulfonate in beagle dogs. *Drug Res.,* **33**, 818-821.

- Tandon, S.K., Flora, S.J.S. and Singh, S. (1987). Chelation in Metal Metal Intoxication XXIV: Influence of various components of vitamin B-complex on therapeutic efficacy of di-sodium calcium versenate in lead intoxication, *Pharmacol. Toxicol.* **60**: 62-65.

- Tandon, S.K., Singh, S. and Flora, S.J.S. (1994). Influence of methionine and zinc supplementation during chelation of lead in rats, *J. Trace Elem. Electro. Health Disease* **8**, 75-77.

- Tandon, S.K., Flora, S.J.S. and Singh, S. (1985). Chelation in metal intoxication XIV : Comparative effects of thiol and amino chelators on lead poisoned rats with normal or damaged kidneys. *Toxicol. Appl. Pharmacol.* **79**: 204-10.

- Tripathi, N., Kannan, G.M., Pant, B.P., Jaiswal, D.K., Malhotra, D.K. and Flora, S.J.S. (1997). Arsenic induced changes in certain neurotransmitters levels and their recoveries following chelation in rat whole brain. *Toxicol. Lett.,* **92**, 201-208.

- Tripathi, N. and Flora, S.J.S. (1998). Effects of some thiol chelators on enzymatic activities in blood, liver and kidneys of acute arsenic (III) exposed mice. *Biomed. Environ. Sci.,* **11**, 38-45.

- Twarog, T. and Cherian, M.G. (1984). Chelation of lead by dimercaptopropane sulfonate and possible diagnostic uses. *Toxicol. Appl. Pharmacol.* **72**: 550-6.

- Walker. E.M., Stone, A., Milligan, L.B., Gale, G.R., Atkins, L.M., Smith, A.B., Jones, M.M., Singh, P.K. and Basinger, M.A. (1992). Mobilization of lead in mice by administration of monoalkyl esters of meso 2,3-dimercaptosuccinic acid. *Toxicology* **76**, 79-87.

- Wieldemann, P., Fichtl, B. and Sizinicz, L. (1982). Pharmacokinetic of [14]C-DMPS ([14]C - 2.3-dimdercaptopropane 1-sulphonate) in beagle dogs. *Biopharm. Drug Dispos.* **3**. 267-274.

- Wildenauer, D.B., Reuther, H. and Weger, N. (1982). Interactions of the chelating agent 2,3-dimercapropane 1-sulphonate with red blood cells in vitro. I. Evidence for carrier mediated transport. *Chem. Biol. Interact.* **42**, 165-177.

- Woods, J.S. (1995). Porphyrin metabolism as indicator of metal exposure and toxicity. In Handbook of experimental pharmacology, Toxicology of metals - Biochemical aspects, eds, R.A. Goyer and M.G. Cherian. Berlin: Springer-Verlag.

- Zheng, W., Maiorino, R.M., Brendel, K. (1990). Determination and metabolism of dithiol chelating agents. VII. Biliary excretion of dithiols and their interactions with cadmium and metallothionein. *Fundam. Appl. Toxicol.,* **14**, 598-607.

- Zvirblis, P. and Ellin, R.I. (1976). Acute systemic toxicity of pure dimercaprol and trismercaptopropane. *Toxicol. Appl. Toxicol.,* **36**, 397-405.

# 15

# Agricultural and Envrionmental Aspects of Poultry Waste Management

*S. C. Talashilkar, A. A. K. Dosani and A. G. Powar*

Wastes of animal origin is one of the major underutilized resources in our country. The poultry is one of the second largest and fastest growing livestock production system in the country and a lot of wastes/byproducts are generated daily in the poultry keeping units. These wastes include poultry excreta in the form of solid and liquid (urine), feathers, beaks, mortalities of chickens, broken eggs etc. Their presence near the poultry unit is a source of nuisance and pollution since they contain pathogenic organisms and produce unbearable offensive smell. The scattered and bulky nature of these wastes and their smell pose collection and transportation problems although many of these are valuable sources of organic matter and plant nutrients. These wastes could not be fully exploited due to the non-availability of a viable technology for their economic recycling. It is therfore, imperative to develop a technology which is cost effective and ecofriendly as well as socially acceptable.

## Fertiliser Value of Poultry Manure

Hall (1950) observed that there are available appreciable quantities of poultry manure mixed with variable amounts of litter. The average recoveries in the excreta from laying birds of the N, P and K in the food are about 70, 75 and 80 per cent, respectively. The recovery of nitrogen is greater than that from large animals and of the total nitrogen in the fresh excreta, 60 per cent is in uric acid and 10 per cent in ammonium salts. The average per cent composition of the fresh excreta found during feeding experiments conducted for two years at Edinburgh is as follows:

**Table 15.1 : Composition of poultry manure (per cent)**

|           | Edinburgh | New Jersey | Pennsylvania |
|-----------|-----------|------------|--------------|
| Water     | 70        | 78         | 76           |
| N         | 1.42      | 1.05       | 1.48         |
| $P_2O_5$  | 1.16      | 0.82       | 0.96         |
| $K_2O$    | 0.58      | 0.51       | 0.47         |

On a dry matter basis, all the three manures contain about 4 per cent $P_2O_5$ and 2 per cent $K_2O$. The figure for N is 4.8 for Edinburgh and New Jersey, but 6.2 for Pennsylvania. Breed and age of bird and feeding however, affect the results. It was observed that fresh poultry manure contained twice as much N and three or four times as much phosphate as FYM, the figures for K were about the same. But, of course, allowance must be made for the inclusion of any litter very often granulated peat which is very inert material and for losses during storage. The loss of nitrogen from a heap of wet manure may be as much as 60 per cent. This can be halved by mixing the manure with litter and allowing it to dry in air. Admixture of superphoshate has been recommended to reduce loss of ammonia and calcium hydroxide had been reported as being a good deodourizer as well as a conserver of N. The fresh manure may also be artificially dried at $100^0$C without serious loss of nitrogen. The quantities available for sale are of course, relatively small, as a source of N, it is equal to other readily available nitrogenous compounds and it should be balanced by the addition of phosphate or potassium for certain crops and soils.

Tinsley and Nowakowki (1959) studied the composition and manurial value of poultry excreta, straw, dropping composts and deep litter. Poultry prine saw dust manure is obatined from farms where birds are kept intensively in laying houses. Vast quantities for their by-products are produced in many countries and added to soil as organic fertilisers. It's value is important and hence on crop yields, depends among other factors, on its composition. Perkins *et al.* (1964) studied nutrient composition of chicken manure for its use as a fertiliser. Chemical composition of dried poultry manure reported by Shennon *et al.* (1973) is as follows, dry matter (82.3-96.1), nitrogen (2.9-6.2%) , ash (20.7-49.7%), calcium (5.1-15.1%), available carbohydrates (2.7-13.9%), uric acid (2.3-11.4%), phosphorus (1.9-3.4%), facial protein content (10.1- 14.8%) per cent) and metabolizeable energy ( 640-1270%Kcal / Kg ). Prasad and Sinha (1981) studied properties of poultry litter. Molecular homogenous fractions of humic acid extracted from poultry litter were characterised by elemental and functional group analysis, molecular weight determination, ultravision and infrared spectroscopy. The divalent and trivalent metal complexes prepared from different fractions of humic acid were characterised by infrared spectroscopy. The molecular homogenous fractions of poultry litter humic acid ranged from 2545 to 40219. Average nitrogen, phosphorus and potassium content of dried poultry manure from country as reported by Gaur *et al.* (1984) is 3.03, 2.6 and 1.4 per cent, respectively. Meraikar and Amarasiri (1988) studied plant nutrient content of animal waste. They observed that N,P and K in poultry manure was highest as compared to cow, buffaloes, cattle, goat, sheep and pig dung at 60$^0$C drying.

Total microbial population, bacteria, actinomycetes, fungi and algae of these samples of poultry excreta were studied by, Nodar *et al.* (1990 a). The physiological groups involved in C, N and S cycles have been determined. The results were compared with the common numbers in soils and organic wastes. Poultry excreta had a high density of micro-organisms. Bacteria, actinomycetes and fungi were also in relatively high density. Algae were in low density. A small percentage of aerobic bacteria was acidophillic or acid tolerant, a lesser number was spore forming and cyanobacteri a were not dected. Most of ther microbial population had proteolytic, ammonificant, anaerobic cellulolytic, denitrificant and anaerobic nitrogen fixing capacities, followed by amylolytics, pectolytics sulphate reducers and anaerobic mineralization of sulphur, whereas, microorganisms favoured by aerobic cellulalytic, aerobic free-living nitrogen fixers, ammonium oxidisers, nitrite oxidisers and sulphur oxidisers were in low densities and sulphide oxidisers were not detected. Nodar *et al* (1990 b) studied microbial composition of poultry manure. The average density of viable micro-organisms in poultry prime saw dust litter was 6.3 x 10$^7$ /g dry material, 1 to 6 per cent of the population were aerobic heterotropic bacteria. Acidophillic bacteria, aerobic spore forming bacteria, actinomycetes and fungi were respectively, 4.8x10$^4$, 8.1 x 10$^4$, 5.2 x 10$^4$ and 8.9 x 10$^4$ CEU/g dry matter. Algae were in low densities (18/g dry matter) and cyanobacteria were not detected. Gale *et al.* (1991) studied the effect of drying on the plant nutrient content of hen manure. They observed that inorganic nitrogen in the manure was 1.93 and 0.20 per cent (NH$_4$N) for wet and dry analysis, respectively. So poultry manure sample should not be dry prior to analysis. Mean values for elements other than nitrogen (P, K Ca, Mg and S) were not significantly different for wet and dry samples. Cummins *et al.* (1993) assessed potential nutrient value of composted poultry mortalities and poultry litter as a fertiliser. The same is as follows: N-40 g/kg, ash-247 g/kg, Ca-23 g/kg, K-23 g/kg, Mg-5 g/kg, P-16g/kg, S-5g/kg, Cu-473mg/kg, Fe-2377 g/kg, Mn-348 mg/kg, Zn-315 mg/kg and B-54 mg/kg. Ferrous sulphate (19-20.5 per cent Fe,) Fe - EDTA (9-12 per cent Fe), Fe- EDDHA ( 10 per cent Fe), pyrite, biotite, and organic manure (FYM 0.15 per cent Fe), poultry and piggery manure (0.16 per cent Fe), sewage sludge have been used as sources of Fe to correct its deficiency in crops. Out of these, ferrous sulphate, Fe-EDTA and FYM are most commonly used (Deore, 1994).

Results obtained from the analysis of 216 samples of composts, organic manure of animal or plant origin and of miscellaneous manure collected between 1990-93 in Taiwan are presented by Liabsheen and Lee Yahnchir (1994). The largest Cu and Zn contents were observed in poultry and pig waste composts. Ni and Cr values were high in 33 and 22 per cent of the pig waste composts and miscellaneous manure, respectively, probably due to the incorporation of Cr-tanned leather waste. Qian Long Qing *et al.* (1994) have analysed crude proteins, amino acids, P, Ca, Cu, Zn, Mn, Mg, Na and K contents of several types of poultry manure collected from Shanghai suburbs, China. Average daily fresh manure production of brolier is 87kg/100 kg of live weight and for laying hens is 73 kg/100 kg of live weight as reported by Sims and Wolf (1994). The elemental composition of poultry waste manure from broiler and layer is as follows, for broiler litter, N-4.3 per cent, $NH_4$-1.1 per cent, P-2.1 per cent, K- 2.6 per cent, S-0.7 per cent, Ca - 2.3 per cent, Mg- 1.0 per cent, Cu-251 mg/kg, Mn-309 mg/kg, Zn-338 mg/kg and for layer litter, N-3.8 per cent, $NH_4$-0.9 percent, P-1.6 per cent, K-1.8 per cent, Ca-3.1 per cent, Mg-0.4 per cent, Cu-473 mg./kg, B-54 mg/kg, Mn - 348 mg/kg, Zn-315 mg/kg.

## Changes Occurring During Preparation of Poultry Manure

The majority of nitrogen excreted in polutry manure is in the form of uric acid that can be rapidly converted into urea and $NH_4N$, if temperature, pH and moisture are adequate for microbial activity (Seigal *et al.*, 1975). Reddy *et al.* (1980) reported that as much as 50 per cent of the total nitrogen in poultry waste is often in $NH_4N$ forms. Hansen *et al.* (1989) studied poultry manure composition and design guidelines for ammonia. They found that ammonia emitted during high rate aerobic composting poultry manure was successfully sampled and measured. The highest SP-mass rate of $NH_3N$ production occurred during the second 12 hours of composting. Total cumulative $NH_3$ N production for 14 days test was 6.4 g/kg of initial compost dry solids for C: N ratio of 20 compared to 19.7 g/kg C: N ratio is 15. Echeandia and Menoyo (1991) conducted an experiment on poultry manure composting. They found that the fresh poultry excreta is blended with pine bark (50:50 basis) to increase C: N ratio to give adequate porosity and sponginess and improve the composting process. The mixture is accumulated in 2 meter high heap and is turned over at an interval of three days for 15 days to sterilise material to minimise volatilisation of $NH_3$. pH attended was 9, CEC 80 m.e/100g and nonhydrolyzable N-1.28 per cent.

Sims *et al.* (1992) studied a composting process using poultry carcasses, poultry manure and two carbon sources *viz*, barley and a pelletizer waste product (RDF) was evaluated for its effectiveness and stabilised the release of N from poultry manure composting was completed after one month. The percentage of organic nitrogen mineralised was 41 and 32 per cent of the straw and RDF compost compared to 60 and 44 per cent for the manure and negatively correlated with C: N ratio (r=0.55*). Cabrera and Chaing (1994) studied effect of water content on denitrification and ammonia volatilisation in poultry litter. Poultry litter is a mixture of excreta, bedding material, waste feed and some soil that is removed from poultry house and applied to soil as fertiliser. Because, litter is commonly stock piled outdoors before land application, losses of inorganic N may occur through denitrification and $NH_3$ volatilisation. This work was conducted to evaluate the effect of litter water content on denitrification and $NH_3$ volatilisation during storage. The results suggest that poultry litter should be stored under dry conditions to reduce nitrogen losses.

Mahimairaja *et al.* (1995) studied dissolution of phosphate rocks during composting with poultry manure using a radioactive 32 P labelled synthetic francolite and North Carolina phosphate rock (NCPR) through laboratory incubation experiments. Francolite or NCPR was mixed with different poultry manure composts at a rate equivalent to 5 mg P/g and the dissolution was measured after 60 and 120 days incubation by a sequential phosphorus (P) franctionation procedure. The use of 32 P labelled francollite showed that in manure systems, phosphate rock (PR) dissolution can be measured more accurately from the increase in NaOH extractable P ($\Delta$NaOH-P) than from the decrease in extractable P ($\Delta$HCl-P) in phosphate rock (PR) treated manure over the control. The dissolution measurements showed the approximately 8 to 20 per cent francolite and 27 per cent of NCPR dissolved during incubation with poultry manure composts in the presence of various amendments. Addition of elemental sulphur to the compost enhanced the dissolution of phosphate rocks. The results provide no evidence for the beneficial effect of proton ($H^+$) produced during the nitrification of $NH_4$ in manure composts on PR dissolution. The low level of dissolution of PR in poultry manure composts was attributed mainly to the high concentration ($4.8 \times 10^m$ mol/L.) of calcium ($Ca^{++}$) in manure solution.

## Effect of Poultry Manure on Crop Yields

The field experiments were conducted by Gunasena and Ahmed (1977) in Iran with potatoes and in Philippines and Sri Lanka with rice, in which, plant height, number of tiller per hill and grain yield were measured. The application of poultry dung increased yield of potato tubers significantly. The yields were 15.5, 14.2, 14.1, 14.3 and 14.7 t/ha for poultry dung, compost, FYM, cattle dung and wheat straw, respectively. Rice yield were also higher with poultry dung (4.72 to 7.47 t grain/ha) than with other forms of organic manure (3.78 to 6.68 t grain/ha). There were no differences in plant growth between 5 or 10 t organic manure per hectare applied, but rice grain yields were higher at higher level of organic manure. N, P and K fertilisers gave positive response in potato and rice. Thus, the judicious use of organic manure alone or in combination with inorganic fertilisers is recommended to maximise crop yields. Koay and Chua (1978) conducted a trial to study the effect of well decomposed chicken manure at 13 t/ha (equivalent to 243 kg N, 430 kg $P_2O_5$ and 172 kg $K_2O$/ha) and treated sewage sludge (equivalent to 243 kg N, 415 kg $P_2O_5$ and 116 kg $K_2O$/ha) and 20 kg N, 20 kg $P_2O_5$ and 28 kg $K_2O$/ ha as inorganic form on yield of okra and they obsered that an application of chicken manure recorded highest green pod yield than the other treatments.

Singh *et al.* (1979) conducted an experiment to study the comparative efficiency of FYM, poultry manure and rice straw with and without zinc on zinc availability to maize cv. Ganga Safed-2 in calcareous soil under green house condition. They reported. that the dry matter yield of maize was recorded maximum in poultry manure treatment. Costes (1983) revealed that maize grain yields were optimum (4.08 t/ha) with application of 10 t chicken dung/ha and 3 kg Zn/ha in trial at Kobacan in 1981. Ponisca *et al.* (1983) conducted experiment to study the effects of chicken dung or cow dung application on maize. Maize cv. DMR-2 was grown in soil treated with 6,9 or 12 t dried chicken dung or cow manure or with 45 kg N, 30 kg P and 30 kg K per hectare. Grain yield increased with increasing fertiliser application from 1.20 t (no fertilisers) to 3.15 t (12 t chicken dung/ha) and 2.67 t (12 t cow dung/ha). Overall crop performance was better with an application of 9-12 t chicken dung per hectare than with cow manure or inorganic fertilisers. Field trials were conducted by Joseph and Kuriakose (1984) with *Eupatorium odoratum* and or glyricidia compost in comparison with cow, goat, pig or poultry manure on growth and yield of rice. All composts in combination with N, P and K application recorded significant results. Highest yield of 5.7 t/ha was obtained with glyricidia + pig manure. Results of two years field study conducted by Maskina *et al.* (1985) on the effect of integrated use of organic and inorganic sources on growth of rice seedling and paddy yield revealed that 120 kg N/ha was significantly superior to 60 kg N/ha in terms of dry matter, plant height and seedling quality. Addition of green manure, poultry manure, Azolla and FYM improved the quality of seedling by 76, 54, 21 and 10 per cent, respectively as compared with nitrogen alone.

Felid *et al.* (1986) compared the anaerobically digested and undigested litter free poultry manure with urea on equal nitrogen basis with maize as the test crop. The major grain yield were not significantly different. That means the manurial values for maize crop were comparable. The field trials were conducted by Maskina *et al.* (1986) during the *Kharif* season of 1984-85. Poultry manure, pig manure and FYM were applied to rice cv. PR- 106 to supply approximately 75 kg N/ha and supplemented with 80 or 120 kg N applied as urea. Rice yield ranged from approximately 3.3 t with no manure to 7 t/ha with poultry manure + 120 kg N through urea. Yield with FYM or pig manure + 80 kg N through urea were similer to those with 120 kg N through urea alone. Yields of following wheat crop given 90 kg N+ 13 kg P/ha were increased by 1.18, 0.77 and 0.66 t/ha on plots with poultry manaure, FYM and pig manure, respectively and were comparable to yields obtained with 120 kg N+ 26 kg P/ha.

Scherer *et al.* (1987) conducted field trials on 1980-83 at two sites in Chapeco, Brazil with 0-12 t poultry manure incorporated in to the soil before sowing maize and they concluded that application of poultry manure gave higher yield. The optimum rate of application was 3 to 6 t/ha. The results of experiments conducted by Savithri (1988) revealed that compost coir pith increased the yields of maize and groundnut when applied at 12.4 t/ha. Recently the raw coir pith based poultry litter containing N-1.3 per cent, P-2.5 per cent and $K_2O$-2.0 per cent increased the grain and pod yields of sorghum and groundnut, respectively in alfisols and vertisols when applied at 6.25 t/ha. Sharma and Madan (1988) conducted experiment on effect of various organic wastes alone and with earthworms on the total dry matter yield of wheat and maize. They reported that maximum yield of maize and wheat were recorded with poultry waste at the two per cent level with and without earthworms. Stefaneson and Pasca (1989) revealed that in 1982-87 in a *Phaseolus vulgaris*/ wheat/maize rotation, wheat and maize grain yields ranged from 3.54 and 4.56 t/ha respectively with no fertilisers to 5. 39 and 6.91 t/ha with 4 t poultry manure per hectare. An experiment was conducted on economic analysis of chicken manure and phosphorus application in Indonesia (Anonymous, 1990). There were five doses of poultry manure *i.e.* 0, 5, 10 and 15 and 20 t/ha and 5 rates of P fertiliser *i.e.* 0, 50, 100, 150 and 200 kg/ha. They recorded that the yield of corn in the treatment receiving no fertiliser was 2328 kg/ha. The yield of corn in the treatment receiving poultry manure applied @ 5 to 20 t/ha was increased from 7085 to 15784 kg/ha. Yields were increased from 6826 to 12083 kg/ha using 50 to 200 kg P per hectare.

Borin and Sartori (1990) conducted field trial on a loamy soil. Maize was given 0-300 kg/ N/ha annually with or without 1.5 t poultry manure/ha (supplying 52 kg Na/ha) or 200 kg N as urea either totally before sowing or in split applications before sowing. Maximum shoot dry matter yield of 20.6 and 19.5 t/ha was acheived when 214 kg N was applied as mineral fertiliser + poultry manure or 152 kg N as mineral fertiliser alone. At higher nitrogen rates, dry matter yield declined but grain yeild continued to increase with nitrogen rates upyo 279 kg nitrogen as mineral fertiliser + poultry manure. Nitrogen use efficiency was more from mineral fertiliser + poultry manure than from mineral fertiliser alone. The higher efficiency of poultry manure attributed to its narrow C:N ratio and readily mineralizable nitrogen. Bhudar *et al.* (1991) conducted experiments at Coimbatore and results revealed the positive influence of poultry manure on the grain and straw yield of rice. They recorded maximum yield of 6.63 and 8.76 t/ha of grain and straw yield of rice, respectively with application of poultry manure. Das et al. (1991) studied in field trials in 1987-88 on two sites with P deficient acid sandy loam soils and differing organic matter status, the effect of appllication of 5 t FYM, poultry manure or pig manure/ ha amended with 28 kg P/ha through different sources on yield of maize and the following mustard *(Brassica juncea)* and groundnut JL-24 crops (in low and high organic matter content soils, respectively). Grain yield of maize (3.56 and 4.75 t/ha, respectively in low and high organic matter soils), seed yield of *B. Juncea* (0.46 t/ha) and pod yield of groundnut (2.18 t/ha) were highest with application of poultry manure + SSP+RP. The effectiveness of amended inorganic 'P' fertilisers followed the trend, poultry manure>pig manure>FYM.

Scherer *et al.* (1991a) counducted field trails at three locations in Santa Catarina. Maize was grown on plots given no fertilisers or 2.7, 4.2 or 4.4 tonnes poultry manure per hectare at location a, b, and c, respectively in preceding year and/ or 1, 2 or 3 sacks urea/ha in the maize cropping year. Lowest grain yields were 4.1, 4.5 and 4.9 t/ha at a, b and c, respectively without fertilisers. Highest yields were 5.6 t at a, (no manure + 3 sacks of urea), 8.0 t at b (manure + 1 sack of urea) and 8.8 t at c (manure + 3 sacks of urea). A field experiment conducted on nitrogen management in maize and wheat sequences cropping system at Rakh, Dhiansar. The results obtained showed that application of poultry manure @ 10 t/ha is more effective in respect of maize grain yield (49.2 q/ha) than FYM @ 10 t/ha) and legume residue @ 10 t/ha (31.6 q/ha). Maize grain yield raised upto 60.3 q/ha with application of poultry manure in conjunction with recommended fertilisers level. Residual effect of poultry manure and also other organic was conspicuous on the productivity of wheat. The poultry manure @ 10 t/ha recorded highest grain yield of wheat *i.e.* 41.1 q/ha than the application of other organic manure (Anonymous, 1992). Saleha (1992) studied the effect of organic v/s. inorganic sources of nitrogen application on fruit qualities of okra var. Pusa Sawani at IIHR Bangalore with fourteen treatment combinations consisting of organic (FYM, poultry manure and horse manure) and inorganic source (ammonium sulphate). He reported that the application of recommended dose of nitrogen (40 kg N/ha) in combination of organic sources improved the quality of okra fruit. Organic manures of different forms were added to test their effects on sodium adsorption and pioneer (sorghum var.) by Gaffar *et al.* (1992). They observed that chicken manure gave the best results for pioneer growth. Yield and yield components were increased by the addition of different treatments. Stem diameter was the most affected parameter.

Suthar (1993) conducted an experiment on influence of organic manure and azatobactor in conjunction with weed management to rabi maize cv. Ganga Safed-2. He reported that application of poultry manure @ 5 t/ha produced the highest plant height (233.20 cm), number of cob/plant (64.82) and length of cobs (15.52cm). The application of poultry manure also recorded the highest number of kernels per cob (373.49). and 100-seed weight (354.74 g). However, it was significantly superior over FYM @ 5 t/ha and no organic manure. Application of poultry manure produced significantly the highest seed and stover yield. The seed yield obtained in respect to the application of poultry manure (5337 kg/ha) and FYM (4748 kg/ha) was higher to the tune of 27.31 and 13.26 per cent, respectively as compared to no organic manure (4192 kg/ha). The per cent increase in stover yield due to application of poultry manure and FYM was to the tune of 29.64 and 16.22 per cent, respectively as compared to no organic manure (5215 kg/ha). Maximum net realisation (Rs. 16,368/- per hectare) and CBR (1:3.29) were recorded in respect to the application of poultry manure @ 5 t/ha. A field experiment was conducted by Datta and Banik (1994) with TRC216-4 rice during the rainy season of 1991 in sandy clay loam soil of Lembucherra. It was concluded that poultry manure and the bio-inoculant combination with poultry manure and rock phosphate gave significantly higher grain yield than from single super phosphate and provided better soil conditions for crop growth in the acid soil. A second application of bio-inoculant at a later stage of growth improved the soil conditions and gave higher grain yield. However, a study on residual effect of the application of poultry manure, rock phosphate and the bio-inoculant will be helpful for the better understanding of the phenomenon.

Madhavi and Suryanarayan Reddy (1994) conducted an experiment of effect on poultry manure on soil fertility and maize yield. They found that grain and stover yield were significantly increased with increasing the fertiliser dose, poultry manure also and their interactions. The grain and stover yields were maximum at recommended dose of fertiliser (47.9 and 56.8 q/ha, respectively, poultry manure @ 4.5 t/ha (51.1 and 58.0 q/ha, respectively) and at their interactions (51.7 and 58.2 q/ha (51.1 and 58.0 q/ha, respectively). However recommended dose of fertiliser + poultry manure @ 4.5 t/ha and 50 per cent recommended dose of fertiliser + poultry manure @ 4.5t/ha were at par with each other. Hence, it can be adopted for maximising grain and stover yield of maize. Field experiments were conducted at Ilo-ilo, Philippines, over two years (1998-90) using rice var. UPLRi-5, with two levels of phosphorus (25 and 50kg $P_2O_5$/ha), two methods of application (broad cast and drilling) and two levels of poultry manure (and 3 t/ha). In addition, in one experiment, phosphorus was added to poultry manure and incubated for 15-20 days. One control and one treatment with only the addition of poultry manure were also undertaken. Rice yield, P-concentration at 8 weeks after sowing, preflowering and maturity and phosphorus uptake at maturity were used to evaluate the treatments. The highest yield was obtained with combined application of poultry manure and phosphorus (Anonymous, 1995). Davis *et al.* (1995) studied the poultry manure and nitrogen fertiliser effect on yield , quality and nutrient recovery of Bermuda grass. Ammonium nitrate @ 0, 100, 200, 300 and 400 Ib N/acre and poultry manure @ 0, 4, 8 and 12 t/acre were applied to them and they found that there was increase in forage yield with increase in dose of poultry manure. The effect of soil and poultry litter management on nitrogen and phosphorus loss in runoff and subsurface flow from four plots of 16 m² area which contains ruslon fine sandy loam soil and 6 to 8 per cent slope was investigated under natural rainfall by Heathman *et al.* (1995). Plots under Bermuda grass (*Cynodon dactylon*) received 11 t litter/ha, which amounts to contribution of approximately 410 kg nitrogen and 140 kg phosphorus per hectare per year. The results revealed that application of poultry litter increased the grass yield upto 8518 kg per hectare compared to the control while the yield in control treatment was 3501 kg per hectare. The results of field experiment condcted by Dosani (1997) revealed that application of poultry manure in graded dose *viz.*, 1,2 and 3t/ha increased the dry pod yield by 2.1, 4.7 and 8.7 q/ha respectively over a number of application of poultry manure. Integrated use of fertilisers and poultry exhibited additive effect on both dry pod and haulm yield of groundnut. Total uptake of major nutrients such as N,P,K, Ca and Mg as well as micronutrients like Zn, Cu, Mn and Fe was increased significantly with increasing doses of fertilisers, poultry manure and their combinations. Fertility status of soil was also found to be improved with increasing doses of poultry manure in lateritic soils of Konkan.

Two field experiments were conducted by Mahimai Raja *et al.* (1995) in New Zealand to examine the agronomic value of poultry manure composted in presence of both phosphate rock (PR) and elemental sulphur S (Sulpho-compost) and PR alone (phospho-compost). Winter cabbage and summer maize were used as test crops. For the first season, winter cabbage, the phospho-compost and sulpho-compost were $\sim$ 12 and 60 per cent as effective as urea and both composts were equally effective as urea for the second seasons maize crop. The greater economic effectiveness of sulpho-compost could be attributed to the improved nitrogen use efficiency increased PR dissolution and improved sulphur nutrition. Distribution of $NO_3$ N in the soil profiles of the field plots indicated greater potential for winter leaching of nitrogen from urea than poultry manure which could be the reason for the improved residual value of the manure reflected in summer maize yields. The results indicated that composting poultry manure with S and PR not only reduces pollution associated with manure application but also, increases the agronomic effectiveness of manure. Rubeiz *et al.* (1995) conducted an experiment on comparison of poultry manure rates as a fertiliser in strawberry and lettuce. When poultry manure (PM) was applied @ 7 and 14 t/ha, there was significant increase in yields of strawberry and lettuce.

## Effect of Poultry Manure on Uptake of Nutrients by Crops

Singh *et al.* (1979) conducted an experiment to study the comparative efficiency of FYM, poultry manure and rice straw with and without zinc on zinc availabilty to maize cv. Ganga Safeda-2 in calcareous soil under green house condition. They reported that zinc was maximum in poultry manure treatment. Arora and Takker (1981) studied the effect of poultry manure and pig manure on the nutrition of wheat at varying rates of N, P and K fertilisers. They recorded the highest uptake of all nutrients by wheat, when poultry manure was used as a source of organic manure at different rates of N, P and K fertilisers. Results of two years field study conducted my Maskina *et al.* (1985) on the effect of integrated use of organic and inorganic nitrogen sources on growth of rice seedling and paddy yield. They showed that nitrogen and zinc contents decreased with seedling age and increased with poultry manure. Nutrient uptake in seedling which were given green manure or poultry manure + 60 kg N/ha were similar to that with 120 kg/N/ha.

A pot experiment with alluvival soil was conducted by Jamaluddin (1988).Treatments included five levels of chicken manure 0, 5, 10,15 and 20 t/ha and five levels of phosphorus 0, 50, 100, 150 and 200 kg/ha. Nitrogen uptake of maize at 28 days after planting in the control was 59.98mg N per pot. Application of 50 to 200 kg P/ha increased N uptake to 177 - 252 mg N/pot. With 5 and 10 t/ha of chicken manure combined with phosphorus at 50 to 200 kg/ha uptake of nitrogen increased significantly. Chicken manure when applied @ 15 and 20 t/ha, the uptake of nitrogen was also increased significantly. The phosphorus uptake in control was 1.69 mg P/pot, with phosphorus applied at 50 to 200 kg/ha, phosphorus uptake increased from 18.47 to 33.58 mg P/pot. In the treatments with no chicken manure had no significant effect on phosphrus uptake. Potassium uptake was 52.73 mg/pot in control. Potassium uptake in the treatment 50 to 200 kg P/ha was increased from 155.9 to 215.65 mg K/pot. Application of chicken manure also increased potassium uptake significantly. Gene and Logsdon (1990) studied the composted product in modern agriculture and they concluded that application of poultry manure corrected zinc and iron deficiencies of corn. Bomke and Lowe (1991) conducted experiment on trace element uptake by two British Columbia forages as affected by poultry manure application. Field experiment evaluated yield response to deep-pit poultry manure application to barley on a clay soil near Prince George and a grass legume forage on a silt clay loam near Chilli wack. In British Columbia substantial dry matter yield increases were measured at manure applications upto 20 t/ha. Sub-samples of both crops and the poultry manure were analysed for Cu, Zn, Ba, Pb, Ni, Cr, Cd, B and Co. Selenium analysis were made on selected crop samples. There was no indication of toxicity problems even at 40 t/ha, the highest application. Copper and zinc concentration in forages were increased by increasing levels of poultry manure and the Mn: Cu ratio tended to decrease with manure application. The experiment was conducted during 1984-86 by Saleha (1992) to study effect of organic v/s inorganic sources of nitrogen application on fruit qualities of okra variety Pusa Sawani at IIHR, Bangalore with fourteen treatment combinations consisting of organic (FYM, poultry manure and horse manure) and inorganic source (ammonium sulphate). He reported that the application of 30 kg nitrogen through poultry manure and 10 kg nitrogen through amonium sulphate recorded significantly highest protein (24.34 and 24.21 per cent at fifth and eighth harvest, respectively), carbohydrates (35.65 and 37.22 per cent at fifth and eighth harvest, respectively) and ascorbic acid content (17.86 and 17.35 mg/100 g at both stages, respectively).

Das *et al.* (1992) studied mineral nutrition of maize and groundnut crop as influenced by phosphorus enriched FYM, poultry manure and pig manure on arid alfisols of Meghalaya. From the results of experiment, it is inferred that phosphorus enriched manure had marked influence on uptake of nutrients of maize and groundnut crop. The uptake of potassium, calcium, magnesium and iron by shoots enhanced spectacularly over control due to addition of poultry manure to both the crops. Gaffar *et al.* (1992) studied the effect of FYM and sand on the performance of sorghum and sodicity of soil. Organic manures of different forms were added to test their effect on sodium adsorption ratio and pioneer (sorghum var.) performance. They observed that protein content were increased by the addition of chicken manure. Suthar (1993) conducted an experiment on influence of organic manure and azatobacter in conjunction with management to rabi maize cv. Ganga Safed-2. He reported that different sources of organic manure did not exert any significant effect on per cent content of nitrogen, phosphorus and potassium of maize but application of poultry manure recorded the highest nitrogen content of 2.9 per cent and potassium content of 2.15 per cent. But uptake of these nutrients significantly increased with the application of poultry manure and FYM. Anonymous (1995) studied increasing productivity of rice through phosphatic fertilisers and poultry manure application in acid upland. It was found that the concentration of phosphorus in rice tissue at different stages and phosphorus uptake at maturity increased with the application of phosphorus and/or manure. The highest uptake was recorded with combined application. The comparison of different organic manure was studied by Dangarwala *et al.* (1995) They observed that poultry manure was a good source in improving zinc uptake by maize, bajra and wheat crops, while FYM improved uptake of iron in maize and wheat cropping sequence. The results also suggested that fodder maize responded greatly to zinc application while bajra to iron application and wheat equally to the application of both, zinc and iron.

Davis *et al. (1995)* studied effect of the poultry manure and nitrogenous fertiliser on yield, quality and nutrient recovery of Bermuda grass. Ammonium nitrate @ 0, 100, 200, 300, 400 Ib nitrogen and poultry manure @ 0, 4, 8 and 12 t/ha were applied. They found there was increase in protein content with increase in dose of poultry manure. They also found that nitrogen recovered from ammonium nitrate was considerably higher (70 per cent ) than from manure (50 per cent). 3 tons/ha of poultry manure with recommended dose of fertilizers has proved to be superior over application of morganic fertilizers alone in respect of dry pod and naulm yield, uptake of micro and micro-nutrients, protein and oil yield of a crop.

## Effect of Poultry Manure on Soil Fertility

The utility of organic manure *i.e.* poultry manure in maintaining the soil fertility has been established since long back. Its application improves various physical properties of soils besides its mineral nutrient content. Hileman (1974) used poultry manure composts to reclaim salt polluted soil. Application of broiler litter compost @ 6 t/acre helped to correct soil salinity. Soil test values for untreated plot were as follows: pH-4.9, phosphorus 7 Ib/acre, potassium -35 lb/acre, calcium 175 lb/acre, sodium 723 lb/acre, magnesium 72 lb/acre and electrical conductivity - $0.46 \times 10^3$ dS/m, while those of treated plot were pH 6.2, phosphorus 72 lb/acre, potassium 40 lb/acre, calcium 410 lb/acre, sodium 50 lb/acre, magnesium 80 lb/acre and electrical conductivity $0.40 \times 10^3$ dS/m. Reddy *et al.* (1980) studied nitrogen, phosphorus and carbon transformation in a coastal plain soil treated with animal manure. The losses of ammoniacal nitrogen through volatilisation were higher in soil treated with animal manure than in the soil treated with beef and swine manure. Poultry manure and swine manure application resulted in accumulation of approximately same $NO_3N$. Accumulation of $NO_3N$ in soil treated with beef manure was approximately half that in soil treated with poultry manure or swine manure. Application of poultry manure to soil increased soil organic nitrogen, soluble phosphorus and soluble organic carbon. $NO_3N$ loss increased as manure decomposition period was increased from 60 to 120 days. Prasad *et al.* (1984) studied effect of poultry manure as a source of zinc and iron and as complexing agent of zinc and iron availability on the rice and wheat yield in calcareous soil. They found considerable effect in available zinc and iron with an application of poultry manure or its equivalent amount of ash and their residual effect persisted upto the second crop. Various treatments produced statistically significant influence on available zinc and iron content. Thus, complexing properties of poultry manure may prevent precipitation and fixation of zinc and iron and keep them in soluble form.

Three manures were compared with urea as source of nitrogen for corn (*Zea mays* L.) on a different field site in each on three year by Beauchamp (1986). The manure and their average ammonical nitrogen: total nitrogen ratios were af follows: liquid poultry manure - 0.89, liquid cattle manure - 0.53 and solid beef cattle manure - 0.09. The manures were applied @ 100, 200 and 300 kg/ha. An additional treatment of liquid cattle manure of 600 kg total N/ha was also included. For comparison with the manure as nitrogen sources, urea was applied @ 50, 100 and 150 kg N/ha. The yield response data revealed that all of the ammonical nitrogen and partly (*e.g* 10-20 per cent) of the organic nitrogen in manure are available for crop growth in the field. Regression analysis of paired yield data, sets of urea and liquid cattle manure or urea with liquid cattle manure indicated that only 75-80 per cent of the ammonical nitrogen fraction applied in these manure was equivalemt to urea nitrogen. Thus it was concluded that the model did not take into account net nitrogen immobilisation and possibly nitrogen losses through deritrification following application. It was also concluded that nitrogen release from the organic nitrogen fraction of solid beef manure differed substantially from that for the other manure. This conclusion was supported by green house data which indicated that net nitrogen immobilisation occurred for the first crop shortly after solid beef manure was applied but, this was followed by net nitrogen mineralization for a second crop as manure decomposition contiuned. Soil $NO_3N$ concentration in mid-June generally increased with urea, liquid poulty manure and liquid cattle manure source of nitrogen at higher rate of application in the field. Lower soil $NO_3N$ concentration with solid beef manure reflected the lower available of nitrogen. Sims (1986) added three different poultry manure to an Eresboro loamy sand in a laboratory study and showed that 30 to 60 per cent of the organic nirtogen was mineralised under the favourable moisture condition in 150 days of incubation. He also showed that from 7 to 37 per cent of the organic nitrogen was mineralised when the temperature of incubations were increased from 0 to $40^0$ C Scherer *et al.* (1987) conducted field trials in 1980-83 at two sites in

Chapeco, Brazil in which 0 to 12 t/ha poultry manure was incorporated into the soil before sowing of maize. They reported that application of poultry manure @ 12 /ha increased available phosphorus and potassium contents without affecting soil pH or organic matter content. The optimum rate of application of poultry manure was 3 to 6 t/ha. Yadav and Jha (1987) conducted an experiment on sugars in the humus of soil as affected by manure and mositure. The soil samples (0 to 15 cm) used were calcifluvent (pH 8.3, organic carbon 0.574 per cent, total nitrogen 0.07 per cent, available $P_2O_5$ - 13.2 ppm, available $K_2O$ 106 ppm, CEC 8.6 C. mol ($p^+$) /kg) from the University experimental farm at Pusa and Haplustalf (pH 6.0, organic carbon 0.487 per cent, total nitrogen 0.047 per cent, available $P_2O_5$- 5.7 ppm, available $K_2O$ 7.3 ppm C.E.C. 5.7 C.mol ($P^+$)/ kg) from the Birsa Agricultural University Experimental farm at Ranchi, Jharkhand. The soils were treated with poultry manure (organic carbon 39.2 per cent, total nitrogen 0.78 per cent, C:N ratio 50: 1) and sewage sludge (organic carbon 42.5 per cent, total nitrogen 0.48 per cent, C: N ratio 88: 1) @ 30 t/ha on oven dry basis and incubated for 130 days at $30\pm1^0C$ under field capacity and submergence. The humic and fulvic acids differed in their sugar contents. In both the fractions of these two soils, relatively greater amount and variety of sugar occurred in the hydrolysates under submerged condition than under the incubation of field capacity moisture. This could be due to biosynthesis of more complex polysaccharides as well as less and incomplete decomposition of organic matter during an anaerobic conditions of incubation prevailing during submergence. The latter possibilities also borne out by the fact that under submergence there was much less $CO_2$ production (479-929 ppm) than that field capacity (598-2098ppm). Some of the sugars like xylose, ribose and galacturonic acid in the humic acids, mostly absent under field capacity moisture were detected more frequently under submergence. Similar was the case with ribose and gluconic acid in the fluvic acid fractions. The influence of soils and manure were variable with no definite trend. It thus appear that sugar distribution and persistence in soil humus may be mainly governed by supply of oxygen.

Prasad and Kumar (1988) conducted an experiment to assess changes in fluvic acid fractions of poultry manure incorporated in calcareous soil from Bihar, after the harvest of rice crop. The soil, Harpur silt loam (Entisol) was calcareous and deficient in zinc (DTPA extractable Zn O55 ppm). The treatments in randomised block design consists of (1) $ZnSO_4$, (2) biogas slurry, (3) poultry manure, (4) composts, (5) sewage sludge, (6) press mud. These organic manures and zinc sulphate were applied at equivalent dose of 2.5 ppm zinc. Field experiments were conducted in the year 1981-82, 1982-83 and 1983-84 with wheat-rice crop rotation. A single application of organic manure was made in November, 1981. They concluded that the nature of fulvic acids of poultry manure changed considerably on their incorporation in soils. The observations of proteinous material associated with fulvic acid extracted from poultry manure suggested that the proteinous materials were resistant to decomposition possibly as a result of their incorporation into fatty acid structure. Fatty acids may be associated with fulvic acids extracted from poultry manure amended soil through esterification of phenolic hydroxyls.

Yadav and Jha (1988) conducted an incubation study for 130 days by adding organic manure *viz.*, poultry manure and sewage sludge to two soils of Bihar from Pusa and Ranchi. The humus carbon at 25, 55 and 130 days stage and the functional groups *viz*, total acidity, carboxyl, total hydroxyl, phenolic hydroxyl, alcoholic hydroxyl carbonyl and methoxy groups were determined in humic acids extracted from soil at the end of incubation. Humic acid carbon and fulvic acid carbon increased due to decomposition of the manure. Poultry manure contributed to more of humic acid carbon while sewage sludge contributed more to fatty acid carbon. Maximum of total acidity, carboxyl, carbonyl, methoxyl groups were contributed by the poultry manure and minimum of total hydroxyl, phenolic hydroxyl groups were contributed by the sewage sludge.

Thakkar *et al.* (1989) showed that application of FYM @ 12 t/ha, poultry manure @ 5 t/ha, or pig manure @ 2.5 t/ha prior to sowing of maize in maize-wheat system on a Fatehpur loamy sand soil corrected zinc deficiency as effectively as an application of 11 kg Zn/ha. Yadav and Jha (1989) conducted an experiment on microbial decomposition of poultry manure and sewage sludge in soil. Different genera of bacteria and fungi were isolated from soils treated with poultry manure and sewage sludge. Pseudomonas dominated in the Pusa soil (Calcifluvent) and flavo-bacterium in the Ranchi soil (Haplustalf). Escherichia was only detected in sewage sludge treatment. *Aspergillus candidus. A terreus, alternaria, Currularia spp,. C. lunata, Fusarium oxysporium, Mucor plumbeus, Penicillium digitatum, P. funiculosa and Trichoderma* spp. were identified. The celluloytic activities of the fungi isolated at 130 days of incubation were measured on modified Richard's nutrient agar and in Reese and Mandels medium with paper strips. Maximum and minimum cellulolytic activity were shown by *Trichoderma* spp. (35.1) and *Currularia lunata* (7.3), respectively. Yadav *et al.* (1989) conducted an experiment on kinetics of carbon mineralization from poultry manure and sewage sludge in two soils at field capacity and submergence moisture. The kinetics of carbon mineralization in calcareous soil (calcifluvent) and red loam soil (Haplustalf) mixed with poultry manure and sewage sludge under field capacity and submergence were investigated under the laboratory conditions. At field capacity, 46-56 per cent and under submergence only 30- 38 per cent added carbon was mineralised as $CO_2$ in 25 days of incubation and the biodegradation of the organic manure during total period of 130 days involved first order reactions. Mineralization potential in the poultry manure treatment was higher than in the sewage sludge. The rate of decomposition of sewage sludge treatments were approximately two times at field capacity and 2.5 times under submergence greater than those of poultry manure treatments.

A field experiment was conducted by Prasad *et al.* (1990) to study the transformation and availability of applied zinc in calcareous soil treated with organic manure *viz.*, sewage sludge, municipal waste, poultry manure, farm yard manure and press mud. Most of zinc existed as residual zinc fractions (41 per cent of total zinc) and organically complexed zinc fractions (3 per cent) in calcareous soil treated with organic manure. The organically bound zinc was significantly correlated with organic carbon. Most of the zinc fractions were correlated positively and significantly with DTPA extractable zinc and negatively with the soil pH. The data of path coefficient analysis showed that the major path by which zinc moved in the treated soil was organic complexed zinc. The organic complexed zinc for wheat and the organic complexed zinc and occluded zinc for rice are the major sources of available zinc in organic manure amended calcareous soil. Application of organic manure influenced the properties and nutrient availability in soils with varied organic matter and exchangeble aluminum status were studied by Das *et al.* (1991b). The pH showed a decreasing trend at higher dose of manure. Humic and fulvic carbon contents did not show any definite trend. Available phosphorous increased after 12 days of incubation and reduced drastically thereafter. Amount of exchangeable potassium increased markedly till 24th day and declined thereafter. The degree of decrease was more pronounced under low organic matter status soil than under high organic matter one. In general, the exchangeable calcium content increased gradually upto 36 days while magnesium content did not show any definite pattern. Overall efficiency of organic manure followed the trend as, poultry manure> piggery manure > farm yard manure. The pH, humic and fulvic carbon content showed differential pattern with nutrient availability at differnt intervals. The contribution of humic acid towards nutrient availability was highest under low organic matter status soil while in case of high organic matter status soil, fulvic acid showed the maximum positive correlation. Bijay singh *et al.* (1992) observed the drastic changes in pH due to the application of organic amendments. The pH increased from 7.6 to 7.9 within twelve weeks after application of poultry manure. Organic manure of different forms were added to test their effects on sodium adsorption ratio and pioneer (Sorghum var.) performance by Gaffar *et al.* (1992). They showed that organic manures were added to reduce the sodicity of the soil. The sodium adsorption ratio (SAR) decreased at the top soil (0 to 60 cm) and increased downward due to leaching of soluble salts. The permeability of soil was improved and consequently the physical conditions. Schilke *et al.* (1993) conducted an experiment to study the influence of incorporated residue cover on $NH_3$ losses from poultry manure amended soil. Poultry manure is commonly applied at the rates determined by nitrogen content of manure. In first experiment, a dynamic flow technique was used to measure $NH_3$ losses from eighteen manure applied to a bare soil surface @ 12 t/ha. In second experiment, three of the eighteen manure were incorporated either immediately, 24 to 12 hours after application. The third experiment compared the same three manure applied to bare soil surface or to corn or soybean residues. Surface application of manure resulted in the loss of from 4 to 31 per cent of the total nitrogen applied in the manure. Incorporation of poultry manure with soil significantly reduced $NH_3$ volatilisation losses relative to poultry manure application to bare soil surface. Ammonia volatilisation was not correlated with individual manure properties, but a multiple regression approach using manure pH and total nitrogen content offered some promise as a means to seggregate measures of the basis of volatilisation potential.

The effect of composted poultry manure on the physical and chemical properties of a loamy sand soil were investigated by Warren and Fonteno (1993) in North Carolina, USA. The soil was amended with 0-50 per cent composted poultry manure (pH 7.5) and maintained at $24^0C/18^0C$, day/night temperature and watered daily for thirteen weeks. Substrate pH increased with increasing rate of composted poultry manure. For most landscape plants, pH was in the recommended range (5.5 - 6.5) at 10 and 30 per cent composted poultry manure rate. The 40 and 50 per cent rates raised pH higher than the recommended level. Cation exchange capacity, available phosphorus and exchangeable potassium, calcium and magnesium increased linearly with increasing rates of poultry manure. Organic matter content was unaffected. Water content increased with the rate of amendment to a depth of 55 cm. Total porosity and unavailable water increased linearly with increasing rate of amendment from 42 to 55.5 per cent and 4 to 30.2 per cent, respectively. Bulk density decreased linerally with increasing composted poultry manure concentrations. Amended soil had a 100 - 116 per cent increase in available water capacity, compared with unamended soil. Air space was reduced by soil amendment. The results supported the use of composted poultry manure to improve the chemical and physical properties of a loamy sand soil. Poultry manure is difficult to handle and apply evenly as compared with granular fertilisers and nutrient content varies. To overcome these problems, ordinary poultry manure was enriched with nitrogen, phosphate and potassium and then granulated. The effect of enrichment and the high temperature used in granulation on the amount and rate of nitrogen release were investigated. The mineralization rate of nitrogen in four organic products, granular enriched poultry manure (GEPM), ordinary poultry manure (PM), composted sewage sludge and wheat straw was determined. The GEPM initially released the most nitrogen compared with PM, sewage sludge and wheat straw. The nitrogen releasing capacities of GEPM and PM were similar indicating that the granulation process did not contribute towards the slow nitrogen releasing ability of the GEPM, wheat straw and sewage sludge hardly released only nitrogen during the entire incubation period i.e., 22 weeks (Alberti and Raath, 1994). Madhavi and Reddy (1994) conducted the experiment of effect of poultry manure on soil fertility and maize yield.

They concluded that the availability of nitrogen, phosphorus and potassium in soil significantly increased with increase in rate of fertiliser or poultry manure or combination of both at 30, 60 days after sowing (DAS) and at harvest. The availability of these nutrients also increased with the age of the crop. The addition of fertilisers at recommended dose increased significantly the available nitrogen, phosphorus and potassium of soil by 10.5, 14.5 and 7.7 per cent more over control, respectively. Poultry manure application @ 4.5 t/ha resluted in higher availability of nitrogen, phosphorus and potassium corresponding to 27.4, 40.9 and 28.9 per cent increase over control at harvest. The nutrient content on poultry manure treated plots were higher in comparison to corresponding plots receiving fertiliser dose alone. In case of their interactions, recommended dose of fertilisers plus poultry manure @4.5 t/ha which was on par with 50 per cent recommended dose of fertilisers plus poultry manure @ 4.5 t/ha resulted in higher available nitrogen, phosphorus and potassium which correspond to 43.4, 65.0 and 43.3 per cent more than in treated without manure and fertilisers, respectively. Davis et al. (1995) studied the poultry manure and nitrogenous fertliser effects on yield, quality and nutrient recovery of Bermuda grass. Ammonia nitrate @ 0, 100, 200, 300 and 400 lb nitrogen/acre and poultry manure @ 0, 4, 8 and 12 t/acre were applied. They found that soil phosphorus increased with an increase in rate of poultry manure application.

The effect of soil and poultry litter management on nitrogen and phosphorus loss in runoff and sub-surface flow from four plots of $16m^2$ area which contains rust on fine sandy loam soil and 6 to 8 percent slope was investigated under natural rainfall by Heathman et al. (1995). Plots under Bermuda grass (Cynodon dactylon) received 11 tonnes litter/ha, which amounts to contribution of approximately 410 kg nitrogen and 140 kg phosphorus per hectare per year. In spring, litter was broadcast on three of the plots, the upper half of one and total area of the other two. One of the total area broadcast plot was tilled to 6 cm, the other remained as no till. The fourth plot served as a control. Relative to the control, litter application increased mean concentration of total nitrogen and total phosphorus in runoff during the sixteen week study for no till (15.4 and 5.8 mg/L) and tilled treatment (16.7 and 6.1 mg/L). However values for the half area application (5.6 and 2.0 mg/L) were similar to the control (5.7 and 1.3 mg/L). Interflow (subsurface lateral flow at 70 cm depth) phosphorus was not affected by litter application, however nitrate nitrogen concentration increased from 0.6 (control) to 2.9 mg/L (no till). In all cases, less than two per cent litter nitorgen and phosphorus was lost in runoff and interflow, maintaining acceptable water quality concentration. Thus, results indicated long term litter management and application rates will be critical to the environmentally round use of this nutrient resources. Rubeiz et al. (1995) conducted an experiment on comparison of poultry manure rates as a fertiliser in strawberry and lettuce. They reported that when poultry manure was applied @ 14 t/ha, available nitrogen and phosphorus were increased by 3.4 and 8.6 g per kg in soil. An incubation study was conducted by Yerriswami and Vasuki (1995) in surface soil (0-20 cm) of hirekumbi series (pH 8.7, organic carbon 0.4 per cent, $CaCO_3$ 8.7 per cent, CEC 48.6 m.e/100 g and DTPA Fe 2.9 ppm). Three levels of $FeSO_4$ viz, 0, 15 and 30 kg/ha along with FYM and poultry manure @ 0,5 and 10 t/ha were tried in factorial randomised block design with three replications. The study was conducted using 500 g of soil taken in plastic containers. The DTPA-Fe was extracted at regular intervals viz, 0, 1, 2, 3, 5, 10, 20 and 30 days. The study revealed that significant differences in the available iron content were noticed from third day of incubation due to application of organic manure. However, increase in DTPA-Fe was only 20 days and thereafter started decreasing in the treatments where only $FeSO_4$ was added. The DTPA-Fe found to increase singnificantly even beyond 20 days in the treatments either FYM or poultry manure was added along with $FeSO_4$. This may be due to the formation of complexation with the added iron by organic compounds present in the organic manure (Tisdale et al. (1993). Of the two manure, poultry manure was found to be more effective in keeping major portion of applied iron in available form and this is attributed to the higher stability of heavy metal complex with phenolic, hydroxy-carboxylic and amino groups present in the poultry manure. Application of graded doses of poultry manure from 1 to 3 t/ha to groundnut crop in laterite soils of konkan improved the nutrient states of soil in grodation without any harmful effect on crop and soil health (Dosani, 1997).

## Pollution Aspects of Poultry Manure

The role of poultry wastes in contamination of groundwater was nitrate nitrogen, the eutophication of surface waters by nitrogen and phosphorus, and the fate of pesticides, heavy metal, and pathogen applied to soil in poultry wastes are the central environmental issues from the agricultural perspective (Magette et al., 1989; Weil et al., 1990 and Edwards and Daniel, 1992). Other environmentally related issues are air quality and odour control, disposal of dead or diseased poultry, food safety and animal health and welfare, also confront the poultry industry. Ground water contamination by $NO_3$-N is an issue of global concern, the causes and related environmental effects of $NO_3$-N pollution have been discussed by Greenwood (1990). Environmental protection agency has established a maximum contaminant level of 10 mg $NO_3$- N/litre to protect the safety of US drinking water supplies (US

Environmental Proection Agency (USEPA), 1985]. The European Economic Community (EEC) (1990) has established a similar standard of 11 mg $NO_3$-N/litre. Concentration of the poultry industry in an area without adequate cropland can also result in the accumulation of soil P to the excessive levels. The N:P ratio of poultry wastes usually results in the addition of P beyond crop removal in harvested biomass, except in extremely P-deficient soils (Sims and Wolf, 1994).

*Pesticides, Antibiotics and Heavy metals in poultry wastes:* Nutrients are not the only constituents of poultry wastes that can an environmental impact. Pesticides used to control insects in poultry houses and heavy metals, antibiotics and coccidostats used as feed additives as for nutritional or disease - related purpose are also of concern. Limited research, however, has been conducted on the fate of these waste constituents following their application to agricultrual soils. The degradation and mobility of pesticides in soils help to minimise pollution problems. One example of a pesticide used in poultry production is cyromazine, an S-trizine larvacide that is mixed with poultry feed and passed through the animal to control fly populations in broiler houses. Preliminary research has shown that heavy manure application and intensive rainfall can cause cyromazine losses in runoff (Pote et al., 1994). Antibiotics and Coccidiostats include compounds such as amprolium, salynomycin, streptomycin, tetracyline and terramycin. Very little research has been conducted on the environmental fate of any of these chemicals after manure of litter containing them is applied to the soil.

Heavy metals concentrations in poultry wastes can be similar to or exceed those reported for domestic sewage treatment plants. Metals are normally added to the poultry diet as salts such as $CuSO_4$, $NaSeO4$ or as acids, such as 3- nitro-4 hydroxy phenylarsonic acid; they may also occur naturally in the grains used in the diets. Malone *et al.* (1992) collected broiler litter samples from 60 poultry farms in Delware and found that Cu and Zn values ranged from 289 to 920 and 315 to 680 mg/kg. Kunkle *et al.* (1981) reported average As, Cd, Cu, Hg, Pb and Se values after five flocks of broiler chickens were 35, 0.5, 319, 0.3, 3.0 and 0.3 mg/kg. It is therefore suggested that research on the fate of metals in the soil amended with poultry wastes is needed to determine if guidelines or regulations similar to those mandated for municipal and industrial wastes are necessary for poultry wastes.

Minchiton *et al.* (1973) studied tha phytotoxicity of poultry manure. Reports from field personnel and growers in Western Australia, Victoria and New South wales indicated the presence of plant toxin in deep litter fowl manure. Manure from other poultry manager systems did not produce any toxic symptoms and not all samples of deep litter manure were toxic. Affected crops have included vegetables, in particular tomatoes, ornamental nursery crops both field and container grown and ornamental cut flower speices. Reports from Western Australia suggested that the toxin was 2-4 -D ingested by fowls fed on contaminated wheat seed. Their work in Victoria indicated that the compound had properties differed from 2, 4-D and the present investigation was carried out to check this possibility to isolate and identify the toxin. From above results, they summarised that examination of samples of deep litter poultry manure which causes growth deformation in vegetable crops resulted in isolating of a potent phytotoxic compound. The chemical properties and symptoms showed that it was not 2, 4-D as suggested by these workers but a nitrogen heterocyclic compound with concentrated attached carboxyl group. Poultry manure trials have shown that an impurity 4-amino-3, dichloro-2, 6-outidine, in coccidiostatclopidol (3, 5-dichloro-2, b-dimethy 1-4pyridinol) causes similar phytotoxicity. Increased potency after poultry ingestion indicated that this impurity is metabolised. The most likely metabolite is 4- amino-3-5 dichloro-b-methy1-picolinc acid. Chemical and physical data of metabolite are identical to that of the toxic compound isolated from original manure samples. Liebhardt and Shortall (1974) conducted experiment on amendment of soil with poultry manure and they found that soil salinity increased when heavy rates of poultry manure were applied to sandy coastal plain soils. Analysis of soils involved in a poultry manure study during 1970, 1971 and 1972 had showed that soil salinity was primarily associated with high concentration of potassium in the soil solution. Although concentration of other elements increased with the application of poultry manure also, the increases were not sufficient to account for the salinity in these soils.

Liebhardt (1976) conducted experiment on nutrient concentration of corn as affected by poultry manure. They found that the concentration of heavy metals increased with an increase in dose of poultry manure from 22 to 224 tonnes per hectare resulted into nutrient toxicity to maize crops. Well and Korontje (1979) conducted an experiment on organic matter decompossition in a soil amended with poultry manure. Organic matter assimilatory capacity of soil takes on special significance when large concentrations of animal wastes were produced and applied to land at disposal rates. Recent work had showed that when poultry manure applied to soil at rates exceeding 20 MT per hectare, poultry manure release phytotoxic quntities of ammonia, nitrites and salts. These substances may also have toxic effects on soil organisms responsible for decomposition process. It is possible that soil ecosystem, like aquatic ecosystem, can have their assimilatory capacities overloaded. In some cases, increasing the rate at which organic material added to a soil may decrease the properties if the added carbon which is evolved as carbondioxide. The overall ability of soil to accept and dispose of the poultry manure did not appear to be seriously impaired even at high rate of manure application for it was estimated that only seven per cent of 393 MT of organic, matter added per hectare remained in the below layer after five year period. Field trials conducted by Well *et al.* (1979) in 1972-76 on davidson clay loam near Orange, Virginia. They applied four rates of poultry manure for growing maize cv. Pioneer 3369A. During spring and summer, the concentration of double salts (upto 4064 ppm) and nitrite nitrogen (upto 60 ppm) were high enough to be toxic to the plants. Both stand establishment and subsequent growth of the maize were very poor on the heavily manure plots. Severe moisture stress was evident throughout the growing season due to the effects of salinity and stunted root system.

## SUMMARY

The implementation of environmentally sound management programme for poultry waste products in agriculture is one of the greatest challenges to poultry industry during the present era of energy crisis and food shortage since poultry wastes contain all essential plant nutrients. The present communication disscusses the agricultural and environmental issues of the said wastes.

## REFERENCES

- Alberti, 1. and Raath, P.J. 1994. The nitrogen releasing capacity of processed poultry manure compared with that of differnet organic material. Peciduous Fruit Grower. 44 (10): 376- 379

- Anonymous 1990. Economic analysis of chicken manure and P-application in Indonesia. *Titan Agronmi* 2: 71-77.

- Anonymous 1992. Nitrogen management in maize and wheat sequences cropping system. *All India Co-ordinated Res: Project for Dry Land Agricultre. pp. 99-100.*

- Anonymous 1995. Increasing productivity through phosphatic fertilizer and poultry manure application in acid upland. *Annals of biology* 11 (1/2): 151-157 [Quoted from Rice Abstr. 19(2): 114].

- Arora, C.L. and Takkar, R.N. 1981. Effect of poultry manure on the yield and nutrient content of wheat. *J. Res. Punjab Agric. Univ.* 18 (3) 257-265.

- Beauchamp, E.G. 1986. Availability of nitrogen from three manures to corn in the field. *Can. J. Soil Sci.* 66 (5): 713-720.

- Bhudar, M.N.; Palaniappan, S.P. and Rangasamy, A. 1991 Effect of farm waste and green manures on low land rice *Ind.J. Agronomy.* 36 (2): 251.

- Bijay Singh 1992. Changes in chemical properties of soil due to application of organic manures. In National training on organic farming sponsored by Directorate of extension, Govt. Inda, New Delhi in Aug. 1995. pp.42

- Bomke, A.A. and Lowe, L.E. 1991. Trace element uptake by two British Columbia Forages as affected poultry manure application. *Can J. of Soil Sci.* **71** (3): *305-312.*

- Borin, M. and Sartori, G. 1990. Nitrogen fertilizer rate source and application date *field Crop Abstr.* **43** (6): *493.*

- Cabrera, M.L and Chiang, S.C. 1994. Water content effect on denitrification and ammonia volatilization in poultry litter . *Soil Sci. Soc. America J.* **58**(3): 811- 816

- Costes, Z.B. 1983. Interaction effect of chicken dung and zinc on yield of IBP var. I corn. *Fld. Crop. Abstr.* **36**(1): *26.*

- Cummins, C.G.; Wood, C.W. and Delaney, D.P. 1993. Composted poultry mortalities and poultry litter.

- Composition and potential value as a fertilizers. *J. Substainable Agric* 4(1): 7-8

- Dangarwala, P.T. and Patel, K.P. 1995. Micronutrient Research in Gujarath, GAU, Anand . *A compendium Soil Res. in GAU. Anand* pp.74.

- Das, M.; Singh B.P.; Ram, M.; Dwivedi, B.S. and Prasad, R.N. 1991. Effect of 'P' fertilizer amended organic matter on P-nutrition of crops under mid attitude of Meghalaya. *Anals of Agricultural Research* **12** (2): 134-141.

- Das, M.; Singh B.P.; Ram, M.; Dwivedi, B.S.; and Prasad, R.N. 1991. Influence of organic manures on native plant nutrient availability in an acid Alfisol. *J. Indian Soc. Soil Sci* **89** (2): 286-291.

- Das, M.; Singh B.R., Ram, M. and Prasad, R.N. 1992. Mineral nutrition of maize and groundnut as influenced by P. enriched manures on acid Alfisols. *J. Indian Soc. Soil Sci.* **40** (3): 580 - 583.

- Datta, M. and Banik, S. 1994. Effect of poultry manure and phosphate dissolving bacteria on rice (*Oryza sativa*) in acid soil. *Indian J. Agric. Sci.* **64** (11): 791-793.

- Davis, A.G.; Parkar, M.B.; Neathery, M.W. and Johnson, H.S. Jr. 1995. Poultry manure and N- fertilizer effects on yield quality and nutrient recovery of Bermuda grass. *Agronomy Abstr.* 1995. *Amer. Soc. Agron.* *pp. 256.*

- Deore, S.K. 1994. Micronutrient and sulphur research in Gujarath *Paper in seminar on recent trend in micronutrients research in soils and plant in Maharashtra, M.A.U., Parbhani* pp.13.

- Dosani A.A.K. 1997. Effect of poultry manure in combination with inorganic fertilisers on yield, quality and nutrient uptake by groundnut. M.Sc. (Agri). Thesis sumitted to Konkan Krishna Vidyapeeth, Dapoli.

- Echeandia, A and Menoyo, A. 1991. Poultry manure composting. *Biocycle.* **32** (6): 47

- Edward, D.R. and Daniel, T.C. 1992. Environmental impacts of on farm poultry waste disposal - *A review Bioresource Tech.* **41**: 91-93.

- Field, J.A.; Reneau, R.B.; Jr. Kroontje, W. and coldwell, J.S. 1986. Utilization of anaerobically digested poultry manure effluent nitrongen as fertilizer. *Transaction of the ASAE* **29** (I): 223 - 228. [Quoted from: Soils and Fertil. Abstr. 50 (1): 511]

- Gaffar, M.O.; Ibrahim, Y.M. and Wahab, D.A.A. 1992. Effect of farm yard manure and sand on the performrance of sorghum and sodicity of soils. *Indian Soc. Soil Sci.* **40** (3): 540-543.

- Gale, P.M.; Philips, J.M.; May, M.L. and Wolf, D.C. 1991. effect of drying on the plant nutrient content of hen-manure. *J. Production Agricultural.* **4** (2): 246 - 250.

- Gaur, A.C.; Neelakantan and Dargan, *K.S. 1984. Organic manures.* I.C.A.R. Pub., New Delhi.

- Gene and Logsdon. 1990. Composted product in modern agriculture. *Biocycle.* **31** (9): 66-67.

- Greenwood, D.J. 1990. Production or productivisty: the nitrate problem? *Ann. Appl. Biol.* **117**: 209-231.

- Gunasena, H.P.M. and Ahmed, S. 1977. Potential of organic manures and plant residues in crop production. *J. National Agri. Soc. of Ceylon.* **14**(3): 69-84. [Quoted from Field crop Abstr. 1980. 33 (1): 37]

- Hall, D.A. 1950. Waste organic compounds. *Fert. and Manures.* pp. 203-204.

- Hansen, R.C.; Keener, H.M. and Hotink, H.A.J. 1989. Poultry manure comparison, design guidelines for ammonia. *American Soc. of Agril. Engg.* **89** (4075): 23.

- Heathman, G.C.; Sharpley, A.N.; Smith, S.J. and Robinson, J.S. 1995. Land application of poultry litter and water quality in Oklahoma, U.S.A. *Fertilizer Research.* **40** (3): 165-173.

- Hileman, L.H. 1974. Using poultry manure composts to reclaim salt polluted soil. *Compost Sci.* **15** (2): 22-23.

- Jamaluddin, D. 1988. Effect of chicken manure and P-in fluvaquent soil on the N, P and K uptake by corn. *Agrikan.* **3** (1): 40-43.

- Joseph, P.A. and Kuriakose, T.F. 1984. An integrated nutrient supply system of higher rice production. *Int. Rice Res. Newsletter.* **10** (2) [Quoted from: Fld Crop Abstr. (1985) 38 (11): 750]

- Koay, S.M. and Chua, S.B. 1978. Effect of fertilizers on vegetative growth and production on okra. *Singapore J. Primary Industries.* **6** (2): 79 - 93.

- Kunkle, W.E., Carr, L.E., Carter, T.A. and Bossard, E.H. 1981. Effect of flock and floor type on the levels of nutrients and heavy metals in broiler litter. *Poult. Sci.* **60**: 1160-1164.

- Lian Sheen and Lee Yahnchir 1994. Metal components of organic manures and the current criteria of regulation. *J. Agril. Res. China.* **43** (4): 412-442. [Quoted from soil and Fertility Abstract, 1996. 59 (7): 787]

- Liebhardt, W.C. 1976. Naturient concentration of corn as affected by poultry manure. *Comm. Soil Sci. and Pl. analysis.* 7(2): 175 - 188.

- Liebhardt, W.C. and shortall, J.G. 1974. Potassium is responsible for salinity in soils amended with poultry manure. *Comm. Soil Sci. and Pl. Analysis.* 5 (5): 385-398.

- Madhavi, B.L. and Suryanarayan Reddy 1994. Effect of poultry manure on soil fertility and maize yield. *National Seminar on Devpts. in soil Sci.* **94**: 285-287.

- Magetto, W.L.; Weismilln, R.A.; Angle, J.S. and Brinsfield, R.B. 1989. A nitrate ground water standards for 1990 farm bill. *J. Soil Water Conserv.* **5**: 491-494.

- Mahimairaja, S.; Bolan, N.S. and Hedley, M.J. 1995. Dissolution of phosphate rock during the composting poultry manure: an incubation experiment. *Fertilizer Research.* **40**(2):93-104.

- Mahamairaja, S; Bolan, N.S. and Hedley, M.J. 1995. Dissolution of phosphate rock during the composting poultry manure: an incubation experiment. *Fertilizer Research.* **40** (2): 93-104

- Mahamairaja, S; Bolan, N.S. and Hedley, M.J. 1995 Agronomic effectiveness of poultry manure composts. *Communication in soil Sci. and plant Analysis.* 26 (11-12): 1843-1861.

- Malone, G.W., Sims, J.T., and Gedamu, N., 1992. Quantity and quality of poultry manure produced under current management programs. *Tech. Rep. Delware Dep. Nat. Res. Environ. control,* Dover.

- Maskina, M.S; Sanhdu, P.S. and Meelu, O.P. 1985. Effect of integrated use of organic and inorganic nitrogen sources on growth and nutrient composition of rice seedling. *Oryza.* 22(1): 11-16. [Quoted from: *Field Crop Abstr* (1987) 40 (2): 83].

- Maskina, M.S.; Khind C.S. and Meelu, O.P. 1986. Poultry manure as a nitrogen source in a rice wheat rotation. *Rice Res.Newsletter.* 11 (5): 44 [ Quoted from: *Field crop Abstr.* (1987) 40 (6) 413).

- Meraikar, S. and Amarasiri, S.L. 1988. Plant nutrient content of animal wastes. *Trop. Agric* 144: 79-87.

- Minchinton, I.R.; Jones, D.L. and Sang, J.P.L. 1973. Poultry manure phytotoxicity. J. *Sci. Food Agri* 24 (7): 1437-1448.

- Nodar, R.; Aceae, M.J. and Carballas, T. 1990 a. Microbial composition of poultry excereta. *Biological waste.* 33: 95-105.

- Nodar, R.; Aceae, M.J. and Carballas, T. 1990 b. Microbial composition of poultry excreta. *Biological waste* 33: 296-306.

- Ponisca, E.P.; Escalades, R.G. and Quirol, B.F. 1983. Effect of animal manure application on the growth and yield of corn. *Annals of Trop. Res.,* 5 (3&4): 110-116, [Quoted from *Fld. Crop. Abstr. 1986. 39 (6): 476].*

- Pote, D.H. Daniel,T.C., Edwards, D.R. and Matrice J.D. 1994. Effect of land-applied caged layer manure on cryomazine loss. *Jour. of Environ. Quality.* **23**.

- Prasad, B. and Sinha, M.K. 1981. Properties of poultry litter. Humic acid fractions and their metal complexes. *Plant and Soil.* **63**: 439-448.

- Prasad, B.; Singh., A.P. and Sinha, M.K 1984. Effect of poultry manure as a source of zinc and iron as complexing agent of Zn and Fe availability and crop yield in calcareous soil. *J. Indian Soc. Soil Sci.* **82** (3): 519-521.

- Prasad, B. and Kumar, M. 1988. Changes in the fulvic acid fraction of organic materials resulting from their incorporation in calcareous soil. *J. Indian Soc. Soil. Sci.* **36**(3): 543-545.

- Prasad, B.; Mehata, A.K. and Sinha, M.K 1990. Zinc fractions and availability of applied zinc in calcareious soil treated with organic materials. *J. Indian Soc. Soil. Sci.* IARI, New Delhi **38** (2): 248-253.

- Qian Long Qing. Xu Da Xin, Sun Zhifeng and Tang Yonglan 1994. Analysis of nutrient content in chicken manure *Agri. Sanghai.* **10**: 37-40.

- Reddy, K.R.; Khaled, R and Overcase, M.R 1980 N, P and C trasnformation in coastal plain soil treated with animal manure. *Agril waste* **2**(3): 225-238.

- *Rubeiz, I.G.; Khawsa M. and Preiwat, M. 1995.* Comparison of poultry layer manure rates as a fertilizer in straw berry and lettuce. *Agron. Abstract. 1995 Amer. Soc. Agron. pp.*263.

- Saleha, A. 1992. Studies on the effect of organic v/s inorganic form of nitrogen on the quality of Okra. *J. Mah. Agric. Uni* **7**(1): 133-134

- Savithri 1988. *In* notes National training on organic farming sponsored by Directorate of Extension, Govt. of India, New Delhi *Report Bull. on MWR* pp.14.

- Scherer, E.E. Nadal, R.D. and Castilhos, E.G. 1987. Utilization of PM and phosphate fertilization in maize crop. *Fld. Crop Abstr* **40**(7) 505.

- Scherer, E.E.; Agostini, D.; Wildner, L.P., Nadal, R.; Silvestro, M. and Sorenson, W.J. 1991. Poultry manure and nitrogen for maize on small farms. *Fld. Crop. Abstr.* **44**(9): 811.

- Schilke, Gartley, K.L. and Sims, J.T. 1993 Ammonia volatalization from poultry manure amended soil. *Biol. Ferti. Soil* **16**(1): 5-10.

- Seigal, R.S.; Hafez, A.A.R.; Azevedo J and Stout, P.K. 1975. Management procedure for effective fertilization with poultry manure. *Compost Science* **16**: 5-9.

- Sharma, N. and Madan M. 1988. Effect of various organic waste alone and with earthworms on the total dry matter yield of wheat and maize. *Bio Wastes.* **25**: 33-40.

- Shernnon, D.W.E.; Blair, R. and Lee, D. 1973. Chemical composition of dried poultry manure. *World's poultry Science. J.* **29** (2): 157.

- Sims, J.T. 1986 Nitrogen transformation in a poultry manure amended soil: Temperature and moisture effects. *J. Environ Qual* **15**: 59-63.

- Sims, J.T. Murphy, D.W. and Handwerkar 1992. Composting of poultry waste: Implication for dead poultry disposal and manure management. *J. Sustainable Agric* **2**(4): 67-82.

- Sims, J.T. and Wolf, D.C. 1994. Poultry management agricultural sicence issues, *Advances in Agronomy,* **52**: 83.

- Singh R.P., Prasad, R.N. Sinha, H. and Singh K.D.N. 1979. Effect of organic amendments on Zn availability to maize and soybean in calcareous soil. *J. Ind. Soci. Soil. Sci* **27**(3): 321-324.

- Stefaneson, M. and Pasca, I.C. 1989. The effect of application of organic and chemical fertilizers on wheat and maize. *Fld. Crop. Abstr.* **42**(7): 588.

- Suthar, J.H. 1993. Influence of organic manure and Azatobactor in conjuction with weed management to rabi maize on Ganga Safed-2. M.Sc. (Agri) Thesis submitted to G.A.U., Anand. Unpublished.

- Thakkar, P.N. Chhiba, I.M. and Mehta, S.K. 1989. Twenty years of co-ordinated research on micronutrients in soils and plants. 1967-87. *Bulletin-1, IISS Bhopal.* pp.12-13.

- Tinsley, J. and and Nowakowski, T.Z. 1959. The composition and manurial value of poultry excreta, straw dropping compost and deep litter II Experimental Studies on Compost. *J. Sci. of Food and Agric* **10:** 150-167.

- Tisdale, S.L.; Nelson, W.L.; Beaton, J.D, and Havlin, J.L.1993. *Soil fertility and fertilizers.* MacMillan Publishing Company, New York.

- US Environmental Protection Agency (USEPA). 1985. National primary drinking water regulations: synthetics organic chemicals, inorganic chemicals and miero-organisms: Proposed rule. *Fed. Regist.* **50:** *46935-47022.*

- Warren, S.L. and Fonteno, W.C. 1993. Changes in Physical and chemical properties of a loamy sand soil when amended with composted poultry litter. *J. Environmental Horticulture.* **11**(4): 186-190.

- Weil, R.R.; Weismiller, R.A. and Turner, R.S. 1990. Nitrate contamination of ground water under irrigated coastal plain soils. *J. Environ. Qual.* **19:** 441-448.

- Well, R.R.; Kroontje, W.and Jones, G.D. 1979. In organic nitrogen and soluble salts in Davidson Clay loam used for poultry manure disposal. *J. Environmental Quality.* **8**(1):86-91.

- Will, R.R and W. Krootje 1979. Organic matter decomposition in a soil amended with poultry manure. *J. of Environmental Quality.* **8**(4): 584-588.

- Yadav, K. and Jha, K.K. 1987. Sugars in the Humus of soils as affected by manures and moisture. *J. Indian Soc. Soil Sci.* **35**(2): 304-306.

- Yadav, K. and Jha, K.K. 1988. Effect of poultry manure and sewage sludge on the humification and functional groups of humic substances. *Ind. Soc. Soil. Sci.* **36** (3): 439-444.

- Yadav, K. and Jha, K.K. 1989. Microbial decomposition of poultry manure and sewage sludge in soil. *Indian Society of Soil Sci.* **37**(4): 301-305.

- Yadav, K.; Jha, K.K.; Prasad, C.R. and Sinha, M.K. 1989. Kinetics of carbon mineralization from poultry manure and sewage sludge in two soils at field capacity and submergence moisture. *Ind. Soc.Soil.Sci.* **37** (4): 240-243.

- Yerriswamy, R.M. and Vasuki, N. 1995. Effect of FYM and poultry manure on availability of applied ferrous sulphate in vertisols (Calcareous). *J. of Mah. Agric. Univ.* **20** (1): 117.

# 16

# Plant Fossils as Marker of Palaeoenvironment

*J. Pandey*

The scientific efforts during last few decades have helped understand the environmental changes through geological past. Among the various approaches used to reconstruct palaeoenvironment, palaeobotanical approach provides the most direct and comprehensive method. Initial studies utilized the data, which were not originally collected for palaeoclimatic purposes, to derive local and to some extent the subregional past climatic scenario. The subject gained momentum after the publication of Sewards essay in 1892 on the fossil plants as test of palaeoclimate. During the International Geological Congress in Moscow in 1937, significance of fossil flora in the interpretation of Lower Gondwana climate was highlighted. The interpretation of palaeoenvironment experienced unprecedented development in the light of palynological evidences. The spore-pollen, being more ubiquitous and abundant than megafossils and can be sampled quantitatively at close stratigraphic intervals, provide high resolution criteria for precise comparisons. Such observations have added numerous lines of evidences in the field of palaeoecology.

Climate, although is the primary force governing world pattern of vegetation, non-climatic shifts also change the expected patterns (Graham et al., 1995). Factors such as earth features (topography, landslides and volcanic erruptions), biologically driven mechanisms (competitive elimination of species, mode of dispersal and pollination and the factors of community succession), and the atmospheric forces, particularly the biological feedbacks of radiatively active trace gases, have had a decisive influence on the distribution of palaeofloras. On a small scale it is often difficult to separate sedimentary control from climatic controls on the distribution of microfossils. One natural factor of distribution of organisms is so fundamental that it subdues several other factors to a greater extent. This is linked with the evolutionary factor which arises from the circumstances that plant world of today has gradually developed from pre-existing gene-pool.

## PALAEOCLIMATIC CONSIDERATION OF PLANT FOSSILS

### The Approach

Two basically different approaches are used for palaeoclimatic derivations from plant fossils. The first approach relied on recognising the plant fossils in terms of similar living species and so interpreting the palaeoclimate on the basis of the climatic tolerance of the latter. This method which is often called floristic analogy or the nearest living relative approach, assume no evolutionary change and interprets ancient environment on the assumption that fossil form had the same environmental tolerance as their nearest living relatives (Spicer, 1993). This assumption based on taxonomy is buttressed by certain features of plant morphology that are associated with modern analogues and are likewise characteristic of taxonomically similar fossil flora. The validity of this approach, however, decreases with increasing geological age of fossils. The second approach use the features of fossil, independent of its biological identity to deduce something about the environment in which it had grown. The first approach (NLR) is mainly adopted for Quaternary and Tertiary floras, while the second that mainly depends on phenotypic plasticity has been widely used for older fossils.

A third and lately adopted approach is the quantitative analysis of palaeobotanical data with a view to reconstruct palaeocommunities. Inferences are made from reconstructed communities with a broad expectation of ecological preference of closely related taxa. This approach has been proved to be more successful with palynofossils where quantitative registration is easily accessible. This approach has great potential for palaeoenvironmental reconstruction particularly if coordinated with sedimentary indicators.

## Plant Megafossils

Ever since the pioneering days in the study of palaeoecology, megafossils have been considered as a basic tool. In addition to the more widely used techniques, such as the NLR and the features of a fossil independent of its biological identity, attempts have also been made towards quantitative assessment of megafossil assemblage. Different methods have been used to determine the number of palaeotaxa per sample, and relative dominance of each taxon in a given assemblage. Such analysis helps estimate a coefficient of correlation for each taxon. However, as megafossils are found in pieces, a sound precision is required in data collection and taxonomic placement of species.

Quaternary climate is relatively well explored by integrating palaeobotanical data with climate model experiments. Of pre-Quaternary, Jurassic-Cretaceous flora have received considerable attention. On the basis of megafossil evidences the Northern Hemisphere of Jurassic and Cretaceous has been divided into two main floral regimes namely Siberian-Canadian and Indo-European palaeofloristic realms. Flora of Jurassic and that of early part of Early Cretaceous are believed to be more globally uniform than at almost any other time in the history of land plants. This was believed to be a response to a climate that was remarkable for its equability.

As an independent fossil material, plant foliage have a great significance. Leaf features have high degree of correlation as per the climate relationship is concerned. The important features of the leaf impressions are leaf margin and major venation pattern, leaf texture and venation density, driptip, leaf base shape and leaf size and shape. Leaves of temperate trees are lobed or toothed margined in comparison to smooth margined leaves of tropical species. According to Wolfe (1979) there exists a strong positive correlation between the mean annual temperature under which a flora grows and the percentage of dicots with entire margined leaves. The Talchir flora predominantly contains leaves of *Gangamopteris* having no mid-rib, a character interpreted to indicate cold temperate climate.

For fossil wood, two types of response are important: (1) Presence or absence of a particular feature(s) in response to a limiting factor. For instance, absence of taxa with storied rays from the high latitudes, probably due to a limiting factor relating to temperature. (2) Variation of wood anatomical characters with climate variables. These include nature of support tissues, growth rings, characters pertaining to vessel arrangement, vessel diameter and density and nature of wood parenchyma. Nature of support tissue of trees give information about the environmental preference of the species. This is particularly true for fossil angiosperms and conifers. Growth rings have been widely used to infer climatic patterns of geological past. The thickness and regularity of growth rings, in addition to the proportion of secondary wood, indicate length of growing season and the competitive success of individual in a population.

It is obvious that, plant features including height, nature of support tissue, tree-ring chronology, and leaf features, have definite environmental correlations. However, the degree of correlation is some time peculiar to a species. For example, *Glossopteris* flora is known to have flourished in the temperate climate but according to the modern climatic indicators, the simple smooth margined large leaves of *Glossopteris* indicate plant characteristics of tropical climate. Similarly, *Lepidodendron*, a Carboniferous arborescent lycopod, had xeromorphic strap-like leaves with sunken stomata and small surface area. The leaves clearly were of a type normally found in dry environment where it is important for plants to limit their water-loss, and yet this plant grew in swamp forests (Spicer, 1993). This extinct Pennsylvanian lycopod (*Lepidodendron*) was about 30 meter in height with a trunk diameter of about 1 meter supported by wood-like parenchymatous bark around the periphery of the stem. The species that typically attain very large size have strong mechanical support and are generally late maturing (K-strategy) with efficient energy capture strategy. Such species could grow only in a habitat characterized by sufficient soil moisture regime and under high atmospheric $CO_2$ and $O_2$ concentrations. In fact, xeromorphy in this plant was a function of inefficient vascular system. Near the base of the trunk which might be nearly a meter across, the water-conducting tissue was restricted to a cylinder, only a few centimeter in diameter.

Interpretations some time also vary with individual bias. Based on short-shoots assigned to genus *Behuninia* from the upper Jurassic of Morrison Formation, U.S.A, three different climatic inferences have been derived by three different groups of workers: (1) According to Jensen (1966) the region where these short-shoots occur at the Fremont junction locality, was probably a flood plain with warm and humid climate. (2) Peterson and Turner-Peterson (1987) proposed the climate as being close to arid with extended times of dryness interrupted by only short periods of moisture, while (3) Tidwell and Medlyn (1992) inferred a moist climate with no seasonality. There are some other examples indicating inconsistent interpretations.

## Plant Microfossils

The widespread occurrence of plant microfossils rendered them to be the potential tool for studying plant evolution and palaeoecology (Tiwari and Tripathi, 1988). The use of spore-pollen data has made possible refinements by introducing quantitive registration with high temporal and spatial resolution. Such analysis has helped reconstructing the vegetational history with obvious reflection on the past environment. They have, of course, many limitations, the most obvious being their uncertain taxonomic affinities.

An examination of the Jurassic palynostratigraphy of Perth Basin, Western Australia, revealed that during much of the Early Jurassic the climate in the Perth Basin was warm to hot and arid, during the Middle and Late Jurassic it was wet tropical to subtropical. The conclusions, although agree with other palaeontological, sedimentological and oxygen isotope studies, are not easily reconciled with high Jurassic Palaeolatitudes proposed for Australia. High percentage occurrence of *Classopollis*, a Triassic-Early Cretaceous pollen, in sediments produced under arid regime (*e.g.* evaporite sequence) suggests that *Classopollis* parent plants had xeromorphic features. This is supported by the morphological features (*e.g.* dense cuticle, sunken stomata, etc.) of associated plant megafossils.

Palynological data have merit in two folds. One lies in the pollen-spore diversity registered at close stratigraphic intervals (quantitative approach), while the other, on the morphographic features of pollen-spores (qualitative approach). Quantitative analysis of palynomorphs with their obvious relationships with parental stock help assessing the degree of environmental favourableness. Several attempts have been made to correlate pollen morphographic characteristics with palaeoenvironmental variables. However, such features appear reliable only after answering such questions as whether the character considered is an element of an evolutionary lineage or a proxy climate signal? If morphographic characters of spores and pollen are sensitive to all sorts of climatic variations, spore pollen from same parental stock if disseminated to different "habitat types" give appearance of misleading affinities. Quantitative analysis of pollen-spore data give information on the totality of plant species and their relative dominance at site. Such reconstruction helps tracing the changes in floristic composition with time and to relate such changes back to the agent behind them *i.e.* climate, geologic and other influences.

An important constraint is the apparent bias that may result from differential pollen production and dispersal capacities of parent plants. Khomutova (1995) for instance, have observed that 95 per cent pollen assemblages in a lake bottom sediments were due to the effect of wind. The pollen of plants growing in the lake scarcely contributed any part in total pollen assemblages, despite their being strongly over grown. This is because of exceedingly low pollen production capacity of lake plants in comparison to that of terrestrial plants and distruction of the water plant pollen as they have thin exines. Wind dispersed pollen are generally found to be over represented in relation to the insect dispersed one and may lead to differential preservation and likely over representation in some cases or under-representation in other. The third aspect that sometime becomes the source of error, is the apparent form-similarity between palynomorphs produced by unrelated plant groups. Such form - similarity often makes taxonomic placement of pollen-spores arbitrary. A correlation between spore-pollen and megafossil patterns can help understanding over or under representation.

## SOURCE OF ERROR: NEED FOR CAUTION

1.  The reliability of reconstruction depends on sample size. As the concept of diversity includes both, species richness and the evenness, for a precise estimate of diversity, multiple, closely spaced samples are required. Batten (1992) has suggested that, for better palaeoenvironmental analysis ideally entire faunal and floral assemblages (not just selected parts), and even, minute organic remains associated with these, should be examined.

2.  A statistical treatment of the data gives more objective comparison. Similar to those of the neoecologists studying with extant vegetation, palaeoecologists have also turned to use various ordination techniques. Such techniques help relate the gradients in species composition to the gradients in environmental conditions. Univariate approach have merit over the multivariate analysis, as the former retains the primacy of ecologically significant trait(s).

3.  Fossil records are strongly modified by postmortem and post-depositional processes. Preservational factors may lead to an erratic picture of species diversity, omitting ecologically preferred elements of a community. Taphonomic studies suggest that considerable efforts must be devoted to understand the sedimentological settings at both local and regional scales if an accurate reconstruction of the physical habitat is to be made.

4.  Much of the palaeoclimatic reasoning are based on the principle of uniformitarianism which relates environmental requirements of fossil flora to those of their taxonomically similar living relatives. The validity of this assumption decreases with increasingly older fossils due to unavailability of modern analogues and to the evolutionary changes in the ecology of organisms that have taken place through time.

5.  There is no doubt that the evolution of certain structures may have been turned in respsonse to a particular climatic pressure, but it does not mean that plants possessing these structures must always be found in the same climate. Further, some plant species have the potential to adapt to similar environmental conditions through different morphological changes.

6.  All the preservable features of a plant or a part of it need not necessarily have a climatic significance. Some features of plants are tightly controlled by genotype, while others are less so, and in that sense, are designated as showing phenotypic plasticity. Further, plants have been capable of changing their physiological resistance to drought, cold and other environmental characteristics without necessarily changing their more obvious structural features.

7.  Non-climatic shifts in vegetation constitute a definite source of error in palaeoclimatic reconstructions. The distribution of plant communities, even under undisturbed conditions, is determined by a number of interrelated factors where, in addition to climate, characteristics of substrate material, availability of primary colonizers and competition between species, have important roles. Contribution of non-climatic factors, particularly biological, in species distribution and community changes, is treated in greater detail below.

# NON-CLIMATIC VARIABLES: THE GAIA HYPOTHESIS

The discussion so for, suggests that it is unrealistic to believe that all sorts of species distribution or community changes are brought merely by climatic factors. This is particularly true at local and subregional scale. It is believed by the contenders of the Gaia that the organisms are indeed influenced by and adapted to their non-living environment but they also modify that environment to make it more hospitable to themselves, and on global scale. Life and its environments are so closely coupled that evolution concerns both, not the organisms or environment separately (Lovelock, 1988). Some of the generalities that have been established in the history of the earth include the following.

## Evolution of Oxygenic Atmosphere

The most important role that the primitive living world had played in the record of the earth's history is the evolution of oxygenic atmosphere and different hierarchies of lives. The primitive atmosphere was almost devoid of free oxygen and so the planet earth was exposed to biocidal ultraviolet radiation. It was the primitive live that had been surviving in much deeper parts of the ocean led to the evolution of oxygen through photosynthetic process. This physiologically driven photolysis of $H_2O$ consequently increased the global atmospheric oxygen level. Increased level of oxygen and subsequent formation of ozone led UV intensity to diminish to the extent that terrestrial life could evolve and survive. Thus, a physiological process of primitive life itself opened the way for more complex forms to emerge and survive.

## Palaeozoic Hyperoxia

Global atmospheric hyperoxia not only led to the evolution of oxygenic respiratory system but also helped morphologically complex forms to evolve and survive. These organisms helped maintain atmospheric concentrations of green house gases and so the global temperature. The involvement of green house effect in regulating past global climate has been emphasized since the pioneering works of Chamberlin (Chamberlin, 1897). Such informations provide substantial evidence to palaeoclimatic interpretations since some of the morphological features have rationale relationship with the atmospheric concentrations of biologically active gases, particularly $CO_2$ and $O_2$. Recent studies (Graham et al., 1995) suggest a marked increase (Late Devonian-Early Carboniferous) and then decline (Late Permian) of atmospheric oxygen and associated shifts in the concentration of carbon dioxide. Increased oxygenation of Devonian and Carboniferous atmosphere influenced the contemporaneous biosphere. High Oxygen level in aquatic systems would have permitted greater exploitation of aquatic habitats and aided the vertebrate invasion of land. The Carboniferous and Early Permian flora included tree ferns, sphenopsids and giant arborescent lycopods. Lignin, that resist microbial decay in many depositional environment and formed dominant structural material of many Carboniferous plants is synthesized by oxygen-dependent biological mechanisms. Thus, the giantic size (a measure of carbon reserve) of these plants with high amount of lignin in their support structures, may be considered as a signature of high atmospheric $O_2$ and $CO_2$ concentrations.

The removal of atmospheric $CO_2$ by plants followed by massive burial of sedimentary organic matter (legnin resist microbial decay) during the Carboniferous and Permian periods could have accelerated mid-Palaeozoic drop in $CO_2$ concentration and so the Permo-Carboniferous glaciation. Thus, the changes in atmopheric composition of biologically active gases, $CO_2$ and $O_2$ had have profound effects not only on the diversification and ecological radiation of Late Palaeozoic groups but also on global climate change.

## Plant Succession

Endogenous effect (autogenic) of plant succession is a major ecological factor shaping or channeling plant communities. Autogenesis have particular significance in secondary succession. Both, intensity and frequency of successional factors (the patterns of reproductive timing and likely colonization of available space, nature of substrate material, nutrient regime, competitive success and level of herbivory) have major impact on species composition and diversity of natural groups. Different seral stages of a developing community differ with each other in both, the species composition and structural homogeneity. In a given climatic zone many early successional plants bear pinnately compound foliage permitting successional plants to reduce their investment in wood that does not participate in active photosynthesis. Similarly, in an *in situ* preserved material the size of the stem gives information about the preferred substrate and successional status of the species. For instance, relatively uniformly sized, conspecific trunks in an area indicate an even aged stand, a characteristic of species that require large gaps in order to colonize successfully. Likewise, spacing of conspecific trunks is an indicator of competition for resource.

Crocker and Major (1955) have described the stages in primary succession at Glacier Bay, Alaska. The local till was alkaline (pH 8.0 to 8.4) and had invaded by the pioneer community of arctic herbs and dwarf willows followed by alder bushes at the mark of 50 years. The alders were slowly invaded by sitka spruce *(Picea sitchensis)*. At the mark of 150 years, two species of hemlock *(Tsuga martensiana* and *Tsuga heterophylla)* invaded and finally a spruce-hemlock climax vegetation appeared. The point of interest is that it was the acid residues of alder leaves responsible for desolving carbonates consequently lowering the pH *vis-a-vis* further community development.

In a time series analysis across Lake Michigan sand dunes, Olson (1958) observed, when very fresh the dunes hold only the specialized grasses, but shortly thereafter, perhaps less than a century, a stand of poplars *(Populus deltoides)* was in place. But dunes of all ages from 300 to 12,000 years support woodlands of black oak *(Quercus velutina)*. Black oaks, once established remain definitely as almost single species stand because old sand dunes are too acidic for all but the acid tolerant oaks. The young dunes where grasses, poplars, pines grow are alkaline with pH above 8. Occasional small stands of poplar or pine on older dunes are due to recent disturbances.

## The Competition Hypothesis

Competition is a potent ecological force that greatly influences populations in natural communities. Competition among the species has not only been the cause of character innovation, origin of new species and evolutionary divergence but also has an important bearing with species extinction. In response to intense competitive pressure the plant species tend to adapt (which would be eliminated otherwise) by altering or adding some new characters which are advantageous to them. Accumulation of new characters gradually leads to evolution of species. Vegetation changes are usually caused by a change in competitive relationship in connection with other ecological factors. Ecological advantage may arise from competitive ability of species that allow them to associate with or to replace their progenitors, or from capacity of the latter to occupy new climatic conditions where they are not confronted with competition from their close relatives. The first plant assemblage establishing itself in a seral stage or in a near climax vegetation, may prevent a species from establishing itself inside an area which is otherwise climatically suitable. McArthur (1972) in his book *Geographical Ecology* has commented that:

'the assumption that most plants occur just where their climatic needs are met. Of course, if this were strictly true flower gardens and arboretums would be impossible, every plant that could grow in a particular place would already be present. There are many European tree species growing and reproducing in the cities, where they are weeded by having the lawns cleaned of "competitors", how many of these have we seen growing in the natural forests? If the answer is only few; it is for non-climatic reasons'.

It is obvious that in the absence of potent competitors some plant species could flourish in a climatic regime where generally they are not found.

Competition also explains the order of species replacement in developing communities. If maple tree, for example, were to prove final visitors, why should they wait for the aspen and pines to do their jobs first? Ecologists for long were not able to answer this question without referring to the habitat. Their answer used to be that the maple had to wait for other plants to improve the habitat for them. But the phenomena of competition explains the apparent wait of maples in a constant habitat. Through his model of adaptive geometry of trees, Horn (1971) suggested that in an ecological succession the first trees that replace the shrubs and herbs of an old field are of multilayer design (the canopies of aspen and pine in above example are of 4 layers). These trees can not grow in the dense shade of their parents because their leaf geometry does not then yield a sufficient excess of net photosynthesis over respiration. Shade adapted trees with fewer effective layers of leaves, therefore, invade. Henceforth, trees of a successional sequence are equipped with an everdiminishing number of effective layers until the climax trees are close to being monolayer.

Thus, the competition hypothesis also force to avoid the tacit assusmption that all sorts of species replacements or community changes are due to climatic forcing. Contribution of such non-climatic driving forces specially when community changes appeared at short temporal scale can not be ruled out. It has particular significance for Quaternary palaeoclimatology where to explore the contribution of such factors is easily accessible.

## SUMMARY

The use of plant fossils as marker of palaeoenvironment has become the subject of global concern. Plants that have lived all sorts of diversified environmental conditions have particular significance for interpreting climatic variations. Plant features, such as height, wood anatomy, nature of support tissues, leaf shape, size and surface features (epidermal outgrowth, cuticle, stomatal size and density) and qualitative and quantitative characteristics of spore-pollen, have definite climatic relations. The palaeobotanical data, however, as the evidence of world climatic patterns, are yet illexplored and incomplete, both spatially and temporally. Even many of the interpretative criteria are not yet vigorously established. The major challenge for palaeoecologists is to weave these evidences based on a part of the totality with high degree of refinements through integrating the micro-and megafossil evidences into a regional, continental and then to the global picture. The subject should be reviewed with careful consideration of field-based sampling strategies and detailed information on depositional and stratigraphic settings.

Sampling with high stratigraphic precision will explore the dynamic aspects of fossil vegetation on short term temporal scale with obvious focus on the contribution of non-climatic factors. Detailed statistical analysis helps to locate the source of error and provide more objective comparisons. Emphasis should be given to select the parameters most promising for interpreting climates with particular reference to those directly linked with energy capture, gas exchange and dispersal. Such features, as provide direct link between form and function, indicate the physical and chemical aspects of the environment in which the plant grew, and provide information about the ecological preference of closely related taxa. Such parameters, if related well with the amount of biologically active gases, help understanding the contemporaneous atmosphere with a broad expectation of the climatic scenario.

## GLOSSARY

K-strategy: life-style in which fecundity is reduced to divert resources to persistence.
Palaeoecology: use of fossils to test ecological hypotheses.
Realm: (biogeographic) latitudinal expanse in which organisms have comparable adaptations.
Till: unsorted mineral deposit left by a retreating glacier.

## REFERENCES

- Batten, D.J. (1992). Stratigraphic and palaeoenvironmental analysis continue to demand the inclusion of high quality palaeontological data. *Cretaceous Research,* 13: 591-595.
- Chamberlin, T.C. (1897). A group of hypotheses bearing on climatic changes. *J. Geol.,* 5: 653-683.
- Crocker, R.L. and Major, J. (1955). Soil development in relation to vegetation and surface age at Glacier Bay, Alaska, *Ecology* 43: 427-428.
- Graham, J.B., Dudly, D., Aguilar, N.M. and Carl Gans. (1995). Implications of the Late Palaeozoic oxygen pulse for physiology and evolution. *Nature,* 375: 117-120.
- Horn, H.S., (1971) The adaptive geometry of trees. *Monogr. Pop. Biol;* 3 : 3–144.
- Jensen, J.A. (1966). Foreward. In: Fruiting organs from the Morrison Formation of Utah, USA (Ed. Chandler, M.E.J.) *Bull. Br. Mus. Nat. Hist.,* 12: 137-171.
- Khomutova, V.I. (1995). Signifieance of zonal, regional and loeal vegetational elements in lacustrine pollen spectra. *Grana,* 34: 246-250
- Lovelock, J. (1988). The Ages of Gaia : A Biography of Our Living Earth. Oxford University Press, U.K.
- MacArthur, R.H., (1972). Geographical Ecology: Pattern in the Distribution of species. Harper and Row Publishers, New York.
- Olson, J.S., (1958). Rates of succession and soil changes on southern Lake Michigan and dunes. *Bot. Gaz.,* 199: 125-170.
- Peterson, F. and Turner-Peterson, C.E. (1987). The Morrison Formation of the Colorado Plateau: Recent advances in sedimentology, stratigraphy, and paleotectonics. *Hunteria,* 2: 1-18.
- Seward, A.C. (1892). Fossil plants as test of climate. London: 1-151.
- Spicer, R.A. (1993). Palaeoecology, past climatic systems and $C_3/C_4$ photosynthesis. *Chemosphere,* 27: 947-978.
- Tidwell, W.D. and Medlyn, D.A. (1992). Short shoots from the upper Jurassic Morrison Formation, Utah, Wyoming, and Colorado, USA. Rev. *Palaeobot. Palynol.,* 71: 219-238.
- Tiwari, R.S. and Tripathi, A. (1988). Palynologial zones and their climatic inference in the coal-bearing Gondwana of Peninsular India. *Palaeobotanist,* 36: 87-101.
- Wolfe, J.A. (1979). Temperature paramters of humid to mesic forests of eastern Asia and relation to forests of other regions of the northern Hemisphere and Australasia, *U.S. Geol. Surv. Prof. Pap.,* 1106: 1-37.

# 17

# Key Elements of Environment-oriented Cost Management (EoCM)

*F. Kolling*

## What is the Principle of EoCM?

EoCM is a Cost Mangement Instrument which focuses on the efficient use of those resource flows that are relevant for the environment, such as material, energy and water. It brings down costs and leads to an improvement of the environmental performance by reducing "non-product output" (NPO), *i.e.* those materials, energy and water which are used in the production process but do not end up in the final product. EoCM does not only identify the costs of treatment and disposal of the NPOs, but also the hidden costs caused by the generation and processing of these NPOs.

To relaise this and guarantee the implementation of the developed measures, EoCM builds on resources which are locally available. The motor of the EoCM process is the innovation team of the company, which is supproted by local consultants. The basic assumption of EoCM is that the knowledge regarding weaknesses of the production process as well as capacity to mitigate them exists to a large extent within the company. Therefore, it is not necessary to bring in extensive technical expertise from abroad, which is expensive and often does not create enough ownership for the "internal take off" of the change process, especially for proper implementation of proposed measures.

EoCM includes tools and training modules which aim at the mobilisation of the knowledge and problem-solving capacities available from within the company. In addition to the technical knowledge of the methodology, it applies techniques of good presentaion, moderation and team-building. It is an instrument for cost management, environmental management and organisational change. Only if these areas are adequately taken into consideration, *a triple win* (economic, environmental, organisational) can be achieved and a successful process of continuous improvement in the company be established.

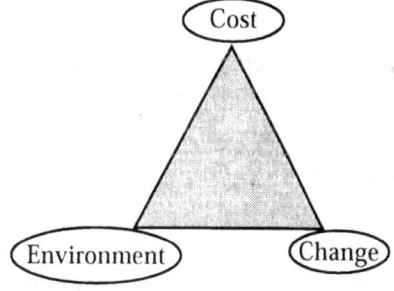

> The three basic principles of EoCM
> **Cost saving**
> **improved environmental performance** and
> **effective organisational change**,
> build a **triangle** which creates synergetic effects, allows tapping the triple win options and leads to a process of continuous improvement in the company

## Why EoCM?

The Pilot Programme for the Promotion of Environmental Management in the Private Sector of Developing Countries (P3U) of the German Technical Co-operation Agency (GTZ) is elaborating an integrated concept for the promotion of environmental management for small - and medium-sized enterprises (SME) in developing countries. As experiences in similar programmes have shown that it is a difficult task to target SMEs in the field of environmental management because the main incentives which exist in industrialised countries are hardly found in the developing countries regarding "green" issues:

- "green" markets or "green" consumer behaviour
- awareness or knowledge about environmental issues by enterpreneurs
- pressure groups of civil society which force the private sector to adopt a proactive behavior
- strict enforcement of environmental legislation.

In response to these problems and based on the fact that measures in the field of environmental management often bring about a considerable potential for cost reductions, the *P3U-concept* aims at assisting enterprises in developing countries in indentifying such win-win options, dispelling fears that environmental measures might involve additional costs. Wihtout a clear economic benefit, only few companies will introduce measures which aim at reducing the negative environmental impact of their activities.

In the framework of this approach, *four different instruments* have been developed that have in *common* that they are :

- simplified
- low-cost or no-cost,
- applicable by a broad range of enterprises, and
- adjusted to the specific requirements of SME in developing countries.

But even under these conditions only few strategies are adopted by a significant number of companies. Institutional resistance to change and risk are the main factors which have not been taken into consideration by most of the approaches, A successful approach has to include strategies on how to overcome this resistance and to obtain more ownership within the companies and respective support from private sector promotion instituions. EoCM helps to identify a third "win"option by leading companies step by step into a process of organisational change and continuous improvement, through regular monitoring of the efficiency and environmental soundness of production process, by means of suitable management instrument and adequate investment in environmentally sound technologies.

By aiming at the triple win, EoCM is a private sector approach which does not depend mainly on the political framework of the respective country, but mobilises the self-interest of the companies in efficient and environmentally sound production.

Improved resource efficiency and pollution prevention are also key success factors for public health, the long-term conservation of national resources as well as economic development and enchanced competitiveness in developing countries.

## Who Developed EoCM?

EoCM is based on the Environmental Cost Management (ECM) methodology developed by Fisher and others in Germany (Fischer, H., 1997). First applied in the textile company kunert, the approach was used in various German companies with significant cost savings and positive environmental results. In 1997, it was applied by P3U for the first time in a developing country. *i.e.* in the food manufacturing company cairns foods in Zimbabwe. This application showed that the approach, in general, can be also successful under the conditions of a developing country, and the results can even be more significant there due to lower overall efficiency and relatively high material costs of production in relation to labour costs.

Nevertheless, quite a few weaknesses in the methodology were detected and a general need to change the approach from an expert-driven approach (as practised in Germany) to a company-based process of step-by step and, hopefully, continuous improvement was identified.

## Pilot Project in CAIRNS-FOODS (November 1997)

Objective: Testing of applicability of ECM in a developing country

Activity:   9 days in-house consultancy by a German ECM expert together with P3U on-the-job training of 2 local expets

Results:

- 33 per cent of total costs were NOP costs
- measures for the reduction of 15 per cent of the NPO -costs were identified (pay back period: 8 - 14 months)
- identification of the need to improve the methodology (especially to give companies more ownership integrate elements of organisational development and include training of communicative skills)
- by the end of 1998, one·third of the identified·measures had been implemented. The annual costs savings amount to 1.5 per cent of total costs (38, 000 US$/a). Due to the difficult economic framework, the more investment-intensive measures are still under consideration.

Based on the experience at cairns, a second, largely modified ECM programme was planned together with the Confederation of Zimbabwean Industries (CZI) and the GTZ-Advisory Service for Private Business (ASPB). This programme includes changes in the methodology and focuses more on the organisational development and communicative skills of the innovation teams. The ECM process is now mainly carried out by the company teams themselves; they are supported by local consultants, who are trained on-the -job to be the future ECM disseminators. The P3U team limited its role to the training and coaching of the teams and consultants. In order to guarantee a high quality of ECM in the future, standards for the training and assessment of consultants and the evaluation are developed together with CZI, ASPB abd the group of local consultants.

## ECM Programme with CZI and 5 Companies (Dec. 1998 - May 1999)

Objective: Generation of success stories' Completion of Handbook based on experience with the modified and improved methodology

Activities: 6-months programme with 5 innovation teams, 8 local consultants and intermittent visits by German experts (ECM and OD) together with P3U

- 5 companies (brewery, battery producer, cardboard factory, plant oil production, tannery), three of them are medium- sized with 100-250 employees and total production costs between 1,5 - 2 Mio. US$/a, two are large companies
- innovation teams of companies are responsible for ECM application (3 members of the middle management)
- top management commitment and financial contribution
- local consultants are trained on-the job"

Results:

- high motivation of all teams and consultants
- high commitment of top-management
- considerable NPO costs identified (10-20 % of total costs)
- high potential for savings identified (first measures in implementation will save 150,00 US$ a)
- change process in companies through training of innovation teams
- institutional scheme for quality control and ECM promotion with CZI and group of consultants

Due to the substantial modification and further development of the methodology and in order to avoid some confusion caused by the former title, the approach was renamed " *Environment-oriented Cost Management*" (*EoCM*).

## Which Actors are Involved in the Application of EoCM

*EoCM* is not only an accounting method. For a company, it is also a strategic instrument to increase productivity and reduce costs, leading to a change process of continuous improvement. For a country or region, it is an instrument to increase productivity and competitiveness of the private sector. Many different actors participate in the EoCM application:

- The *innovation* teams in the company, which are composed by experts from different professional disciplines and working areas (production, accounting, Qality and environmental management, eventually maintenance)
- The *local consultants* which are trained on-the job and form part of the innovation teams
- The network of innovation teams of the participating companies as well as relevant local institutions interested in the dissemination of EoCM
- The local *counterpart insitution* who should be related to the private sector, have an interest in promoting EoCM in a sustainable manner and guarantee the quality of EoCM application
- The local *consultancy companies* who offer EoCM as a service to companies and therefore have an interest in promoting EoCM together with the counterpart insitution and protecting their knowledge against unqualified competition
- The *external team of facilitators* which initalises the EoCM dissemination by building up knowledge and strengthening supportive structures in the country. It should combine economic and environmental know-how with the capacity of moderating innovation-processes. Its input is becoming less important during the process of EoCM application and diffusion.

## Which Benefits can be Expected from EoCM

EoCM - like various Environmental Management (EM) tools - aims at win-win situations, *i.e.* an economic benefit and an improvement of the company's environmental performance.

The difference in comparison to other EM tools: EoCM initialises a *dynamic process of continuous improvement* within the company, because it systematically adding elements of organisational development to technical and economic changes. Thus EoCM adds a third dimension, *organisational change* or development, to a *triple win* approach.

EoCM provides *short term benefits* for the company (cost saving because of quickly implemented technical and organisational measures, positive environmental effects) and a *long-term improvement of productivity and environmental performance* through an enhanced motivation of employees and an increased efficiency of the organisational structure.

EoCM requires the support of external experts, but once initialised it becomes part of the company's culture and an *integrated management tool.*

EoCM can strengthen existing or facilitate the establishment of standardised *environmental management systems*. It generates basic information, helps to build awareness and create structures which can be used as first steps in an ISO 9000, ISO 14001 or EMAS process

EoCM focuses on material, energy and water flows *not on rationalisation*. Unlike most of the other cost management tools, it does not primarily aim at the reduction of labour (costs). Therefore it avoids two kinds of social conflict: with the employees (employment) and with public opinion (environmental impact).

EoCM has a lot in common with *quality management*. The application and monitoring of process and product standards is, at least in the long run, one important condition for the optimisation of the material, energy and water streams and the achievement of sustained competitiveness.

## What Limitations has EoCM?

EoCM is not an instrument to primarily assess environmental impact. It is an instrument to reduce those costs which are arising for the company from inefficient use of environmentally relevant inputs, such as materials, energy and water. External or "social" costs, such as mitigating negative environmental impacts caused by production or the product itself, are not considered as long as they are not paid for by the company.

EoCM is limited to the site where production takes place. It does not take into account the whole production chain "from the cardle to the grave". Inefficiency and environmental impacts in raw material production and product distribution or use are not a subject of this method (as long as it is not part of the company's business). The product design is considered only as far as its influence on the efficiency of production is concerned. However the boundaries of the company at the input and output side may be taken into consideration (providers of raw materials, product packaging) and inputs and NPO can be assessed qualitatively with regard to their environmental impact. In addition, measures which increase the negative environmental impact of the company are against the rationale of EoCM and should not be adopted.

EoCM does not take into account the following environmental costs:

- environmental destruction by the production of purchased raw material
- efficient or decreased use of scarce, non-renewable resources
- the environmental impact of tranposting and processing of raw meterial (as long as it is not part of the company's business)
- the impact of the product itself (*e.g.* on consumer health)
- the treatment of the used product after consumption and disposal.

EoCM analyses the costs caused by Non- Product-Output in one company or production site, including if integrated in a group approach of different companies. It is applicable in service companies as well, but has main advantages in industrial production. It is applicable in medium and large companies, but would not be recommendable for small enterprises without a determined organisational structure, a separate accounting department and a layer of middle management. For the latter target group, P3U has developed other tools, such as the Resource Management Module (RMM) and the Good Housekeeping Guide (GHK).

## What is Non-Product Output (NPO)?

A large part of the materials used ends up in the desired final product. The other part turns into solid waste, waste water and air emissions. Almost all energy used ends up as waste heat These outputs are summarised as "non-product output" (NPO).

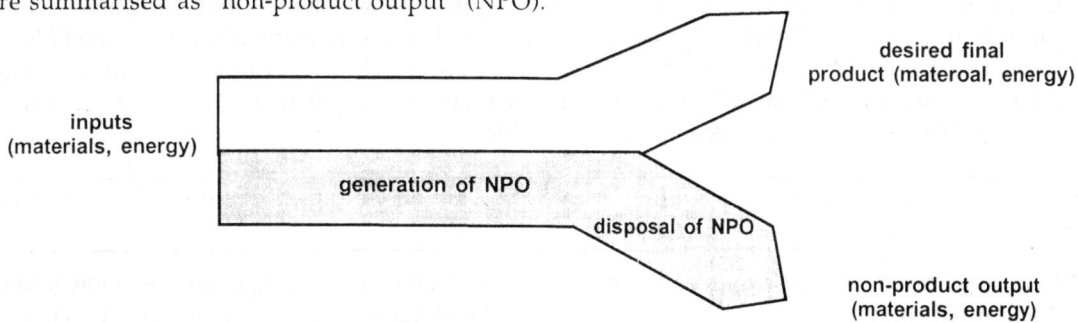

NPO = Material, Energy and Water which is used in the production but does not end up in the final product.

This is valid also for all by-products, especially if their selling price does not cover their production costs. are:

- solid waste, waste water and energy losses in the production process. These output contain all auxiliary materials and part of the raw materials that are inputs to production
- disposal of raw materials or finished goods, that are no longer of use or cannot be sold anymore
- semi-finished or finished goods of insufficient quality which have to be reprocessed
- rejects due to insufficient qulity which have to be eliminated or sold at a low price
- heat losses in steam or electricity generation
- solid waste and waste water from office buildings
- solid waste from packaging of the materials used in production
- losses of finished goods and energy during distribution
- by-products sold at a price which does not cover their production costs
- over-fillings/over-application of inputs, including packaging, which are not paid by the customer and sometimes even reduce the quality of the final product.

The generation and disposal of NPO are non value-adding activities and therefore cause unnecessary costs for the company. Additionally they can block production capacity (*eg.* in the case of reprocessing), thus resulting in a loss of production and and opportunity costs.

Normally, the "mental image" of production does not include NPO. The whole management and accounting system is oriented at the product output. In most of the companies NPO-related costs are not allocated to specific production steps, but accounted as a separate cost centre (energy, water, disposal costs), or they just disappear amongst other issues. Hence, there is no exact allocation of where in the production process NPO are generated. In decision-making processes NPO are of no relevance, because nobody does exactly know their costs. Production managers are not interested in reducing costs for which they are not accountable. The environmental department, may be the only division of the company to deal with NPO, is isolated because other divisions are not aware that a lot of money is going down the drain with the NPO.

## What are Potential Cost Saving effect of NPO Reduction?

The result of ECM applications in Germany have shown a range 1-5 per cent cost reduction to be achieved by technical or organisational measures with limited investment. In Zimbabwe, the food processing company CAIRNS could reduce its total annual costs by 1.5 per cent by implementing only one third of the measures identified during an ECM application.

Companies with low resource efficiency have a higher saving potential than companies which have already undertaken efforts to increase their efficiency. In each company, the prevention of NPO has a certain optimum where the economic bebefit of measures reaches a maximum. The further status quo of the company is away from this optimum, the higher is the saving potential. A complete prevention of NPO is neither technically nor economically feasible.

> The objective of applying EoCM is not the complete prevention but the optimisation of the amount and handling of NPO.

In general, the resource-efficiency of industrial production in developing countries is lower than in industrialised countries. At the same time, the share of material costs is higher because of relatively low labour costs. In the five companies of the Zimbabwe Programme, labour costs do not exceed 10 per cent of total costs. The saving potential which can be expected in a medium-size company in a developing country is likely to be in the range of 10-20 per cent If only 10 per cent of this potential can really be saved, the company will reduce its total costs by 1-2 per cent.

Cost savings through NPO reduction represent a full net profit. In input-limited companies the reduction of NPO can lead to an output increase and thus a considerable growth of the total turnover and market share. In addition, the quality of the product can often be imporved due to product and process innovation

> In a company with a profit of 5 per cent  return on sales before taxes, a cost reduction of only 1 per cent of the total cost leads to a 20 per cent  increase of profit.

## What effects can be expected on the Environmental Performance?

Reduction of NPO flows has a direct positive impact on the company's environmental performance. There are less solid materials, waste water and air emissions released into the environment. Measures which generate cost savings but lead to a negative enviornmental impact are not compatible with the rationale of EoCM, and consequently have to be excluded or compensated by other measures. Nevertheles, EoCM does not guarantee the elimination of all negative environmental impact caused by the company. It focuses on win-win-situations, where the reduction of NPO is related to an economic benefit for the company.

## What other effects are likely to Benefit the Company?

EoCM  can also improve the workers safety and health and increase the motivation of all company members to act more consciously with regard to the environmental aspects of their work. As it makes the production process more transparent and involves different areas of the company, it improves the communication between the environmental division and the rest of the company. Product quality can often be improved due to process and product innovation.

## What is the EoCM Cycle?

EoCM is not just another "change project", where an external consultant comes into the company, asks a lot of questions and after a while delivers a thick final report full of suggestions that nobody will ever implement. EoCM  means a change of culture within the company, which leads to a process of continuous improvement and organisational learning.

EoCM is based of the assumption that most of the relevant knowledge regardung inefficient use of materials, energy and water, including the respectve problem solving capacities, can be found within the company. The EoCM cycle is the adequate  instrument to mobilise this knowledge. The first steps are diagnostic activities which aim at identifying:

- where the NPO are generated (flow analysis)
- how much they cost (cost allocation) and
- why they occur (analysis of causes).

In the second part of the EoCM cycle, the energy and problem-solving capacity of both the teams, including the consultant, and the company have to be mobilised to find out.

- whether, to what extent and how the NPO can be reduced (development of measures), and
- how to implement the carefully selected  measures.

As a last step of the cycle, the success of the measures has to be evaluated and  made sustainable. As in every process of change, the organisation needs time to assimilate structural change and build a common consensus about it. Showing the benefit of EoCM  helps to convince the resistant members of the company.

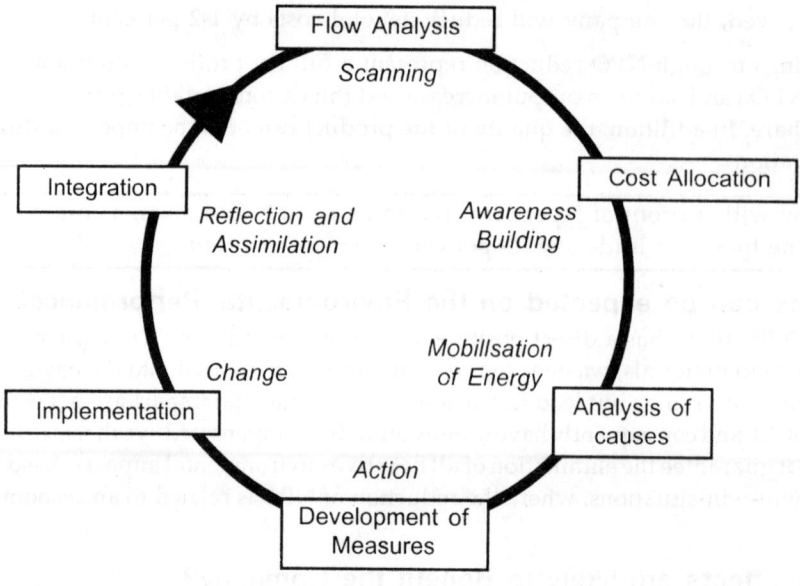

In a company which has been operating in a highly specialised sector for decades, the accounting manager saw through EoCM' the production process for the first time and understood its complexity. When the team started analysing causes of material losses, he was surprised by the fact that the supervisors and the workers already knew most of the reasons. Some of them had been working in the company for more than ten years, but nobody had ever asked them for their opinion.

## The "Cycle of Change"

These six steps can only be integrated into the company sucessfully, if the company is going through a internal change process at the same time. This "cycle of change" (the inner circle in the figure) reflects the state of organisational willingness and ability to implement EoCM within the company. For the success of EoCM it is important that the company has gone through every step of the cycle; that the organisation is observing the problems ("scanning"), is aware of the consequences and can be mobilised to prepare action to tackle them. Without this awareness building process and the mobilisation of relevant parts of the company, there will be a high resistance to implement the developed measures in the daily business.

The internal change process will not necessarily take place at the same time of the steps of EoCM. There will always be parts of the company which are not following this process. The task of the Innovation-Team is to convince and integrate a "critical mass" within the company, applying communicative skills which are trained during the EoCM programme. In this way, EoCM will become part of the company culture and structure - the internal "take off" of the process.

EoCM can also be applied step-by-step by elaborating measures only for certain divisions of the company or selected NPO, such as energy, soild waste or water. It can work in sequences over a determined period of time: after half a year of working on energy, the team starts working on water or another NPO. A comprehensive approach, however, is preferable in order not to duplicate work or reduce one NPO by increasing another. It can also can be applied in parallel at different production sites of the company, if an intensive exchange of experiences and results between the participants is provided. Important is that the technical and communicative skills trained in the EoCM process are available in the company, as in the form of these skills the EoCM approach is already institutionalised even before it is reflected in the organisational structure of the company.

## Which Communicative Skills are required in EoCM Process?

A main factor of success in the EoCM application is the building of awareness and ownership for the programme within the company. Without the support of the different levels of decision-making, production and support activities, the methodology will not lead to a continuous process of improvement. Therefore communication is crucial for the implementation and sustainability of EoCM. This includes the clear and concise presentation of the methodology, the task as well as the results, by using a common language and good visualisation. Commitment can only be achieved by information and motivation and tangible success and benefits.

Therefore, in all five Zimbabwean companies some form of in-house training and discussions on a reward system were held.

Like in any process of change, there are obstacles to overcome. The forces of change have to find arguments and strategies to convince the resistant members of the organisation. EoCM offers a common language to facilitate communication between the relevant company members: the flow chart and cost analysis are instruments to understand the problem of NPO from a different perspective. By translating them into costs, accountants, production manager, machine operator and top manager can communicate and co-operate more effectively.

The centre of an EoCM implementation in a company is the EoCM team. Teambuilding, moderation skills, efficient communication, distribution of work and time management are crucial for the successful analysis of NPO and the development and implementation of measures in the company.

## What Type of Quality Assurance System is Applied for the Diffusion of EoCM?

P3U is interest in diffusing its instruments as fast and extensively as possible; however, aspects of quality assurance, authorisation by P3U (*e.g.* copyright), an appropriate feedback of experience with the application of the current concept as well as the communication of the result of the implementation of EoCM have to be ensured.

Therefore, the instruments can at present only be applied by trainers and consultants who are duly qualified and authorised by P3U. A list of these trainers and consultants can be obtained from P3U.

The responsibility for quality assurance as well as the copyright- are with GTZ P3U. A licence for using EoCM may be negotiated by interested and trained institutions with P3U.

Since the trainers will also be ambassadors for environmental management and the P3U approach, a minimum of environmentally oriented behaviour and the respective know-how are considered indispensable. We expressly do encourage the qualification of *female* trainers. For these reasons, any participation in training measures on P3U concepts is subject to the approval by P3U.

## Conditions for the Applications of P3U Instruments

1. In case you want to use the EoCM, you have to ask for an agreement with P3U on the modalities.

2. Only if you are authorised trainer or consultant you are permitted to hold workshops and trainings.

3. Regarding these workshops and trainings, you are requested to obtain the formal approval from P3U in good time, submitting details on the programme, cooperation partners, trainer (s), venue, date, participants and training concept; with regard to the further development of the instruments, the latter is of special importance if you are planning to modify the basic module.

4. At the end of the training programme, the event has to be adequately evaluated by the participants by means of the questionnaire developed by P3U (monitoring and evaluation).

5. The trainer is requested to analyse this quantitative and qualitative evalution by summarising the results of the questionnaires and submit this analysis to P3U together with the original questionnaires.

6. The trainer is also expected to write a summary report on the workshop in order to give a feedback of learning experiences to P3U and the EoCM network.

In exchange, the trainers will be informed on or involved in further P3U activities, and will be included in the P3U list of consultants/trainers and the EoCM network, thus being recommended as well.

# 18

# Chemical Toxicity and Health Hazards

*Y. C. Tripathi, G. Tripathi and P. Verma*

## Introduction

The living world is heavily dependent on chemicals. Natural and synthetic chemicals have become an integral part of human life. Use of various types of chemicals in household needs, health care, protection of crops and grains, cottage industries and personal hygiene has been common since the development of civilization. One of the bad consequences of modernization, technological progress and industrial revolution has been the release of a large number of chemicals into environment. Many activities of the modern society like automobile movement, electric power generation, processing of chemicals and petroleum, manufacturing of agrochemicals, plastics, dyes and other products, unsafe disposal of wastes and discharge of solid particles and gaseous pollutants are causing a variety of health and environmental hazards. Contamination of air, water, soil and food has become a threat to the existence of many plant and animal communities of the ecosystem and may ultimately threaten the very survival of the human race. For many of the chemicals, the toxicity may not be known at the stage of production. So many chemicals in liquid waste effluents find their way to water supplies, chemicals from industrial and autoexhausts are breathed and residues from agricultural pesticides are consumed with food.

Natural exposure to toxic chemicals may occur where water dissolves the chemicals in percolation through the ground. Among the toxic substances encountered through breathing are chemically active dusts like lead, gases like chlorine, carbon monoxide and solvent vapour mainly hydrocarbons and chlorinated hydrocarbons. Some gases are irritating at low concentrations. At higher concentrations hydrogen sulfide may be fatal. Allergic reactions may occur after chemical contact depending on individual sensitivity. Direct contact with acids, alkalis, detergents and solvents can cause danger of burns or long term skin problems. The use of pesticides in agriculture and discarding wastes into air, soil and water constitute major pathways of human exposure to toxicants. These practices release hundreds of millions of tons of potentially hazardous substances into the environment each year. Almost all industrial processes and urban activities involve the release of at least trace quantities of half a dozen metals in different forms contributing to the increase of metallic ions in lakes and streams day by day. Chemicals may concentrate in certain tissues of plants, animals and fishes and may result in manifold increase over the initial concentration through ecological cycling and biomagnification.

Though chemicals are hazardous, their proper use has fast effect and apparently improves quality of life. The use of DDT in public health for over 30 years as control of malaria-carrying mosquitoes in more than 100 countries has saved approximately 50 million lives and averted more than 1 billion human illness. Nitrogen fertilizers are necessary to increase the crop production, but an overabundance will also result in a buildup of nitrates in the ground water. Chlorine used to destroy pathogens in drinking water and swimming pools and to oxidize wastes but when inhaled is extremely toxic. Too much fluoride to natural water will mottle tooth enamel. While food additives are sometimes questionable, many are beneficial in lengthening shelf life or improving the nutritive qualities. During the last few decades, public anxiety over chemical pollution has made the study of their hazardous effects as one of the principal areas of research.

## Heavy Metal Toxicity

Heavy metals are neither degraded nor metabolized. They are the examples of ultimate persistence. Most of the elemental metals do not easily enter living organisms, but they can form both inorganic and organic compounds. These compounds differ markedly in their access and effects on living organisms. Nonetheless the essential toxicity of metal compounds is characteristic of the metal, modified by the degree to which a specific compound reaches specific tissues. Heavy metals like copper, cadmium , cobalt, silicon, zinc, nickel, lead, arsenic and mercury resulting from industrial effluents, fossil fuel burning, domestic sewage discharge and land run-off, can cause toxicity to aquatic organisms and human beings (Goyer, 1986). Impacts of some of the important heavy metals have been discussed as follows.

Heavy metals are the trace elements most commonly encountered in the environment cause toxicity when accumulated in high doses in human body (Table 18.1). Cadmium is used in a wide range of industrial processes

**Table 18.1 : Unhealthy effects of heavy metals**

| Heavy metal | Body part/function affected | Toxicity symptoms |
|---|---|---|
| Aluminium | Stomach, Brain, Bone | Gastrointestinal irritation, Colic, Rickets, Convulsions |
| Arsenic | Cell and Cellular metabolism | Gastroenteritis, Low vitality, Loss of body hair, pain sensation, Skin colour changes dark |
| Cadmium | Renal cortex of kidney, Blood vessels, Brain | Hypertension, Kidney damage, Loss of sense of smell, |
| Copper | Blood, Artery, Hair, Stomach | Anaemia, Depigmentation of hair, Reduced arterial elasticity, Irritation of Gastrointestinal tract |
| Lead | Bone, Liver, Kidney, Pancreas, Heart, Brain, Nervous system | Weakness, Fatigue, Pallor, Abdominal troubles |
| Mercury | Nervous system, Appetite, Pain Centre, Cell membrane | Loss of appetite and bogy mass, Tremors, severe emotional disturbances, loss of sense of pain, Inflammation of gums, Convulsions |
| Silver | Liver, Kidney, Spleen, Bone marrow, Skin, | Discolouration of skin, Destruction of bone marrow, Argyria |

including electroplating to impart corrosive resistance to ironware. It is a very deadly poison. Cadmium chloride is used as pigments, as components of batteries and as photographic materials. It is also used as a plastic stabilizer. Cadmium sulphate in a 1per cent solution, is a constituent of a shampoo used in the treatment of seborrhoeic dermatitis and dandruff. Cadmium accumulates in liver and kidney. It is associated with hypertension, cirrhosis of the liver, pulmonary complications and lung cancer. Its accumulation induces calcium deficiency in concentration even at lower levels. Therefore, elderly people and pregnant women exposed to cadmium are at greater risk. Respiratory and pulmonary damage is reported from the breathing of cadmium vapour or its particulates. Cadmium does not affect the central nervous system and cannot cross the placental and the mammary glands. Cadmium enters the aquatic environment from mining and metallurgical operations and electroplating industries. Metallic and plastic pipes may also introduce cadmium in water. Automobile tyres are a source of cadmium pollution in the environment.

Organic acids used in day to day cooking such as vinegar (acetic acid), imli (tartaric acid) and lemon (citric acid) can dissolve cadmium from the thin electroplated layer and cause poisoning. Accidental cases of cadmium poisoning can also occur from cadmium fumes and dust. It must be kept in mind that inhaled cadmium is about six times more dangerous than ingested cadmium. Cadmium is found in significant amounts in unfiltered cigarettes, about twenty unfiltered cigarettes a day can yield 6 mg of cadmium, of which the smoker may retain upto 65 per cent. Symptoms of cadmium poisoning includes muscles ache and pain and in more serious cases, decalcification and bone fracture.

Cadmium ingested through intake of water as well as rice causes chronic poisoning manifesting in the form of a complete syndrome specially in menopausal women. The initial symptoms and signs are sensation of constriction around the throat, a nasty taste in the mouth, irritation of the upper respiratory tract manifested by troublesome cough and reddening of eyes. The prominent respiratory symptoms are difficulty in respiration, pain in chest, malaise, shivering and profuse sweating.

Silver has both medicinal and non medicinal uses. Its main non-medicinal uses are in jewellery, coins, silverware, tableware and manufacturing of mirrors and electrical wiring. Silver and its salts have been used as medicines for various ailments throughout the history. During the nineteenth century it was prescribed for the treatment of digestive disorders including stomach ulcer. Later small sticks of compressed crystals of silver nitrate began to be used for cauterization, notably of throat lesions, because of its astringent properties. Application of astringent often arrests secretions or discharge, so it is often applied to lesions which are discharging secretions. The toxicologically important compounds of silver are silver nitrate, silver lactate, silver cirate, silver acetate and the silver halides. Dressings soaked in 0.5 per cent silver nitrate have been extensively used in the treatment of burns. Silver is also used in dentistry for dental fillings.

Silver salts because of their germicidal properties, are also used as drinking water disinfactants. Such treated water may contain upto 50 micro gram per litre. In humans, more than 50 per cent of the body burden of silver goes in the liver, elimination of which is mainly via faeces. The concentrations of silver in kidney, liver and spleen of normal human have been reported to be about 0.4, 0.7 and 2.7 mg/kg respectively on a dry weight basis (Agrawal, 1997). Fifty miligram or more of callargol (a silver salt) has been reported to be lethal after intravenous injection in therapeutic purpose. Autopsy findings in such cases have included watery lungs, and destruction of bone marrow, liver and kidney. Nose drops occur been due to poisoning with silver iodide. Silver nitrates has been used by quacks to induce abortions. In case of intrauterine administration of approximately 25g of silver nitrate causes rapid death of mother. Argyria is chronic poisoning with silver in small doses administered slowly. Silver bound to body protein is deposited widely in the body tissues resulting in blue-grey patches on skin. The pigmentation results mainly from photo-activated reduction to metallic silver in the dermis. Hence the distribution of patches are on the areas exposed to light. Anti-smoking lozenges contain silver acetate and ammonium chloride claimed to reduce the smoking desire at a recommended dose of six lozenges per day. It has been reported to cause argyria in several cases. Occupational handling of silver objects, especially if repeated minor injury is involved, may give rise to so called local argyria which is bluish-gery discoloration of the skin at the exposed site.

Aluminium, the most abundant metal in biosphere has so far demonstrated no biological function. However, it gains access to human body *via* the gastrointestinal tract, lungs and olfactory tract. It has been observed that aluminium accumulates in the human brain with ageing and abnormal levels of industrial exposure leads to aluminosis (an occupational disease). Aluminium has been implicated over the last two decades as a potential neurotoxic factor in different pathological conditions and detrimental effects have been proved. The potential role of aluminium has also been suggested in the aetiopathogenesis of Alzheimer's disease, a common form of dementia beginning in middle age or later. Defective memory and loss of other intellectual functions has also been suggested (Perl, 1985). Copper which is essential for all forms of life, its deficiency and excess both cause health problems. Copper deficiency results in anaemia, loss of hair pigment, reduced growth and arterial elasticity whereas Wilson's disease occurs with excess of copper. Irritation of the gastrointestinal tract is another effect of copper toxicity. Water containing a high dose of zinc could cause growth depression and anaemia. It could decrease liver copper and interfere with iron metabolism.

Mercury is the most toxic heavy metal resulting in a number of serious incidences due to poisoning. It is used in manufacturing chlorine and caustic soda, production of batteries and fluorescent tubes, pharmaceuticals and fungicides. Mercury ultimately enters into the water environment resulting in fish mortality. Marine organisms readily concentrate mercury. It finds applications in chlor-alkali industry, electrical appliance and pesticide industries. Liquid mercury appears to have little effect, but mercury vapour is readily absorbed into blood stream producing severe damage to central nervous system. The solubility of methyl mercury in lipids is a major factor regarding its toxicity, as it readily crosses the blood/brain barrier and the placental membrane.

Lead finds a widespread use in our consumer society. Environmental contamination by lead is attributed to industrial discharges like battery manufacturing units, run-off from contaminated land mass, atmospheric fall-out, sewage effluents, PVC plastics, paints and glazing of ceramics. It is associated with hypertension, cirrhosis of the liver, pulmonary complications and lung cancer. The uses of lead most commonly associated with poisoning are lead glazed pottery, solder, plumbing, paint and an additive to petrol. The main damaging effects of lead poisoning are on the haemopoietic system leading to anaemia, on nervous system leading to irreversible brain damage and on the renal system. In mild form, lead effects the central nervous system, manifest in the form of hypertension, irritability and impaired motor skills. Young children being particularly susceptible, the damage showing up in behavioural and educational abnormalities leading to mental retardation. Lead poisoning can produce irreparable brain damage in children and deformity in unborn babies. Arsenic, on account of its criminal and wartime applications is well known for its toxicity. It is used mainly in agrochemicals, ceramics and glass, chemical and pharmaceuticals. The symptoms of acute arsenic poisoning is severe gastro-enteritis and in chronic poisoning, loss of weight and hair and skin lesions. Poisoning by arsenic compounds used in insecticides and herbicides leads to loss of appetite and body mass, gastrointestinal disorders and skin cancer. Arsenic is a metabolic inhibitor and cause iron deficiencies.

There are several salts of barium almost all of which are poisonous except barium sulphate. Some of these are barium carbonate, barium nitrate, barium chloride, barium hydroxide, barium sulphide, barium chlorate and barium acetate. Barium carbonate and barium chloride are most often responsible for poisoning in man. Barium salts are used in a number of industrial processes, but their use in day to day life is the major cause of poisoning. Barium sulphide in a cream is used as a hair remover. Barium carbonate and barium sulphide are often used as rat poisons. Barium sulphate contaminated with other soluable salts of barium may prove to be poisonous. The salt contaminated with barium chloride shows symptoms of nausea, vomiting, occasional diarrhoea and muscular paralysis in poisoned people. In 1963, more than 100 people fell ill in Israel following the ingestion of sausage made from turkey contaminated heavily with barium carbonate. The main symptoms of patients were diarrhoea, vomiting, generalized weakness, paralysis, dryness of mouth, tightness in the throat, dyscrasia, headache and muscular twitchings.

## Toxic Non-Metals

Selenium, a nonmetallic element closely related to sulphur and found commercially in steel and copper alloys and metal bluing solution is used for making stained glass, ink and even cosmetics.. A suspension of selenium disulphide has been used as a shampoo in the treatment of seborrhoea, which is a kind of skin disease. Selenium sulphide in 2.5 per cent aqueous solution is still used as a shampoo for the treatment of dandruff. Though it is absorbed through unbroken skin, but if absorbed it may cause motor neuron disease. Naturally, it occurs in the surface soil in certain areas and is readily absorbed by plants, including grains and vegetables growing in these areas. Herbivorous animals feeding on these plants may accidentally get poisoned by selenium. In south Dakota (USA) where the selenium content of soil is high, it could have been the cause of blind staggers in cattle causing impaired gait and vision. In addition, the animals show wasting stomach upsets, liver damage, bizarre growth, loss of hair and hooves and sometimes sterility. Similar symptoms may occur in man as well as outside the recognized endemic areas. Many selenium compounds are very irritating or even corrosive to the skin, mucus membranes and respiratory tract. Many pesticides containing selenium compounds have been abandoned on account of their human toxicity. Because of the finding that selenium is a naturally occurring antioxidant in the body and may be anticarcinogenic, it is being consumed in megadoses as a dietary supplement. However, the Centre for Disease Control (CDC) in USA reported 12 persons with nausea, vomitting, nail changes, fatigue and irritability from excessive selenium intake. About half of the patients experienced hair loss and about one-third lost their nails. Other symptoms includes watery diarrhoea, abdominal cramps, dryness of hair, paresthesis and garlic breath odour. In industrial situations a worker may slowly absorb selenium in his system thus suffering from chronic selenium poisoning or chronic selenosis. Acute selenium poisoning produces primarily central nervous system effects including convulsions. The initial symptoms are nausea, vomiting and a metallic taste in the mouth, dizziness and extreme lassitude.

Chlorination of drinking water for disinfection has been called the single most important public health measure ever undertaken as it is effective against most pathogenic bacteria. But it produces toxic byproducts. The most important byproduct is a class of organic molecules called trihalomethane. Chloroform, the most common example of this class cause cancer in rats and mice. Lifetime consumption of chlorinated water have a higher rate of bladder cancer than users on nonchlorinated water. Gastrointestinal cancers have also been associated with chlorinated surface waters in some epidemiological studies, but in other studies there has been no significant association. Fluoride is sometimes added to drinking water to partially protect against dental decay. Aluminium is also added in the form of alum to flocculate and remove organic matter that may cause odour or taste problem. Florine is another element which may contaminate water either by industrial effluents or by nature such as fluorine containing rocks. If ingested upto a certain dose, it is good for teeth and bones, but beyond the threshold limit, it makes teeth chalky and brittle. Much higher doses of fluoride can cause bone disease (Leverett, 1982).

Iodine is needed by the thyroid gland to make thyroxine hormone. Iodine defficient diet may lead to the enlargement of thyroid gland known as goitre. The daily requirement of iodine is about 150 micrograms/day in adults, of which the thyroid gland takes up about 70 micrograms and rest is used for some other essential purposes. Some commercial preparations containing iodine are povidone-iodine and tincture of iodine are basically used as antiseptic and disinfectants. Higher concentrations of iodine in such preparations may lead to excessive tears, tightness in the chest, sore throat, headache, irritation of the respiratory tract and water logging in the lungs. Iodine is a powerful irritant and vesicant, which can cause skin eruptions. Symptoms may occur through inhalation, skin or eye contact or ingestion. Iodine vapour may cause brown staining of the cornea. About 3-4 g of elemental iodine or 30-250 ml of strong tincture can kill a person.

Arsine is one of the most poisonous gases known which can kill outright. Even brief exposure to moderate concentrations can cause serious illness. In several industries there is a rough and ready practice of producing zinc chloride to provide a soldering flux by putting zinc scrap in hydrochloric acid. The zinc scrap may contain arsenic as an impurity, and when arsenic acts with hydrochloric acid, it forms arsine. Arsine is a cumulative poison that excrete much more slowly from the body than it is absorbed resulting in gradual accumulation of the poison in the body which can be very dangerous. The hazards of arsine gas exists in various industries including the refining of metal, the manufacture of corrosive acids, galvanizing and electroplating. Use of wall papers coloured with pigment which contained Scheele's Green (a popular name of cupric arsenite) yields arsine in the home when acts upon by a mould. The deadly poison arsine hemolyses all the red blood cells of the body. This liberates haemoglobin which ultimately finds its way in the urine which becomes dark.

Acetylsalicylic acid is used for relief from pain. Ordinary disprin which is available in the market for pain relief contains 350 mg of acetylsalicylic acid. If too much tablets are ingested, one can get salicylate poisoning. The symptoms of high fever, thirst and profuse sweating are seen in salicylate poisoning. It is surprising to note that although, acetylsalicylic acid is normally used to control high temperature, in case of an overdose, it produces high fever itself.

Cyanide enters the environment as hydrogen cyanide gas which is generally used as a fumigating agent for destroying rodents. It also finds use in various chemical synthesis, in electroplating and metal cleaning industries. Carbon monoxide, a component of some fuel gases is a significant air pollutant. The initial effect of carbon monoxide poisoning involves the loss of awareness and judgement which have been found to be responsible for many automobile accidents. With increasing exposures to its higher levels, various metabolic disorders takes place which ultimately leads to death.

## Industrial Toxicants

There are atleast 18 types of industries which have been identified for causing pollution. Some of these are associated with pesticide, fertilizer, paper, refineries, paints, dyes, leather tanning, sodium potassium, cyanide, basic drugs foundries, batteries acid and alkalies manufacturing. Toxic emissions in atmosphere cause various hazardous effects on human health (Table 18.2). The pesticide industry is a big health hazard. According to one study, some one in the third world is poisoned by pesticides every minutes and that some one could possibly be an Indian every minute, considering the enormous population of India. A wide range of products are manufactured by various chemical industries. These chemicals

**Table 18.2 : Hazardous effects of toxic emissions in the atmosphere**

| Emissions | Source | Hazardous effects |
|---|---|---|
| Carbon monoxide | Automobile, Petroleum industry, Forest fires | Deprives oxygen, Respiratory problems, Impairment of Central Nervous System |
| Carbon dioxide | Automobile, Fuel combustion for heating, Energy production | Increase in earth's temperature, Rise in sea levels, |
| Oxides of sulphur | Burning of sulphur containing fuel like diesels, Industries | Irritation of respiratory system, Reduction in brain ability to control muscle movement, Increased eye blinking |
| Oxides of Nitrogen | Fuel combustion in motor vehicles and furnaces, Forest fire Corrosion | Increased acute respiratory infections and bronchitis, Morbidity in children, Brown haze in urban air, |
| Hydrocarbons | Partial combustion of carbonaceous fuel, Industrial processes, Disposal of solid waste, | Production of photochemical smog and irritants in air, Premature aging, Soreness, Coughing, Breathing problems Tightness in chest, Carcinogenic |
| Chlorine | Industrial, Refrigerators, Water purification plants, Organochlorine Pesticides | Decrease in ozone layer, Skin cancer |

may be inorganic substances like sulphuric, nitric, hydrochloric, hydrofluoric and phosphoric acid and their salts and organic substances like fertilizers, pest controlling agents, hydrocarbons, plastics, man-made fibres, paints and lacquers, pharmaceutical products, adhesives, detergents, cosmetics, polishing powders and leather and textile accessories. The major emissions of these chemical industries are gases and vapours of organic chemical compounds such as hydrocarbon and their halogen derivatives, aldehydes, ketones, carboxylic acids and nitrogen and sulphur (amines, mercaptans, disulfides), gases and vapours of inorganic chemical compounds such as hydrogen sulfide, hydrochloric acid, fluorine compounds, sulfur dioxide and hydrogen phosphide and toxic powders such as fluorides and carbides, iron alloys, arsenic and asbestos (Francis, 1994). It is worth-while to point out that the prolonged inhalation of sulphur dioxide is known to damage respiratory system causing asthma, tuberculosis etc. These oxides are readily absorbed by plants and cause damage to have the second highest level of sulphur dioxide in the city. People in the vicinity are afflicted with chronic lung ailments and defoliation of vegetation is conspicuous. Oxygen availability in the atmosphere decreases as industries, vehicles and internal combustion engines throw out carbon monoxide, carbon dioxide, sulphur dioxide and other gases disturbing the ecological balance. Some gases produce both acute irritation by a single high level exposure and chronic lung disease by repeated exposure of low level. The nitrogen oxides are extremely irritating to the eyes and upper respiratory tract. Exposure to the concentrations above the threshold limit causes cough and chest pain immediately.

Health problems like chest pain, cough, dyspnoea and abdominal discomfort are the major health hazards suffered by workers in chemical plants. Serious problems are involved in the use of chemicals, especially those commonly encountered in the production of dyestuffs and their intermediates. These problems include sensitization for a few of the compounds and the ablity to cause cancer. The petroleum industry regularly discharges hydrocarbons, other organic compounds, sulphur dioxide and fine dust. It is assumed at present that one third of production losses by the petroleum industry pass into the atmosphere as hydrocarbons (Sundareson, 1984). The day to day increasing use of spray gun containing chlorofluorocarbons as propellant previously regarded as neutral in its effect, is now identified to be responsible for irreversible damage to the environment. The chlorofluorocarbon molecules are broken down by the strong ultraviolet radiation in the stratosphere releasing chlorine atoms which breaks down ozone molecules by a catalytic process. The gas rises into the stratosphere and damages the zone belt surrounding the earth. Extensive studies have shown that chlorine at high concentration is irritating and damages the skin, eyes, nose, nasal, sinuses, throat, larynx and larger air tubes. It may cause chronic inflammation of the sinuses and continued hoarseness. Workers suffer from ulcers in the centre section of the nose and seriously affected by the skin infections. Methyl isocyanate (MIC) is a toxic gas that reacts quickly with water and causes the lungs to swell and eyes to develop cataract. The leakage of MIC from pesticide manufacturing plant of Union Carbide at Bhopal on 2-3 December 1984 resulted in the death of more than 2500 residents of the city and acute health problems in 20000-50000 others.

The risk of exposure to several chemicals like catalysts, dye, stabilizers, plasticisers, monomers are very common in plastic industries. Many health hazards are involved in the manufacturing of epoxides. Liquid epoxy resins are sensitizers and irritants. It is generally considered that they are extreme irritants and may have anesthesic and sensitizing effects. Some epoxy compounds are nonvolatile and when heated, extremely irritating to upper respiratory tract, skin and eyes. They can burn the skin also. If lung irritation is severe enough, they may lead to pneumonia and pulmonary edema. Ethylene oxide is extremely irritating. Skin and eye contact can cause severe burns leading to death of tissues involved. Excessive vapour can cause severe lung irritation, which can lead to lung infections. Nitric acid is an another hazardous chemical which is extremely corosive and attacks the eyes, skin and mucuous membranes. The fumes contains nitrogen dioxide which is highly toxic. Exposure to high concentrations can lead to serious lung disease. Sulphuric acid is quite volatile when concentrated and gives of sulphur trioxide gas and sulphuric acid mist, both strongly irritating to the respiratory tract. Acute respiratory effects are similar to those of hydrochloric acid. Lung scarring pulmonary fibrosis and emphysema may follow acute reactions.

A variety of solvents used to make proprietary blends are widely known by their trade names such as Chlorox (chlorine bleach), Freon (CFC) and Arctic (methyl chloride) etc. The most common solvents are alcohols (methanol, isopropyl alcohol), ketones (acetone, methyl ethyl ketone) aliphatic hydrocarbon like hexane, aromatic hydrocarbon like benzene, toluene, xylene and halogenated hydrocarbon such as trichloroethane, methylene chloride and CFCs etc. Most of the solvents are hazardous. Some are inflammable, others explode easily, some are corrosive and most are toxic. Human health effects due to exposure to solvents can include damage to the skin, liver, blood, central nervous system and sometimes the lung and kidneys. Some solvents are irritants, while others are capable of causing cancer. Inhaling solvent vapours, even for very short periods, can lead to lung and throat irritation, pulmonary edema, dizziness, light headedness, blurred vision, nervousness, sleepiness or insomnia, nausea, vomiting, disorientation, confusion, irregular heartbeat and even unconsciousness and death (Andrews and Snyder, 1986). Solvents can affect the body's ability to manufacture blood, while some can damage the immune system. Some of them are suspected of causing both defects also. The solvent acetone is familiar as finger nail polish remover. The widespread use of fingernail polish and remover in the home makes acetone a common source of childhood poisoning. Ingestion of acetone causes central nervous system depression, high blood sugar levels and high levels of acetone in blood. Skin application of acetone can increase the permeability of undamaged skin, potentially enhancing absorption of other dangerous chemicals. It also causes peeling, splitting or brittleness of exposed fingernails (EPA, 1988). The most common symptom of acetone allergy is dermatitis.

Water resources have become repositories for the disposal of industrial effluents and other waste materials (Rao, 1979). Pollution of water resources by various industrial toxicants (Table 18.3) has resulted in menace to

### Table 18.3 : Contamination of water resources by Industrial effluents

| Water contaminants | Source |
| --- | --- |
| Metal Electroplating | Heavy metals, Fluorides, Cyanides, Acids, Alkalies, |
| Chemical plants | Abrasives, Plating salts, Oils, Phenols. |
| Chrome tanning | Acids, Alkalies, Phenols, Amines, |
| Pesticide Industry | Lime, Sulphide, Chromium, Organic matters |
| Pharmaceutical units | Organochlorine and Organophosphorous chemicals, Heavy metals |
| Petroleun refinery | Organic solvents and residues, Mercury and other heavy metals |
| Plastic industry | Oil, Phenols, Heavy metals, Ammonia salts, Acids, Caustics Hydrocarbons |
| Paint Industry | Chlorine compounds |
| Paper mills | Organic solvents, Synthetic pigments, Heavy metals |
| Textile Units | Cellulose fibre, Free chlorine, Rresins, Starch, Caustic soda, Other organic matter |
| Farm drainage | Starch gums, Dyes, Acids, Alkalies, Free Chlorine, Sulphide, Soap and Detergents |
| /Sewage | Phosphates, Nitrates, Copper pesticides, Organic matter of high BOD |

aquatic environment affecting biotic communities and human beings through food chain. Heavy fish mortility has been reported from various rivers and reservoirs due to pollution by toxic industrial chemicals. Pollution of oceans and rivers has largely affected the quality of life forms. Serious deterioration in fresh water quality of rivers causing a widespread public health problems. Consuming water contaminated by toxic effluents give rise to various ailments. For instance, vinyl chloride from plastic industry found to cause a rare form of liver cancer, excess of nitrate in drinking water cause infantile methaemoglobinaemia and pesticide contaminated water cause damage to the nervous, digestive, cardiovascular and blood formation systems (Bindra, 1971). The world's supply of water already threatened by rising level of pollution limiting the economic and agricultural development and harming a wide range of ecosystem.

## Hazards of Synthetic Agrochemicals

The growing demand of food as a result of the increasing population has led to a substantial increase in the production and application of agrochemicals like fertilizers and pesticides resulting in continued contamination of air and water environments. Use of synthetic chemicals as fertilizers and pesticide is an essential adjunct to modern agriculture providing the most effective and economically viable means for increasing production and controlling thousands of species of insects, weeds, fungi and nematodes. The technological advancement in agriculture is brought about through the increased production of new high yielding varieties of crops by means of the application of synthetic fertilizers mainly nitrogenous and phosphatic as plant nutrients and pesticide chemicals for crop protection. However, only 20-30 per cent of the applied nitrogen fertilizer is actually used by the plant and the balance is lost to the environment due to denitrification and leaching. This hardens the soil and poisons the habitat and renders the soil gradually less productive, to overcome which additional quantities of fertilizers are added to maintain the production levels. They contribute to air and water pollution and adversely affect fish, wildlife and human beings.

Excessive use of nitrogen fertilizers has resulted in increased levels of nitrates in ground water in most countries of developed and developing world. These levels will continue to rise for many years to come if optimum use of nitrogenous fertilizers is not followed in agriculture. In addition to nitrogenous fertilizers, other source of nitrate and nitrite pollution are industrial wastes, poultry farms in a limited area, dumping of domestic solid waste, seepage and run off from septic tanks, tinned food etc. Drinking water is the major sources of intake of nitrate. In order to provide safe drinking water, Government of India launched the programme of water quality survey in different states. High nitrates have been reported in some districts of the state like Maharashtra, Tamil Nadu, Haryana, Rajasthan, Karnataka and Andhra Pradesh. Many other water quality surveys conducted in recent past had also indicated nitrate pollution in ground as well as surface water. In Nagpur and Satara districts of Maharashtra about 70 per cent of wells surveyed had nitrate concentration exceeding permissible limit of 45 mg/ l in respective districts. A survey of Nagaur district of Rajasthan covering about 1000 water samples also showed higher levels of nitrates in ground water. Due to increased levels of nitrates in water bodies, nutrient enrichment occurs resulting in enormous growth of aquatic filamentous green algae leading to eutrophication. This huge algal growth creates unaesthetic conditions in water body. Health effects due to high nitrate in water and food uptake of animals and human beings are equally significant. Nitrates as such are not toxic to health and about 85 per cent of ingested nitrates are rapidly absorbed from gastrointestinal tract in normal healthy individuals and excreted by the kidneys. However, conversion of nitrates into nitrites may cause potential health hazards. Nitrate has become one of the key environmental issues because of its implications on human and animal health that causes methaemoglobinemia in infants which may lead to death of a child. Recently, epidemiological studies have correlated the intake of excessive nitrates with occurrence of gastric cancer and formation of congential malformations. It is assumed that nitrate gets reduced to nitrite in gastro-intestinal tract due to microbial activity and nitrite formed reacts with secondary amines and amides producing carcinogenic N-nitroso compounds which act on the blood hemoglobin to form methemoglobin. The same process can occur in the stomach of ruminants so that livestock can also be affected by nitrate poisoning.

Ambitious use of pesticides chemicals as insecticides, fungicides, herbicides (Glaston, 1979), acaricides, nematicides, rodenticides, molluscides have caused severe environmental degradation and serious health problem during the last few decades. Their continuous use affect the ground water sources through seepage into the soil. As a result, rivers, streams and ponds have become highly polluted with these harmful chemicals affecting drinking water. Many form of life such as fishes, birds and other animals have been affected by this pollution. Being destructive of life they cause severe ecological problems on dissemination in the environment. Development of pesticidal resistance among pests is one of them. On account of bulk application of chemical pesticides after the second world war, the power of resistance of pest species has increased dramatically (Mehrotra, 1983). Organochlorine and organophosphorous compounds are most predominant in agriculture and public health care. The organochlorine pesticides cover a wide range of chemicals including aldrin, endrin, dieldrin, chlordane, heptachlor (cyclodiene series), endosulfan, kelthane, methoxychlor, chlorobenzenzilate, chlorfenson (halogenated aromatic series), benzene hexachloride, lindane (cycloparaffin series), strobane and toxaphene (chlorinated terpene series). They are thermally and chemically stable having prolonged protective action against pests. At the same time they create a danger of contaminating the environment and agricultural products, thereby causing health hazards. Toxicity due to these chemicals causes damage to the nervous, digestive, cardiovascular and blood-formation systems. They also cause tremor of the limbspolyneuritis, encelphalopolyneuritis and neurovegetative syndroms. The most common form of toxicity are headache, dizziness, paraesthesia of the limbs, vascular liability and neurocirculatory disturbances. Liver and kidney damage are observed in long exposure to such chemicals (Wang and Mac Mohan, 1979). Important biochemical and physiological activities like microsomal enzyme induction, protein synthesis, lipid synthesis, excretion and liver function are affected. They are most frequently manifested as dyspnoea, high heart rate, oppression and pain in the heart, increased heart volume. Blood and capillary disturbances have also been reported that appear as thrombopenia, anaemia, haemolysis and capillary disorders. Acute toxicity of organochlorine pesticides is demonstrated by gastrointestinal symptoms like nausea, vomiting, diarrhoea and stomach pain. A number of chlorinated pesticides such as DDT, BHC etc. have been characterized as carcinogens/mutagens. Excessive DDT has caused hepatic disorders. Cases of cancer, deformalities, diseases of the liver and nervous system from pesticide poisoning have been identified in cotton growing districts of Maharashtra and Karnataka. They have a tendency to accumulate in tissues lipids when the food containing their residues is eaten. Their residues in food are a great danger to the health of future generation (Gupta, 1977). Most of the pesticides interfere with the central nervous system and inhibit the system and the activity of enzymes involved in muscular response. DDT affects the CNS and its high doses cause symptoms such as distorted sensitivity in the tongue, lips, face and hands accompanied by hypersusceptibility to stimuli, irritability, dizziness and tremors (Ramachardran, 1973). Organophosphorous pesticides including dichlorovos, tetrachlorovos (phosphoric acid derivatives), metafos, methyl parathion, metathion, trichlorometaphos, bromophos, fenthion, cyanophos, phoxim, diazinon (phosphorothioic acid derivatives); malathion, papthion, dimethoate, formothion, amiphos, imidan, benzphos, sayphos (phosphorodithioic acid derivatives) and chlorophos (phosphonic acid derivatives) have very strong biological activity, not only for insects and acarids, but also for warm blooded animals and humans. Poisoning is not only due to ingestion or inhalation but also due to absorption through the intact skin. The symptoms of chronic poisoning include headache, weakness, feeling of heaviness in the head, decline of memory, quick onset of fatigue, disturbed apetite, loss of apetite and loss of orientation (Korsak and Sato, 1977). Tremors, psychic disorders and paralysis also develop in certain cases. Organophosphorous pesticides are rapidly absorbed through the mucous membranes of the digestive tract, the respiratory system and the skin and are conveyed by the blood to various body tissues.

Some pesticides especially metal-based ones (arsenic, copper and mercury) are well recognised agents of chemically induced autoimmunity. Several pesticide chemicals are known to be extreme skin sensitisers. Allergic rhinitis and asthma are also result of acute hypersensitivity on the part of the immune system in which abnormally high levels of an antibody is produced. In India, the water of Yamuna on which an estimated 57 million people depend, contains many pesticides at levels which far exceeds limits considered fit for human consumption. The average daily intake of DDT by an Indian is estimated to be 0.27 mg. The report of UN sponsored global monitoring programme revealed the presence of DDT and BHC residues in the human breast milk at least four times higher than those in other developed countries. Seven out of eight chillies studied contained 100 to 160 times the permissible levels of malathion and other pesticides. Out of 104 samples of cereals, pulses, milk, eggs, meat and vegetables analysed, 108 contained pesticides, 88 had traces of more than one pesticide and 69 had residues more than the permissible limit (Rahmani, 1999).

# Atmospheric Toxicants

Carbon monoxide produced almost entirely by artificial processes is the major individual pollutant in the atmosphere. It is estimated that approximately 80 per cent of carbon monoxide comes from automobiles. Atmospheric levels of carbon monoxide in urban areas exhibit a positive correlation with the density of vehicular traffic. Many geophysical and biological processes like volcanic action, natural gas emission, electrical discharge during storms, seed germination and marsh-gas production are also known to produce carbonmonoxide. Forest fires, burning of agricultural waste and coal, operations used in iron and steel production, regeneration of catalyst in petroleum industry, furnace operations in wood, pulp and paper industries are the other sources of carbon monoxide emission in the air. Increased level of carbon monoxide in the atmosphere have several detrimental effects on human health. It displaces oxygen from haemoglobin to produce carboxyhemoglobin. The reduction in awareness, a probable cause of automobile accidents being the first discernible effect of carbon monoxide. Progressively higher exposures cause impairment of central nervous system functions, changes in cardiac and pulmonary functions, drowsiness, coma, respiratory failure and finally death. Carbondioxide produced by the combustion of carboniferous substances such as coal, petroleum products and wood in industry, automobiles, breathing of large human and animal population and households is not directly toxic for human beings and animals. But due to structure of carbon monoxide, it has the property of absorbing infrared rays and converting them into heat. Consequently, a slight increase in the carbon dioxide content of the earth's atmosphere considerably increase the heat-retaining capacity of the air. Normally, the earth's surface disseminates into the universe again a large part of the entering sunlight, in the form of infrared heat rays preventing the temperature on the earth from constantly rising under the influence of solar radiation. Due to increase in carbondioxide content of the atmosphere, a large part of this refeleted infrared radiation is got absorbed and so remaining on earth thereby raising the temperature. The increase in temperature can change the climate of the earth considerably in the long run. A rise in average temperature throughout the world by 2-3 degree centigrade would very probably result in the melting of large quantities of polar ice and so lead to a rise in the sea level and to the loss of large tracts of land.

Oxides of sulphur consisting primarily of two colourless gaseous compounds, sulphur dioxide and sulphur trioxide are the other atmospheric toxicants harmful to plants and animals. Acute exposure to high levels of the sulphur dioxide kills leaf tissues whereas its chronic exposure causes bleaching or yellowing of the normally green portions of the leaf called as chlorosis. Sulphur dioxide gets converted in the atmosphere to sulphuric acid. In the areas surrounding large industrial sources of the gas plants could be damaged by sulphuric acid aerosols appeared as small spots where sulphuric acid droplets get impinged upon the leaves. In humans, the sulphur dioxide appear to cause irritation of the respiratory system. Mucus secretion is also affected by exposure to the sulphur dioxide contaminated air thereby increasing eye blinking and is also thought to affect central nervous system. Persons who already have respiratory weakness are particularly susceptible to high levels of sulphur dioxide in the atmosphere. Inhalation of sulphur dioxide, sulphur trioxide, carbon disulphide etc. has been shown to increase the incidence of coronary diseases. It also changes the blood chemistry and reduces the brain's ability to exert control over muscle movement. The three oxides of nitrogen normally encountered in the atmosphere are nitrous oxide, nitric oxide and nitrogen dioxide. Nitrous oxide, a colourless, odourless gas is produced by microbiological processes is relatively unreactive and probably does not significantly influence important chemical reactions in the lower atmosphere. Acute exposure to nitrogen dioxide having a reddish brown colour and a pungent choking odour, can be quite harmful to human health varying with the degree of exposure. A level of 50-100 ppm brings about inflammation of lung tissue for a period of 6-8 weeks. Exposure up to 150-2000 ppm of the gas brings about 'bronchiolitis fibrosa obliterans', a condition fatal within 3 to 5 weeks. Death generally results from 2-10 days after exposure to 500 ppm or more of nitrogen dioxide. It is suspected to accelerate tumour growth and decrease the resistance of the body to diseases. Exposure of plant to several ppm of nitrogen dioxide brings about leaf spotting and breakdown of plant tissue. Exposure to 10 ppm of nitric oxide causes a reversible decrease in the rate of photosynthesis. Fumigation of bean and tomato plants with 10 ppm nitric oxide results in an immediate 60-70 per cent decrease in the rate of photosynthesis as measured by carbondioxide absorption.

Chlorine is found in atmosphere as element itself, as hydrogen chloride, as chlorine containing organic compounds such as perchloroethylene and as inorganic chlorides. The most common sources of chlorine in the atmosphere are from which it is manufactured or used to produce other chemicals. Hydrogen chloride is evolved in numerous industrial chemical processes. The main effects of chlorine and its compounds are respiratory irritation from chlorine, corrosion by hydrogen chloride and damage to vegetation from chlorine and hydrogen chloride. DDT and PCBs, the persistant chemicals are considered to be worldwide atmospheric contaminants. Being inert and essentially harmless at ground level, CFCs have found many uses. As freon, they are the cooling agents in refrigerators and in automobile airconditioners. They are the foaming agents in the rigid foams used to insulate refrigerators and to protect fast foods, and in the flexible foams used for mattresses, sofa cushions and car seats. They are essential and seem to be irreplaceable in cleaning computer chips. They serve as dry cleaning solvents and are very popular as propellants in spray cans. The average residence time of CFCs in atmosphere is between 60-75 years depending on latitude. They are so inert in the lower atmosphere that they can float unhindered into the stratosphere, where the chlorine in the CFCs combine with ozone to generate molecular oxygen and chlorine oxide. The latter is then broken down by an oxygen radical regenerating chlorine that break down another molecule of ozone. Decrease in ozpone layer will lead to increase in skin cancer in humans.

Hydrocarbons and photochemical oxidants are also present in the atmosphere. An analysis of urban air has identified 56 different hydrocarbons. These are non toxic and do not pose any hazards at the level they are present in the atmosphere. However, they react with nitrogen oxides in the presence of sunlight and cause photochemical smog. Smog and its specific components produce physical, chemical and biological effects. It causes chemical damage to rubber, clothing, paints and exposed surfaces. The photochemical reaction results in the formation of ozone and other oxidants. These oxidants in the short run cause soreness, coughing, difficulty in breathing and tightness in chest. In the long run, they lead to impaired lung-function and an increased susceptibility to respiratory infection. Benzene is a cause of leukemia in rubber and chemical industries workers and is present in the air from refinery operations and gasoline combustion (Majumdar *et al.*, 1995). Lead and lead salts produced in the atmosphere by automobile emissions, combustion of coal and fuel pesticides damage the nervous system causing deadening of the nerve sense receptors. It is a cumulative poison and can be absorbed through the skin and by ingestion. It causes nervous disorders in children including decrease in Intelligence Quotient (IQ) and hyperactivity and kidney damage leading to high blood pressure in both children and adults. A burning feeling of feet is noticed in cases of lead poisoning. It also causes anaemia and therefore prevents absorption of vitamin cyanocobalamine resulting in malnutrition. Lead poisoning also causes bleeding.

Chemicals present in indoor air resulting from synthetic and natural materials used for carpeting, foam insulation, wall covering and furnitures may cause various health problems. Glue used in some plywood gives off formaldehyde. Latex carpet is a source of phenylcyclohene. Photocopying machine and computer printers are a source of toxic organic substances such as toluene. Many commercial products such as furnitures, polishes, glues, cleaning agents, cosmetics, deodorizers, pesticides and solvents used in the home contribute to the toxicity of indoor air. Headaches and eye irritation are common as a result of poor air quality at homes and work places (Nero, 1988).

## Toxic Food Additives

Chemicals added deliberately to impart some desirable quality or property to the food stuffs and to improve their shelf-life, stability, appearance, colour, texture and flavour are called 'additives' Functionally these are acidulants, antioxidants, bleaches, colours, emulsifiers, flavours, flavour enhancers, preservatives, stabilizers and thickeners, sweeteners, tenderisers, anticaking and moisture-retaining agents. Salting meat was the first of many preservation techniques to keep meat from spoiling. In the early 1900s, boric acid, formaldehyde, lead salts and salicylic acid were used as common but toxic food additives.

Carbonates and phosphates of calcium and magnesium, silicates of calcium, magnesium, aluminium and sodium, silicon dioxide, metallic soaps are added to table salt, onion powder to keep them free-flowing. Sorbitol is added to pastries and packaged cakes and glycerine to lozenges for preventing them from drying out and becoming hard. Newer additives like dimethyl- and polysiloxane are used to prevent foaming in edible oils and fats while deep frying and as release agents in confectionery. The safety of synthetic food additives has always been a subject of debate and discussion.

In order to build sensory qualities like colour, texture, flavour and temperature into the food, additives are incorporated. Food colours, when properly added to the food products, enhance its aesthetic appeal. Edible food colours may be natural or synthetic. Pigments occurring in plant and animal tissues *viz.*, yellow or orange red coloured carotenoids in carrot, orange, peaches, tomatoes, banana skins, corn and apricot; chlorophyll as a geen pignment in leaves; red, blue and violet pigment anthocyanins in beetroot, plums, raspberries, cabbage and black grape skins, yellow pigment flavonoids in leaves and petals of plants. Among permitted synthetic colours, azo dye such as tartrazine, sunset yellow, carmisine, amaranth, chocolate brown, red, violet, black reythrosine etc form the main group (Blumenthal, 1990). The colouring agents make even synthetic foods resembles the real ones. Making use of this fact food manufacturers add colours to foods, canned fruits and soft drinks. It is claimed that azo dyes are potentially carcinogenic (Ames, 1983). Synthetic colours may produce adverse allergic reactions in certain sensitive individuals. Tartrazine has been shown to increase histamine levels in the blood resulting in allergies. Colour have also been used in association with flavours to increase the variety and range of products. Saffron, paprika, sandalwood and turmeric are used as colouring as well as flavouring agents. During the past few years, a number of approved colours has fallen from 11 to 8 and their maxium limit has also been reduced.

Flavouring agents include all spices and natural fruit flavours as well as artificial flavours such as vaniline. Synthetic flavours are obtained from raw materials from natural sources, petrochemicals or coal-tar. Vanilla extract is the commonest flavouring agent used to flavour sweets, ice-creams, chocolates, cakes, pastries and custards. Saffron from stigmas and styles of the flowers of *Crocus sativus*, chocolate brown cmpound from cacoa beans, turmeric from *Curcuma longa,* pista colour from Pistachio nut, peppermint from *Mentha spicata* are common examples of colouring and flavouring compounds. Synthetic flavours like monosodium glutamate (MSG) are used to intensify, strengthen or alter the flavour or smell of food items. Chinese food containing a large amount of MSG develops 'Chinese restaurent syndrome' among regular visitors in which they suffer from chest pain, headache, a burning sensation in arms and neck and retinal diseases (Olney, 1982). The other flavour enhancers are guanosine 5'-disodium phosphate, inosine 5'-disodium phosphate, sodium 5'-ribonucleotide. They are mainly used in crispies, snacks and slow frozen potato products.

Preservatives are incorporated in food products to improve their shelf-life and prevent spoilage. Some additives like mono- and diglycerides retards the salting of bread due to which the bread loses its 'bounce' or springiness, an indicator of freshness. Preservatives are also used to restrict the growth of microorganisms and consequently reduce the risk of food poisoning. Antioxidants are used mainly to retard or prevent oxidative rancidity in fats and oils and to minimize the oxidative destruction of vitamins and essential fatty acids. Certain additives such as lactose and sulphites are known to cause allergic manifestations in some people. Infant weaning foods are artificially flavoured to make them acceptable to children, even milk contains a variety of flavouring substance, from pineapple, raspberry to coffee flavours. Ice cream with emulsifiers is more creamy than icy, coloured and flavoured. Sodium carboxymethyl cellulose is a common ingredient in ice-creams and amino azotoluene, a yellow colour used in butter have been recently found to be cancer causing substance. The possible presence of potentially carcinogenic polycyclic aromatic hydrocarbons in mineral oil used in chewing gum and in the processing of confectionery is a matter of concern (Cohen, 1987).

Certain chemicals are sometimes added to foodstuffs for fraudulent purpose. Lead chromate (a yellow colour) is added to turmeric powder, asbestos is used as a contaminant in talcs used to polish pulses and rice, amaranth, a red food colour and dimethyl stilbestrol, a hormone used to fatten up poultry and cattle for slaughter, potassium aluminium sulphate used to give tang to pickles, copper or zinc salts used to intensify the colour of green vegetables like peas are some of the examples of additives used for fraudulent purpose.

Some foodstuffs naturally contain poisonous substances. For instance, wild mushrooms contain phylloidine, a polypeptide which is not destroyed even after cooking. Selenium containing vegetables from plants grown in selenium rich soils, or spinach and amaranth leaves which contain large amounts of oxalic acid often cause food poisoning. Bitter almonds and rangoon beans sometimes contain excessive amounts of glucosides which on hydrolysis yield poisonous cyanides. Erucic acid occurring naturally in mustard and rapeseed oil is often responsible for inflammation of heart muscles. Khesari Dal contains poisonous derivatives of the amino acid alanine and excessive use of this pulse can cause crippling lathyrism. Excessive use of insecticides, rodenticides, fungicides, germicides, antiseptics, hormones during farming may leave some residue in the food stuffs which when enter the body cause various harmful effects in humans (Concon, 1988).

## Hazards of Domestic Chemicals

Ethylene glycol is familiar to almost every car owner as automobile antifreeze but it is also used in a wide range of other products such as polyester, cosmetics, paints, ink, glues, wood stains, tobacco products and automobile brake fluid. It is a popular industrial solvent used for manufacturing countless other chemicals. Cosmetics, particularly those with a creamy texture, often contain such chemicals. Chronic exposure to this chemical cause headache and throat irritation. If large amounts are inhaled or swallowed, convulsions and coma will also occur. Other signs of overexposure to the solvent include irregularities of the eye, such as rapid eye movement, paralysis of eye muscles and blurred vision. Symptoms like high blood pressure, rapid heart beat and shallow rapid breathing are experienced after 24 hours and irreversible kidney damage caused after 24-72 hours (Linnanvuo-Laitinen and Huttumen, 1986). Hydroquinone is a skin bleaching agent, an artificial suntan agent and an important ingredient in photographic developer. The consumer or hobbyist can come into contact with hydroquinone either by using one of several skin-bleaching products, freckle remover, or suntan lotions or by using a photographic developer containing the compound. Ingestion of moderate amounts of hydroquinone can cause ringing in ears, nausea, dizziness, a sense of suffocaton, increased respiratory rate, vomiting pallor, muscle twitching, headache, difficulty in breathing, blue fingers, delirium and collapse (Sax, 1988). Prolonged exposure can lead to discolouration of the eyelids, clouded eye lenses and eye colour changes. Anemia and loss of skin pigmentation have also been associated with chronic exposure. Hydroquinone has recently been found to cause bladder cancer in mice and short term tests reveal that the compound may also be a mutagen.

Efforts are being made to create environmental awareness in public through various ways including enactment of laws. Unfortunately, due to lack of proper implementation of policies and strict enforcement of Acts, the degradation of environment continued unchecked (Tripathi and Tripathi, 2000). Depletion of forest, population growth, vehicular emission, use of hazardous chemicals and various other undesirable human activities are mainly responsible for degraded scenario of environmental health all over the world. Infact, hunger, ignorance, ecological degradation, hopelessness, fiscal crisis etc are retarding the progress of environmental cleaning programmes in different parts of globe specially in underdeveloped and developing world.

## SUMMARY

It has been estimated that over five million chemical substances have been identified; about 70,000 of these are marketed, may be half of them in quantity. Several thousand new ones are found every year and about a tenth of new discoveries reach the market. Not only are the numbers of substances growing rapidly in the chemical revolution but the quantity produced is increasing in a proportion resulting in various health hazards. The problem of industrial waste disposal and river pollution, confront the public health authorities in every countries. Indiscriminate discharges of these pollutants lower the oxygen content of the stream and are offensive to eye and nose, dangerous for aquatic life and unsuitable for horticultural and agricultural purposes. The industrial effluents containing compounds of mercury, copper, iron or nitrogen etc. are considered harmful to marine life and have been found to enter the aquatic and human food chain through bio-accumulation and bio-magnification. It is obvious that the civilization will continue to require increasing amount of fuel, transportation, industrial chemicals, fertilizers, pesticides and countless other products. It will also continue to produce waste products of all descriptions. Environmental toxicology will undoubtedly continue to be a subject of major concern among various socities of the world. Protection of human health and environment from chemicals and pollution of all kinds has increased during the last few decades. Regulations have become more complex and difficult to interpret. Whatever pesticides and chemicals introduced deliberately into the environment poseing threat to health and environment.

## REFERENCES

- Aggrawal, A. (1997). Silver. *Science Reporter* **34**: 40-43.
- Ames, B.N. (1983). Dietary carcinogens and anticarcinogens. *Science* **221**: 1256-1264.
- Andrews, L. and Snyder, R. (1986). Toxic effects of solvents and vapours. In *Casarett and Doull's Toxicology: The Basic Science of Poisons*, 3 rd edition (Eds. Klaassen, C.D., Amdur, M.O. and Doull, J.) Macmillan., New York .
- Bindra, O.S. (1971). The pesticidal pollution of water. *Everyday Science* **16**: 1.
- Blumenthal, D. (1990) Red No 3 and other colourful controversies. *FDA Consumer* **24**: 18-21.
- Cohen, Leonard A. (1987) Diet and cancer. *Scientific American* **257**: 42-48.
- Concon, J.M. (1988) *Food Toxicology, Part B: Contaminants and Additives*, Marcel Dekker, New York
- Environmental Protection Agency (1988) *Updated Health Effect Assessment for Acetone*, EFA-600/8-89-085, Cincinnati, Ohio.
- Francis, B.M. (1994). *Toxic Substances in the Environment*, John Wiley & Sons, Inc. New York, pp. 61-92.
- Galston, A.W. (1979). Herbicides: A Mixed Blessing. *Bioscience* **29**: 85-94.
- Goyer, R.A. (1986). Toxic Effects of Metals, In *Casarett and Doull's Toxicology: The Basic Science of Poisons*, 3rd edition (Ed. Klaassen, C.D., Amdur, M.O. and Doull, J.), pp. 582-635, Macmillan, New York.
- Gupta, P.K. and Gupta, R.C. (1977). Debate on DDT. *Pesticides* **11**: 16.

- Kornhauser, A., Vrtacnik, M. and DeSilva, E. (1997) Information support for toxic waste management. *Nature & Resources* **33**: 2-17.

- Korsak, R.J. and Sato, M.M. (1977). Effects of chronic organophosphorous pesticide exposure on the central nervous system. *Clinical Toxicology* **11**: 83.

- Leverett, D.H. (1982). Fluorides and the changing prevalence of dental caries. *Science* **217**: 26-30.

- Linnanvuo-Laitinen, M. and Huttumen, K. (1986) Ethylene glycol intoxication. *Clinical Toxicology* **24**: 167-174.

- Maujumdar, S. K., Miller, E.W. and Brenner, F.L. (1995) *Environmental Contaminants, Ecosystems and Human Health*, Pennysylvania Academy of Sciences, Easton, Pennsylvania, pp. 507.

- Mehrotra, K.N. (1983). Benefits and hazards of pesticides to society. *Pesticide Information*, 38.

- Nero, A.V. (1988). Controlling indoor air pollution. *Scientific American*, **258**: 42-48.

- Olney, J.W. (1982). Toxic effects of glutamate and related compounds in the retina and the b r a i n . *Retina* **2**: 341-359.

- Perl, D.P. (1985). Relationship of Aluminium to Alzheimer's Disease. *Environ. Hclth. Persp.* **63**: 149-153.

- Rahmani, A.R. (1999). Fatal foods. *Down to Earth*, Jan, 15, 34-35.

- Ramachandran, M. (1973). DDT and its metabolites in human body fat in India. *Bull. World Health Organisation*, **49**: 637.

- Rao, K.L. (1979). *India's water wealth*, Orient Longman Limited, New Delhi.

- Sax, N.I. (1988). Hydroquinone. *Dangerous Properties of Industrial Material Report*, January/February, pp.51-60.

- Sundareson, B.B. (1984). Hazards of Industrial effluents. *The Financial Express*, 15th April.

- Tripathi, G. and Tripathi, Y.C. (2000). Current status of environmental pollution in India, In: *Industry Environment and Pollution* (Eds., Goel P.K. and Kumar, A.), pp.317- 343, ABD Publishers, India.

- Wang, H.H. and MacMohan (1979). Mortility of workers employed in the manufacture of chlordane and heptachlor. *J. Occup. Med.* **21**: 745.

# 19

# Environmental Legislation: Indian Context

*Kshemendra Mani Tripathi, N. K. Chaubey, and V. Tripathi*

## Introduction

The post second world war witnessed rapdid industrialization by the developed and the developing nations. As a result environment is the casualty. The anthropogenic and non-anthropgenic source of pollutants brings environmental changes and consequently may become cause of pathogensis of several disease states. The consequence of diseases account for a considerable economic burden to governments worldwide. Unitl 'seventies' no concrete International law emerged regarding environment protection. It was in 1972 that United Nations Conference on Human Environment[1] was held at Stockholm. The motto of Stockholm Conference was "world has just one environment", hence measures must be taken at the global level to prevent environment pollution and ecological imbalances. After the Stockholm conference, a number of Treaties/Conventions took place, *viz.* The World Charter for Nature, 1982; The Bio-Diversity Convention, 1987; The Montreal Protocol (Ozone treaty), 1987; The Kuala Lumpur Conference, 1992. Apart from all these conventions the representatives of 170 nations met at Rio-de-Janerio in the United Nations Conference on Environment and Development, 1992. Rio was chosen as the venue for 'Earth Summit'[2] ('Earth Summit' projected the necessity that sustainable development of the Earth is simply not an 'action' it is in fact a 'requirement' which is increasingly imposed by the limits of the nature to absorb the punishments which humanity has inflicted on it to effectively highlight the consequences of man's recklessness and to devise strategies to combat the ecglical disasters. The other point of discussion, which the countries discussed in Stockholm, was whether environment protection and economic development were consistent or antithetical to each other.

In India there was growing need for statutory enactment to tackle the problems of environmental pollution. In 1974, Water Act was passed for the prevention, control and abatement of water pollution Then the two acts, Air Act, 1981 and the Environment Protection Act, 1986 were passed as India's obligation to multilateral treaties and conventions. These Acts dealt specifically with their objects of environment protection. Thereby, after the Bhopal Gas Disaster, the government passed the Public Liability Insurance Act, 1991 to provide for mandatory insurance to the victims of any future industrial accidents. In order to fulfil the international obligations and also to meet the challenges like Bhopal Gas Disaster the National Environment Tribunal Act, 1995 was passed to provide a separate forum for environment cases and to impose strict liability on the ecociders.

## INDIAN STATUTORY RIGHTS

### A. Water (Prevention and Control of Pollution) Act, 1974

In the year 1974, the Water Act came into force in pursuance of Article 252 (1) of the Constitution, consequent on resolution passed by all the Houses of Legislature of the States of Assam, Bihar, Gujarat, Haryana, Himachal Pradesh, Jammu & Kashmir, Madhya Pradesh, Rajasthan, Tripura and West Bengal.

The Water Act, 1974, which tends to provide legal control of water Pollution, was passed with the following objects:

1. To provide for prevention and control of water pollution and maintaining or restoring of wholesomeness of water (in streams and wells of sewer on land.)
2. To establish Central and States Boards with a view to carrying out the above purposes, and
3. For conferring on and assisting to such boards powers relating there to for matters connected.

Section 3 of the Act establishes a Central Board for Prevention and Control of Water Pollution and similar Boards in the States. These Boards are empowered to control pollution primarily through standards laid down by them and the issue of consent orders, stiff penalties have been provided by the Act, namely, imprisonment which shall not be less than six months but which may be extended to six years and fines.

Under the existing enactment the affected groups could not go to the court directly without the sanction of the Board. This was a major defect in implementing the provisions of the Act and stands against the declared goals.

However, apart from legislation of 1974, attempts for legal control of water pollution were made by other legislations also. Section 277 of the Indian Penal Code which lays down that whoever voluntarily corrupts or fouls the water of any public spring or vesorvior, so as to render it less fit for the purpose for which it is ordinarily used, shall be punished with imprisonment of either description for a term which may extend upto three months or with fine which may extends upto Rs. 1,000, or both. Section 278 lays down that whoever voluntarily vitiates the atmosphere in any place so as to make it noxious to the health of the person, in general dwelling or carrying on business in the neighbourhood or passing along a public way, shall be punished with fine which may extend to Rs. 500.

There is a provision in Factories Act, 1948 with regard to the disposal of water and effluents by factories. Section 12 provides that:

1. Effective arrangement shall be made in every factory for disposal of water and effluents due to manufacturing process carried therein, and
2. The State Govenment may make rules prescribing the arrangement to be made under sub-section (1) or requiring that the arrangements made in accordance with sub-section (1) shall be approved by such authority as may be precribed.

Under Section 133 of the Criminal Procedure Code, 1973, the Magistrate has been given power to order that any unlawful observation or annoyance should be removed from any public place a from any way, river or channel which is or may be lawfully used by public. The Supreme Court decision in Municipal Council, @ Ratlam v. Vardichand clearly shows that Section 133 can be really potent in curbing pollution.

## Scheme of the Act

The Water Pollution Act consist of 64 sections comprised within eight chapters. Chapter 1 (Sec. 1&2) contains preliminary provisions, including definitions. The most important definitions are those contained in following provision: Section 2 (e): 'Pollution,; Section 2 (j): 'Stream'; and Section 2 (k): 'Trade Effluent'.

Section 47 of the Act provides for offences by companies, i.e.,

1. Where an offence under this Act has been committed by a company, every person who at the time of the offence committed was in-charge of and responsible to the company for the conduct of the company, as well as the company, shall be deemed to be guiltly of the offence and shall be liable to be proceeded and punished accordingly: provided that nothing contained in this sub-section shall render any such person liable to any punishment provided in this Act if he proves that offence was committed without his knowledge or that he exerted all due diligence to prevent the commission of such offence.

2. Notwithstanding anything contained in the sub-section (1), where an offence under this Act has been committed with the consent or connivance of, or is attributed to any neglect on the part of

any Director, Manager, Secretary, or other officer of the company, such as director, Manager, Secretary or other shall also be liable to be proceeded against and punished accoordingly.

*Explanation*: For the purpose of this 'section'

a) 'Company'means any body corporate, and includes a firm or other association of individual

b) 'Director, in relation to firm means a partner in the firm.*/

## Offences by Government Department

Section 48 of the Act states, if any offence has been committed by any Government Department, then in that case the Head of the Government Department shall be deemed to be guilty of the offence and shall be liable to be proceeded against and punished accordigly. But the punishment to the Head of Government Department is subject to exemption if he is able to prove that offence was committed without his knowledge or due to diligence had been exercised to prevent such commission of such offence.

## B. Water (Prevention and Control of Pollution) Cess Act, 1977

The preamble of Water (Prevention and Control of Pollution) Cess Act says that 'an Act to provide for the levy and collection of a cess on water consumed by persons carrying on certain industries and by local authorities, with a view to augmenting the resources of the Central Board and the State Boards for the prevention and control of water pollution constituted under the Water (Prevention and Control of Pollution) Act, 1974. Thus, this Act can be said to be an Act which supplements the Water (Prevention and Control of Pollution ) Act, 1974.

Section 3 of this Act provides for levy and collection of cess. Sub-section (1) says that there shall be levided and collected a cess for the purpose of the Water (Prevention and Control of Pollution) Act, 1974 and utilization there under. Sub-section (2) says that the cess under sub-section (1) shall be payable by-

a) every person carrying on specific industry, and

b) every local authority shall collect cess on the basis of water consumed by such person or local authority, as the cess may be, for any of the purposes specified in column (1) of Schedule II, at such rate, not exceeding the rate specified in the corresponding entry in column (1) thereof, as the Central Government may by notification in the Official Gazette, from time to time specify. 'Specified Industry'means any industry specified in Schedule 1.

Section 7 speaks of Rebate and says that where any person or local authority, liable to pay the cess under this Act, installs any plant, for the treatment of sewage, or trade effluent, such person or local authority shall, from such date as may be prescribed, entitled for a rebate of 70 per cent of cess payable by such person or local authority.

## Certain other Features of Cess Act, 1977

The Boards set up under the Act have to lay down standards of pollution. The Board is empowered to take samples of effluents under prescribed conditions and following the presecribed procedure. The Boards are endowed with the jurisdiction to pass 'consent' orders for putting trade and sewage effluents into the streams. Appeals against the order of the State Board can be given to such authority as the State Government may think fit to constitute. The Government has also been given the power of revision over the order of the Board.

For the contravention of the standards laid down by the State Board for violation of the provisions relating to the consent by the Board, stiff penalties have been provided, like-when a person commits an offence for which he had been convicted earlier the court can publish his name in newspapers. The cost of such publication should be met by such perosn. No court can take congnizance of any offence under the Act except on a complaint made by or with the previous sanction of the State Board.

The State Board can also apply to the Court for restraining apprehended pollution of water. So also in the case of emergency the court's aid could be sought by the State Board for removal of the polluting matter or for remedying or mitigating the pollution caused.

No civil court shall have jurisdiction to any suit or proceedng in respect of any matter which an appellate authority under the Act is empowered by or under the Act of determine. No injunctions shall be granted by any court or other authority in respect of any action taken or in pursuance of Water Act or Rules.

## C. Air (Prevention and Control of Pollution) Act, 1981

It was not before the year 1972, when India participated at the United Nations Confernece on Human Environment held in Stockholm, that some concrete measures were taken by India regarding environment protection. The same is true with the enactment of Air (Prevention and Control of Pollution) Act, 1981. Prior to year 1981, there was no concrete effort to legally control air pollution. Although, there are instances when the States in the British Rule had brought about first ever pollution control law. The Bombay Nuisance Act, 1912 to control smoke emission. Unfortunately, the provisions of the Bombay Nuisance Act could not be effectively enforced.

The Air (Prevention and Control of Pollution) Act of 1981 was enacted by the Parliament by invoking of the Central Government's power under Article 253 to make laws implementing decisions taken at international conferences.

The Air (Prevention and control of Pollution) Act covers/extends to the whole of India. The Preamble of the Act reads as follows: "An Act to provide for prevention, control and abatement of air pollution, for the establishment, with a view to carrying out the aforesaid purposes, of boards, for conferring on and assigning to such Boards connected therewith."

## Scheme of the Act

The Air pollution Act consists of 54 sections comprised within 8 chapters. Chapter (section 1 & 2) contains preliminary provisions, definitions. The most important definations are those contained in following provisions: Section 2 (i): "air pollution". Section 2 (j): emission"; Section 2 (k): "industrial plant"; Section 2 (m): "occupier";

## Central and State Pollution Control Boards

Section 3 and 4 of the Air (Prevention and Control of Pollution) Act provides that in the States, where there is already existing a Central Board for the Prevention and Control of Water Pollution shall also exercise the power and functions for the prevention and control of air pollution. (Section 3 of Water) (Prevention and Control of Pollution) Act, 1974.

Section 4 clarifies that in the States where a States Pollution Control Board has already existed then such Board shall be the State Board for Prevention and Control of Air Pollution under the Act.

## Power and Functions of Boards

Chapter III of Air (Prevention and Control of Pollution) Act, 1981 deals with powers and functions of the Boards. under section 16 of the Act, the main function of the Central Board shall be to improve the quality of air and to prevent, control and abate air pollution.

## Prevention and Control of Air Pollution

Prevention and control of air pollution is dealt in Chapter IV of the Act. Section 19 of the Act deals with declaring of 'air pollution control area or areas'. The State Government may, after consultation with the State Board, notify such 'area'. The State-Government has the prerogative to either extend or reduce any air pollution control area or may even create new air pollution control area. The new 'control area may be merged into one or more existing control areas or any part or parts thereof.

The State Government has also the use of fuel, or any burning of material, after consultation with State Board, in any 'air pollution control area'. It may do so by notifying in the Official Gazette.

Section 20 of the Act deals with giving instructions to the concerned authority in-charge of registration of motor vechicle under the Motor Vehicles Act, 1939, in order to make sure that standards for emission of air pollutants from automobiles laid down by the State are compiled.

## Penalties and Procedure

The provisions relating to penalties and procedures are dealt under Chapter VI of the Act. Section 37: the provisions under this section say that any failure to comply with the provisions of Section 21 or Section 22 or directions issued under Section 31 A (closure, prohibition, regulation, stoppage of electricity, water, etc.) are punishable with imprisonment for a term which shall not be less than one year and six months but which may extend to six years and with fine.

Where the failure continues, an additional fine is also leviable which may extend to Rs.5000 for every day of continuing failure after the conviction for the first such failure.

Where the above failure continues beyond a period of one year after the date of conviction, the offender shall be punishable with imprisonment for a term which shall not be less than two years which may extend to seven years with fine.

## D. Environment Protection Act, 1986

It was back in the year 1972 that National Committee on Environmental Planning and Co-ordination (NCEPC) was set by the Department of Science and Technology to identify and investigate problems of preserving or improving the human environment and also to propose solutions for environmental problems. Earlier, the enactment of Water and Air Pollution Control Acts were dealt with specific subjects *viz* air and water. It was only in the year 1980, which saw the setting up of the Tiwari Committee so as to review and to recommend legislative measures and administrative machinery for ensuring environmental, protections. Recommendations of the Tiwari Committee witnessed setting up a new Department of Environment, which became a part of the new Ministry of Environment and Forest in January, 1985.

## Objects of the Act

The Environment Protection Act came into existence due to certain environment hazards which were left uncovered in earlier environment legislation, *viz*, Water Act and Air Act. Existing laws generally focused on specific types of pollution or on specific categories of hazardous substances. There were inadequate linkages in handling matters of industrial and environmental safety. Control mechanisms to guard against slow, insidious build up of hazardous substances, especially new chemicals, in the environment are weak. Because of multiplicity of regulatory agencies, there was need for an authority which can assume the lead role for studying, planning and implementing long term requirements of environmental safety and to give direction to, and co-ordinate a system of speedy and adequate response to emergency situations threatening environment[4].

## Powers of the Central Government

Chapter II of the Act deals with general power of the Central Government so as to take measures in protecting and improving environment, and preventing, controlling or abating environment pollution. Section 3 rests power in the Central Government to which it has the prerogative to take all such measures which are necessary or expedient for environment protection. Under Section 3(2) (viii), the Central Government can lay down procedures and safeguards for the handling of hazardous substances;

- examination of such manufacturing processes, materials and substances as are likely to cause environmental pollution.
- carrying out and sponsoring investigations and research relating to problems of environmental pollution;
- establishment or recogniation of environmental laboratories and institutions to carry out the functions entrusted to such environment laboratories and institutes under such Act;
- preparation of manuals, codes or guides relating to the prevention, control and abatement of environmental pollution.

Section 6 gives authorisation to the Central Government, by giving notification in the official Gazettes to frame rules in regard to any matters referred under Section 3 of the Act.

## Prevention, Control and Abatement of Environmental Pollution

Chapter III of the Act imposes certain restrictions and directions on the persons who are handling any industry, operation or processes, *viz.*, under Section 7 of the Act there is a prohibition on the person who is carrying on industry, operation etc. preventing him from discharging or emission of environmental pollutants in excess of than the standard laid down.

Secondly, Section 8 requires the compliance of certain procedural safeguards in case any hazardous substance being used in any process, operation or industry.

Thirdly, Section 9, lays down certain measures to be taken and intimated by the person in charge of any industry, etc. and secondly, the action to be taken by the agencies responsible under the Act. That is to say that if the person apprehends any accident or unforeseen act or event in consequence of excess discharge of environmental pollutant". Henceforth-

- he shall intimate the facts of such occurrence or apprehension of such occurrence; and
- be bound, if called upon, to render all assistance, to such authorities or agencies as may be prescribed.

Fourthly, Section 10 gives power to the Central Government to enter and inspect any place for the purpose of performing any function entrusted under the legislation. This section also enjoins upon the person carrying on any industry, operation or process or handling any hazardous substances to render all assistance to the Central Government, and any failure on the part of the concerned person, shall be held against him and he shall be punishable under this Act.

Section 11 of the Act empowers "the Central Government or any officer empowered by it in this behalf, shall have power to take, for the purpose of analysis, sample of air, water, soil or other substances from any factory premises or other place in such manner as may be prescribed".

The Environmental Protection Act is special in comparison to other environmental legislation in context to setting up of environmental laboratories or recognise a laboratory or institute as an environmental laboratory. The Central Governments under Section 12 of the Act is authorised to recognise one or more laboratories or institutes as laboratories to carry out the function as entrusted upon it. Simultaneously, the Central Government may make rules specifying the functions of the laboratories, procedures to be followed in carrying out the tests, or any other such matter which is necessary or expedient to do so.

Section 15 specifies the penalties to be imposed on those who contravene any of the provisions of the Act or the Rules under Section 15 (1) any contravention of rules or orders or directions, or each such failure be punishable with imprisment for a term which may extend to 5 years or with fine which may extend to one lakh rupees or with both, and in case the failure or contravention continues, with additional fine which may extend to Rs. 5000/ for every day during which such failure or contravention continues after the conviction for the first such failure or contravention. As per section 15(2), if the contravention continues as referred under sub-section (1), the terms of imprisonment may extend to seven years.

## E. Public Liability Insurance Act, 1991

The Public Liability Insurance Act, 1991, was passed to provide relief to the members of the general public who became victims of industrial accidents. This legislation expressly excludes the 'workmen' from its purview since they are entitled to relief under the Workmens' Compensation Act, 1923. For the purpose of fixing liability for payment of compensation under the Public Liability Act, 1991, no distinction has been made between public sector and private sector or between an individual or government official. National as well as multinational companies are equally liable. Any person who has control over handling of any hazardous substance would be liable to pay compensation under the Act.

## Scheme of the Act

The PLIA consists of 23 sections and a schedule. Short title and commencement are dealt in Section 1, while section 2 contains several definitons. The substantive provisions are mainly contained in Section 3 and 4.

## F. National Environment Tribunal Act (NETA), 1995

The Supreme Court of India, in number of cases, pointed out the difficulties involved in adjudicating the environmental disputes which mainly included judicial delay and lack of expertise in handling of the environmental justice. The judiciary suggested to constitute a separate forums₅ (court suggested set up a "Enviornment Court" and directed the Government of India to set up a "Ecological Sciences Research Group", duly constituted by neutral scientific experts of respective fields, which would assist the courts in complex environment cases) to settle the 'litigation relating to environment. The NETA tries to fill this gap in the administration of environmental justice.

The NETA, 1995 provides strict liability for damages arising out of any accident. Section 3 (3) of the Act provides the apportionment of compensation on the 'equitable basis' among those who are responsible for the pollution. The present legislation, intesestingly, follows 'no-fault' principle in case of payment of compensation.

## Concluding Observations

The irony of Indian Environmental legislations is that it has primarily adopted a system of criminal sanctions to preserve natural resources and regulate their use. Civil compensation recovered through private citizens suite plays a peripheral role in the overall regulatory strategy.[6]

The judiciary (the Supreme Court and High Courts) has given the thought that environmental degradation is a social problem, hence, environmental awareness is must. In one of the judgement[7], the court has accepted in principle that through the medium of 'education awareness' of the environment, and its problems related to pollution, should be taught as a compulsory subject. The court also directed that since higher education was to be tackled by the Central Government-the University Grant Commission shall take appropriate steps to introduce a course on environment in the Universities. The efforts made by the judiciary is a laudable one, especially in the absence of any specific right to environment in the Constitution. Judiciary has tried to evolve a new fundamental right to environment through its various judgements. Simultaneously, it has also tried to evolve fundamental right to environmental education, fundamental right to live in clean environment, fundamental right to right to know/ information, fundatmental right to compensation, etc. hence, widening the scope of enviromental protection in India.

## REFERENCES

- For principles enumerated in the Conference-see: Environment Law (Documents)- International Environmental Law; Vol. II; Part one; compiled by CEERA research team, National Law School of India University, Bangalore, 1998.

- see Ashok Jain- 'Law and Environment; Ascent Publication, New Delhi, 1998. Also see for Principles Enumerated at Earth summit: International Legal Material; Vol. IV, July 1992.

- AIR 1980 SC 1622.

- Published in the Gazette of India, Extraodinary, Pt. II, See I dated 26.5.1986. (See particularly-M.C. Mehta v. Union of India, AIR 1987 SC965.)

- See also-Foundation v. Konkan Rly. AIR1992 BOM 4716.

- For detailed discussion, see- 'Environment Law and Policy in India- case, Material and Statues': Armin Rosencranz, Shyam Divan, Martha L. Noble; N.M. Tripathi Pvt. Ltd. 1992.7.

- M.C. Mehta v. Union of India, AIR 1992 SC 382.

# 20

# Biodiversity Crises in the Geological Past and Present

*K. L. Shrivastava*

In the Earth science, as part of the principle of uniformitarianism, the present has been treated as a key to understand the past. Sciences like Actuo-Paleontology are entirely based on the principle of uniformitarianism. As human beings, we belong only to a fraction of the geological time, thus are unable to understand a mass extinction and / or biodiversity crises episode which might have remained spread over certain spans of the geological times; most likely we are now a part of it.

Assuming that the principle of uniformitarianism can also be implemented *vice versa*, a study of biodiversity crises in the geological history must be of great help to understand the present aspects of the environmental biology.

In the present article, an attempt has been made to connect various segments of biodiversity crises in the geological times; both the well defined once and those which are not so well identified. In the light of biodiversity crises in the geological times the present time of biodiversity has also been discussed.

## Major Biodiversity Crises and Mass Extinctions

Paleontologists recognize six mass extinctions in the geological past. The number was until recently believed (Wilson, 2000) to be five but one more Late Proterozoic to early cambrian times has been added.

**Late Proterozoic - Early Cambrian (900 Ma to 500 Ma):** A series of biodiversity crises occurred during the initial radiation of animals during the Late Proterozoic and Early Cambrian. This is being treated as first known marine biodiversity crisis.

The earliest fossils appeared almost 3500 Ma ago, but until about 650 Ma the fossil record of life was limited to the microscopic remains of various unicellular organisms embedded in chert and the structures these microbes formed. Many microbial communities secreted calcium carbonate or trapped passing sedimentary grains. These activities produced finely laminated mats, domes, and columns known as stromatolites. Curiously, many stromatolites are very distinctive and some morphologies are restricted to particular intervals of time. About 900 million years ago the number of different types of stromatolites began a precipitous decline. This diversity crisis is believed to be due to the first appearance of burrowing and grazing animals. Today stromatolites are limited to high salinity bays, mainly.

**Late Ordovician ( ~ 438  Ma):** The first one out of the five great mass extinctions of the Phanerozic, time namely the Late Ordovician major diversity crisis had relatively less effect on the hisroty of life than any of the other major crises. It eliminated about sixty one per cent of marine genera. The limited impact on marine ecosystem may reflect that although all marine groups were effected, no major groups of animals became entirely extinct. Hence, ecological communities were able to reform relatively quickly. The Late Ordovician extinction occurred in several steps over one or two million years. A global cooling and major glaciation event coincide with the extinction interval. Resultant changes in sea level, so habitat area, are believed to have initiated the extinction.

**Late Devonian ( ~ 355 Ma):** The Late Devonian biodiversity crisis had a relatively greater long term effect, and this extinction lasted over several million years without any well defined extinction peaks. It culminated in the extinction of fifty five per cent marine genera. As the terrestrial ecosystems were in the developing stage, there is no indication of a correlative extinction on land. Tropical, shallow-water and reef ecosystems were affected more severely and coral dominated reef ecosystems which were so far dominating, did not recover untill Triassic. Presence of low oxygen waters is evident by formation of black limestones and shales Such dysaerobic waters may have been incursion from the deep ocean onto the shallow marine shelves. There is some evidence of an extraterrestrial impact too, near the extinction interval in the form of small glassy spherules.

**Permo-Triassic Boundary ( ~ 250 Ma):** During Late Permian - Early Triassic crisis, over a span of two to three million years, some forty nine per cent marine families and seventy two per cent genera disappeared. As per one of the estimates some ninety per cent marine species became extinct. On land vertibrates show extinction of some seventy five families. Shallow-water forms have been more severely affected than deeper-water species. Mobile forms like bivalves and gastropods were less heavily affected than attached life forms. Insects experienced the only major extinction event in their history. Plants show little evidence of mass extinction across Permo-Triassic boundary except interesting change in pollens and increase in fungal spores.

Permo-Triassic boundary shows pronounced physical change. Pangea, the single land mass, gradually started withdrawing, the sea lead to the exposure of much of Pangea during the latest Permian. It resulted into climatic instability and sea rise by perhaps 180 m or so. Also, in Siberia, the largest flood basalt erupted to caused severe climatic disruptions. This boundary also shows sharp changes in ocean chemistry (shift in C, S, O, Sr isotopes). Thus, climate must have been showing rapid cooling and warming both, one after other.

Possibly, a multitude of causes were involved in the extinction during Permo-Triassic boundary, including the loss in habitat area, and climatic effects of sea level drop, oceanic anoxia and the impact of the Siberian volcanism.

**End of Triassic ( ~ 205 Ma):** After suffering a series of Permo-Triassic mass extinctions marine communities show low diversity upto five million years but could be fully rejuvenated by Middle Triassic. The end Triassic mass extinction eliminated twenty three percent of both marine and terrestrial vertebrate families. Cephalopodes were particularly hard hit. There was a single episode rather then several phases of extinction, although not necessarily a catastrophic event.

Possible extinction could occur because of climatic change and a drop in sea level. At the end of this mass extinction the earliest dinosaurs radiated. Without its clear relationship with the extinction, some evidences of an extraterrestrial impact has been found near the extinction horizon.

**Cretacous - Tertiary boundary or K/T/ boundary ( ~ 65 Ma):** K/T boundary or Cretaceous-Tertiary mass extinction is the best known of all the mass extinctions. Some forty seven percent of marine genera disappeared during K/T boundary mass extinction but only fourteen percent of vertebrate families were affected. The oceanic ecosystems particularly were disrupted and almost all the marine groups experienced some degree of extinction. Foraminifera and alike skeletal microfossils were very hard hit. The large rudistid and inoceramid bivalves disappeared. The ammonite cephalopods have been decimated after very hay days just before. On land, the dinosaurs were completely wiped out and large animals suffered the most. Mammals did not experience much extinction. Also fresh water species like Crocodiles and Turtles were among least affected.

There was a dramatic change in plants of K/T boundary, fern spores became far more common for a brief duration and Early Cenozoic floras were quite different from those of the Late Cretaceous.

To establish the possible cause of K/T boundary mass extinction is a point of debate among geologists. A large extraterrestrial object (Comet or Meteorite) might have hit the planet earth. This theory is supported by availability of high irridium concentration at K/T boundary. Also, shocked quartz as an indication of impact is present at K/T boundary. Geologists have now evidence of an extraterrestrial impact at more than 100 boundary sections around the globe, including the Chixulub Crater (Mexico) and the Shiva Crater in the Indian ocean.

As extinction started well before the impact horizon so it does not seem a sole cause. The scientific debate is still on. The impact must have produced a dust cloud that would have circled the globe after several months, blocking the sunlight, so cooling the globe possibly, acid rain, unchecked wildfires and the direct effects of the blast (earthquake, tidal waves etc). must have exacerbated the extinction.

The constant reign of calcareous and siliceous organisms on the ocean floor provides such a record that provides persuasive evidence for very rapid extinction. Other evidences suggest that some species might have begun disappearing before the impact, but still the major cause of the extinction appears to be the impact.

Aftermath of K/T boundary shows creative aspects including

(i)   Both, flowering plants and mammals rapidly diversified and established themselves as the predominant group on land.
(ii)  Fish expanded, replacing the ammonite cephalopods.
(iii) Scleractiman corals took over as reef-builders in place of rudistid bivalves.

## Other Major Biodiversity CRISES and Mass Extinctions

Eocene/Oligocene ($\sim$ 36.5 Ma): The Eocene/Oilgocene extinction has some evidence for an extraterrestrial impact. However, current evidence suggests that the extinctions covered a period of perhaps 10 million years, and thus involves more than an impact. Calcareous and siliceous microplankton underwent a series of extinctions, as did some shallow-water marine invertebrates, particular molluscs. On land, plants provide evidence for at least two periods of global warming followed by global cooling, with the final cooling event being particularly severe. Vertebrates show a marked drop in diversity from the Mid-to Late Eocene, largely among crocodiles, turtles, and several mammal groups. Many of the mammals that disappeared in North America were considered archaic forms and were replaced by species better adapted to the less forested terrain that appeared at this time. Thus, there is considerable evidence that the extinctions and faunal replacements were intimately linked to climatic changes. Of particular interest are suggestions that the climatic changes were linked to the initial development of ice in Antarctica and the changing patterns of oceanic circulation caused by continental drift. Finally, it is worth remembering that much of our ability to reconstruct these complex patterns of change, particularly on land, reflects the relatively short interval since the Eocene.

Pleistocene ($\sim$ 1.6 Ma): The earth experienced numerous episodes of extensive continental glaciation, global cooling, and drops in sea level during the Pleistocene. Although cooling and glaciation have been invoked as causing earlier extinction episodes, the extinctions associated with glaciation were relatively minor. The major Late Pleistocene extinction focused on large terrestrial mammals. In North America, 37 genera of large mammals disappeared, South America lost 46 genera, Europe lost 13 genera, and an uncertain number of genera were lost in Africa and Asia. The extinctions occurred at different times on different continents, at times at least roughly coincident with the first appearance of moden human beings in each area. The association between the appearance of humans and extinction led to one of the two most common explanations for these extinctions: the overkill hypothesis. According to this hypothesis the spread of human beings into new regions led to overhunting. In support of this hypothesis, the disappearance of many birds on Pacific islands also tracks the migration of groups across the Pacific. The alternative mechanism for the extinctions is climatic and environmental changes associated with the end of the last glaciation. The difficulty, however, is that continental glaciation has waxed and waned for several million years with no apparent effect in the biota. It is not clear why such environmental changes would only cause extinction at the close of the last glacial episode. Some regional marine extinctions did occur during the Pleistocene, but thesee were relatively minor.

## Minor Biodiversity Crises or Background Extinctions

As dramatic as these major mass extinctions appear, they account for less than ten percent of species extionctions during the Phanerozic. Most species disappeared during the intervals between major events, as so-called background extinctions. Some became extinct in limited diversity crises that affected only a few groups or a limited region, others simply disappeared in ones and twos. Possibly, this suggests some dichotomy between mass and background extinctions. Does the selectivity of mass extinctions somehow differ qualitatively as well as quantitatively from background extinctions? To search the answer some research suggests that during mass extinctions some groups might have disappeared not because they were poorly adapted during background times, but simply because the regions or environments in which they lived suffered preferential extinction. David Raup, a well known paleontologist, has proposed that most extinction horizons, mass extinctions as well as most smaller events, are due to extraterrestrial impacts. In his views smaller extinctions reflect smaller objects; larger extinctions reflect the impact of larger objects.

## Present Context

Researchers of biodiversity agree that the present time is in the midst of the latest mass extinction. As per some estimates, half the species of plants and animals would be gone by the end of the twenty first century.

The quenching of the life exuberance will be more consequential humanity than all the present day global warming, ozone depletion and pollution combined. Firstly, humanity's food supply comes from a danagerously narrow sliver of biodiversity. Secondly, only a few hundred wild species have served to stock our natural pharmaceuticals, including antibiotics, anticancer agents, pain killers and blood thinners etc. Third one is to consider the survival. The biosphere gives us renewed soils, energy, clean water and air to breathe. The more species compose wild communities, the more stable and resilient becomes the planet as a whole. Lastly is to consider the ethics. Every species is a masterpiece, exquisitely adapted to the particular evinornment in which it has survived for thousands to millions of years. Religion and science, both advocate that who are we human beings to diminish or destroy biodiversity and thus the creation? The profligancy of twentyth century has led humanity into bottle neck of over population and shrinking natural resources. To that end it is important to accept the challenge and responsibility of global conservation. This time of human beings will certainty be judged by the amount of biodiversity, we carry through the bottleneck with us. Surely nothing can be more important than to secure the future of the rest of the life and thereby to safequard our own.

Biodiversity crises alongwith mass extinctions or background extinctions have occurred episodically throughout the history of life. Six well defined major mass extinctions and biodiversity crises have been indentified so far. Late proterozoic and Early Cambrian, almost 900 Ma to 500 Ma ago, was the first one, which occurred in a series of biodiversity crises to wipe out most of the early life from the seas. The great Phanerozic biodiversity occurred at the end of Ordovician, around 438 Ma. It occurred in several steps to eliminate about sixty percent of marine genera. The Late Devonian crises (355 Ma), culminated extinction of fifty five percent of marine genera as the terrestrial ecosystems were in the developing stage. Permo-Triassic boundary (250 Ma), the fourth major crisis was responsible for disappearence of ninety percent marine life and seventy five land vertibrate families. It resulted in the loss of habitat area, climatic effects of sea level drop, ocean anoxia and the impact of the Siberian volcanism. In a single episode rather than in at the series, end of Triassic (205 Ma) diversity crisis occurred, as fifth major event. It shows loss of life, climate changes, a drop in sea level and impact of extra terrestrial objects. The K/T boundary (65 Ma) is perhaps the most discussed diversity crisis in the history of life. It was possibly triggered by comet or meteoritic impact. Dinosaurs wiped out. Aftermath K/T boundary shows the better creative evolution. Discussions are still on to recognize Eocene/oligocene boundary (36. 5 Ma) as seventh major biodiversity crises and mass extinction event.

Present time is possibly, a part of eighth major episode which started some 1.6 Ma ago as Pleistocene biodiversity crisis. Numerous episodes of continental glaciations, global cooling and drop in sea level focussed on large disaappearence of terrestrial mammals. The association between the appearence of man and extinction has given rise to many hypothesises. In short, it is clear from the geological past that mass extinctions occurred most commonly due to set of environmental stresses that push biota and ecosystem beyond their ability to adopt. Decreased environmental heterogenity also appears linked to reduced biotic diversity. It suggets that as human continues to modify the climate, increased rate of extinction can be expected. By the end of twenty first centuary, half of the species of plants and animals are likely to disappear. To that end, it is important to accept the challenge of global conservation for the existence of human beings.

## SUMMARY

Biotic diversity crises have occurred episodically throughout the history of life in the geological times, ranging from minor, regional events affecting only a few lineages to extensive global mass extinctions removing a larger part of the planet's biota. Late Ordovician (~438 Ma), Late Devonian (~355 Ma), Permo-Triassic boundary (~ 250 Ma), end of Triassic (~205 Ma), and Cretaceous-Tertiary boundary (~65 Ma) have been treated as major mass extinctions and episodes of biodiversity crises. 900 Ma to 500 Ma time has now been considered as earliest and sixth mass extinction and biodiversity epidose.

Seventh biodiversity time namely, Eocene -Oligocene boundary (~36.5 Ma), has yet to gain the full status of mass extinction.

Present time, possibly is the eighth mass extinction episode in the history of life. This episode has yet to be recognized as part of Pleistocene mass extinction and biodiversity crisis. Whatsoever may be the fact, we are about to witness loss of half of the species of plants and animals by the end of the twenty first century. This situation is critical. If humans continue to modify the climate , increased rate of extinction can be expected.

## GLOSSARY

**Actuopaleontogy** : A branch of Paleontology which deals the study of fossible on the basis of living biota.

**Background extinction** : Relatively constant disappearance of low numbers of species

**Biodiversity** : Number of taxa present during an interval of time.

**Mass extinction** : Globally, major loss of biodiversity (both marine and terrestrial) in brief interval of geological time.

**Phanerozoic time** : Geological time of the last 545 Ma to present.

**Proterozoic time** : Geological time of the last 2500 Ma to 545 Ma.

**Uniformitarianism** : Geological processes and their products forming on the earth today are essentially the same as those of the past.

## ACKNOWLEDGEMENT

I am deeply grateful to my Guru Prof. B.S. Paliwal, Dean of Faculty of Science, JNV Univeristy and those whose references have been cited.

A great assistance have been extended by Miss Manju Sharma, Dr. Beena Tripathi, Mr.Virendra

Gaur, Dr. S.K. Ojha. Mr. Vijay Gaur, Mr. Sameer Naval and Mr. Narendra Chaudhary of my research team. The assistance is gratefully acknowledged.

## REFERENCES

- Donovan, S.K., Ed. (1989) Mass Extinction. New York: Columbia Univ. Press.
- Erwin, D.H. (1993). The Great Paleozoic crisis: Life and Death in the Permian. New York: Columbia Univ. Press
- Erwin, D.H. (1998). Diversity crises in the Geological Past in Encyclopedia of Enviornmental & Biology, vol. 1, 507-516.
- Humphries, C.J. Williams, P.H. and Vane Wright, R.I. (1995). Measuring biodiversity value for conservation. Ann. Rev. Ecol. Syst. 26, 93-112.
- Jablonski, D. (1995). Extinctions is the fossil record in estimating extinction rates (J.H. Lawton and R.M. May eds.) Oxford Univ. Press.
- Raup, D.M. (1991). Extinction: Bad Genes or Bad Luck? New York: Norton.
- Signor , P.W. (1990). The geological history of diversity. *Ann. Rev. Ecol. Syst.* **21**, 509-539.
- Stanley, S.M (1986). Earth and life through time W.H. Freenan and Comp. New York, 690 p.
- Walliser, O.H. ed. (1994). Global Bio-Events and Event Stratigraphy, Springer - Verlag. Berlin:
- Wilson, E.O. (2000). Vanishing before our eyes. Time vol. 155 No. 16 A, 29-34.

# 21

# Ecological Perspectives of Baya Birds in the Western Ghats, Karnataka

*K. L. Naik and B. B. Hosetti*

A large number of common public may not be knowing much about weaver birds. But the rural people identified these birds with different vernacular names. These birds are known to mankind due to their attractive nests. The bottle nests hang on trees, twigs or in agricultural lands, during their breeding season in monsoon months.

Nests of weaver birds are specially well known amongst rural women of western India. A common myth among the rural women is that if a nest of the baya is hung in the house, all milking cattle would yield bountiful milk. Rather oversized nests are selected for hanging in their homes. Further there is also a belief that there is a relation between the size of the nest and the quantity of milk produced by the cattle. *i.e.* the bigger the nest, the more would be the quantity of milk produced. It is for this reason that many of the rural houses have baya nests suspended. Half built nest are used as efficient "Sieves" and also used as caps by children during local festivals. Half built nests are also used for house decoration, baskets making and as fuel (Sharma, 1995). These birds are widely found all over India.

## Systematic Position

| | | |
|---|---|---|
| Phylum | : | Chordata |
| Class | : | Aves |
| Order | : | Passeriformes |
| Family | : | Ploceidae |
| Genus | : | *Ploceus* |
| Species | : | *philippinius* |

More than 95 species of weaver birds are known to occur in the world. But India possess only four species and they are mentioned below.

| | Scientific Name | Common Name |
|---|---|---|
| i) | *Ploceus philippinus* | Baya weaver bird (most common) |
| ii) | *Ploceus benghalensis* | Black throated weaver bird (rare) |
| iii) | *Ploceus manyar* | Streaked bird weaver bird (very rare) |
| iv) | *Ploceus megarhynchus* | Finns baya (not found in Western Ghats) |

## Literature Survey

Late Dr. Salim Ali was a pioneer ornithologist of India, prepared a detailed checklist of birds of Indian subcontinent. According to him Indian landmass possess four species of baya birds. Those include, *Ploceus bengalensis, P. manyar, P. megarhynchus* and *P. phillipinus.* Out of these four species *P. Phillipinus* is a resident and local migrant bird of Karnataka state. In India, the economic status of birds in relation to agriculture depredation was first reported by Mason and Maxwell Lefroy (1912). The other workers on this line include D'Abreu (1920) ; Mukharjee (1969) ; Ali and Rippley (1973). Though a good amount of literature is available on birds of the area still there are many places which are not visited by any Ornithologist .

Baya are important birds known for their skill of weaving bottle nests and their care for rearing young ones. A typical normal nest of a baya bird can be divided into three parts, stalk, body (egg chamber) and entrance tube (Jasse, 1897 ; Ambedkar 1964 ; Crook, 1964 ; Sharma 1985). The nests building by the baya birds is so powerful that even strong showers will not damage them (Pittie, 1996). The bayas construct their hanging nests on a variety of supporting trees and objects in protected areas. The deviation in morphology of a normal nest are referred as abnormal nests (Sharma 1995).

Mathew (1976) persued research in the ecobiology of a baya from Guddappah district in Andhra Pradesh. His observation on feeding pattern in the field revealed that the major component of their food was rice (65 per cent). The stomach contents of nesting birds revealed 22.37 per cent rice and 34.89 per cent grass-hoppers. This signifies the importance of baya in the biological control of insects in cropland. Sharma (1995) observed that multistoreyed nests are common in Rajasthan, and Ambedkar (1984) reported up to six storeyed nests.

## Keys for Identification

(i). *Ploceus philippinus:* Size- Sparrow, Length-15 cm (6 inches)

**Field Characters:** Female and male in non breeding plumage, looks like the hen house sparrow, dark-streaked fulvous below. Stout conical bill, short square cut tail. Breeding male has bright brown yellow crown and upper parts dark brown streaked with yellow. Yellow breast, cream buff colour on under parts. Flocks found in the open cultivated areas, along irrigation channels and protected places.

**Distribution:** Throughout India, Bangladesh, Pakistan, Sri lanka. These are residents and local migratory. Three races are recognized based on size and details of colouration.

**Habits:** Flocks, of considerable size, found in the paddy fields and other crop lands. Occasionally these cause damage to ripening crops. Roosts in enormous numbers in reed-beds bordering tanks, etc. The seasonal and local movements are largely governed by paddy and cereal cultivation which provide both nesting and food materials These birds also feed on insects and wild grass seeds.

**Call:** A sparrow like chit-chit-chit more loudly during cool hours of the day. In breeding season males fallow up these by a long drawn joyous chee-ee uttered in chorus, accompanied by flapping of wings while weaving their nests in a colony.

**Nest:** A swinging retort shaped structure with long vertical entrance tube, compactly woven of strips of paddy, bamboo and rough-edged grasses, suspended in clusters from twigs usually over water. Blobs of mud, collected when wet, are stuck inside the dome near the egg-chamber. Eggs 2 or 3, pure white. Male alone fabricate the nest and female alone incubates the eggs. Each male builds 3-4 nests in a season and female also pairs 3-4 times in a season.

(ii). *Ploceus benghalensis:* Size: Sparrow

**Field characters:** Male in breeding plumage has brilliant golden yellow crown, white throat and a black band separating it from the fulvous-white under parts. In non-breeding male and female, crown is brown like rest of upper plumage, black pectoral band less developed. A prominent supercilium, a spot behind ear, and narrow moustachial streaks, yellow. Flocks found around cultivated crops, reedy margins of tanks and extensive tall grass areas.

**Distribution:** Polygynous, colonial, on the whole similar to those common baya and streaked weavers. During courtship male bows low before visiting female, presenting golden crown at her. Flaps wings deliberately and sings softy tsi-tsisik-tsisik, tsik like chirp of cricket or subdued speaking of unoiled bicycle wheel.

**Nesting:-** Season -June to September (Depends on monsoon).

**Nest:** Similar to the streaked bayas, some-what smaller and normally with short entrances tube. Built in reed-beds in marsh with some of the growing reeds incorporated into the dome as to support singly or in scattered groups of 4-5, sometimes large colonies. Eggs are 3 to 4, white indistinguishable from those of the other two weavers.

*(iii). Ploceus manyar:* Size: Sparrow.

**Field characters:** Differs from the baya in having the breast fulvous, boldly streaked with black in both sexes and at all season. Crown of head in breeding males yellow, in females it is brown. Flocks, in swampy tall reed-beds of *Ipomea aquatica.*

**Distribution:** India, Bangladesh, Pakistan, Sri lanka, etc.

**Habits:** Similar to the baya's except that it is more inclined to tall coarse grassland and swampy reedy tank margins. In addition to the normal *chit-chit-chit,* the breeding male has pretty song *ti li lili, tililee-kititi lileekiti,* etc., utter in courtship chase and in invitation to a female to an available nest.

**Nesting:** Season February- September, varying with local monsoon conditions. Nests similar to baya but not so free swinging. Usually also smaller and with short entrance tube. Attached directly to tips of several arching bulrush or grass blades or some emergent aquatic plants. Small colonies in marshy reed-beds. Eggs 2 to 4 pure white.

*(iv). Ploceus megarhynchus:* Size: Sparrow

**Field character:** Adult male in breeding plumage with head and nape bright yellow constructing brown ear-coverts. Back dark brown streaked. Rump yellow, below bright golden yellow. Female possess head and nape pale canary or brown heavily diffused yellow or fulvous white. First year breeding males similarly colored. In non-breeding plumage sexes alike and difficult to separate from common baya.

**Distribution:** Resident in the Kumaon terai and West Bengal affects marshes with extensive strands of *Imperata* and *Saccharum* grasses sparsely dotted with silk cotton trees.

**Habits:** Gregarious at all time moving in floks in the grassland.

**Food:** Rice and other grains. Nestlings feed on insects.

**Call:** Louder and harsher than that of the baya. A high-pitched alarm note. Male song rendered as *wit -t.t-trr wheeze whee whee.* Birds sing in chorus.

**Nesting:** Season is May to August. Nest built in colonies on tree tops 9 to 10 above the ground level or in marshy reed beds. Unlike other weavers nest is supported, not suspended and made by coarse grass. Males have an elaborate wing beating display. Eggs 2-3, white, male polygynous. Both sexes participate in feeding the young ones.

## Habitat Selection for Nesting by Weavers
Two types of sites are preferred for nesting by weaver birds.

(a). Vegetational areas

(b). Non vegitational areas

A variety of trees, shrubs, herbs, grasses, reeds, etc. constitute the vegetational sites. Such sites have been recorded by many workers like Ali (1931); Kirkpatrick (1950); Ambedkaar (1968); Davis (1971) Naik and Hosetti (2000). Besides traditional vegetational habitats, telegraph and power lines (Ambedkar 1970) are non-vegetational sites liked by birds belonging to *Ploceus philippinus.*

Why certain plants and their particular branches are selected for nesting by weaver birds is still not crystal clear. According to Davis (1985) those plants, which have prominent thorns, prickles or similar devices which may deter predators are selected by weavers. In some cases, trees themselves not being spiny but when surrounded by thick brambles, may be patronized by weavers. Many unbranched tall trees like palms have smooth or very rough trunk, the long swaying leaves which not only keep away predators but also provide a convenient source of leaf strips for weaving.

Salim Ali (1931) advocated that nests on trees projecting or standing inside water are less liable to be attacked by the terrestrial animals. Safety factor again favours the presence of nest colonies of weavers on the sides of irrigation and open wells surrounded by vegetation. Inner sides of open wells, vertical banks of rivers and irrigation channels are comparatively safer places. The tress growing in flowing or stagnant water offer safer sites for nesting. Perhaps it is owing to this safety factor, that the nests are often suspended from branches hanging over water.

## Orientation of Nests

There is a definite orientation pattern of nests with respect to the stem of the host tree, generally the entrance chamber of the nest faces towards the outside while the egg chamber faces the stem (Plate-1). Due to this particular orientation of the nest, the entrance tube always remain oriented towards the outer side. Flying routes of the bird are so managed that the host stem or other vegetation growing nearby do not pose any hindrance.

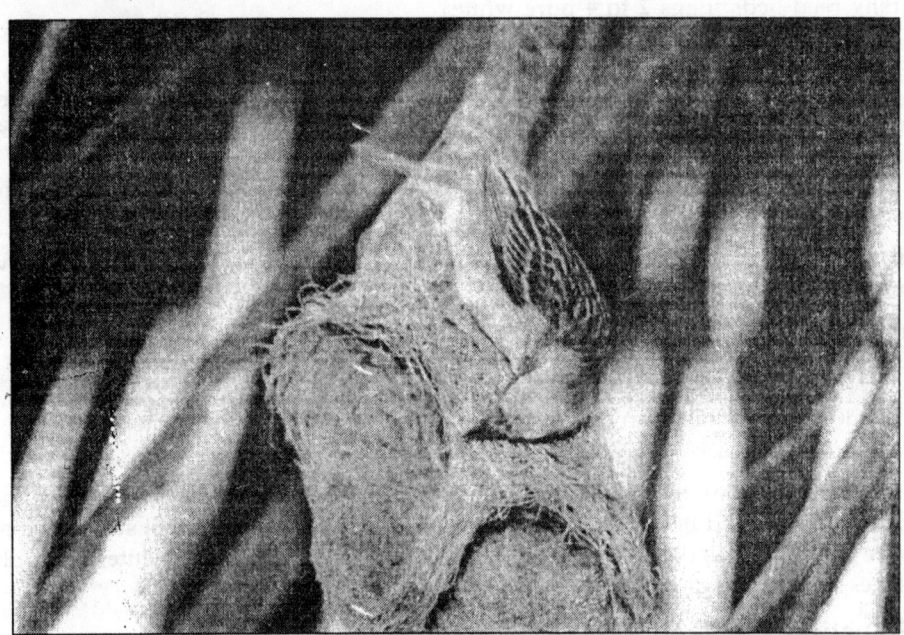

**Plate 21.1 :** A cock of Ploceus philippinus actively constructing the nest

Orientation of nests is different in wells and non vegetational areas, where they are oriented in relation to the nearest surface. The egg chamber half is kept facing towards the closest surface while the entrance chamber half is maintained towards the opposite direction. The entrance tube thus kept away from the vertical wall or surface to facilitate free-flying movement.

*P. philippinus* hangs its nest according to the direction of the prevailing wind direction. When egg chamber faces the wind direction, the eggs are safe within. But, if a nest built with the egg-chamber side facing away from the wind is strongly tilted by the wind, the eggs would roll into the entrance tube and fall down (Davis, 1971).

## Selection of Twigs

The selection of twigs is also one of the important factor for nest weaving. Twigs which are generally thin pliable and pendant to horizontal branches (leaves in case of Palms) are selected by *P. phillipinus* to suspend its nest. Twigs having a thickness more than a human thumb are generally avoided, possibly because they can't be accommodated in the grip of claws during the knitting of fibres in nest initiation. Strongly upwarding branches are generally not preferred. Twigs which are sufficiently tough so as to support the weight of nest are selected. Their terminal or bulb terminal portions are used to anchor the hanging nests.

## Orientation of Nesting in Study Area

We have studied the orientation of nest by weaver bird, *Ploceus philippinus* in Western Ghat area of B.R. Project. The study area is located in the foothills of Western Ghats near B.R. project (13⁰ 42' 00'' Longitude & 75° 38' 20'' latitude). The study area was divided into three imaginary zones, considering B.R. Project as its center. The three zones spread in north, (Zone-1) northeast (Zone-2) and southeast (Zone-3) direction each in about 20-km$^{-2}$ area. All the three zones surveyed for orientation of nests by colonies of *Ploceus philippinus* (Map 1).

B. R. Project area is a part of Malnad (Heavy rainfall receiving area) located under the foothills of Western Ghats of Karnataka range. The crops of the area include paddy, ragi, sugarcane, jowar and plantation crops. Paddy is grown two to three crops annually and the area is rich in water sources and vegetation. Perhaps due to the availability of plenty of food sources, protection, and suitable habitat conditions, various members of Plocidae have inhabited this area, those include weaver birds, munias and sparrows (Jasse, 1897). In the present chapter, the breeding season 1999 for baya, *Ploceus philippinus* started from August and terminated in October was chosen, to observe diverse type of orientation pattern of their bottle nests. The study area include three imaginary Zones, Zone I (B. R. Project), Zone II (Bhadravathi) and zone III (Shimoga) respectively. In each of the above mentioned three zones an area of 20 km$^{-2}$ was surveyed. Bottle nests of baya colonies were located and their nest orientation pattern was recorded in various habitats and trees are printed in Table 21.1.

The onset of rainy season of the area is mainly influenced by the activity of southwest monsoon that operates usually for 4 months from June to September. Any variations in the south west monsoon is found to influence directly on the nesting behaviour and orientation pattern of the baya birds, specially in *Ploceus philippinus* as pointed out earlier (Ambedkar, 1958). Our study on orientation pattern of nest of *Ploceus philippinus* revealed that the first year male without breeding dress and sexually mature adults constructed their nests mainly in 3 types of orientations. The nests were oriented lateral, central, and peripheral sides of trees.

Among the three types of orientations, lateral orientation was most common and the number of nests oriented laterally were 28. This accounts about 71 per cent of the total lateral orientations. Again out of the total lateral orientated nests, maximum nests were directed towards the east side. The reason behind constructing the nests on east side may be attributed to seek protection from southwest monsoon. It means in order to avoid any damages to be caused by the strong winds and rain, most of the cocks preferred to construct their nests towards the eastern direction. But this rule does not hold good in case of the situations like open wells and step wells, vegetation growing on vertical bank and sloppy areas. This indicates the intellectual experience of the baya birds to seek protection from possible natural hazards. This particular observation also supports the investigation made by Frank Finn (1990).

In contrast to the statement made above, there were other laterally oriented nests, they include 12 nests in the north east (NE), 3 in west (W), 8 in central north east (CNE), 2 in north east west (NEW),

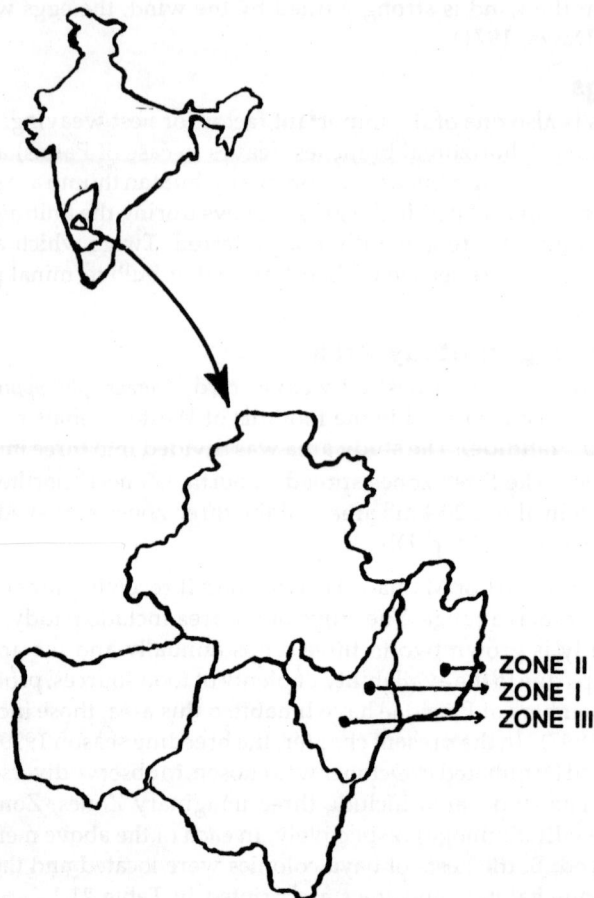

ZONE II
ZONE I
ZONE III

Map showing study area Zone I B.R. Project, Zone II Bhadravathi and Zone III Shimoga, Shimoga District of Karnataka State.

12 in north (N), 6 in north west (NW), 5 in S south(S), 5 in south east (SE), 2 in north east (NE) & 3 in south north (SN) direction were recorded respectively. The tabulation revealed that the orientation towards west side was negligible. Inspite of their experience we could find orientation of a few nest in the west direction also. That is, inside the open wells and in highly protective habitats or in other areas, such an activity may be attributed to the constructions by inexperienced yearlings or it may be due to assured protection in that area.

Hence in such situations and in case of present study, the monsoon that prevailed in southwest direction could not direct the orientation of the nests instead, it was the habitat and the vegetation which have become the causative factors for the orientation by weaver cocks. Additionally, it is worth to note that in all the situations invariably the egg chamber was facing towards the stem side of the host tree and the entrance tube was towards the opposite side . This arrangement is made, perhaps to ensure further protection to the eggs and the young ones from the predators and falling out during hanging by the wind action . It is also because the swinging action may deter the enemies to get in or it may not be convenient for them to enter in.

**Table 21.1 : Orientation of nest colonies by Ploceus philippinus in the area of Western Ghat, B.R. Project**

| Host Plant | No. of colonies showing different types of lateral orientation with orientation diagrams | | | | | | | | | | | | No. of colonies showing central | No. of colonies showing Peripheral | Total |
|---|---|---|---|---|---|---|---|---|---|---|---|---|---|---|---|
| | E | N-E | W | C-N-E | N-E-W | N | N-W | S | S-E | N-E-S | S-N | C-N | | | |
| Bomboosa bomboos | 10 | 6 | 1 | — | — | — | 2 | 1 | 1 | — | — | — | — | — | — |
| Cocos nucifera | 16 | 2 | — | 2 | 1 | — | — | 1 | 1 | — | — | — | 12 | 2 | 08 |
| Phoenix sylvestris | 2 | 2 | — | 1 | — | — | — | 1 | 1 | — | — | — | 1 | 2 | 08 |
| Butea moncsperma | 05 | — | 1 | — | — | — | 2 | — | 1 | — | — | — | 1 | — | — |
| Acacia catachu | 2 | 1 | 1 | 1 | — | 1 | — | 2 | 1 | 1 | — | — | 2 | — | 12 |
| Eucalyptus sps. | 1 | — | — | — | — | — | — | — | — | — | 1 | 1 | — | 2 | 05 |
| Feronia elephantum | 09 | 2 | 2 | — | 1 | — | — | — | 2 | — | — | — | 2 | — | — |
| Ipomea terrestris | 3 | 2 | 1 | 3 | — | 4 | 1 | — | 3 | 1 | — | 1 | 2 | 2 | 23 |
| Lantana aculeata | 2 | 1 | 1 | — | 1 | 3 | 2 | — | — | — | — | — | 2 | 2 | 14 |
| Total | 28 | 12 | 3 | 8 | 2 | 12 | 6 | 5 | 5 | 2 | 3 | 3 | 19 | 10 | 121 |

E=East, W=West, N=North, S=South, C=Central colony, P=Peripheral colony, ↑ =Direction of SW monsoon, O=Tree canopy

■ Nested part of canopy in respect of SW monsoon.

In Zone III of our study area a colony of *Ploceus manyar* was also recorded. The Nests were constructed on emergent aquatic plants in the Navile tank. There was a vast growth of *Ipomoea aquatica* along the periphery and littoral zone of the tank and the water depth was in the range of 3-4 meters. The number of nests recorded were 14, these were constructed in highly protective area and *P. manyar* birds constructed their nests and hung them to the tips of the Ipomea plants, in such a way that the stalk was covered by bunch of beautiful flowers (Plate-21.2).

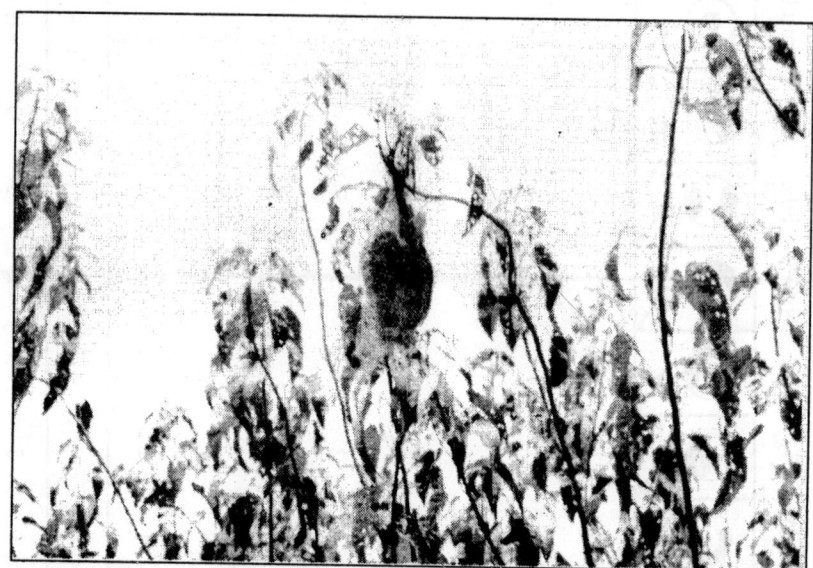

**Plate 21.2 :** A beautiful nest hung amidst Ipomea aquatica plants in a wetland

This type of nesting may be made for attracting the females. In no other parts of our study area these colonies are recorded. Among three species recorded *P.manyar* ranks third in terms of abundance. *Ploceus megarhynchus* was not recorded in any of our visits in the study area. Comparative study on the abundance of baya birds, revealed that *P. manyar* is found to be endemic to specific wetlands and it may be included under the category of endangered species, in Karnataka.

*Ploceus benghalensis* also not recorded in the study area, but a few colony of birds showing relation to benghalensis were observed near the Sahyadri college campus adjacent to bypass road. The nests were hung to *Ipomoea aquatica* plants and these were more or less similar to the *P.benghalensis* as explained by Salim Ali (1996). However the only difference was in the head region where instead of brilliant golden yellow it was dull red. The authors are not clear weather this particular species is a sub species of *P.benghalensis* or some other new species not recoded earlier. Further studies for this species is needed.

## Nesting Patterns

A typical completed nest is a bottle shaped structure and can be divided into three parts *viz.* a stalk, middle body and the entrance tube

The nest has a entrance tube slightly shifted towards the ante-chamber side due to which more bulging appears towards the egg chamber. Due to this position of the entrance tube, a completed nest can be divided into two equal halves across the chin-strap only (longitudinally).

## Abnormal Nests in Study Area

Besides typical nests, which are otherwise called as normal nests, various other types of abnormal nests were constructed by sexually mature male birds and yearlings during breeding season. Many variations can be seen in nests of bayas, which make the nest abnormal. The variations may be broadly categorized into two: The first category of abnormality is in the structure of nest or any part of it. Abnormal structure may appear due to deposition of parts, formation of additional parts, elaboration of normal parts and abolition of normal parts (Sharma, 1995). The second category of abnormality is regarding position of nests or any part of it. In this case, there might be many kinds of abnormalities. When one type of abnormality is present in the nest, it may be called as simple abnormal and when there occurs more than one type of abnormalities, it may be referred as mixed or complex abnormal nest.

Perhaps due to the availability of plenty of food sources, protection and suitable habitat conditions various members of plocinae have inhabited this area, those include weaver bird, munias & sparrows (Naik *et al.*, 2000).

A total of 795 nests were studied from four zones, to know the trends of abnormalities in the study area and the findings are printed in Table 21:2. It is clear from the data that there is a trend towards bistoreyed nests followed by the multistalked nests. Why and how and under what conditions abnormal nests are constructed by the baya weaver bird, is an interesting and complicated aspect.

**Table 21.2: Abnormal Nests of Ploceus Philippinus in B.R. Project, Area of Western Ghat**

| Zone | Year | Total Number of nests observed | Structural Abnormality | | | | | | Orientational Abnormality | | | | | | | Pseudostoreyed Nests | Bistoreyed Nests | Chain storeyed Nests | Mixed abnormal nests | Total number of abnormal nests |
|---|---|---|---|---|---|---|---|---|---|---|---|---|---|---|---|---|---|---|---|---|
| | | | Bell jar Shaped | Buttressed | Blind | Closed | Stalkless | Multistalked | Chained | Meshed | Fused | Branched | Symmetrical | Stomach | Completed nest with Double opening | | | | | |
| Zone A | 1999-2000 | 248 | 2 | 4 | - | - | 2 | - | 3 | - | 1 | - | - | 1 | - | - | 13 | 2 | - | 28 |
| Zone B | 1999-2000 | 166 | - | - | 1 | - | 1 | 7 | - | - | - | - | - | - | - | 1 | 8 | - | - | 18 |
| Zone C | 1999-2000 | 229 | 1 | 1 | 1 | - | 6 | 3 | 4 | - | - | - | - | 2 | 1 | 1 | 15 | 2 | - | 37 |
| Zone D | 1999-2000 | 152 | - | 3 | - | - | 4 | 6 | 2 | 4 | - | - | - | - | - | 2 | 10 | - | 31 | |
| | Total | 795 | 3 | 8 | 2 | 0 | 13 | 16 | 9 | 4 | 1. | 0 | 0 | 3 | 1 | 4 | 46 | 4 | - | 114 |

Zone A = B.R. Project, Zone B=Bhadravathi, Zone C= Shimoga, Zone D. Holehonnur of Shimoga District, Karnataka State, INDIA

Though bistoreyed nests are common in this area, field observations revealed that more than four storeyed nests are not present in the study area (Plate 21.3). Multistoreyed nests were noticed in those areas where comparatively long monsoon periods prevailed (Davis,1985). In Karnataka the monsoon period is too short to fabricate 6 to 10 storeyed nests. Hence, extensive storeification cannot be expected and long chains of nests are very rare in this area as it is also evidenced elsewhere by Ambedkar (1956).

Multistalked nests were also common in this area. Presence of two or more stalks provide extra attachment and strength to the nest, which make a hanging nest prone to simple harmonic motions on windy days. Hence to minimize such a pendulous motion more than one pinnae are used for stalking the nest. Moreover, length of stalks is also kept smaller. Sometimes the gap between two stalks is blocked by a woven mesh due to which a nest becomes a wide stalked nest. This device is again equally good to minimize the simple harmonic motion. Stalkless, nests are also seen in the area and such nests are equally liked by females. The other type of abnormal nests like Belljar, Buttressed, Blind Closed,

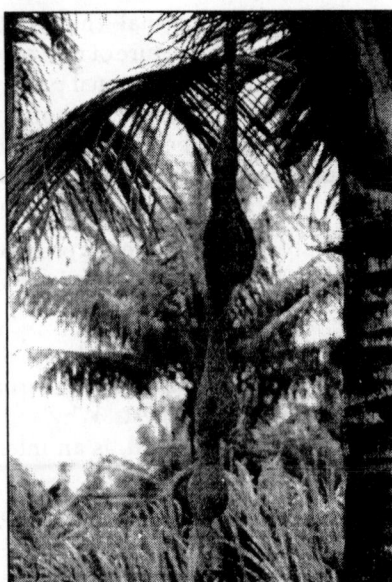

**Plate 21.3** : Four storey nest constructed by Ploceus Philippinus an a coconut tree

Chained, Meshed, Fused, Branched, Symmetrical, Stomach shaped, completed nest with double opening are also cited but in negligible in numbers.

Out of the total 795 nests 248 in Zone A followed by 229 in Zone C, 166 in Zone B and minimum of 152 nests in Zone D were observed respectively. The numbers was maximum in Zone A, this is because the area bound with rich habitat sources like irrigation channels and slopy area. The plants present in this zone are thorny, which might have attracted the birds and also act as deterrent to predators. In some cases trees themselves not being spiny but when surrounded by thick brambles, may be selected by *Ploceus philippinus*. Many unbranched trees like palms and coconuts are tall also selected by *Ploceus philippinus*. Hence in this zone the number of nests was maximum. Tallest coconut tree where nests were fabricated in Zone C. It was at a distance of around 80 ft. from ground level. This area is surrounded by thick vegetation and crop lands and additionally irrigation channel is flowing nearby. Maximum abnormal multistoreyed nests were found on a coconut tree which is the tallest (Plate 21.3). But in Zone D the number of nests was minimum. This is because of the area is poor in habitat sources which possessed open cultivation, the plants situated in this area are easily accessible to the predators. The study on nesting pattern by the baya in Western Ghat area revealed that 14.3 per cent of the nests were abnormal of which 14.03 per cent were multistalked and 40.35 per cent bistoreyed. It is confirmed that the area is found to be the most habitable for the baya birds.

## Breeding Biology

The male baya birds are polygynous. These build the nest and the female takes no part in the work except in scantily lining the bed in egg chamber after she has accepted the nest. In the early stages of a nest fabrication females are not cited. When some of the nests have reached the helmet stage (half-built) a party of females visit the colony to inspect the nests. The birds hop from one helmet to another perching on the initial ring (or) chin strap, pulling a strip here and another there, obviously examining the structure critically. All the while they are engaged in the scrutiny, the owner males flutter excitedly, clinging outside the nest giving their wing beating displays and and warding off competing males. Some nests are approved by females, others rejected. Those that fail to find tenants are often discontinued construction and go for building a new one. Once a nest is approved by her, the female softens to the owners advances and permits, and even invites, copulation by the impetuous suitor. The act takes place on the chin strap and seals the pair bond. The male thereafter hurries to complete the egg chamber and complete the nest for her occupation. As soon as she is settled on the eggs he commences to build a second nest close by to invite another female. It is true for the female also. In a season a male will fabricate 4-5 nests and a female also pairs 4-5 times to reproduce new progeny (Mathew 1976).

Bayas are popular with bird fanciers and with itinerant entertainers at country fairs. They readily learn to perform a variety of clever tricks such as retrieving a ring thrown into a well before it touches water, threading tiny beads with a needle, plucking and bringing back leaves from a chosen tree to their master, and picking up the correct numbered card among the several spread in front. Many of the tricks require much skill and seeming intelligence and the birds quite obviously enjoy performing such orders.

# REFERENCES

- Ali, S. (1931): The nesting habits of the Baya ( *Ploceus philippinus*) *J. Bombay Nat. Hist, Soc* **34**: 947- 64.
- Ali, S.(1996): The book of Indian Birds, 12^TH edition, Bombay Natural History Society, Oxford University Press, Mumbai.
- Ali and Repley (1973): Hand book of the Birds of India and Pakistan. Oxford University Press.
- Ambedkar V. C (1956): Notes on the Baya weaverbird, *P.philippinus* (linn), *J. Bombay Nat. Hist, Soc* **53**: 381- 389.
- Ambedkar, V. C. (1958): Notes of the baya breeding season of 1957. *J. Bombay nat. Hist. Soc.* **55**: 100-106.
- Ambedkar , V.C . (1964): Some weaver birds: A contribution to their breeding biology, Ph.D. Thesis, University of Bombay, Mumbai , India.
- Ambedkar , V.C . (1968): Observation on the breeding biology of finns baya in the Kumaon Terai. *J. Bombay nat, Hist.. Soc.* **65**(3): 596-607.
- Ambedkar , V.C . (1970): Nest of baya, *Ploceus philippinus* (Linn) On Telegraph wires. *J. Bombay nat, Hist. Soc.* **66**: 624.
- Ambedkar, V. C. (1984): Some notes on the breeding of common baya (*P. philippinus*) *J. Bombay nat. Hist. Soc.* **81**: (3): 701-2.
- Crook, J.H (1960): Studies on the reproductive behaviour of the baya weaver bird *P.philippinus* (linn). *J. Bombay, Nat, Hist, Soc.* **57**: 1-44.
- Davis J.A. (1985): Blind or closed nests of baya weaver bird, *J. Bombay, Nat. Hist, Soc.* **82**: 628-660.
- Davis J.A. (1971): Baya weaver bird nesting on human habitations. *J.Bombay, Nat. Hist, Soc.* **68**: 246-8.
- D. Abreu, E.A. (1920): Some insect prey of birds in the Central Provinces. Report of the third entomological meeting held at Pusa, February 1919.3: 859-871.
- Frank Finn. (1990): Garden birds of India. Royal Publications, Delhi.
- Jesse,W. (1897): Bird nesting in and around Lucknow, *Ibis*, 7: 554-562.
- Kirkpatrick, K.M. (1950): Peculiar roosting site of the House Swift (Micropus affinis). *Bombay Nat. Hist. Society*, **49**: 551-52.
- Mason C.W. and Maxwel Lefroy, (1912): The food of birds in India Mem. Agr. Dept. India, Entomological Series 3.

- Mathew, D. N. (1976): Ecology of the weaver birds, *Bombay Nat. Hist. Society*, **73** : 249-250.
- Mukherjee, A.K.(1969): Food habits of weaver birds of the Sunderban, 24 Parganas district, West Bengal, India, part-I *J. Bombay Nat. Hist. Soc.* **68**: 37-64.
- Naik K.L., and B.B. Hosetti (2000): Abnormal nesting of baya bird in the B.R. Project Area of Western Ghats, Karnataka *Journal of Field Ornithol* (in press).
- Naik K.L., Naveed A, and B.B. Hosetti (2000): Orientation of nests by Weaver Bird *Ploceus philippinus* in the B.R. Project area of Western Ghats Karnataka 3:Ind. *J. Environ & Eco Plan L:* 147-151. (1)
- Pittie, A. (1996): Black breasted weaver birds, *News letter for bird watchers*, **36**. Nov-Dec, 115
- Sharma, S. K. (1985): A study on qualitative aspects of abnormal nesting in Baya weaver bird *Ploceus philippinus*. (linn) *J. Southern Forest Ranges College*, Coimbatore **60**: 50-54.
- Sharma S. K. (1995): Ornithobotany of Indian weaver bird, Himanshu Publications, Udaipur, Rajasthan.

# 22

# Acetylcholinesterase Enzyme: A Tool for Monitoring Environmental Toxicity in Mammals

*Mahira Parveen and Santosh Kumar*

Pesticides are unique group of compounds whose prime importance is to prevent, control and eliminate pest and whose extensive use resulted in green revolution in the country. These pesticides not only hit the target animals but also affect adversely the nontarget organisms. Many pathological changes in organisms associated with environmental toxicity are well established even due to sublethal doses of pesticides. Acetylcholinesterase (AChE; EC 3.1.1.7) is a polymorphic enzyme which is distributed in the whole vertebrate series. AChE hydrolyses the neurotransmitter acetylcholine at cholinergic synapses and plays an important role in cholinergic transmission (Katz and Thesleff 1957). The hydrolysis of acetycholine at the nerve ending is necessary for the continuous impulse transmission and contraction of muscles.

When toxicant is added to animal system it binds with AChE enzyme and forms enzyme inhibitor (EI) complex. Due to the formation of this complex AChE is unable to hydrolyze the neurotransmitter acetylcholine causing its accumulation at synaptic junction. This results in continuous contraction of muscles followed by paralysis and ultimately death. It is now well established that organophosphates and carbamates are the potent inhibitors of AChE enzyme. Besides these compounds some other organic compounds are also known as AChE inhibitors.

## Inhibition of AChE in Mammals

Enzymes are amongst the most fundamental material which make life possible. The enzyme cholinesterase belongs to esterases which is a subgroup of hydrolytic enzyme which are found in many tissues throughout the body. AChE has clinical importance in diagnosis. Many drugs temporarily alter the cholinesterase activity and some insecticides depress its activity measurably. Test for the activity of enzyme in the plasma and other tissues may be useful in detecting over exposure to these agents. For the biochemical estimation two methods were extensively used. One is proposed by Hestrin (1949) and later modified by Metcalf (1951), another method is of Ellman *et al* (1961) and later modified by Voss and Sachsse (1970), Nostrandt *et al* (1993) and Venkataraman *et al* (1993). The AChE and its inhibition have been investigated in liver, blood, erythrocytes, serum, plasma, brain and other tissues of mammals. However, the work on AChE in the heart tissue is meagre.

## Liver

Low amounts of cholinesterase is found in patients having the liver disease in human beings. Ellman *et al* (1961) determined AChE enzyme activity by taking liver tissue and treating it with substrate acetylcholine. They found that the AChE and BuChE activities were 1.07 and 0.65 µm/mim/gm respectively. Purshottam and Srivastava (1989) injected rats intraperitoneally with phenobarbital (PB) which is microsomal enzyme inducer and studied its effect on AChE activity of Liver microsomes. They also studied the effect of Soman on AChE of control and PB pretreated animals. They found that PB pretreatment did not affect AChE activity. IN PB treated liver microsomes it became 25.2 nm/min/mg protein from control of 22.0 nm. However, Soman administration to PB treated rats inhibited ChE activity greatly where it declined to 4.12 nm. they found that Soman administration to PB untreated rats significantly inhibited the activity of liver microsomal AChE and only 2.97 n, (14%) activity remained with respect to control. In a similar study Purshottam and Kaveeshwar (1992) reported that Soman which is a OP compound and used as a potent chemical warfare agent inhibits cholinesterase in the liver microsomes even if administered its sublethal dose at 0.5 and 2 hours period. The inhibition of ChE was greatly enchanced and only 18 per cent of the initial level remained.

Tomar et al (1995) found 66.5 per cent inhibition of AChE in the liver of goat Capra capra on 75 mg/kg malathion exposure. 150 mg/kg dose caused 71.3 per cent inhibition indicating dose dependent inhibition. Nandakumar and Udayabhaskar (1980) developed a rapid colorimetric method for quantification of dimethoate and its oxygen analogues using pig liver acetone powder as enzyme source. They used various dimethoate and its oxygen analogues using pig liver actone powder as enzyme source. They used various dimethoate concentrations ranging from 1 to 10 ug and reported 8.50 to 58.58 per cent inhibition suggesting linear relationship between pesticide concentration and cholinesterase inhibition.

Inhibitory effect of thiocholine compounds (Murphy 1966) and dialdrin (Bhatia et al 1972) on rat liver AChE has also been reported, whereas Siva Kumar (1989) described recovery of AChE activity after a period of 45 days in rat liver due to the acute neurotoxicity of OP compounds.

## Blood

Pesticides also inhibit AChE in the blood. Carakostas and Landis (1991) described a modification of Ellman's assay's technique for ChE activity and determined ChE activity in blood of rat. Briefly,the modification involved changes in the incubation time ($T_i$) total reaction time (Tf), the interval of time between specific absorbance readings used to determine the reaction rate (Tr) etc. They reported activity of blood ChE as 5710 IU/l from Ellman assay whereas three modifications gave 3728, 3004 and 2710 IU/l.

Dikshith et al (1991) found inhibitory effect of methyl parathion and HCH+methyl. parathion on the RBC of Rattus norvegicus. They observed that 2 mg/kg/day methyl parathion led 62 per cent decrease of AChE at 7th day which enhanced with the increase in exposure period.

Srivastava and Raizada (1996) reported 13-37% inhibition of AChE as effect of dimethoate on RBC of Rattus norvegicus. Venkataraman et al (1993) determined blood AChE activity in rat by using acetylthiocholine iodide (ATI) and butyryl thiocholine iodide (BTI) as substrate. They stated that for pseudocholinesterase (PuChE) BTI is more suitable than ATI because ATI might be reacting with AChE and other substances alongwith PuChE in samples. Potter et al (1993) observed the effect of various taxicants on blood ChE of human. The mean value of ChE activity was 4-70 KU/l which inhibitled by 1.48 per cent due to Insecticide + herbicide, remain unchanged due to fumigators and slightly increased (+4.04 per cent) with herbicide.

Shtenberg and Rybakova (1968) and Voss and Sachsse (1970) reported strong inhibition of AChE activity in the blood of large number of mammals including human beings due to OPs ans carbamates. According to Smith and Muir (1977) in rat 17 per cent blood ChE activity was regenerated within 10 min after soman infusion, whereas in guineapig no reactivation was detected.

## Erythrocytes

Mammalian erythrocyte AChE is well studied. Carakostas and Landis (1991) determined AChE as 4880 IU/l by Ellman's method, whereas its three modifications gave as 3323, 2607 amd 2357 IU/I. Nostrandt et al (1993) studied the inhibition of AChE in the erythrocytes of rat due to the effect of carbaryl by his radiometric modified method and compared it with that of Ellman's method. They found percentage inhibition from 19 to 68 in erythrocyte AChE activity and claimed that result observed by his modified method are more reliable than Ellman's method. Mice erythrocyte membrane and synaptosome AChE activities are greatly inhibited by dimethylsulfoxide (DMSO), which is used as cryoprotective drug to treat burns (Jagota 1992). With the in vitro exposure of DMSO concentrations ranging from 0.13 to

0.91 mM they obtained 28 to 92 per cent inhibition and suggested that DMSO is toxic in nature as it inhibits AChE almost completely. AI-Jafari *et al* 1995 investigated inhibitory effect of an anticaner drug cyclophosphamide (CP) on human erythrocyte membrane bound AChE. They found a remarkable inhibition of AChE and reported that CP inhibits AChE in a concentration dependent manner. Seto and Shinohara (1987) determined the inhibitory effect of paraquat and dichlorvos on AChE activity of human erythrocytes. They found that the degree of inhibition against the AChE activity in human stroma by dichlorvos was increased during the preincubation time from 0 to 100 min, indicating an irreversible inhibition. On the contrary the degree of AChE inhibition by paraquat and diquat did not change over a period of 100 min showing reversible inhibition indicating that inhibition is more produced with dichorvos than that of paraquat. Ellman *et al* (1961) reported AChE activity in bovine erythrocytes as 0.033 to 0.083 U/min.

## Serum

Serum AChE estimation has been established as an important parameter for the diagnosis of toxicity. Venkataraman *et al* (1993) compared pseudocholinesterase activities of rat serum by using two different substrates acetylthiocholine iodide (ATI) and butyrylthiocholine iodide (BTI). They held that activity was more with ATI than that of BTI. Purshottam and Kaveeshwar (1992) studied the effect of soman on ChE of serum of rat after 1/2 and 2 hour periods. On 0.22 mg/kg soman administration it declined to 33% of its initial value which was totally inhibited at 2 hour exposure. Rao *et al* (1993) worked on toxicity of a liquid insect repellent N.N-diethylphenylacetamide (DEPA) in rats. Administration of 825 mg/kg dose by gavage caused the decline in AChE to 1472 nm from control value of 1658nm/min/ml. Ansari *et al* (1990) investigated the serum AChE activity in cattle and buffalo infested with a tick species *Boophilus microplus*. Treatment of infested cattle and buffalo with synthetic pyrethroids, cypermethrin and fenvelerate resulted in inhibition of AChE significantly. Estimation of serum AChE might help in clinicobiochemical diagnosis of tick toxin and pyrethroid toxicity in cattle and buffalo treated with these pyrethroids against tick toxin. Dose dependent inhibition in Serum AChE of goats due to OP compounds as reported by Tomar *et al* (1995) is inhibited due to exposure of phosphate ester insecticide, nerve gases or succinylcholine, muscle relaxant (Garry and Routh (1965). Exposure of OP pesticides to agricultural works declined serum AChE at the end of work day as compared to that beginning of work day (Carillo & Cervantes 1993). Human serum acetylcholinesterase (Venkataraman and Nagarani 1994) and butyrylthiocholinesterase (Adams and Whittaker 1949) hydrolyze butyrylthiocholine (BTC) at a faster rate than acetylthiocholine (ATC). Clark and Rattner (1987) found that orthene inhibits serum ChE activity of bats. *Myotis lucifugus* and mice, *Mus musculus*. ChE activity in control bats, is found to be 3.2 times higher than in mice.

## Plasma

Plasma AChE shows considerable changes in toxic conditions. Purshottam and Srivastava (1989) evaluated the effect of acute toxicity of the OP compound soman on rat plasma ChE activity. ChE activity was unchanged in the plasma of PB-treated rats as compared to control, whereas soman administration greatly decreased the AChE. However, this value was not significantly different from that of PB treated rats receiving soman dose of 0.22 mg/kg. PB treatment did not protect this enzyme from inhibition by soman. Miyamoto *et al* (1976) fed albino rats with 10 and 3 mg/kg/day sumithion for consecutive six months and found a significant depression of ChE activity. Padilla and Hooper (1992) compared the inhibition of plasma ChE due to paraoxon, aldicarb and carbaryl. Carbaryl produced 41 per cent inhibition whereas aldicarb and paraoxon produced 61 per cent and 64 per cent inhibition respectively. Nostrandt *et al* (1993) reported 26-60 per cent inhibition due to carbaryl doses. Carakostas & Landis (1991) developed 3 modified methods of Ellman's method and determined plasma ChE of rat as 766 IU/I from Ellman's method and 800, 806 and 807 IU/1 from modifications.

AChE activity in plasma of human beings exposed to fumigators, insecticide+herbicide and herbicide only in the agricultural fields is determined by Potter *et al* (1993). With all the toxicants they found statistically significant (50%) decrease in plasma ChE activity which is exposure related. Venkataraman and Nagarani (1994) found ChE activity in human plasma with ATC as 14.02 μm whereas with BTC it was 18-94 μm. The inhibitory actions of sumithion, DFP (Nakagawa *et al* 1977) and dichlorvos (Nakagawa *et al* 1977), Boyer *et al* 1977) on ChE in human plasma indicates that $1X 10^{-5}$ concentration of dichlorvos completely inhibits ChE.

## Brain

There are several reports on the effects of organophosphates (Kozar *et al* 1976) and carbamate (Nostrandt *et al* 1993, Takahashi *et al* 1994) on AChE activity in brain regions of mammals. Padilla and Hooper (1992) studied the inhibition of brain by carbaryl at different durations of incubation and dilution of brain ChE reactivation at 37°C was approximately 2- fold faster than the same sample at 23°C. Dilution of tissue caused considerable ChE reactivation. Inhibition of AChE of rat treated with carbaryl ranged 45 to 72 per cent; whereas aldicarb induced 47 to 63 per cent inhibition. Highest degree of inhibition (75%) is obtained with paraoxon. Nostrandt *et al* (1993) compared carbaryl induced inhibition of rat brain ChE activity estimated by Ellman's method and radiometric method. The activity of AChE was gradually decreased with the increase in dose, and only 19 per cent AChE remained in brain at 75 mg/kg dose. Carr and Chambers (1996) reported brain AChE as 20.1 nm/min/mg protein at 30°C and 21.1 nm at 37°C incubation temperature. Naidu *et al* (1987) obtained significant inhibition of rat brain AChE activity (82-92.4%) with various doses of dichlorvos (30-90 mg/kg). Purshottam and Kaveeshwar (1992) administered sublethal dose of soman (0.22 mg/kg/) intraperitoneally and assayed ChE in three different regions of brain after 0.5 and 2.0 hr periods of administration. Cerebellum showed very less inhibition (6%), however cerebrum (44%) and brain stem (47%) were inhibited almost equally. Singh *et al* (1990) and Singh and Agarwal (1990) studied AChE in developing rat brain and held that the enzyme activity depends both on the nutritional status and the development age. Mahon and Brink (1970) added 3.0 mm pentyl enetetrazol (PTZ) to homogenates of brain of different postnatal ages and registered 80 per cent inhibition.

Dikshith *et al* (1991) used 2 mg/kg/day dose of methyl parathion (MP) for 7, 15 and 30 days exposure to female rats *Rattus norvegicus* and observed a significant recovery with the increase in exposure period. Mahaboob Basha and Nayeemunnisa (1993) made a comparative study of methyl parathion on various brain regions of 7 day old albino rats. Their result indicated highest AChE inhibition *i.e.* 44.8 per cent in cerebral cortex followed by 37.6 per cent in brain stem and least AChE inhibition *i.e.* 31.8 per cent in spinal cord. Fixation of tissue by formaldehyde caused inhibition of rat brain AChE as 76 per cent, 70 per cent and 44 per cent in cortex, striatum and cerebellum respectively (McGeer and McGeer 1989). The brain of rats treated with methanol resulted in a significant decrease in AChE showing 40.6 per cent inhibition as compared to control (Sureshbabu *et al* 1992). Chiappa *et al* (1995) exposed male rats with 15, 30 and 60 mg/kg doses of chlorpyrifos and recorded 6 to 30% inhibition in dose dependent manner. Similar trend of inhibition is observed in different brain regions of rabbit intoxicated with physostigmine, 2-5 butyl phenyl methyl carbamate (BPMC), isoprocarb, 2-isopropylphenyl methyl carbamate (MIPC) and propoxur, 2- isopropoxyphenyl methyl carbamate (PHC) (Takahashi *et al* 1994). More than 72 per cent inhibition occurred in diaphragm and aorta.

Guhathakurta and Bhattacharya (1988) purified AChE from the cerebellum of Indian goat, *Capra Capra* and determined the AChE activity in cerebellar homogenate, purified enzyme and polymaleinic anhydride (PMA) bound AChE. In purified fraction AChE highly increased to more than 40-fold. The further study of inhibitory effect of parathion on PMA bound AChE indicated the inhibition of AChE with all the concentrations and the results established that AChE can be purified and successfully immobilized to PMA. Similarly, Jayanthi and Balasubramanian (1991) purified AChE enzyme from the brain basal ganglia of monkey, *Macaca radiata* by a three step affinity purification followed by gel filtration on sephadex G-75 or G-25 and got it purified to 170-fold. This purified enzyme was also inhibited by all the AChE inhibitors. Prostigmine, eserine and diisopropylfluorophosphate (DFP) exhibited 100 per cent, 96 per cent and 81 per cent inhibiton respectively. These authors suggested that the peptide lacks the binding sites for inhibitiors. Several other OP compounds such as O-alkyl-S hexythiosphosphorates, (Maslova and Reznik 1976), malathion (Kurtz 1977b) and parathion (Vijayan and Brownson 1975; Robinson et al 1978) are also potent inhibitors of ChE in different brain regions.

## Heart

The inhibition of heart AChE has been less reported. Cardiotoxic responses of dichlorvos in rats may be directly related to the inhibition of ChE activity (Naidu *et al* 1987). 30-90 mg/kg doses of dichlorvos caused 55.6-88.9 per cent inhibition alongwith changes in ECG and heart rate. Parveen (1997) observed 25.7 to 56.0 per cent inhibition in heart AChE of rats with 3.0 to 7.0 mg/kg doses of dichlorvos. Dichlorvos was administered intraperitoneally to rats for 96 hours (Parveen and Kumar 2001). Sublethal exposure of carbaryl for 96 hours to rats caused significant inhibition in heart AChE. 100-400 mg/kg doses inhibited enzyme in a range of 21.8 to 54.8 per cent. Heart AChE in rats is also reported to be greatly inhibited in the artificially produced myocardial infarction by isoprenaline hydrochloride (Gaur 1997).

## Accumulation of Acetylcholine Due to inhibition of AChE

As a result of inhibition of AChE the substrate acetylcholine (ACh) does not hydrolyze resulting in its accumulation in the tissue. Accumulation of ACh occurred in rat brain regions after treatment with 15mg/kg intravenous dichlorvos (Stavinoha *et al* 1976). Striatum had the highest rate of accumulation of ACh while the cerebellum had the lowest. ACh accumulation in rat brain due to DMSO (Jagota 1992), methanol (Sureshbabu *et al* 1992) and methyl parathion (Mahaboo Basha and Nayeemunnisa 1993) has also been reported. ACh accumulation in heart of rats, *Rattus norvegicus* due to dichlorvos (3-7 mg/kg) results in the paralysis of heart muscles (Parveen 1997 Parveen and Kumar 2001). ACh contents in heart are gradually enhanced with the increase in dose as well as increase in exposure period.

## Inhibitory Power of Toxicants

The inhibitory power of toxicants is determined with the help of $I_{50}$ of toxicant for AChE. $I_{50}$ is the numerical value which gives the concentration of toxicant at which 50 per cent inhibition of enzyme occurs. It clearly indicates the inhibitory power of toxicant, i.e. if $I_{50}$ value is lower, then the toxicant is a strong inhibitor and *vice versa*. By calculating the $I_{50}$ value Rahman *et al* (1989) compared the effect of some biphenyl derivatives (1) p-phenyl-phenyl-N-ethyl carbamate (2) P-(4-nitrophenyl) phenyl-N-methyl carbamate (3) P-4-(nitrophenyl) phenyl-N-ethyl carbamate (4) 0, 0-dimethyl-O, P-nitrophenyl phosphate and (5) o,o-diethyl-o, p-nitro pheny phosphate on AChE of vaious vertebrates (fish, pigeon and rat) and honey bee. They determined the concentration of biphenyl derivatives responsible for 50 per cent AChE inhibition in rat brain. $I_{50}$ values indicated that biphenyl derivatives of phosphate esters are more active against rat brain AChE in comparison to that of carbamic acid esters. All the biphenyl derivatives of carbamate esters have almost same inhibitory potential against rat brain, and their relative toxicity against rat brain is compound no. 4>3>1>2>5. Inhibitory concentration $I_{50}$ of cyclophosphamide (CP) for human erythrocyte AChE is noticed as 511.3 µm (Al-Jafari *et al* 1995). The $IC_{50}$ of CP for human erythrocyte AChE was 25 per cent of the value indicating that human erythrocyte AChE is more sensitive to CP than that form chicken brain. $IC_{50}$ of paraquat (PQ) was 25 µM and diquat (DQ) 1.5 mM for human erythrocyte AChE (Shinohara and Seto 1986, Seto and Shinohara 1987). Both the compounds showed negative cooperativity, as their Hill coeffcients were 0.83 for PQ and 0.95 for DQ. The Hill coefficient nH is calculated with the help of Hill plot and gives the cooperativity of an enzyme in the presence of inhibitor. The inhibitory powers and Hill coefficients of dichlorvos and carbaryl computed as 30 $\mu$m and $1.4 \times 10$ $\mu$m respectively suggests the ratio of inhibitory powers of dichlorvos and carbaryl as about 1:46.6. Dichlorvos strongly inhibited AChE of rat heart in comparison to that of carbaryl. Hill coefficient for dichlorvos (0.91) and carbaryl (0.95) suggests negative cooperativity between these inhibitors and AChE enzyme.

## Kinetic and inhibitory Constants of AChE in Mammalian Tissues

The kinetic constants Michaelis Menten constant(km) and Vmax are determined with the help of Lineweaver-Burk double reciprocal plot and Michaelis Menten equation whereas inhibitory constants are calculated by Dixon plot. Km, Vmax and Ki can be used for biomonitoring the toxic level of these compounds. Nishioka *et al* (1976) assumed that the further binding of carbamate molecules to the reversible complex and / or the carbamylated enzyme is significant with high inhibitor concentrations. They further held that Kd and K2 are obtainable with a rather low carbamate concentration range whose product by Ki is in the order of 0.2-1.0/min. The enzymes are nowadays extensively used for the clinical diagnosis of pathological condition in mammals in general and human beings in particular. Several pesticides have synergistic effect. Their inhibitory effect in mammals is well reported but the kinetic and inhibitory parameters are less studied.

### Erythrocytes

Shinohara and Seto (1986) studied the *in vitro* inhibitory kinetics of AChE by paraquat, which has been widely used for an immediate acting herbicide toxic for animals and was orally used by human beings for suicide. Their results established paraquat as a competitive inhibitor with the help of kinetic behaviour. The human erythrocyte AChE showed competitive and noncompetitive nature of inhibition due to cyclophosphamide (CP) as Km increased and Vmax reduced (Al-Jafari *et al* 1995). Km had increased by 78 per cent after the exposure of CP. Bovine erythrocyte AChE gives the km as $1.48 \times 10^{-4}$ M (Aarseth *et al* 1968), $1.40 \times 10^4$ M with ATCH and $2.0 \times 10^4$ m with ACh (Ellman *et al* 1961). Affinity constants for methyl carbamate and dimethyl carbamate range 0.034 to $17.9 \times 10^3$M and 0.008 to $72.9 \times 10^3$M respectively for bovine AChE (Obrien *et al* 1966). This indicates that methyl carbamates hydrolyze much faster than dimethyl carbamates. The *in vitro* inhibitory kinetics of dimethyl sulfoxide (DMSO) for mice erythrocyte AChE indicates different Km and Vmax values for bound and solubilized fractions (Jagota 1992). Fixed concentrations of DMSO (0.64 and 1.27mM) competitively inhibited AChE.

### Synaptosomes

Bound and solubilized fractions of mice Synaptosome AChE showed different Km values but similar Vmax values for both (Jagota 1992). The ki determined by the Dixon plot indicated the competitive inhibition of AChE due to 0.64 and 1.27 mM concentrations of DMSO by giving the Ki of 0.11 mM.

### Serum

Km for serum AChE has been determined as $7.5 \times 10^{-7}$m (Purshottam and Kaveeshwar 1993). Administration of semipurified enzyme from electric el upto 3000 unit in 3 mg protein produced no adverse effect on animals after two weeks. In order to observe whether enhanced level of serum enzyme in the injected rats was indeed the exogenous enzyme, they calculated Km and Vmax of electric eel AChE. Vmax of the ChE in the Serum of uninjected rats was not affected by the increasing substrate concentration from 10 to 400 $\mu$l, which is characteristic of pseudocholinesterases Km of the serum of enzyme injected rats is similar to the Km of the electric eel AChE *i.e.* $6.2 \times 10^{-7}$m.

### Brain

The Km of rat brain AChE at $37^0$ C assay temperature has been reported as 111.9 $\mu$m (Carr and Chambers 1996). Decreasing the incubation temperature of rat AChE from 37 to $30^0$ C resulted in a significant decrease in Km and a small decrease in the Vmax. The Ki values for paraoxon and chlorpyrifos-oxon also increased significantly with the rise in incubation temperature form $30^0$ C to $37^0$C. Pentylenetetrazol (PTZ) enhanced rat brain AChE Km from $1.22 \times 10^{-4}$ M to $8 \times 10^{-3}$ M (Mahon and Brink 1970).

## Cerebellum

Guhathakurta and Bhattacharya (1988) isolated and purified the AChE from carebellum, since this region possess maximum AChE activity. Purified enzyme expressed Km as $3.3 \times 10^{-5}$ M with a slight change in Km to $3.0 \times 10^{-5}$ M with polymaleinic anhydride (PMA). Purified AChE was a highly stable and active enzyme which could be used for the purpose of immobilization.

## Cerebrum

The Km for cerebrum of rat brain has been recorded as $2.2 \times 10^{-4}$ M (Patocka and Bajgar 1969).

## Optic lobes

Optic lobes of rabbits of 0 to 364 days exhibited Km values ranging from 1.33 to 6.66 M and Vmax ranged from 0.26 to 7.14 (Dawood & Sharief 1995).

## Retina

The efficiency of the retinal AChE is prefixed in the neonatal development and no further structural development appears necessary for the retina during this stage (Dawood and Sharief 1995). The Km and Vmax shows similar trend to that of optic lobes during the stages.

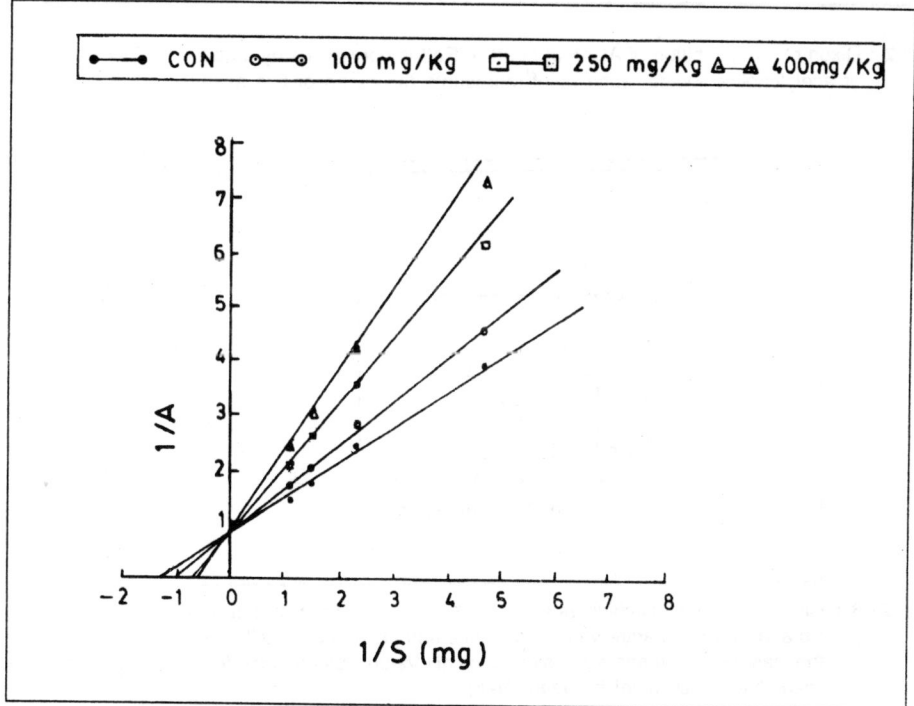

**Fig. 22.1 :** Line weaver burk plot of inhibitory effect of various doses of car baryl on AChE of heart of *Rattus norvegicus* treated for 96 hours AChI is used as substrate. Each point is the mean of five assays.

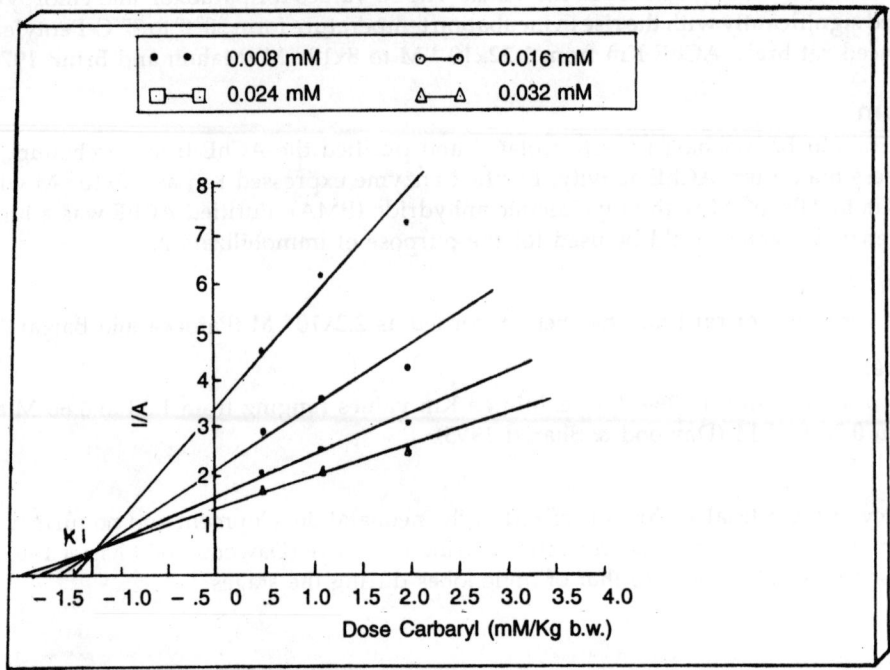

**Fig. 22.2 :** Dixon plot of inhibition of AChe of heart of *Rattus norvegicus* by carbaryl for four concentrations of acetylcholine iodide. each point represents the mean of five assays.

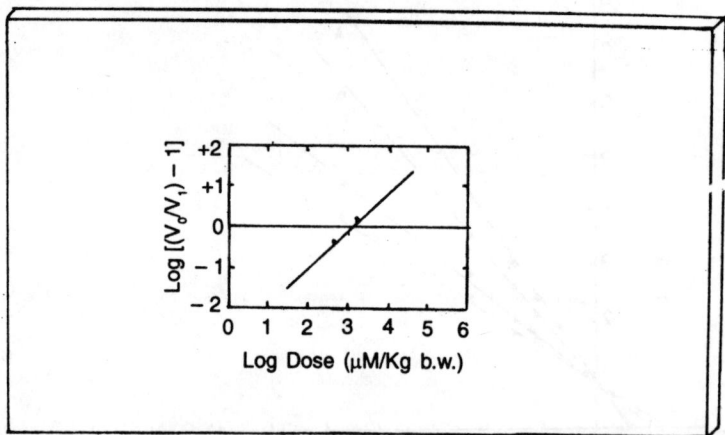

**Fig. 22.3 :** Hill plot of the acetylcholinesterase inhibition in heart of *rattus norvegicus* by carbaryl. The Vo and Vi are the activity in the absence and presence of inhibitors. By data analysis with the least square linear regression, each nH Value was obtained from the slope of the fitted linear line. Each point is mean (N=5)

## Heart

The heart of rat exhibits Km of $2.69 \times 10^{-3}$ M which gradually increased with the increase in dose while Vmax remained constant for all the doses (Parveen 1997). The carbaryl gave Ki as 1.30 mM indicating competitive nature inhibibtion.

**Table 22.1 : AChE Activity and effect of pesticides on AChE in mammalian Tissues**

| Tissue / Animal | Method | AChE Activity | ACh Content | Pesticide (Dose / duration) | % Inhibition | % increase in ACh | Author |
|---|---|---|---|---|---|---|---|
| **1. LIVER** | | | | | | | |
| (i) *Rattus Norvegicus* | Ellman *et al* 1961 | 1.07 ml/l/minx 104/gm | – | – | – | – | Ellman *et al* 1961 |
| (ii) Rat | Ellman *et al* 1961 | 22 µm/min | – | Soman *in vivo* (0.5 & 2.0 hrs.) | –82 | – | Purshottam and Kaveeshwar 1992 |
| (iii) Rat | Ellman *et al* 1961 | 26.6nm/rrin/mg protien | – | MEPA *in vivo* SPB DEPA + SPB | –65 –23.9 –16.2 | – | Rao *et ai* 1993 |
| (iv) Rat | Ellman *et al* 1961 | 22.0 nm/min/mg protein | – | Phenobarbital (PB) PB + Soman Soman | +14.5 –81.2 –86.5 | – | Purshottam and Srivastava 1989 |
| (v) Goat | Augustinson 1957 | 38.73 µm/mg protein | 75 mg/kg 150 mg/kg | Malathion *in vivo* –66.5 –71.3 | – | – | Tomar *et al* 1995 |
| (vi) Pig | – | 30 µm/l/mg/hr. | – | Dimethoate *in vitro* (1 to 10 µg) | –8.50 to –58.58 | – | Nandakumar and Udayabhaskar 1980 |
| **2. BLOOD** | | | | | | | |
| (i) Rat | Ellman *et al* 1961 | 5710 µm | – | – | – | – | Carakostas and Landis |
| (ii) Rat | 3 modified assays Voss and Sachsse 1970 (improved) | 3728, 3004 & 2710 13.24 µm/ml/ 20min (ATI) 6.32 (BTI) | – | – | – | – | Venkataraman *et al* 1993 |
| (iii) *Rattus norvegicus* | Hestrin 1949 | – | – | – | – | – | Srivastava and Raizada 1996 |
| (iv) Rat (female) | Hestrin 1949 | 1.33 µm/ml/min | – | Methyl parathion (7,15 & 60 days) HCH + MP (7, 15 30 days) | –62, –76 & –71 –75, –71 & –75 | – | Dikshith *et al* 1991 |
| (v) Human | Thomson *et al* 1988 | 2.29–2.55 KU/l | – | Herbicide Insecticide+ Herbicide Fumigators | –4.89 –4.63 –4.7 | – | Potter *et al* 1993 |
| **3. ERYTHROCYTES** | | | | | | | |
| (i) Rat | Ellman *et al* 1961 3 modified assays | 4880 IU/l 3323, 2607 and 2357 | – | – | – | – | Carakostas & Landis 1992 |
| (ii) Rat (Male) | Ellman *et al* 1961 Radiometric assay | 1.3 µm/min/ml 0.80 µm/min/ml | – | Carbaryl 37.5 mg/kg 37.5 mg/kg 75 mg/kg 75 mg/kg | –36 –62 –32 –81 | – | Nostrandt *et al* 1993 |

Contd....

| Tissue / Animal | Method | AChE Activity | ACh Content | Pesticide (Dose / duration) | % Inhibition | % increase in ACh | Author |
|---|---|---|---|---|---|---|---|
| (iii) Mice | Ellman et al 1961 | – | – | DMSO 0.13 mM 0.91 mM | –28 –92 to –95 | – | Jagota 1992 |
| (iv) Human | Ellman et al 1961 | – | – | CP in vitro 1.33 to 1.67mm in vitro | –38.8 to 76.7 | – | Al–Jafari et al 1995 |
| (v) Human | Ellman et al 1961 | – | – | Paraquat (359 µm) Dichlorvos (113µm) | –70 –67 | – | Seto and Shinohara 1987 |
| (vi) Bovine | Ellman et al 1961 | 0.0333–0.083 U/min | – | – | – | – | Ellman et al 1961 |
| **4. SERUM** | | | | | | | |
| (i) Rat | Voss and Sachsse 1970 | 15.99 µm/ml/20 min (ATI) 10.74 µm (BTI) | – | – | – | – | Venkataraman et al 1993 |
| (ii) Rat | Ellman et al 1961 | 0.70 µm/min/ml | – | Soman in vivo (0.22 mg/kg) 1/2 hr. & 2 hr. | –33 | – | Purshottam and Kaveeshwar 1992 |
| (iii) Rat | Ellman et al 1961 | 1658 nm/min/ml | – | DEPA | –11.2 | – | Rao et al 1993 |
| (iv) Cattle and buffalo | Bergmeyer 1974 | 120.6 µm/min/l | – | Cypermethrin + fenvelerate on Boophilus infected Cattle calves | –0.033 | – | Ansari et al 1990 |
| (v) Goat | Augustinson 1957 | 626.91 µm/min/l | – | Malathion (24 hrs) 75 mg/kg 150 mg/kg | –54.7 –60.7 | – | Tomar et al 1995 |
| (vi) Human | – | 7.6–13.7 µm/ 3min/ml | – | – | – | – | Garry and Routh 1965 |
| (vii) Human | – | 4.85 KU/l | – | Begining of work day After work day | –1.4 –7.2 | – | Carillo and Cervantes 1993 |
| (viii) Human | – | 11.26 µm (ATC) 16.10 µm (BTC) | – | – | – | – | Venkataraman & Nagarani 1994 |
| **5. Plasma** | | | | | | | |
| (i) Rat | Ellman et al 1961 | 0.6 µm/min/ml | – | Aldicarb(0.34 mg/kg) Carbaryl (75 mg/kg) Paraoxon (0.3 mg/kg) (75 mg/kg) (37.5 mg/kg) (75 mg/kg) | –61 –41 –64 –61 –47 –74 | – | Padilla and Hooper 1992 |
| (iii) Rat | Radiometric Assy | 0.28 µm | – | – | – | – | Carakostas & Landis 1992 |
| | Ellman et al 1961 3Modified assays | 766 IU/l 800,806,807 IU/l | | | | | |
| (iv) Rat | Ellman et al 1961 | 704 µm/min/ml | – | Soman in vivo | –67 | – | Purshottam and Srivastava 1989 |
| (v) Human | Thomson et al | 2.29–2.55 KU/l | – | Herbicide | +2.47 | – | Potter et al 1993 |

Contd....

| Tissue / Animal | Method | AChE Activity | ACh Content | Pesticide (Dose / duration) | % Inhibition | % increase in ACh | Author |
|---|---|---|---|---|---|---|---|
| (vi) Human | 1988 | 14.02 μm (ATI) 18.94 μm (BTI) | — | Insecticide + Herbicide Fumigators | -1.2 — -2.0 | — — — | Venkataraman & Nagarani 1994 |
| **6. BRAIN** | | | | | | | |
| (i) Rat | Ellman et al 1961 | 17.6 μm/min/gm | — | Carbaryl (75 mg/kg) Aldicarb (0.34 mg/kg) Paraoxon(0.34 mg/kg) | -45 to -72 -45 to -63 -75 | — | Padilla and Hooper 1992 |
| (ii) Rat | Ellman et al 1961 Radiometric assay | 6.1 μm/min/gm 5.9 μm | — | Carbaryl 37.5 mg/kg 75mg/kg 37.5 mg/kg 75 mg/kg | -36 -58 -55 -81 | — | Nostrandt et al 1993 |
| (iii) Rat | Ellman et al 1961 | Cerebrum 110.8 Cerebellum 49.6 Brain stem 193.3 with midbrain | — | Soman in vivo (0.22mg/kg) | Cerebrum -6 Cerebellum -44 Brain Stem -47 with mid brain | — | Purshottam and Kaveershwar 1992 |
| (iv) Rat | Ellman et al 1961 | 202 nm/min/mg protein | — | DEPA SPB DEPA + SPB | -3.9 -29.7 -18.3 | — | Rao et al 1993 |
| (v) Rat | Ellman et al 1961 | 2 μm to 8.9 um | — | Pentylenetetrazol in vitro (3.0 mM) | -19.3 | — | Mohan and Brink 1970 |
| (vi) Rat | Ellman et al 1961 | 3.19 μm/min/gm | — | Dichlorvos 30 mg/kg 50 mg/kg 70 mg/kg 90 mg/kg | -82.5 -88.6 -92.4 -92.4 | — | Naidu et al 1987 |
| (vii) Rat | Ellman et al 1961 | 5.17 units/gm | — | | — | — | Singh et al 1990 |
| (x) Rat | Ellman et al 1961 | 20.1 (30°c) 21.1 (37°c) | — | | — | — | Carr and Chambers 1996 |
| (xi) Rat | Hestrin 1949 | 21.30 μm/gm/min | — | Methyl parathion (2mg/kg/day) 7 day 15 day 30 day HCH + Methyl parathion 7 days 15 days 30 days | -37 -76 -35 -23 -28 -28 | — | Dikshit et al 1991 |
| (xii) Rat | Hestrin 1949 | Cerebral Cortex 39.42 brain stem 56.45 spinal cord 27.9 | 0.71 μm/gm 1.31 μm/gm 0.65 μm/gm | Methyl parathion (1mg/kg) | -44.88 -37.64 -31.8 | +38.02 +41.98 +36.92 | MahaboobBasha & Nayeemunnisa 1993 |

Contd....

| Tissue / Animal | Method | AChE Activity | ACh Content | Pesticide (Dose / duration) | % Inhibition | % increase in ACh | Author |
|---|---|---|---|---|---|---|---|
| (xiii) Rat | Hestrin 1949 | – | – | Dimethoate (3.75,7.5 15 & 30 mg/kg) Maternal brain fetal brain | –22 to 70 –30 to –42 | – | Srivastava and Raizada 1996 |
| (xiv) Rat | Snug and Ruff 1983 | Cortex472nm/h/gm Striatum 2113nm/h/gm Cerebellum 302nm /h/gm | – | 15 mg/kg 30 mg/kg 60 mg/kg Formaldehyde | –6 –25 –30 –78 –72 –48 | – – | Mc Geer and Mc Gear 1989 |
| (xv) Rabbit | Ellman et al 1961 | Cortex 18 µm/mg/ min Hypothalamus 4.1 Mid brain 19.3 Medula oblongata & pons 14.3 Cerebellum 10.7 Diaphragm 1.7 aorta 1.6 | – | Physostigmine (3.13 µm/) PHC (50 µm/kg) MIPC (200 µm/kg) BPMC(200 µm/kg) | 65.5/71.1/65.5/ 77.2 64.5/70.9/78.0/84.3 73.0/85.4/74.6/83.4 69.9/79.0/74.1/74.8 59.8/63.5/76.6/71.0 88.2/94.1/94.1/94.1 100/93.7/93.7/93.7 | – | Takahashi et al 1994 |
| (xvi) Goat (Capra capra) | Ellman et al 1961 Purified | Cerebellum 1.05 µm/min/mg protein 48.30 µm | – | – | – | – | Guhathakurta & Bhattacharya 1988 |
| (xvii) Monkey (Macaca radiata) | Ellman et al 1961 | 0.45 µm/min | – | DFP Eserine Physostigmin | –81 –96 –100 | – | Jayanthi & Balasubr amanian 1991 |
| **7. HEART** (i) Rat | Ellman et al 1961 | 3.19 µm/min/gm | – | Dichlorvos 30 mg/kg 50 mg/kg 70 mg/kg 90 mg/kg | –55.6 –70 –86.4 –88.9 | – | Naidu et al 1987 |
| (ii) Rat | Hestrin 1949 | 4.72 µm/mg protein/hr. | 74.05 µm/gm | Carbaryl (96 hrs) 100mg/kg 250 mg/kg 400 mg/kg | –21.8 –42.1 –54.8 | +2.14 +17.1 +24.7 | Parveen 1997 |
| (iii) Rat | Hestrin 1949 | 0.225 µm/mg protein/hr | 4.5 µm/gm | Isoproterenol (48 hrs.) | –22.2 | +44 | Gaur 1997 |

**Table 22.2 : Kinetic Constants $K_m$, $V_{max}$ and Inhibitory Constant ki for inhibition of AChE enzyme during pesticide toxicty in various tissues of mammals**

| Tissue / Animal | Method | Control Km | Control Vmax | Pesticide | Km/Vmax | Ki | Author |
|---|---|---|---|---|---|---|---|
| **1. ERYTHROCYTE** | | | | | | | |
| (i) Human | Ellman et al 1961 | 76μm | 5.3ml | Paraquat | 290 μm | 4.2 μm | Shinohara & Seto 1986 |
| (ii) Human | Ellman et al 1961 | 132μm | 73.8 μm/hr/mg Protein | CP | +78%/−54.5% | – | Al-Jafari et al 1995 |
| (iii) Bovine | – | $1.48 \times 10^{-4}$M | – | Methyl carbamate | – | Ka 0.034 to17.9x $10^3$M | Aarseth et al 1966 |
| (iv) Bovine | – | – | – | Dimethyl carbamate | – | 0.008 to 72.9x $10^3$M | Obrien et al 1966 |
| (v) Bovine | Ellman et al 1961 | $1.4 \times 10^4$ (ATACH) $2.0 \times 10^4$ (ACH) | – | – | – | – | Ellman et al 1961 |
| (vi) Mice | Ellman et al 1961 | Bound 0.5m Solubilized 0.33mM | 0.67mM/mg protein/min 0.59mM/mg | DMSO | – | 0.11mM | Jagota 1992 |
| **2. SYNAPTOSOMES** | | | | | | | |
| (i) mice | Ellman et al 1961 | Bound 0.2mM Solubilized 0.15mM | 0.4mM/mg 0.4mM/mg | DMSO | – | 0.11mM | Jagota 1992 |
| **3. SERUM** | | | | | | | |
| (i) Rat | Ellman et al 1961 | $7.5 \times 10^{-7}$M | – | – | – | – | Purshottam & Kaveeshwar 1993 |
| **4. BRAIN** | | | | | | | |
| (i) Rat | – | 65.0 μm(30°C) 111.9 μm (37°C) | 65.3nm/min/min/ protein 68.6 | Paraoxon Chlorpyrifos-oxon Paraoxon Chlorpyrifos-oxon | – | 397.2nM/min(30°C) 4477.9nM/min 854.7nM/min (37°C) 7528.1nM/min | Carr andChambers 1996 1996 |
| (ii) Rat | Ellman et al 1961 | $1.22 \times 10^{-4}$M | 1.37μm/gm/min | PTZ | $8 \times 10^{-3}$M | $4.7 \times 10^{-3}$M | Mahon & Brink 1970 |
| **5. CEREBELLUM** | | | | | | | |
| Goat (Capra Copra) | Ellman et al 1961 | $3.30 \times 10^{-5}$M(free) $3.0 \times 10^{-5}$M(bound) | – | PMA | $3.0 \times 10^{-3}$M | – | Guhathakurta & Bhattacharya 1988 |
| **6. CEREBRUM** | | | | | | | |
| (i) Human | – | $2.2 \times 10^{-4}$M | – | – | – | – | Patocka and Bajgar 1969 |
| **7. OPTIC LOBES** | | | | | | | |
| (i) Rabbit of 0-364 days age | Hestrin 1949 | 1.33 to 6.66 M/mg protein/hr | 0.26 to 7.14 | – | – | – | Dawood & Sharief 1995 |
| **8. RETINA** | | | | | | | |
| (i) Rabbit of 0-364 days age | Hestrin 1949 | 3.33 to 4.00m/mg protein/hr | 0.50 to 5.50 | – | – | – | Dawood & Sharief 1995 |
| **9. HEART** | | | | | | | |
| (i) Rat (Rattus vegicus) | Hestrin 1949 | $2.69 \times 10^{-3}$M | 1.25 A/mg protein 30min | Carbaryl (96hrs.) 100 mg/kg 250 mg/kg 400 mg/kg | $3.66 \times 10^{-3}$M 5.232M 6.315 | 1.30mM | Parveen 1997 |
| (ii) Rat Rattus norvegicus | Hestrin 1949 | $3.0 \times 10^{-3}$M | 1.25 A/mg protein/ 30min | Isoproterenol (48hrs.) | – | – | Gaur 1997 |

## SUMMARY

The pesticides particularly organophosphate and carbamate are generally affecting the cholinesterase system as they are cholinergic inhibitors. AChE is a predominate enzyme in those organs which contain cholinergic nerves. The brain, heart, liver, blood are under the control of cholinergic and adrenergic component of autonomic nervous system. The effect of pesticides on these systems have been studied by a number of investigators, however they have restricted to the biochemical estimation of AChE and its inhibition. On the other hand, a few investigators demonstrated the kinetics of AChE by using various plots and kinetic constants. The AChE seems to be the most sensitive parameter for the monitoring of intoxication due to pesticides, toxic compounds and drugs to the mammals.

## REFERENCES

- Aarseth, P., Barastad, J.A.B., Rogne, O. and Oksnes (1968): Histochem. 15: 229 as quoted by Mahon and Brink (1970). Inhibition of AChE by Pentylenetetrazol. *J. Neurochem.*, **17**: 949- 953.

- Adams, D.H. and Whittaker, V.P. (1949): The cholinesterase of human blood. 1. The specificity l of the plasma enzyme and its relation to erythrocyte cholinesterase. *Bicochem. Biophys. Acta.*, **3**: 358-366.

- Al-Jafari., A.A. Duhaiman, A.S. and Kamal, M.A. (1995): Inhibition of human acetylcholinesterase by cyclophosphamide. *Toxicol.*, 1-6.

- Ansari., M.J., Kumar A., Prasad, R.L. Basu, A., Sahai, B.N., Sinha, A.P. (1990): Clinico-biochemical use of serum acetylcholinesterase following treatment with synthetic pyrethroids, cypermethrin and fenvalerate, in cattle and buffalo experimentally infested with Boophilus microplus. *Ind. J. Exp. Biol.*, **28**: 241-244.

- Bhatia, S.C. Sharma, S.C and Venkita Subramanian, T.A. (1972): Effect of dieldrin on certain enzyme systems of rat liver. *Brit. J. Exp. Pathol.*, **53** 419-426.

- Boyer, A.C., Brown, L.J., Slomka, M.B. and Hine, C.H. (1977): Inhibition of human plasma cholinesterase by ingested dichlorvos: Effect of formulation vehicle. *Toxicol. Appl. Pharmacol.*, **41**(2): 389-394.

- Carakostas, M.C. and Landis, M.A. (1991): Modificaton of an automated method for determining plasma and erythrocyte cholinesterase activity in laboratory animals:. Vet. Hum. *Toxicol.*, **33**: 450-456.

- Carillo, L.L. and Cervantes, M.L. (1993): Effect of exposure to organophosphate pesticides on serum cholinesterase levels. Archives Envir. *Health*, **48** (5): 359-363.

- Carr, R.L. and Chambers, J.E. (1996): Kinetic analysis of the *in vitro* inhibition, aging and reactivation of brain acetylcholinesterase from rat and channel cat fish by paraoxon and chlorpyrifos-oxon. *Toxicol. Appl. Pharmacol.* **139**, 365-373.

- Chiappa. S., Padilla S., Koenigsberger C, Moser V and Brimijoin S. (1995) Slow accumulation of acetylcholinestrase in rat brain during enzyme inhibition by repeated dosing with chlorpyrifos. *Biochem. Pharmacol.* **49** (7) 955-963.

- Clark, D. R. Jr and Rattner, B.A. (1987): Orthene toxicity in little brown bats (*Myotis lucifugus*): Acetylcholinesterase inhibition, coordination loss and mortality. *Environ. Toxicol. Chem.*, **6**(9): 705-708.

- Dawood N. and Sharief D. (1995) Orientation in the catalytic efficiencies of acetylcholinesterase in the optic lobes and retina of *Oryctolagus cuniculus* during the different stages of postnatal development. *J. Ecobiol.* **7**(3) 213-217.

- Dikshith, T.S.S., Raizada, R.B., Singh, V., Pandey, M. and Srivastava, M.K. (1991): *Ind. J. Exp. Biol.*, **29**: 149-155.

- Ellman, G.L., courtney., K.D. Andres, V. Jr and Featherstone, R.M. (1961): A new and rapid colorimetric determination of acetylcholinesterase activity. Biochem. Pharmacol., 7:88-95.

- Garry, P.J. and Routh, J.I. (1965): A micro method for serum cholinesterase. *Clin. Chem.*, **11**(2): 91-96.

- Gaur, M. 1(1997): A comparative study of the AChE enzyme kinetics of normal and infarcted heart of vertebrates. Ph.D. Thesis, Barkatullah Unversity, Bhopal.

- Guhathakurta, S. and Bhattacharya, S. (1988): Immobilization of puried goat-cerebellar acetylcholinesterase for inhibition studies in a column. *Ind. J. Exp. Biol.*, **26**: 44-47.

- Hestrin, S. (1949): The reaction of acetylcholine and other carbonylic acid derivatives with hydroxyl amine and its biological application. *J. Biol. Chem.*, 180:249-261.

- Jagota, S.K. (1992): Inhibition of acetylcholinesterase of mice erythrocytes and synaptosomes by dimethylsulfoxide. *Ind. J. Med. Res.* **(B) 96:** 275-278.

- Jayanthi, L.D. and Balasubramanian, A.S. (1991): Isolation of a tripeptide showing weak acetylcholinesterase activity from a soluble from of monkey basal ganglia acetylcholinesterase by limited trypsin digesion. Ind. J. Biochem. Biophys., **28:** 100-108

- Katz B. and Thesleff S. (1957) A study of "desensitization" produced by acetylcholine at the motor endplate. *J. Physiol. (Lond.)* **138,** 63-80.

- Kozar, M.D., Overstreet, D.H., Chippendale, T.C. Russel, R.W. (1976): Changes in acetylcholinesterse activity in three major brain areas and related changes in behaviour following acute treatment with diisopropyl flourophosphate. *Neuropharmacology*, **15:** 291.

- Kurtz, P.J. (1977b): Dissociated behavioral and cholinesterase decrements following malathion exposure. *Toxicol. Appl. Pharmacol.*, **42** (3): 589-594.

- Mahaboob Basha, P. and Nayeemunnisa (1993): Methylparathion induced alterations in GABAergic system during critical stage of central nervous system development in albino rat pups. J. **Exp. Biol.** 31: 369-372.

- Mahon., P.J. and Brink, J.J. (1970): Inhibition of AChE *in vitro* by Pentylenetetrazol. *J. Neurochem.*, **17:** 949-953.

- Maslova, M.N. and Reznik, L.V. (1976): Inhibition of cholinesterase activity in the rat brain by organophosphorus inhibitors with different degrees of hydrophobicity. *Ukr. Biokhim Zh.* **48(4):** 450-454.

- McGeer, E.G and McGeer. P.L. (1989): Effect of fixatives on rat brain acetylcholinesterase activity. *J. Neurosci. Met.* **28:** 235-237.

- Metcalf, R.L. (1951): In Methods in biochemical analysis (ed. D. Glick). Interscience publishers *Inc., New York,* 5.

- Miyamoto, J., Hosokawa, S., Kadota, T., Kohda, H., Arai, M., Sugihara, S. and Hirao, K. (1976): Studies in cholinesterase inhibition and structural changes at neuromuscular junctions in rabbits by subacute administration of sumithion. *J. Pestic. Sci.,* **1** (3): 171-178.

- Murphy, S.D. (1966): Liver metabolism and toxicity of thiophoshate insecticides in mammalian, avian and piscine species. *Proc. Soc. Exp. Biol. Med.*, **123:** 392 - 398.

- Naidu, K.A., Vishanathan, S. and Krishnakumari, M.K. (1987): Cardiotoxic effects of Dichlorvos (DDVP) in albino rats. *Ind. J. Physiol. Pharmacol.*, **31** (1): 19-24.

- Nakagawa, M. Kobayashi, H., Kajima, S., Uemura, A. and Uchtyama, M. (1977): Comparison of inhibitory actions of organophosphate pesticides on cholinesterase and lecithincholesterol acyltransterase in human plasma. *Chem. Pharm. Bull. (Tokyo),* **25 (10):** 2530-2534.

- Nanda Kumar, N.V. and Udaya Bhaskar, S. (1980): Colorimentric determination of dimethoate by quantification of cholinesterase inhibition. *J. Food Science and Technol.*, **17:** 153-155.

- Nishioka, T., Fujita, T. and Nakajima, M. (1996): kinetic constants for the inhibition of AChE by phenyl carbamates. *J. Pestic. Sci.,* **1** (3): 239-247.

- Nostrandt, A.C., Duncan, J.A. and Pandilla, S. (1993): A modified spectrophotometric method appropriate for measuring cholinesterase activity in tissue from carbaryl treated animals. Fundam. and Appl. *Toxicol.*, **21:** 196 _203.

- Obrien, R.D., Hilton, B.D. and Gilmour, L. (1996): The reaction of carbamates with cholinesterases. *Mol. Pharmacol.*, **2** :593-605.

- Padilla, S. and Hooper, M.J. (1992): Cholinesterase measurements in tissues from carbamate-treated animals; Cautions and recommenations. Proceedings of the U.S.-EPA Workshop on cholinesterase Methodologies, pp. 63-81. Office of Pesticide Programs U.S. Envir. Protection Agency, Washington, D.C.

- Parveen M. (1997) Various aspects of inhibition of AChE in heart of *Rattus norvegicus* by carbaryl. Proc. Awarded paper in MAPCOST 94-97.

- Parveen M. and Kumar S. (2001) Effect of DDVP on the histology and AChE Kinetics of the heart muscles of *Rattus norvegicus J. Environ. Biol.*22(3) in press.

- Patocka, J. and Bajgar, J. (1969): *FEBS Leftt.* ,**2**: 195.

- Potter, W.T., Garry, V.F.,Kelly, J.T.Tarone, R., Griffith, J. and Nelson,R.L. (1993): Radiometric assay of red cell and plasma cholinesterase in pesticide appliers from Minnesota. *Toxicol. Appl. Pharmacol.*, **119**: 150-155.

- Purshottam, T. and Kaveeshwar,U. (1992): Effect of soman administration on B-esterases in blood, liver microsomes and brain regions of rats., *Ind. J. Physiol. Pharmacol.*,**36**(3): 197-200.

- Purshottam,T. and Kaveeshwar,U. (1993):Comparative efficacy of exogenous acetylcholinesterase administration on soman and dichlorvos toxicity in rats. *Ind. J. Exp. Biol.*, 31 ̄365-368.

- Purshottam, T. and Srivastava, R.K. (1989): Role of carboxylesterase in protection against soman toxicity, *Pharmacology*, **38**: 319-326.

- Rahman, M.F., Siddiqui, M.K.J., Anjum, F., Qadri, S.S.H. (1989): Acutotoxicity and antiacetylcholinesterase potentional of some biphenyl derivatives to non-target species. *Ind. J. Exp. Biol.*, **27**: 138-140.

- Rao, S.S., Kaveeshwar, U.and Purkayastha, S.S. (1993): Acute oral toxicity of insect repllent N, N-diethylphenylacetamide in mice, rats and rabbits and protective effect of sodium pentabarbitol. *Ind. J. Exp. Biol.*, **31**: 755-760.

- Robinson, C.P., Smith, P.W., Crane, C.R., McConnell, J.K. Allen, L.V and Endecott, B.R. (1978): the protective effects of ethylestrenol against acute poisoning by organophosphorus cholinesterase inhibitors in rats. *Arch. Int. Pharmacodyn. Ther.*, **231** (1): 168-176.

- Seto, Y. and Shinohara, T. (1987): Inhibitory effects of paraquat and its related compounds on the acetylcholinesterase activities of human erythrocytes and electric eel *Electrophorus electricus.* Agric. Biol. Chem., **51 (8)**: 2131-2138.

- Shinohara, T. and Seto, Y. (1986): *In vitro* inhibition of acetylcholinesterase by paraquat. Agric. *Biol.Chem.*, **50** (1): 255-256.

- Shtenberg, A.I and Rybakova, M.N. (1968): Effect of carbaryl on the Neuroendocrine system of Rats. Fd, Cosmet. Toxicol. Vol. 6. pp. 461-467. Pergamon Press. Printed in Great Britain.

- Singh,U.K. and Agarwal,K.N. (1990):Acetylcholinesterase activity in developing rat brain during undernutrition. *Ind. J. Biochem. Biophys.*, **27**: 329-331.

- Singh, U.K., Agarwal, K.N. and Shanker, R. (1990): Effect of undernutrition on succinate dehydrogenase and acetylcholinesterase in developing rat brain *Ind. J. Exp. Biol.*, **28**: 868-870.

- Sivakumar (1989): Recovery of acetylcholinesterase (AChE) from different regions of brain liver and kidney of rat, *Rattus norvegicus* exposed to phorate. M. Phil. dissertation, Univ. of Madras.

- Smith, A.P. and Muir A.W. (1977): Antinodal action of the oxime HS6 at the soman poisoned neuromuscular junction of the rat and guinea-pig. *J. Pharm. Pharmacol.*, **29** (12): 762-764.

- Snug, S.C. and Ruff, B.A. (1983) Molecular forms of sucrose extractable and particulate acetylcholinesterase in the developing and adult rat brain. *Neurochem.* Res. **8**: 303-311.

- Srinivasan, R., Karozmar, A.G., Bemsohn, J. (1976): Rat brain acetylcholinesterase and its isozymes after intracerebral administration of DFP. Biochem. *Pharmacol.*, **25**: 2739.

- Srivastava, M.K. and Raizada R.B. (1996) Developmental effect of technical dimethoate in rats: Maternal and fetal toxicity evaluation. *Ind. J. Exp. Biol.* **34**, 329-333.

- Stavinoha, W.B. Modak, A.T. and Weintraub, S.T. (1976): Rate of accumulation of acetylcholine in discrete regions of the rat brain after dichlorvos treatment, *J. Neurochem.*, **27** (6): 1375-1378.

- Sureshbabu, R., Uma, R., Sembulingam, K. and Namasivayam, A. (1992): Acetylcholine and cholinesterase levels in the brain of methanol trated rats. *Ind. J. Physiol. Pharmacol.*, **36** (4): 289-290.

- Takahashi,H. Kakinuma, Y. and Futagawa, H. (1994):Non-cholinergic lethality following intravenous injection of carbamate in secticide inrabbits. *Toxicol.*, **93**: 195-207.

- Tomar, M.S., Dhanotiya, R.S., Shilaskar, D.V. and Dixit, N.K. (1995): Effect of malathion on enzymes of goat liver and serum. *J. Environ. Biol.*, **16** (2): 151 -155.

- Venkataraman, B.V. and Nagarani, M.A. (1994): Species variation in the specificity of cholinesterases in human and rat blood sample. *Ind. J. physiol. Pharmacol.*, **38** (3): 211-213.

- Venkataraman, B.V., Nagarani, M.A., Andrade, C. and Joseph, T.(1993): Improved colorimetric method for cholinesterase activity. *Ind. J. physiol. Pharmacol.*, **37** (1): 82-87.

- Vijayan, V.K. and Brownson, R.H. (1975): Polyacrylamide gel electrophoresis of rat brain acetylcholinesterase: Isoenzyme changes following parathion poisoning. *J. Neurochem.*, **24**: 105-110.

- Voss, G. and Sachsse, K. (1970): Red cell and plasma cholinesterase activities in microsamples of human and animal blood determined simultaneously by a modified acetylcholine/DTNB procedure. *Toxicol. and Appl. Pharmacol.*, **16**: 764-772.

# 23

# Toxicity Assessment for Environmental Safety

*Ram Chandra and Sandeep Kr. Misra*

## 1. Introduction

With the increased worldwide industrialization over the past 25 years, and with the concomitant higher demand for chemicals, both the developing and developed nations face increasing ecological and toxicological problems from the release of toxic contaminants to the environment. In response to these expanding stresses on the environment and in the belief that there is no single criterion by which to adequately judge the potential hazard (either to the environment or man) of a given substance, a multitude of biological assay procedures have been developed, proposed and used to assess toxicant impacts. Due to our newly acquired awareness of the long term effects of chemicals discharged into receiving waters, research efforts are being diverted at short-term bioassay tests in an attempt to alert monitoring agencies as well as dischargers of toxic conditions.

Pollutants are defined as a substance that occurs in the environment, which has deleterious effects on living organisms. As industrial pollutants and toxicants such as herbicides, insecticides, fertilizers and exhaust fumes affect aquatic biota systems at different levels and in many ways, it is acknowledged that the battery approach utilizing several different short-term biological tests would be preferred in any monitoring scheme. In some studies investigators have employed a battery of ecological and health effect tests to estimate the toxicity and mutagenicity of industrial effluents. Ecological effect tests are conducted to measure mainly the acute toxicity of chemicals to aquatic organisms representing various trophic levels of the food chain. These tests help in the estimation of chemical toxicity in natural and man modified ecosystems. Bacteria, algae, zooplankton, benthic invertebrates, and fish have been used in these tests. Bacteria and enzymes may be exposed to a wide range of toxic, organic and inorganic compounds in natural waters, soil and in sewage treatment process. The toxicity of the compounds depend on environmental parameters as well as on the microorganism or enzyme systems being tested. The compounds may be metabolically altered to nontoxic metabolites or may exert a direct toxic action on microbial populations and this may adversely affect the operation of the plant. Toxicant action is concentration dependent. For example, phenol can be metabolized at low concentrations but becomes toxic at higher concentrations. Toxicant action also depends on the presence of other chemicals in solution. A toxicant is an agent that can produce an adverse response effect in a biological system, seriously damaging its structure or function or producing death. The adverse response may be defined in terms of a measurement that is outside the normal range of healthy organisms. A toxicant or foreign substance (*i.e.* xenobiotic) may be introduced deliberately into the aquatic ecosystem, impairing the quality of the water and making it unfavourable for aquatic life. Pollutant or toxic agent is used occasionally to indicate an agent that can produce adverse effects. However, these toxicants as they encompass adverse abiotic changes, such as extremes in temperature and pH, decreases in dissolved oxygen, and increases in suspended solids or sedimentation. Pollution means the introduction by humans, directly or indirectly, of substances or energy into the aquatic environment resulting in such deleterious effects as harm to living resources, hazards to human health, hindrance to aquatic activities including fishing, impairment of quality for use of water and reduction of amenities.

Industrial waste is one important source of environmental pollution and effluents may be classified as water pollutants because they may be toxic and also change the temperature, pH and salinity of a receiving water in which they enter. However, effluents usually contain one or more chemical toxicants that vary in composition over time.

Toxicity is a relative property reflecting a chemical's potential to have a harmful effect on a living organism. It is a function of the concentration and composition/properties of the chemical to which the organism is exposed (*i.e.*, externally and internally) and the duration of exposure. Traditionally, toxicity data have been used in comparing chemical substances or the sensitivities of different species to the same substance. Information about the biological mechanisms affected and the conditions under which the toxicant is harmful is also important for this comparison. (Parkhurst 1979)

Toxicity tests are therefore used to evaluate the adverse effects of a chemical on living organisms under standardized, reproducible conditions that permit comparison with other chemicals or species tested and comparison of similar data from different laboratories. (Processing of third international course held at edinturg U.K. 1985)

Toxicity can be divided into the broad categories direct and indirect. Direct toxicity results from the toxic agent acting more or less directly at sites of action in or on organisms, indirect toxicity occurs as a result of the influence of changes in the chemicals, physical and/or biological environment (*e.g.* Changes in the quality and/or quantity of food organisms or habitat changes and/or losses). Direct toxicity is largely the result of internal biochemical changes, whereas indirect toxicity is more a function of changes in general organism viability produced by factors external to the organism.

## Basic Requirement and Terminology for Toxicity Assessment

The basic requirements and desirable conditions for toxicity tests are :

(a)   Abundant supply of water of desired quality.
(b)   Adequate and effective flowing water system constructed of non-polluting or absorbing materials.
(c)   Adequate space and well planned holding, culturing and testing equipment and facilities.
(d)   Adequate source of healthy experimental organisms.
(e)   Appropriate lighting facilities for plant toxicity tests.

The facilities, equipment and water supplies needed for effective tests depend on the type of tests and their objectives. For effluent and monitoring compliance tests requiring receiving water as the dilution water, use water immediately upstream and outside the zone of influence of the waste. When studies require the use of laboratory grade water, use a water supply free from pollution and one that provides for acceptable survival, growth, and reproduction of the aquatic test organisms to be studied.

The most important requirements for designing a toxicity testing programme are defining objectives of the study and establishing quality control practices, to ensure that the data are of sufficient quality to address the objectives and to ensure credibility.

Following general terminology can be used in toxicity assessment :

**Dose:** Amount of toxicant that enters the organism. Dose and concentration are not interchangeable.

**Exposure time:** Time of exposure of test organism to test solution.

**Acute Toxicity Test:** A test designed to determine mortality over a relatively short period of time, generally 48-96 hours.

**Chronic Toxicity Test:** A test in which there is long term exposure to a toxicant, often for the entire reproductive life-cycle (egg to egg) or for a portion of the life-cycle that includes sensitive life-stages. A chronic toxic effect can be measured in terms of reduced growth, reduced reproduction, etc., in addition to lethality.

**Lethal Concentration (LC):** Toxicant concentration estimated to produce death in a specified proportion of test organisms. Usually defined as median (50%) lethal concentration, $LC_{50}$, *i.e.* concentration killing 50 per cent of exposed organisms at a specific time of observation, for example, 96-h $LC_{50}$. Any desired LC value *e.g.* $LC_5$, $LC_{95}$ can be calculated for particular needs.

**Effective Concentration (EC):** Toxicant concentration estimated to cause a specified effect in a designated proportion of test organisms. The effect is usually sublethal, such as a change in respiration rate or loss of equilibrium, but is defined in quantal terms, *i.e.*, a particular individual either shows the effect or does not show it. The exposure time also is specified, for example, the 96 h $EC_{50}$ for loss of equilibrium is the effective concentration for 50 per cent of the test organisms in 96 h, for this kind of effect.

**Inhibiting Concentration (IC):** Toxicant concentration estimated to cause a specified percentage inhibition or impairment in a qualitative biological function. For example, an $IC_{25}$ could be the concentration estimated to cause a 25 per cent reduction in growth of test organism, relative to the control. This term should be used with any toxicological test that measures a change in rate, such as respiration, number of progeny, increase in number of algal cells etc. (the term $EC_{50}$ is not appropriate for such changes because it is limited to quantal measurements).

**Asymptotic LC50:** Toxicant concentration at which $LC_{50}$ approaches a constant for a prolonged exposure time.

**Medium Tolerance Limit (TLm):** Test material concentration at which 50 per cent of test organism survive for a specified exposure time. This term has been superseded by median

**No Observed Effect Concentration (NOEC):** In a full or partial life-cycle test, the highest toxicant concentration in which the values for the measured response are not statistically significantly different from those in the control.

**Lowest Observed Effect Concentration (LOEC):** In a full or partial life-cycle test, the lowest toxicant concentration in which the values for the measured response are statistically significantly different from those in the control.

**Maximum Allowable Toxicant Concentration (MATC):** Toxicant concentration that may be present in a receiving water without causing significant harm to productivity or other uses. MATC is determined by long-term tests of either partial life cycle with sensitive life stages or a full life cycle of the test organism.

**Chronic Value (ChV):** Geometric mean of the NOEC and LOEC from partial and full life-cycle tests and early life-stage tests.

**Acute to chronic ratio:** Numerical relation ship between acute and chronic toxicity that is applied to acute toxicity test values to estimate toxicant concentration that is safe for chronic or long term exposure of a test organism.

**Static test:** Test in which solutions and test organisms are placed in test chambers and kept there for the duration of the test.

**Renewable test:** Tests in which organisms are exposed to solutions of the same composition that are renewed periodically during the test period (with renewals usually at 24 hr intervals). This is accomplished by transferring test organisms or replacing test solution.

**Flow-through test:** Test in which solution is replaced continuously in test chambers throughout the test duration.

**Bio-concentration:** The process whereby living organisms acquire toxicants from water by diffusion or transport through gills or integument or by absorption to the body surface and store it in or on their bodies at concentrations higher than in the environment.

**Bio-concentration factor (BCF):** The ratio of a toxicant in an organism to its concentration in water.

**Depuration:** Loss of a chemical from an organism; often reported as a rate function.

**Bio-accumulation:** The process whereby living organisms acquire and store a toxicant after absorbing it from all sources.

**Bio-accumulation Factor:** The ratio of concentration of a toxicant in an organism to its concentration in food and water.

## Standard Procedures

A variety of test methods have been developed by the American Public Health Association (APHA), U.S. Environmental Protection Agency (USEPA), American Society for Testing and Materials (ASTM), International Standardization Organization (ISO), and Organization for Economic Co-operation and Development (OECD) to evaluate the potential toxicity and hazard of materials to organisms. Doudoroft *et. al.* (1951) first recognized the need to develop uniform, standardized test procedures to maximize the comparability of data from tests. The advantages of using standardized test procedures were summarized by Davis (1977) as follows:

(a) Allows selection of one or more uniform and useful tests by a variety of laboratories.
(b) Facilitates comparison of data and results and thus increases usefulness of published data.
(c) Increases accuracy of the data.
(d) Allows replication of the tests.
(e) Allows the test to be easily initiated and conducted by a variety of personnel (if the procedure is well documented).
(f) Legal advantage if procedures are accepted by the courts.
(g) Useful for routine monitoring purposes.

Davis. (1977) stated that the initial step to standardization is a thorough knowledge of the various chemical, physical and biological factors that affect toxicity test results. Standardization can then be achieved by :

(i) Adoption of detailed test protocols and minimize or standardize disturbing effects.
(ii) Use of a standard test species.
(iii) Use of reference toxicants or "disease free" certified test animals, plant or seed.

A standardized method (protocol) with reference toxicants and standard test species theoretically maximizes comparability, replicability, and reliability and thus is essential for answering questions on relative toxicity and sensitivity or replicability of tests (*Buikema et. al.*, 1982). The effectiveness of a test method can be judged according to the five Rs- Relevance, Reproducibility, Reliability, Robustness and Repeatability (Calow, 1993).

Although there is an obvious need for standardized toxicity test protocols, there is also a danger in over standardization because it "may stifle innovative and creative work" do not recognize work that does not coincide with their own priorities" (Davis, 1977). For example, a standardized toxicity test may not be appropriate for answering specific questions about a particular body of water for assessing the hazard of a particular chemical to an indigenous fish community in a specified body of water, it may not be useful to employ standard test species that are not normally present in that body of water. Furthermore, it is desirable to conduct the tests under the physical and chemical conditions characteristic of that body of water. (*Water et. al.*, 1989)

Toxicity test protocols typically specify the exposure if test organisms to fixed concentrations of chemical compounds for a definite period of time. However, chemicals rarely, if ever enter the environment at a constant concentration and rate (Cairns and Thompson, 1980). Most chemicals enter the aquatic environment sporadically in "pulses", intermittently as "sludge", or as a one-time "spill", creating episodic exposures. Therefore, the toxicant is present in high concentrations for a relatively short period of time and is usually diluted to lower concentrations with time.

In these cases mortality is function of a changing toxicant concentration and the length of exposure. Generally, although there are marked exceptions (*e.g.* acids) organisms can tolerate high concentrations for longer periods of time (Buikema *et al.*, 1982). A typical standard test, in which all test conditions are kept constant or maintained optimally, may be inappropriate for predicting responses in a changing natural system. In that case, site-specific studies should be conducted.

The objectives of a study will determine which toxicity test and which experimental design are most applicable. If the results are to be used to compare the toxicity of one chemical to another, rigid standardization is necessary. However, if the data are to be used to describe or predict the behaviour of the chemical in a specific water system, there is a danger in over standardization and there are many advantages to customizing the choice of test(s). Some methods have been widely accepted and are now standardized or in the process of being standardized.

It is necessary to be a standard operating procedure (SOP) for the international validity and acceptance of published data for the any hazardous compound. Therefore, each test has own SOP. The importance of SOP and other factors is for the international trade. The OECD is similar one important organization of 24 of the most highly industrialized nations in the world and undertook a programme to develop guidelines for test procedures acceptable to its 24 member states and to develop the principles of good laboratory practice. This latter, commonly referred to as GLP, is also a most important document. It sets out an international consensus concerning the organizational process and the conditions under which laboratory studies should be planned, monitored, recorded and reported. The purpose of GLP is to promote the validity and quality of test data. GLP also includes provisions for quality assurance (QA) to ensure that by means of external checks, the studies have infact been carried out in strict compliance with the principles of good laboratory practice.

The technical and toxicological information that could be called for in the safety evaluation of a chemical by a competent authority is now quite comprehensive. It ranges from melting points, partition coefficients, flammability, through to acute and sub acute toxicity to mutagenicity tests and rodent bioassays for carcinogenicity. In deciding test requirements, the sixth amendment has adopted a pragmatic approach and calls for a limited base set of data for all new chemicals. However, depending upon the tonnage to be placed on the market, the competent authority may call for additional tests. At levels greater than 1000 tons per annum the requirements would normally include a wide range of tests, such as fertility test and a rodent bioassay for carcinogenicity. Specifying a particular test for legislative purposes can only be done if the test procedure is well established so that its protocol can be defined in great detail. The establishment of definitive guidelines for technical procedures and toxicity tests proved to be difficult, controversial and costly undertaking. The OECD working through National Governments, which had in some cases already established guidelines, and with the help of hundreds of experts spent years and millions of dollars in the accomplishment of this enormous task. The final production was a massive compilation of guidelines on the conduct of all the technical and toxicological procedures commonly used by member states in a chemical safety programme. These guidelines, together with the principles of GLP and QA have proved to be a major contribution towards a uniform international approach to chemical safety programmes.

OECD consists following important tests which is commonly used in our country. Physical-chemical properties test of different toxic chemicals toxicological evaluation by different test model

## Effect on Biotic Test Systems
- Alga growth inhibition test.
- *Daphina* sp. acute immobilization test and reproduction test.
- Fish acute toxicity test.
- Fish prolonged toxicity test.
- Avian dietary toxicity test.
- Avian reproduction test.
- Earthworm acute toxicity test.
- Terrestrial plants growth tests.
- Activated sludge respiration inhibition test.
- Fish early life stage toxicity test.

## Degradability Tests

- Ready biodegradability.
- DOC Die-away test.
- $CO_2$ evolution test.
- Modified MITI test.
- Closed bottled test.
- Modified OECD screening test.
- Manometric respiratory test.
- Inherent biodegradability.
- Simulation test: aerobic sewage treatment.
- Inherent biodegradability in soil.
- Bio-accumulation.
- Static fish test.
- Flow through fish test.
- Biodegradability sea water.

## Health Effect

- Acute oral toxicity.
- Acute dermal toxicity.
- Acute inhalation toxicity.
- Acute dermal irritation/corrosion.
- Acute eye irritation/corrosion.
- Skin sensitization.
- Repeated dose oral therapy.
- Sub-chronic oral toxicity.
- Repeated dose dermal toxicity.
- Sub-chronic dermal toxicity.
- Repeated dose inhalation toxicity.
- Sub-chronic inhalation toxicity.
- Teratogenicity.
- Reproduction toxicity.
- Teratokinetics.
- Reproduction toxicity.
- Teratokinetics.
- Acute delayed neuro toxicity.
- Sub-chronic delayed neurotoxicity.
- Carcinogenicity studies.
- Chronic toxicity studies.
- Combined chronic toxicity/carcinogenicity studies.

**Table 23.1 : U.S. Regulatory agencies having involvement with toxicology**

| Agency | Agency Description | Coverage |
|---|---|---|
| Food & Drug Administration (FDA) | A unit of the department of heath and human services. | Drugs and foods Food additives and cosmetics |
| Environmental Protection Agency (EPA) | Independent agency, not a part of a cabinet department | Pesticides, industrial chemicals, air pollutants, industrial waste |
| Occupational Safety & Health | Unit of the department of labour. | Occupational Exposure |
| Consumer Product Commission (CPSC) | Independent commission | Consumer products |

The U.S. EPA was created in 1970. It is the federal agency responsible for the administration of environmental protection laws in the United States including the Toxic Control Act., U.S. Public Law 94-469. TSCA was created by the U.S. Congress in 1976 to "protect human health and the environment by requiring testing and necessary use restrictions on certain chemical substances and for other purposes". This law became effective in the U.S. on January 1, 1977 and is codified in Title 40 of the U.S. Code of Federal Regulations.

The U.S. Food and Drug Administration (FDA) has published a guideline that describes an acceptable format for organizing and presenting toxicology data required in the non-clinical section of the application. These guidelines pertain only to organization of existing data, not specific study requirements.

## Categories of Toxicity Test

There are three categories of tests commonly used to predict the chronic effects of toxic chemicals or aquatic organisms the first categories life cycle toxicity tests, measure the effects chronic exposure to a chemical has on reproduction, growth, survival and other parameters over are or more generation of a population of test organisms. The second category, test on most sensitive life stages, measures the effects chronic exposure to a chemical has chronic exposure to a chemical has on the survival and growth of the toxicologically most sensitive life stages of a species, for example, eggs and larvae of fishes.

The third category, functional test, measure the effect of chemicals on various physiological functions of individual organisms.

**Life Cycle Test**: In life cycle tests, groups of test organisms are exposed to a series of concentrations of the test chemical. The test are initiated with eggs, larvae, or juveniles and are continued until the test organisms have reproduced. The test can continue through several generations, its desired chemical concentrations range from the those having significant adverse effects on survival growth and reproduction to at least one not having any significant effect on these parameters compared to controls.

The species of aquatic animals that can be used in life cycle toxicity test are limited to those which can complete their life cycles under laboratory conditions. Mc Kim(1985) has listed those species most commonly used for life cycle toxicity tests.

A species form of life cycle toxicity studies are population toxicity experiments. The most commonly performed population toxicity experiments are tests with algal although also other species invertebrates like *Daphnia* are used. In these experiments either effects on the exponential on the logistic growth of population are studies population dynamics concepts can also be incorporated in tests with cohorts *i.e.* in test in which a fixed number of individuals are exposed from the juvenile through the adult period. In these tests separate measure of age specific survival and fecundity are linked together and used to estimate the intrinsic rate of natural increase according to the enter safetequation.

$$X = O \, ^1X^m X^e \, ^{-r}m^x = \overset{\sim}{\underset{}{\Sigma}} = 1$$

In this equation l X is the probability of survival to age X, mx represents the number of female off spring per female of age X, born during the time internal X to X+1 and pm is the growth constant of an exponentially increasing population *i.e.* the intrinsic rate of natural increase. Example of these procedures are given by Daniels and Allen (1981) and Allen and Daniels (1982).

**Tests with Sensitive Life Stages**: Because of the considerable time and expense involved in conducting life cycle toxicity tests, especially with vertebrates, methods have been developed for utilizing tests with the most sensitive life stages of aquatic organisms, primarily fishes, to predict chronic toxicity threshold concentrations. The life stages of fishes most sensitive to chemical toxicants are generally early life stages (Mc Kim 1985, Van Leeuwen *et al.*, 1985). It should be noted that early developing stages of fish eggs in ocean surface if not in the uppermost micro-layer in the water itself, or are deposited at the bottom of rivers or estuaries, at least heavy metals and chlorinated petroleum hydrocarbon are concentrated in the oceanic surface microlayer. Thus, the risk of serious exposure of fish eggs to oil, air, pollutants or sediments contaminants increases by their position.

It has been found that estimates of chronic toxicity threshold concentrations calculated from embryo larval toxicity test do not differ significantly from those calculated from entire life cycle toxicity test (Mc Kim 1985) fish embryo larval toxicity test are iniated by exposing groups of fertilized eggs or embryos, generally in a flow through toxicant delivery system, to a series concentrations of the test chemical. The range of concentrations used should span the expected effects and include concentrations producing no significant effects. Cold water species like rainbow trout (*Salmo gairdneri*) are generally exposed for 60-90 days. Warms water species like zebrafish (*Brachydanio rerio*) are exposed for 8-28 days. Parameters to be measured include survival, growth and teratogenesis (Van Leeuwen *et. al.,*1986).

Aside from the time and expense saved in using embryo larval tests to estimate chronic toxicity thresholds, an additional advantage is that they can study a much larger number of species than life cycle toxicity tests. Thus, estimates of chronic toxicity thresholds can be made for a much wider variety of species from a much wider range of habitats and trophic levels than are possible with life cycle toxicity tests. Although embryo larval tests as compared to life cycle studies reduce the time to produce information on toxicity of chemicals, they remain laborious. A further reduction of the exposure time, *i.e.* short-cut methods are needed because fish toxicity data are still very scarce. In a study of the differences in susceptibility of early life stages of rainbow trout to pollutants it was concluded that early try was the most sensitive stage for was the most sensitive stage for six pollutants. Eggs were relatively resistant. These differences in susceptibility could be explained by alternations in chemical and biotransformation process during embryonic development (Van Leewen *et. al.,* 1987).

**Functional Tests:** Fish and other aquatic organisms are known to aquatic respond physiologically and behaviorally to exposure to sublethal concentrations of toxic chemicals. Some of these functional responses are a result of the mode of action of the toxicant. While others are adaptive responded by the organisms to the toxicant. Among the types of functional responses that have been measured in fish and in invertebrates exposed to toxic chemicals are changes in blood biochemistry, histology, swimming performance, avoidance, respiration, enzyme activities, sensory perception and disease resistance. Good reviews on the use of function responses of fish in environmental toxicology are provided by Mehrle and Meyer (1985) and Mayers and Hendricks (1985).

Many of these functional responses are sensitive indicators of sublethal toxic effects: however, their usefulness in environmental risk analysis for chemicals is limited by several factors. First, many of the effects are transitory and gradually disappear as the animal acclimates to the stress. Second, the variability in sampling tends to be large, reducing the precision of the analysis. Last, there have been few, if any, studies undertaken to determine the relationship between functional responses measured in individual organisms and the effects of the toxic chemical on survival, growth and reproduction at the population level. Interpretation of these response at the population level or above is thus precluded.

## Types of Toxicity Tests: Their Uses, Advantages and Disadvantages

Toxicity tests are classified according to (a) duration – short-term, intermediate, and/or long-term, (b) method of adding test solutions – state, renewal, or flow-through, and (c) purpose – effluent quality monitoring, single compound testing, relative toxicity, relative sensitivity, taste or odor, or growth rate, etc. (Aman 1955)

Short-term toxicity test are used for routine monitoring suitable for effluent discharge permit requirements and for exploratory tests. These acute definitive tests typically use mortality as an end point or other discrete observations to determine effects due to the toxicant (*i.e.* $LC_{50}$ or $EC_{50}$ values). These tests also may be used to indicate and long-term tests, rather than longer-duration tests, are used to obtain toxicity data as rapidly and inexpensively as possible. They are valuable for estimation of overall toxicity, for screening test solutions or materials for which toxicity data do not exist, for assessing relative toxicity of different toxicants or wastes to selected test organisms, or for relative sensitivity of different organisms to different conditions of such variables as temperature and pH. The results of these tests can be used to calculate acceptable concentrations for very short exposures, such as those that might occur as organisms pass through an effluent zone of initial dilution or a mixing zone. (CRC Handbook 1895)

Toxicity tests of intermediate duration typically are used when longer exposure duration are necessary to determine the effect of the toxicant on various life stages of long-life-cycle organisms, and to indicate toxicant concentrations for life-cycle tests.

Long-term toxicity tests are generally used for estimating chronic toxicity. Long-term testing may include early-life-stage, partial-life-cycle, or full-file-cycle testing. Exposures may be as short as 7 d to expose specific portions of an organism's life cycle, 21 to 28 d to several months or longer for traditional partial-life-cycle and full-life-cycle tests with fish.

To establish a successful testing programme, consider the following: Use caution when static tests are used for evaluation of solutions with high BOD and/or COD levels or high bacterial populations. These tests can be conducted successfully with incorporation of rigorous dissolved oxygen monitoring and acceptable aeration. Volatile or unstable toxicants may decrease in concentration during the test, resulting in an underestimation of the exposure concentration causing an effect on the test organisms. Metabolic product, such as ammonia, may increase to undesirably high concentrations resulting in stress or death of test organisms and overestimation of the concentration that causes a toxic response. Toxicant concentration may be reduced by sorption on sediments, test chamber walls, by the food provided for the test organisms, or by combination with the mucus or metabolic products of the test organisms and in their bodies.

Flow-through toxicity tests are desirable for high-BOD or COD samples and for those that contain unstable or volatile substances. Organisms with high metabolic rates are difficult to maintain under static exposure conditions, whereas flow-through tests provide well-oxygenated test solutions and continuous removal of metabolic wastes. Use flow-through toxicity tests whenever there is evidence or expectation of rapid degradation of the test solution. Such a change is indicated when the survival time of test animals in a fresh solution is significantly shorter than in a corresponding 2-d-old solution (provided that adequate DO is present throughout both tests). Flow-through toxicity tests are also desirable for industrial effluents and chemicals that are removed appreciably from solution by precipitation, by test organisms, or by other means.

The $LC_{50}$ values may be useful measures of acute toxicity but they do not represent concentrations that are safe or harmless in aquatic habitats. Concentrations of wastes that are not demonstrably toxic in 96 h may be toxic at longer exposure periods in a receiving water. thus the 96-h $LC_{50}$ may represent only a fraction of long-term toxicity. When estimating safe discharge rates or dilution ratios for effluents or other pollutants on the basis of acute toxicity evaluations, use acute-to-chronic ratios determined primarily from life-cycle tests; however, NOEC values determined from shorter-duration chronic toxicity tests can be used. Even the provision of an apparently ample margin of safety can fail to accomplish its purpose when there is cumulative toxicity that cannot be predicted from acute toxicity results.

No single, simple acute-to-chronic ratio is valid for all wastes or toxicants. However, research on effluents has shown that acute-to-chronic ratios for whole effluents often are around 10. An acute-to-chronic ratio of 20 commonly has been used for non-persistent chemicals while a factor of 100 has been used for persistent chemicals. The constituents of a complex waste responsible for acute toxicity may be, but are not necessarily, the constituents responsible for chronic or cumulative toxicity demonstrable in diluted waste that is no longer acutely toxic. The chronic toxicity may be lethal after a long exposure period or it may only cause impairment of function. Knowledge of acute toxicity of a waste often can be very helpful in predicting and preventing acute damage to aquatic life in receiving waters as well as in regulating toxic waste discharges.

## Short-term Toxicity Tests:

a) *Range-finding toxicity tests:* For effluents or materials of unknown toxicity conduct short-term (usually 24-h or 48-h), small scale range-finding or exploratory tests to determine approximate concentration range to be included in definitive short-term tests. For effluents with low or slow-acting toxicity, 48 or 96-h tests may be necessary. Expose test organisms to a wide range of concentrations of the substance, usually in a logarithmic ratio, such as 0.01, 0.1, 1, 10, and 100 per cent of the sample. Attempt to include concentrations that will kill all organisms and others that will kill very few or no organisms. For short-term, definitive tests, select a geometrically spaced series of concentrations between the highest concentration that killed no, or only a few, test organisms and the lowest concentration that killed most or all test organisms. (*Fava et. al.,* 1989)

b) *Short-term definitive tests:* Because death is an important, easily detected adverse effect, the most commonly used tests are for acute lethality. These tests are most appropriate for routine monitoring and checking conformity with NPDES requirements. If it is not possible to perform a range-finding toxicity test before a definitive acute toxicity test, using a concentration series with a 0.5 (100, 50, 25, 12.5, 6.25%) or 0.3 (100, 30, 10, 3.1%) dilution factor may be appropriate. (Weber 1988)

Short-term tests may be static, renewal, or flow-through. Exposure periods for these tests usually are 48 h or 96 h. static or renewal tests often are used when the test organisms are phyto or zooplankton because these organisms are easily washed out in flow-through tests. Static and renewal tests are considerably less expensive to perform than flow-through tests. Overnight express mail shipments of samples often make static and renewal tests the method of choice for regulatory compliance testing.

Test solutions may be renewed daily if required because of oxygen demand, if the toxicant is unstable or volatile, or in the case of whole effluents, daily variation in the composition of the effluent. Renewals also may be less frequent. If the test material has high BOD and/ or COD level or is relatively unstable, use test vessels with maximum surface area-to-volume ratio, or use the renewal or flow-through technique. (*Peltier et. al.,* 1985)

Test duration is determined by the toxicant and the test objectives and usually is the same for different groups of organisms. For short-life-cycle organisms such as phytoplankton, the usual exposure time can cover many generations. Determine test duration, in part, by the length of the life cycle. Generally, expose fish and large invertebrates in static and static renewal tests for 96 h and in flow-through tests for an equal period unless composition of the toxicant is variable. In this case longer exposure may be useful to assess impacts of toxicant variability. Expose *Daphnia* and *Ceriodaphnia* for 48 h. Short-term tests have been limited arbitrarily to 96 h, but longer tests sometimes are desirable because death does not always occur within the 48-h or 96-h period. When some test animals, though still alive, are dying or evidently affected after 96-h exposure, prolong the test or express the results of the as a 48-h or 96-h $EC_{50}$, defining the observed effect. If tests are continued for longer periods, the test organisms may need to be fed.

Special tests may be conducted on altered or treated samples of effluent to obtain additional toxicity information. For example, effluent dilution water mixtures may be aged 24 to 48-h before adding the test organisms, to determine changes in toxicity. When special tests are conducted, describe methods in detail.

**Intermediate-Term Toxicity Tests:** No sharp time separation exists between short- and intermediate- or between intermediate- and long-term tests. Usually tests lasting 10 d or less are considered short-term while intermediate tests may last from 11 to 90 d. the length of the test organism's life cycle helps to determine what is short-term, intermediate, or long-term for that species.

Intermediate-length test may be static, renewal, or flow-through, but flow-through tests are recommended for most situations.

**Long-Term, Partial- or Complete-Life-Cycle Toxicity Test:** With few exceptions, use flow-through tests with exposure extending over as much of the life cycle as possible. Continue tests from egg to egg or beyond, or for several life cycles for smaller forms. Determine the maximum concentrations of toxicant not producing harmful effects with continuous exposure. The overall objective of this type of test is to determine NOECs or chronic value (Ch V) of effluents, toxicants, or wastes. Use life-cycle tests whenever possible to determine acute-to-chronic ratios and the effects on growth, reproduction, development of sex products, maturation, spawning, success of spawning and hatching, survival of larvae or fry, growth and survival of different life stages, deformities, behavior, and bio-accumulation, although bio-accumulation (or bio-concentration) often is determined with more mature animals in specially designed tests.

In life-cycle or partial-life-cycle tests, ensure that water quality factors such as temperature, pH, salinity, and DO follow the natural seasonal cycle unless the test objective is to study one of these factors. It may be essential that the natural annual cycle be duplicated if the development of sex products, spawning, and development of eggs and larvae are to be normal. Whenever possible, do not let toxicant concentrations vary by more than ±15 per cent from the selected concentration because of uptake by test organisms, absorption, precipitation, or other factors.

In these tests, select five or more concentrations on the basis of short- or intermediate-term tests and set up the exposure chambers at least in duplicate. Vary exposure chambers, spawning chambers, and other equipment to meet the needs of the different organisms.

**Short-term Tests for Estimating Chronic Toxicity:** Tests are available to estimate long-term effects of a toxicant or effluent after a relatively short (7-d) exposure. End points for the tests, called chronic estimator or rapid bio-assessment tests, include lethality, reproductive potential, and growth. Tests estimating chronic toxicity frequently are being included as biomonitoring requirements in discharge permits. The long duration of life-cycle or early-life-stage chronic tests increases the cost and reduces ability of laboratories to conduct long-term tests successfully as the demand for testing increases, the EPA has published a number of short-term chronic estimation toxicity test methods for fresh- and saltwater invertebrates and fishes. These tests were designed to evaluate effluent toxicity and may not be appropriate for other testing requirements such as pre-manufacturing testing, development of water quality criteria, etc. (*Hollste in metal*, 1979) *Robinson et. al.*, 1989.

**Special-purpose Toxicity Tests:**

  (a) *Relative sensitivity to a toxicant:* To rank the sensitivity of different species to a toxicant, use a standard water and standard exposure conditions. Select exposure conditions (*e.g.*, temperature, DO, pH, $CO_2$, light and salinity) in a favorable range for the test species and keep conditions constant throughout the test.

  (b) *Relative sensitivity of various toxicants to selected species:* These tests resemble sensitivity tests because the selected test conditions, dilution waters, and test species are kept constant and standard. Prevent any change in sensitivity of test organisms during the tests. If possible, select species from several different groups; an alga, microcrustacean, macrocrustacean, insect, mollusk, or fish.

  (c) *Toxicity reduction evaluation:* Use acute and chronic toxicity tests to determine the toxicant in the effluent. A toxicity reduction evaluation (TRE) is a approach that first, characterizes the acute or chronic toxicity of an effluent, second, identifies the toxicant(s) of concern (this phase often is termed Toxicity Identification Evaluation (TIE), and third, confirms toxicity. This approach is then used to evaluation the removal of the toxicant(s) by pretreatment or changes at the wastewater treatment plant. EPA guideline manuals for performance of TIEs and generalized TRE protocols for municipal and industrial facilities are available. Other TRE protocols are available.

(d) *Flesh tainting tests: Caution: Performs such tests only when there is assurance that the intake of potentially substances through consumption of organism is safe. In cases where sufficient information on the substances is not available, replace consumption with smell.* Use these tests to determine the maximum concentrations of wastes and materials that do not taint the flesh of edible aquatic organisms. Expose organisms that are large enough to supply portions for a taste panel. Set up exposure tanks as for other flow-through tests. Perform range-finding tests over a wide concentration range to determine the concentrations for a more definitive series of tests. (Surber 1962)

After exposure, prepare test organisms for taste testing. Clean, prepare for cooking (without seasoning), wrap in aluminum foil, and bake in an oven. When organisms are cooked, divide them into portions, wrap in aluminum foil, assign a code number, and distribute to a taste panel while still warm, along with samples of unexposed organisms similarly cooked, wrapped, and coded. Record the observations of the panel on a prepared form and determine the highest concentration of test material not causing detectable tainting based on either taste or smell. Several tests mat be necessary.

(e) *Growth-rate determinations:* Growth rate is an important response of both algae and fish to toxicants and environmental factors. This section discusses the topic with respect to fish. Always report details of the method of feeding fish in growth studies.

## Three techniques are available :

*Unrestricted food supply*: Provide attractive and palatable food (usually live food such as Daphnia, tubificid worms, or brine shrimp) uninterruptedly in greater quantities than fish can consume. It is desirable to make a mass balance on food consumed by weighing food introduced and uneaten food removed.

*Intermittent satiated food supply:* Provide all the attractive food that fish can consume at time of feeding once or twice daily. After fish cases to feed, remove all uneaten food.

*Uniformly restricted food supply*: Once or twice per day, provide all fish with an amount of food that they will consume completely and without exception. Ideally, hold fish separately in individual aquariums or compartments. For fish held together, feed so that all fish have an equal opportunity to consume food. Uniformity of temperature and DO helps to ensure equal feeding of a group of fish.

While growth studies usually have been conducted with unrestricted and intermittent satiated feeding techniques, it is recommended that each study include at least one series using uniformly restricted food supply. Only this technique can reveal whether growth rate differences are not the result of the effect of the toxicant on appetite or food consumption rate. The presence of an abundant food supply can obscure toxic effects. For example, fish exposed to toxicants such as cyanide or pentachlorophenol increase food consumption rate to compensate partially for loss of efficiency of food utilization caused by the toxicant. This may not be possible in natural conditions where food supply may be limited.

Ideally, include a series of tests with different, uniformly restricted food ration with the lower ration near that which results in no growth (or loss of weight) in the control. This is the maintenance level. Determine the effect of the variable under study at any level of food availability and consumption by relating observed growth rates to, for example, toxicant concentration, at each feeding level.

Juvenile fish may gain enough weight in 1 to 3 weeks to determine growth rate satisfactorily. Longer exposure with weighing at intervals of approximately 10 d are needed to determine long-term effects such as acclimation or accumulative toxicity.

Report results as specific growth rates computed as follows :

$$\text{Growth rate} = \frac{\text{Weight gain (g)}}{\text{Time interval (d)}} \times \frac{1}{\text{Mean weight(g)}}$$

where:

Mean weight = [weight at start of time interval (g) + weight at end of time interval(g)÷2

Determine dry weight wet weight, and fat (lipid) content of fish at the beginning and end of a test. Weight gain due to increased fat content is not universally considered true growth: some investigators consider that true growth occurs only when there is an increase of protein. However, fat storage is important ecologically and bioeneregitaclly because fat can be used as an energy source during periods of malnutrition, reproduction, and overwintering survival. Fat content also is important in the dynamics of toxicant uptake, storage, and depuration. Fat and water content should typify that of the target species.

## Selection of Toxicity Test Organism

Selecting Test Organisms: The prime consideration in selecting test organisms are: their sensitivity to the factors under consideration; their geographical distribution, abundance, and availability within a practical size range throughout the year; their recreational, economic, and ecological importance and relevance to the purpose of the study; their abiotic requirements and whether these requirements approach the conditions normally found at the study site; the availability of culture methods for rearing them in the laboratory and a knowledge of their physiological and nutritional requirements; and their general physical condition and freedom from parasites and disease. To select a best species consider available information on sensitivity, consult with local authorities in pollution control or fish and wildlife agencies, or determine sensitivity with short-term tests. Select the test species based on the considerations listed as well as organism size and life-cycle length. For testing of early life stages of organisms, species having a short life cycle are most cost effective, but some tests require larger organisms with long life cycles (e.g. bioaccumulation or in situ biomonitoring studies).

For studies to determine effluent effects, select species representative in the area impacted. In most cases, use of laboratory-cultured species is preferable to use of those collected from the field. Laboratory-cultured organisms, either from in-house cultures or purchased from commercial bio-assay organism suppliers, are of known age and quality (those taken from the field may already have been selected or biased for the more resistant members of the population). This allows for use of the most sensitive life stages throughout the year. Their use may also be more cost-effective and allows for better quality assurance and control. For each series of tests, use organisms from a single source. Choose organisms that are nearly uniform in size, and for fish, with the largest individual not more than 50 per cent longer than the shortest. Use organisms of the same age group of life stage. Optimally, conduct reference toxicant tests on cultured stock and on lots of acquired or collected organisms, report time, place, source, and culture history for cultured organisms and method of collection, transportation, handling and acclimation of acquired or collected organisms, and their response to reference toxicants.

Knowledge of their environmental requirements and food habits is important in selecting test organisms. Methods for laboratory holding and culturing are well described for a number of standard test species. When the purpose of the testing is site-specific, it may be necessary to collect certain life stages of selected organisms from the field for testing.

## Common Terrestrial Animals Used in Toxicity Testing

(a) Monkey

(b) Rats, mice

(c) Guinea pigs, Rabbits

(d) Earthworm

### Aerial Organism

These are mainly birds.

## Aquatic Organism

*Phytoplankton:* The phytoplanktons are primary producers in the aquatic community and as such are at the base of aquatic food chains, because of this, they must be tested in bioassay that predict and determine the potential effects of a substance on the aquatic environment. (Mount 1988, 1989)

Common Organisms

- Algae
- Phytoplankton
- Zooplankton.

Collecting Test Organisms: Preferably, use standard laboratory-reared organisms. In special instances, such as when it is important to incorporate genetic variability from wild populations, use species indigenous to the receiving water. This is particularly important for organisms with recreational, commercial, or ecological significance.

In designing a test, consider any unusual past conditions to which the organisms may have been exposed (pesticides, effluents from industries, waste treatment plants, return flows, etc.). Interactive effects of a new toxicant mixed with those presently being discharged to the receiving water may be important. Do not collect test organisms from polluted areas where they are in poor condition, diseased, parasitized, or deformed, or where they have unusually high body burdens of chemicals, avoid testing organisms with questionable histories.

Many smaller invertebrates and fish can be collected along the shore in dip nets, in coarse plankton nets, or by hand. Catch larger species that occur near shore in seines. Traps, nets, and trawls are valuable tools for collecting organisms, but may be selective for some species. Other trawls are effective for collecting benthic species and midwater trawls for pelagic species. Various dredges are available to collect benthic species from different types of bottoms or to collect different sizes of organisms. Commercially important species such as lobster, blue crab, and dungeness crab may be taken by the researcher in traps or deep-water trawls or may be purchased from commercial suppliers if proper care is taken before purchase. Species that colonize surfaces, such as barnacles, may be harvested from hard surface submerged in the water insure that organisms are not damaged during collection, transfer, and transport.

When seining or using trawls, make short hauls. Avoid collecting significant amounts of plant materials, mud, sand, or gravel in net or in bag of seine because these will injure the animals. Always leave seine bag in the water end of haul, stretch out wings of seine, open bag entrance, dip out organisms with a bucket or hand net, and transfer directly to prepared holding tanks. Do not expose delicate, easily damaged species to air. Take out larger, more hardy species with soft mesh dip nets. Do not collect too many animals at one time. After bringing a trawl up to the boat, bring it over the side without delay and avoid letting the catch hit the boat. Immerse that portion of net containing specimens in a tank of water open trawl and remove desired animals by dipping with a bucket or a hand net with small soft mesh. Have adequate quantities of clean water available in tanks before beginning a haul. Transfer organisms to tanks as rapidly and carefully as possible. (Rand *et. al.,* 1995)

If organisms are to be transported any distance by boat, hold in aerated live boxes. If they are transported by truck, put them in large baffled and insulated tanks filled with water from area in which they were collected. Aerate the water and maintain at temperature of collection. Determine water temperature, salinity, DO and pH at the collecting site. Do not handle organisms more than necessary. Make transfers with suitable containers or hand nets, or for small organisms, by large-bore pipettes. Use hand nets made of soft material with several layers around the net rim and free from sharp points or projections. Clean and sterilize all equipment before use. Avoid overcrowding of organisms during transport. Aeration, oxygenation, water exchange, and cooling may reduce distress. Avoid cold shock as much as overheating.

**Handling, Holding, and Conditioning Test Organisms:** Inspect organisms closely and frequently to determine stress, unusual behavior, parasites or disease, changes in color, or failure to eat. Avoid crowding. Provide adequate flow-through water so that characteristics such as DO, pH, $CO_2$, salinity, hardness, and $NH_3$ are favorable. Check temperature and DO frequently. Do not let metabolic products accumulate. Generally, use a flow-through rate of 6 to 10 tank volumes/d. usually, greater amounts pf flow-though water are required for smaller organisms on a weight-volume basis. For small organisms, use a water flow of at least 3 L/d/g. When brood stock are being held, periodic or continuous treatment for parasite and disease control may be required.

Clean tanks and equipment thoroughly and often, removing or flushing out all growths and wastes, preferably daily but at least twice per week. Remove all uneaten food within 24 h. use different nets and other equipment for different groups of organisms and clean and sterilize them between uses. When handling is necessary, clean hands and nets before touching organisms. Cover tanks and containers to prevent organisms from jumping out. Shield tanks with curtains or by some other means to protect organisms from unnecessary disturbances and noise. Provide photoperiods and light intensities favorable to the organisms begin acclimation to test conditions at a suitable interval in advance of testing.

It is of utmost importance that animals be kept in excellent condition before the tests. Make no abrupt changes in environmental conditions: preferably follow natural seasonal variations in environmental conditions such as temperature and daylight patterns. Many water supplies are supersaturated with gases, especially in winter when very cold water is brought into the laboratory and warmed. Because there is a danger of gas bubble disease, keep incoming water in an open system and let it cascade over baffles or otherwise aerate it to bring dissolved gases into equilibrium

**Culturing Test Organisms:** The advantage of cultured test organisms over field-collected animals is that the age, life history and existing conditions are documented and thus the responses of these organisms are more consistent between tests lots. For organisms used extensively in effluent biomonitoring programmes, EPA has developed a series of test methods that are adaptable to most laboratories. Culturing test organisms requires strict adherence to standard protocol 7-d/week monitoring, and an adequate facility.

*6.5(a)* Facilities, Construction Materials, and Equipment: Do not use construction materials in contact with dilution water that contain leachable substances or adsorb significant amounts of substances from the water. Use tempered glass, fiberglass, or stainless steel and silicone sealant as construction material for fresh water system. Do not use rubber or plastics containing toxic fillers, additives, stabilizers, plasticizers, etc. fluorocarbon plastic, nylon, and their equivalents usually are acceptable. Test the toxicity of all materials before purchasing large quantities. Clean, soak, and flush all new tanks, troughs and similar equipment with dilution water for several days before use. Use a glass or titanium interface between the water and heating elements for marine waters and glass or stainless steel for fresh waters.

Provide adequate space for test organisms, holding facilities, water storage reservoirs, and water supply systems. Provide distribution of hot and cold water mixing facilities to obtain any desired temperature. Aerate or vigorously mix to prevent gas supersaturation caused by heating dilution water.

use oil free pumps if possible. If air pumps are not oil-free, they should have water seals and filters to prevent oil from entering air lines and contaminating tanks. When large volumes of air are needed, use low-pressure blowers. Do not locate air intakes in shops or furnace rooms or near outlets from chemical exhaust hoods, chemical laboratories, or vehicle exhausts.

Provide acclimation and culturing tanks with temperature control and aeration. Design holding facilities for ease of cleaning and prevention of bacterial growths. For holding and culturing fish and many macroinvertebrates, preferably use round or oval tanks of at least 1 to 3 m diameter. Provide a standpipe drain in the centre, threaded below the tank floor so that, when the standpipe is removed, the opening is flush with the tank bottom. Slope tank bottom gently to center. Use tanks with smooth surfaces to facilitate cleaning to prevent injuries to organisms, and to insure that no material will collect in cornerscracks, and crevices. Introduce water into a circular tank as a jet along the edge and above the surface to create a circular movement of water around the central standpipe. Fit another pipe, with half-moon cutouts at its base, over the standpipe and screen, so that the out-flowing water passes up through the outside pipe, then down the standpipe. This results in a circular current and a certain amount of self-cleaning. Square or rectangular tanks may be used for special purposes or when space is scarce. Provide standpipes at one end for draining, with threads for securing the pipe on the underside. Ensure that corners are rounded and that surfaces are smooth.

**Multi Species Test:** When the test organism are used from more than one species or genus. It may be community or population. There is inter relationship between two genus, or population. The pollution incident which may directly affect just one component of the community can ultimately give rise to a more widespread change in the community. An important implication of these interactions for environmental toxicology is that a concentration of a chemical which may be harmless to a species which we consider, for one reason or another to be important, may nevertheless eventually prove disastrous by affecting other more susceptible vital components of the community.

Multi species test are more realistic approach in any ecosystem. Because in the multispecies test of any community reflect the indirect toxic effects, such as changes in competition predation, community function and structure, ecosystem energy flow and nutrient cycling. The only way to obtain the information relatively unbiased is to follow a more ecologically realistic approach *e.g.* follow the effects of exposure in natural ecosystems of man made system especially designed to mimic aspects of natural systems (multi species test) microcosms model ecosystems, mesocosms, enclosures, limno-corals etc. (*Fava et. al.*, 1989)

A multi species test inevitably will be the product of a compromise between the irreconcilable wishes with respect to replicability and resemblance of natural systems. Only effects on those properties and interactions test system allow direct extrapolation to the field prediction of effects accuring in other aspects can only be accomplished by mechanistic mathematical modelling. In this respect the results of multi species test do not differ from standard toxicity test. The mechanisms involved can be clarified by simplified process experiments in microcosms. In this view, multi species test should not be considered as a regular part of sequential scheme for toxicity testing. Therefore, is no need for standardization of multi-species test protocols. (*Good felow et. al.*, 1989)

Besides, above in recent years aquatic toxicity testing has been applied to a variety of different regulatory and scientific purposes including toxicity testing of municipal and industrial effluents as part of monitoring/permit compliance in aquatic ecosystem where multispecies exists in natural condition. (Warren 1971)

(i)    The derivation of national and site specific water quality criteria for individual chemicals.

(ii)   Product safety evaluation

(iii)  Chemical persistence studies

(iv)  Effluent interaction studies

(v)  Testing of Leachates and sediments

(vi)  Toxicity reduction evaluation (TRE) programs to identify constituents causing toxicity in effluent.

## Different Toxicity Test Models

*Daphnia* Micro-bioassay: *Daphnia* belongs to the cladocera group of crustaceans and plays an important role in aquatic food chain. Daphnids have a short generation time and genetic uniformity, they are easy to culture and maintain, have a high fecundity rate, a small size and also show high severity to many aquatic pollutants. Test with daphnids can be performed at low experimental cost. These factors make *Daphnia* sp. an important and generally accepted organism for aquatic pollution studies. For the better result and under standing of any toxic compound in aquatic ecosystem it is prerequisitic step solubility, vapour pressure, stability, dissociation constant and biodegradability should be known. Moreover, structural formula of compound, degree of purity, water partition coefficient of test compound also help for planning and interpretation of results. Commonly used water free species is *Daphnia magma* and two types of bioassay are in general use.

(a)  Static bioassay

(b)  Continuous bioassay

For the data evaluation the percentage immobilization in each test chamber at specified time period is plotted against the concentration. These data are plotted on logarithmic probability paper and time is fitted to a point causing 50 per cent immobilization which is known as $EC_{50}$ value. The $EC_{50}$ value and 95 per cent confidence limit may be calculated by a simple monographic method of litchfield and Wilcoxan, 1949 or by the method of probit analysis of Finney, 1971 and samolloft 1983.

**Bioassay Toxicity Test with Fish:** A bioassay is a test in which organisms are used to detect the presence or the effect of physico-chemical factors in the environment. Fish bioassay is used for acute toxicity as well as chronic toxicity test both. Any representative fish species may be used for the toxicity testing inhabiting in marine or fresh water ecosystem approved by standard procedure for example. Fresh water test fish is *Chirhinus mirgala, Channa punctatus* (Gopal *et.al.*,1975). The results are expressed as tolerance limit, median lethal concentration, median effective concentration, effective dose. For the median tolerance limit (TLm, $LC_{50}$, $EC_{50}$, $Ed_{50}$), the interpolation of straight line graph between survival percentage of test fish and test concentration is plotted and the test concentration is plotted and the concentration at which 50% survival is observed.

Apart from survival biochemical parameters (haematological) and behavioural parameters such as movement, surfacing activity, convulsion, distance travelled, hanging duration are also recorded at the onset of each interval as a symptom of toxicity at the individual level. (Brown 1957 and *Baldwin et. al.*, 1981

**Algal Bioassay:** Algae being a primary producer and important step of food chain in aquatic system is also used for detecting the fate of any toxic compound in aquatic ecosystem. The commonly used fresh water algae are *Scenedesmus* species, *Chlorella sp., Nostoc sp.*, etc. for the data recording following parameters can be measured. (Walsh 1983)

(a)  *Bio-mass:* This is difference in weight of fresh weight and dry weight of tested organism at different time. This is calculated in grams per litre of culture medium.

(b)  *Chlorophyll:* The total chlorophylls are extracted from 10 per cent (w/v) homogenate aliquotes in 95 per cent acetone at 0-4°C for 20 hours. Chlorophyll a and b contents are estimated by a spectrophotometric method (Arnon, 1949).

(c)  *Protein:* Total protein contain is also estimated by spectrophotometric method (Lowry *et al.*, 1951).

(d)  *Morphological:* Visible charges are recorded under light microscope.

Data interpretation can be done for their phyto-toxic properties (Kallquist, 1984)

**Table 23.2 : Format for Tabulation of raw data for acute effect**

| Conc. of pollutants In culture medium | Replicates | Fresh weight/cell no./optical density etc. |
|---|---|---|
| Control | 1 | ..................................... |
|  | 2 | ..................................... |
|  | 3 | ................................ .... |
|  | 4 | ..................................... |
| 1 | 1 | xxxxxxxxxxxxxxxxxxxxxxxxxx |
|  | 2 | xxxxxxxxxxxxxxxxxxxxxxxxxx |
|  | 3 | xxxxxxxxxxxxxxxxxxxxxxxxxx |
|  | 4 | xxxxxxxxxxxxxxxxxxxxxxxxxx |
| 2 | 1 | *********************************** |
|  | 2 | *********************************** |
|  | 3 | *********************************** |
|  | 4 | *********************************** |

**Duckweed for Toxicity Testing:** Duckweed (*Lemna minor*) is a wide spread, free floating source of food for water found in animals and provide shelter and support for small aquatic invertebrates. It is fast growing and reproduces faster than other vascular plants, because it is a floating microphyte duckweed may be particularly susceptible to surface active chemicals. The advantage of using duckweed instead of an algae are that test solutions can be renewed daily and background algae in receiving water or effluent can be removed for frond production or chlorophyll measurement. However, the Lemna species has limitations only for surface active toxicants in aquatic ecosystem. The test duration should be not less than 10-15-days. Data recording is done by total frond enumeration, visual appearance, chlorophyll content, protein and bio-mass. In the morphological studies (root length, chlorosis necrosis) and multiplication of test plants is also considered. Result is presented in form of $EC_{50}$, $LC_{50}$, as described in algal toxicity test model (Dot & Grothe 1989)

**Seedling Growth Inhibition Test:** Plant seed undergo rapid changes in metabolism, nutrient transport and cell division during its germination. Therefore, seed growth is one of the important and simple test system for soil contaminants. The contaminants may inhibit biochemical changes, stunting of seedling growth, foliar injury of radicals, inhibition of hypocotyl elongation, lowering of fresh and dry weight of seed lings and root growth inhibitions.

Seeds and seedling occupy little space and they do not create logistic problems for full scale field studies. These arguments and simplicity of experiments strongly support for successful bioassay of growth inhibition test. The test is also approved from *EPA (1975)*, OECD (1981) and U.S. Department of Health and Human Services (1984).

Date recording and result interpretations are done as in other models in form of $EC_{50}$, $LC_{50}$.

**Cytological Tests:** During the last few decades toxicologists and cytogeneticists have introduced few higher plants such as barley *(Hordeum vulgare)*, broad bean *(Vicia faba)*, garlic *(Allium sativum)*, *Tradescancia sp.* and Onion *(Alluim cepa)*. Among these tests systems common onion test *(Allium cepa)* Chauhan, 1985, have been well accepted and utilized due to the morphology of chromosome.

The use of chromosomes as monitoring organelles helps to determine whether a compound is cleistogen or not, although, chemicals that induce mitotic aberrations do not affect DNA directly, nevertheless abnormal chromosome segregation should not be considered genetically insignificant.

For the toxicity testing root tips are investigated for chromosomal aberration after proper growth.

Chromosomal aberrations include chromosome and chromatid breaks, fragmentation, chromatid exchanges, formation of dicentric chromosomes, spindle formation during the mitotic cell division. The appearance of severe chromatin (nuclei) and chromosome condensation and stickiness are considered cytotoxic effect of chemical. This test may be very useful for several environmental chemicals specially pesticides, industrial effluent sludge, domestic sewage sludge or any other chemical industrial pollutants of soil.

**Toxicity Testing using Microorganisms:** Since bacteria are involved primarily in the mineralization of organic substrates and in the recycling of mineral nutrients. Their activities are essential to self purification processes in aquatic environments they have relatively short life cycles and respond rather quickly to change in the environment. They are stable and easily maintained at low cost. Relatively large number of cells are exposed to the toxicants under study. These characteristics make bacteria a suitable to for rapid screening of toxicants in natural water. There are three commonly used methods for bacterial toxicity testing. (Daw Jon 1951)

**(a): Motility Test:** Flagelllar system of bacteria are excellent sense organs of any toxic compound. Flagella being as locomotive organs of bacteria/microorganisms the response of any toxic compound can be recorded as motility test. For example *Spirillum volutaus* has been shown the dose response toxicity with zinc by Ghose *et al*, (1996) Fig 23.1.

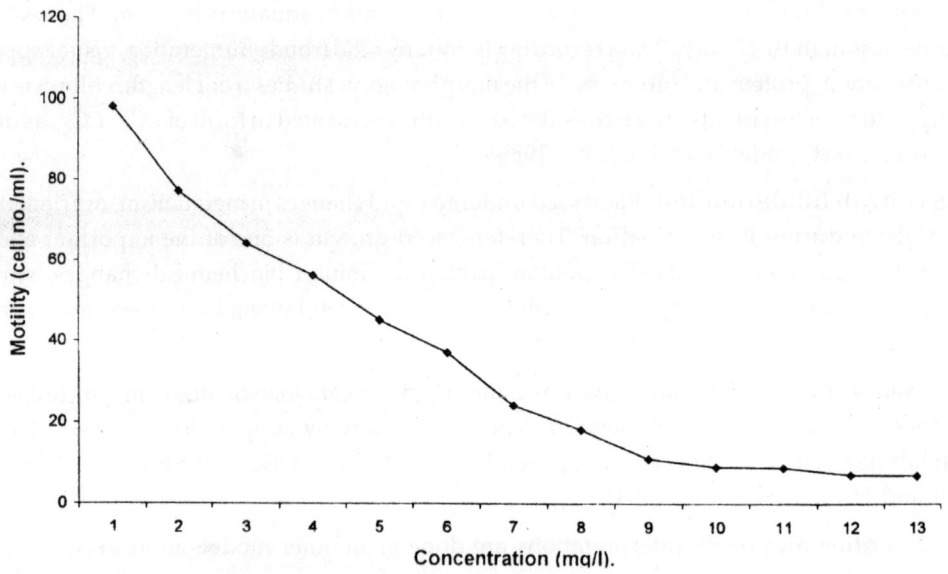

**(b): Growth Inhibition Test:** Bacterial assay for chemical toxicity in aquatic environments are based on measurement of growth inhibition/respiration or viability of cell. Sewage microorganisms as well as bacteria belonging to Genera *Psudomonas, Klebsiella, Aeromonas, Citrobacter sp.* has been suggested for these assay. One particular bioassay is based on nitrifying ability of *Nitrobacter* in sewage treatment plant. These bacteria have been proposed as bioassay microorganisms to measure the toxicity of heavy metals and industrial waste. Nitrite disappearance or nitrite formation is monitored in these tests. The toxicants concentration ($ED_{50}$) that causes 50 per cent inhibition of nitrite conversion to nitrate can be obtained from plot of relative metabolic rate of *Nitrobacter* as a function of toxicant concentration.

The growth inhibition test can be done either using water sample dissolved with test compound by measuring the optical density (OD) at 660 nm or agar plate method by measuring inhibition zone or test compound. The toxicants under investigation is introduced into a mixture containing buffering agent, nutrients, growth substrates and bacterial seed inoculum. Where a mixture of 1 ml of seed bacteria (may be taken from many sources municipal waste water, activated sludge soil, mixture of pure culture) 4 ml of phosphate buffer (dissolve 0.85 g $KH_2PO_4$, 2.18 g $K_2HPO_4$, and 3.34 g $Na_2HPO_4.7H_2O$ in 100 ml dist. water) 20 ml of dilution water from a biochemical oxygen demand (BOD) test, 4 ml of stock buffer from the BOD test, 10 ml of a nutrient broth and 4 ml of aqueous solution of test toxicants is incubated in a cotton plugged 250 ml round flask for 16 hrs at $22\pm2^0C$, the turbidity is read at 530 nm against a blank of unseeded control. The results can be plotted in form of graph concentration Vs optical density (OD) and concentration Vs growth inhibition zone size respectively as shown in Figs. 23.2 and 23.3 growth inhibition can be expressed in term of percentage by using following formula.

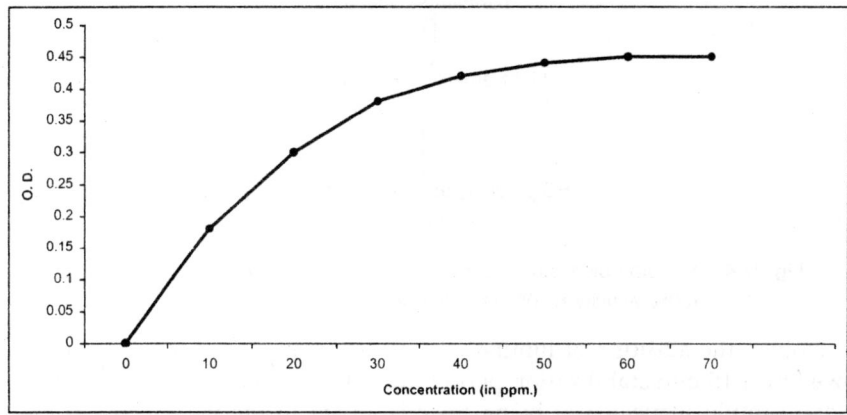

**Fig. 23.2 :** Growth curve showing the effect of toxicants of various concentration

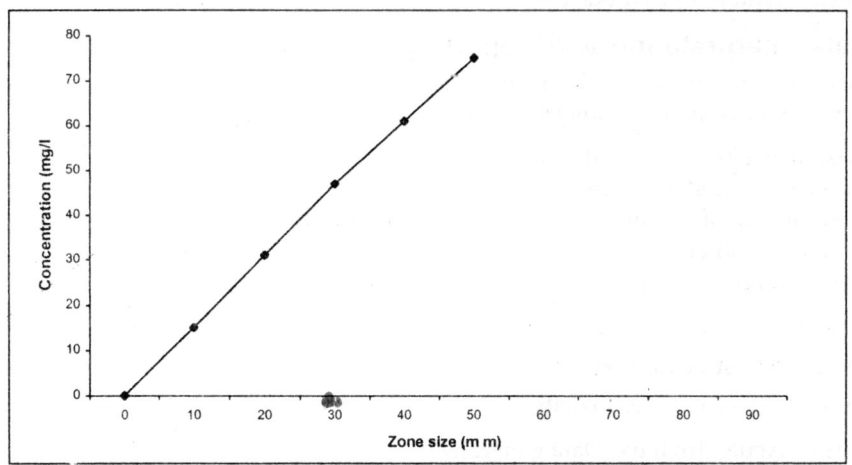

**Fig. 23.3 :** Showing the effect of toxicants concentration on growth zone inhibition

$$\frac{\text{Absorbance of test bottle}}{\text{Asorbance of seed control (unseeded)}} \times 100 = \% \text{ of controls}$$

**Microtox Bioassay:** Microtox bioassay was developed by Beckman Instruments Inc. for assessing acute toxicity in aquatic sample. The bioassay is based on the measurement of activity of a luminescent bacteria. *Photobacterium phosphorium* or *Vibrio fitcheri* which emits light under normal metabolic conditions. Any stimulation or inhibition of metabolism affects the intensity of the light output. By accurately measuring the light output, in control and toxicant treated sample $EC_{50}$ values can be determined as mentioned below in Fig 23.4

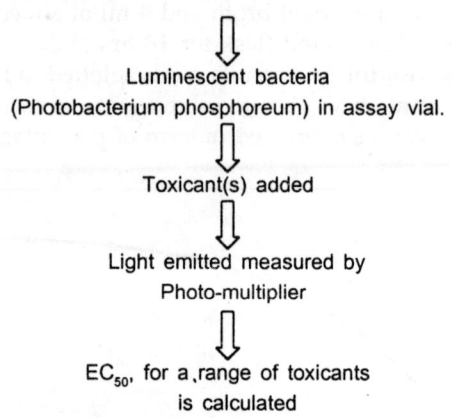

Luminescent bacteria
(Photobacterium phosphoreum) in assay vial.

Toxicant(s) added

Light emitted measured by
Photo-multiplier

$EC_{50}$, for a range of toxicants
is calculated

**Fig 23.4 :** Microtox bioassay A control containing no toxicant(s) is considered 100% activity or 0% inhibition in calculating $EC_{50}$ values.

The test involved the addition of luminescent bacteria into a vial of pre-cooled (15°C), diluent solution followed by a 15 min stabilization period immediately after, a known amount of toxicant(s) or environmental sample suspected of being toxic is added to the vial, which is placed in a light compartment where it is adjacent to a photomultiplier tube total light emissions are recorded over a fifteen minute period and displayed on digital meter by testing a range of concentrations, an $EC_{50}$ value can be obtained. (Britton and Dutka 1986)

## Toxicity Data Interpretation and Reporting of Results:

Various statistical methods are used for analysis data of acute and chronic toxicity tests. Statistical method of analysis have both advantages and disadvantages.

The precision of a biological test is limited by a number of factors including the normal biological variation among individuals of a species. Studies with a randomly selected species do not give accurate information on toxicity of a compound to other species and test with one species yields an estimate of the toxicity only to others of that species of similar size, age and physiological condition, in water with the same or similar characteristics and under similar test conditions.

Data analysis may be divided under two broad heads.

1. Data analysis of acute toxicity.
2. Data analysis of chronic toxicity.

**Data Analysis of Acute Toxicity:** Data generated in acute toxicity tests are quantal, *i.e.* responses are measured with yes/no type observations (*e.g.* did exposure cause immobilization, death, or not ?)

Continuous measurements that are measured in quantitative or graded tests, such as length, weight or number of young produced, usually are not utilized as end points in an acute toxicity test. Acute toxicity test results generally are characterized by the median lethal concentration ($LC_{50}$) when mortality is the test end point, or median effective concentration ($EC_{50}$) when a sublethal effect is the end point. For example, a 96 h $LC_{50}$ value of 15 per cent effluent means that over a period of 4-day test, 50 per cent of the test organisms are killed when exposed to a solution containing 15 per cent effluent and 85 per cent dilution water. In comparing $LC_{50}$ values the higher $LC_{50}$ value is less toxic because a greater concentration is required to produce 50 per cent mortality. It is important to recognize that the $LC_{50}$ is the median response of a given test population and is an estimate to the true median lethal concentration of that test material for the entire species. Whenever an $LC_{50}$ value is given, some measure of the variability of the test population should also be provided. Therefore, the 95 per cent confidence limit around the $LC_{50}$ value is very important. The 95 per cent confidence limit define an interval such that if it was possible to calculate 95 per cent confidence limits repeatedly with test organisms from the same population, 95 per cent of the calculated intervals will include the true $LC_{50}$. LC or EC values other than 50% may also be used to characterize waste toxicity (Table 23.3 & 23.4). (Snedecor 1980)

**Table 3 : Effect of different dilutions of distillery effluent on growth inhibition of *Lemna minor* after 96 hrs.**

| S No. | Effluent dilution | No. of fronds |
|-------|-------------------|---------------|
| 1 | 0 | 90 |
| 2 | 25 | 76 |
| 3 | 50 | 65 |
| 4 | 75 | 58 |
| 5 | 100 | 46 |

Note $IC_{50}$ =100%

**Table 4 : Effect of different dilutions of distillary effluent on mortality of *Tubifex* after 24 hrs.**

| S No. | Effluent dilution (%) | Mortality |
|-------|----------------------|-----------|
| 1 | 10 | 0 |
| 2 | 20 | 5 |
| 3 | 30 | 12 |
| 4 | 40 | 30 |
| 5 | 50 | 40 |
| 6 | 60 | 45 |
| 7 | 70 | 50 |
| 8 | 80 | 65 |
| 9 | 90 | 85 |
| 10 | 100 | 100 |

Note ; $LC_{50}$ =70%

**Calculation of $LC_{50}$:** Numerous procedures are available for analysis of quantal toxicity data. $LC_{50}$ calculations include parametric procedures such as probit analysis and logit method. Non-parametric methods are the Spearman-Karber method, white numerical interpolation and the binomial distribution. No single method is most appropriate for all data sets, but graphical interpolation and binomial distribution methods are used most often. (Kopperdhal 1976)

**Estimating LC$_{50}$ by Probit Method using Graphical analysis:** This method involves manually ploting dose, response and then drawing a base fit regression line by eye. Experimental data from hypothetical toxicity test subjected to probit analysis is given in Table 23.2. (Bliss 1934)

**Table 23.2 : Experimental data from hypothetical toxicity test subjected to probit analysis.**

| Concentration Of waste % | No. of test organisms | 2 h | 4 h | Number of test organisms dead at 6 h | 8 h | 24 h | 48 h | 72 h | 96 h |
|---|---|---|---|---|---|---|---|---|---|
| 10 | 10 | | 1 | 4 | 7 | 9 | 10 | 10 | 10 |
| 10 | | | | | | | | | |
| 7.5 | 10 | | 0 | 1 | 2 | 6 | 9 | 9 | 10 |
| 10 | | | | | | | | | |
| 5.6 | 10 | | 0 | 0 | 0 | 2 | 7 | 7 | 8 |
| 9 | | | | | | | | | |
| 4.2 | 10 | | 0 | 0 | 0 | 0 | 1 | 4 | 4 |
| 4 | | | | | | | | | |
| 3.2 | 10 | | 0 | 0 | 0 | 0 | 0 | 1 | 1 |
| 1 | | | | | | | | | |
| 0 | 10 | | 0 | 0 | 0 | 0 | 0 | 0 | 0 |
| 0 | | | | | | | | | |
| LC$_{50}$, % Estimated From graph | | 10 | 10 | 9 | 7.1 | 5.2 | 4.7 | 4.5 | 4.4 |
| LC$_{50}$, estimated By probit analysis 95% confidence limits | | – | – | 8.96 | 7.02 | 5.27 | 4.70 | 4.46 | 4.34 |
| | | – | – | 7.60 | 5.82 | 4.53 | 3.95 | 3.87 | 3.49 |
| | | – | – | 10.5 | 8.42 | 6.12 | 5.59 | 5.14 | 5.40 |
| Slope of probit Line | | – | – | 10.9 | 8.42 | 10.1 | 7.03 | 9.54 | 11.3 |

To construct the graph percentage mortality as the ordinate is plotted against concentration as the abscissa on probit paper. Death is plotted on a probit or probability scale and concentration on a logarithmic scale. Because the probit scale never reaches 0 or 100%, any such points are plotted with an arrow indicating their true position.

**Confidence limits of the LC$_{50}$:** Confidence limits of the LC$_{50}$ should be calculated and reported with the LC$_{50}$. A preliminary estimate of significant difference between two LC$_{50}$'s obtained from duplicate tests can be accomplished by examining confidence limits for overlap. In general if there is no overlap the LC$_{50}$'s are significantly different. However, the LC$_{50}$'s still may be different if the confidence limits overlap. Test for significant differences can be determined more exactly by the formula. (Berkson 1953)

$$F_{1.2} = \frac{1.96 \text{ SE diff}}{LC_{50 \ 1.2}}$$

$$= \text{antilog } \ddot{O}(\log f_1)^2 + (\log f_2)^2$$

where,

f= factor for 95% confidence limits, of LC$_{50}$

If the ratio (greater LC$_{50}$/smaller LC$_{50}$) exceeds the value for f$_{1.2}$, the LC$_{50}$'s are significantly different.

If $LC_{50}$'s calculated from duplicate tests are significantly different, test the populations to determine if they differ in length, weight, age, or sex. Use parameteric statistical tests such as Student's t test and ANOVAs to determine if such differences in populations are significant and, therefore, could influence the $LC_{50}$s. If assumptions of analysis of variance are not met, then nonparametric tests for significant differences may be used. The Mann-Whitney U test or equivalent is a nonparametric test that is analogous to the two-sample t test and ANOVA with two classes.

The confidence limits about the $LC_{50}$ do not describe variability of the $LC_{50}$ under conditions other than those tested. The limits indicate the accuracy of the estimate of replicate tests at the same time under the same conditions.

**Other Methods of Analyzing Results:** The graph for estimating the $LC_{50}$ can be constructed with an arithmetic scale for percentage mortality. However, the probit scale is preferred because it usually gives a straight line. Logits are also used instead of probits as they give equivalent results. (Bliss 1934)

*Plotting Toxicity Curves:* Most tests provide information on mortality at times before the final selected time. Such information can be used for plotting toxicity curves. LC from a graph plotted can be estimated for each observation time. A toxicity curve gives an overall picture of test progress and indicates when acute lethality has ceased. This is indicated by the curve becoming asymptotic to the time axis. The $LC_{50}$ for an exposure time in the asymptotic part of the curve (asymptotic $LC_{50}$) also can be termed the "threshold" or incipient $LC_{50}$.

## Data Analysis of Chronic Toxicity:

A chronic toxicity test is made to determine the long term effect of relatively low concentrations of a chemical or a waste on the viability of test organisms. Data generated in chronic toxicity tests may be quantal, quantitative or a combination of the two. Results in chronic toxicity tests often are analyzed statistically to determine the lowest observed effect concentration (LOEC), the no observed effect concentration (NOEC) and the chronic value (Ch V). Statistical significance generally is assumed to mean significantly different at $P=0.05$. The chronic value (Ch V) is calculated as the geometric mean of LOEC and NOEC. Chronic toxicity limits may specify either NOEC or Ch V as the end point. The term maximum acceptable toxicant concentration (MATC) often is used interchangeably with the chronic values (Ch V). Similar to acute toxicity data, lethal concentration (LC) or effective concentration (EC) values can be used with chronic toxicity data to describe chronic toxicity tolerance levels. Recently the concept of inhibiting concentration (IC) has been introduced to characterize effects in chronic tests. This has been defined as a point estimate of the toxicant concentration that would cause a given percent reduction in a non-quantal biological measurement such as fecundity or growth.

**Methods for Analyzing Chronic Toxicity Data:** NOEC's and LOEC's are determined by hypothesis testing (Dunnet's test, Bonferronis T-test, Steel's Many-one Rank test, Wilcoxon Rank Sum-test) and LCs, ECs and ICs by point estimation techniques (probit analysis or interpolation method).

**Plotting the Data:** Many anomalies and trends in test results are not obvious unless the data is plotted. Chronic toxicity test data should be plotted before making statistical analysis for proper interpretation of results.

**Reporting Toxicity Results:** Results from toxicity tests should be reported as completely as possible so that any conclusions can be evaluated independently. Result should include the following.

## Use of Toxicity Data

Toxicity test are useful for a variety purposes that include determining :
(a) Suitability of environmental condition for aquatic life.
(b) Favourable and unfavourable environmental factors, such as DO, pH, temperature, salinity or turbidity.

(c) Fate and their effect on metabolic system of any toxic compound in tested animals in case of terrestrial ecosystem. Similarly the effect of any air pollutant may be noted for aerial life e.g. Bird, insect or plants.

(d) Effect of environmental factors on waste toxicity.

(e) Toxicity of waste to a test species.

(f) Relative sensitivity of aquatic organisms to an effluent for  toxicant.

(g) Amount and type of waste treatment needed to meet water pollution control requirements.

(h) Effectiveness of waste treatment methods.

(i) Permissible effluent discharge rate.

(j) Compliance with water quality standards effluent requirement and discharge permits.

## REFERENCES

- Allen J.D. and R.E. Daniels (1982). Life table evaluation of chronic exposure of Eurytemore affines (Cope poda) to Kepone. *Mar. Biol.* (Berlin) 66: 179-184.

- Aman C.W. (1955). The relation of taste and odor to flavor. *Taste odor control J.*, **21** (10):1.

- American Society for Testing and Materials. (1987). Standard practice for conducting bioconcentration tests with fishes and saltwater bivalve molluses. E-1022-84, Annual Book of ASTM Standards, Vol. 11.04. americal Soc. Testing & Materials, Philadelphia, Pa.

- American Society for Testing and Materials (1990). Practice for evaluating an effluent for flavor impairment to fish flesh, ASTMD 3696-89, American Soc. Testing & Materials, Philadelphia, Pa.

- APHA (1992): Standard methods for the Examination of water and waste water 18th Edition. American Public health Association 1015 fifteenth street. NW washington . DC 20005

- Arnon DI (1949). Copper enzymes in isolated chloroplasts I. Polyphenol oxidase in Beta vulgaris. *Plt. Physiology*, **24**, 1-16.

- Baldwin R.E., D.H. Strong & J.H. Torrie (1961). Flavor and aroma of fish taken from four fresh-water sources. *Trans. Amer. Fish. Soc.* **90**: 176.

- Berkson, J. (1953). A stastically precise and relatively simple method of estimating the bioassay with quantal response based on the logistic function. *J. Amer. Statist. Assoc.* **48**: 565.

- Bitton G. and Dutka B.J. (1986) Toxicity testing using microorganisms Vol 1 CRC Press Inc. Boca Raton, Florida

- Bliss, C.I. (1934). The method of probits. *Science* **79**: 38.

- Botts, J.A., J.W. Braswell. J. Zyman, W.L. Goodfellow & S.B. Moore (1989). Toxicity Reduction Evaluation Protocol for Municipal Wastewater Treatment Plants. EPA-600/2-88-062. Risk reduction engineering lab., Off., Research and Development, U.S. Environmental Protection Agency, Cincinnati, Ohio.

- Brown M.E. ed. (1957). The physiology of fishes. Vol. 1, Metabolism. Academic Press Inc., New York, N.Y.

- Buikema A.L. Jr., Niederlehner B.R. and Cairns J. Jr. (1982). Biological monitoring Part IV Toxicity testing. *Water Res.*, **16**: 239-262.

- Calow P. (1993). General principles and overview. Handbook of ecotoxicology vol. I (ed.) P. Calow pp. 1-5 Cambridge M.A. Blackwell Scientific.

- Cairns J. and Thompson R.W. (1980). A computer interfaced toxicity testing system for stimulating variable effluent loading. 2 Symposium on Process Measurements for Environmental Assessment (Eds.) P.L. Leuin, J.C. Harris and K.D. Devewitz pp. 183-198. Cambridge, M.A.: Arthur D. Little.

- Chauhan L.K.S., Dikshith T.S.S. and Sunderraman V (1985). *Mut. Res.*, **171**, 25-30.

- CRC Handbook of Toxicology (Eds.) M.J. Derelako and M.A. Hollinger (1995). Published by CRC Press, New York.

- Daniels R.E. and J.D. Allen (1981). Life table evaluation of chronic exposure to a pesticide. *Can J. fish Aquat. Sci.* **38**: 485-494.

- Davis J.C. (1977). Standardization and protocols of bioassays. Proc. 3 Aq. Tox. Workshop, Nova Scotia 2-3 Nov. 1976. Pp. 1-14.

- Dawson, E.H. and B.L. Harris (1951). Sensory methods for measuring differences in food quality. *Agr. Inform. Bull.* **34**, U.S. Dep. Agriculture, Washington, D.C.

- Dot, J. & D.R. Grothe (1989). Use of fractionation/chemical analysis schemes for plant effluent toxicity evaluations. In G.W. Suter II & M.A. Lewis, eds. Aquatic toxicology and Environmental Fate: Eleventh Volume. ASTM STP 1007. American Soc. Testing & Materials. Philadelphia, Pa, p 123.

- EPA (1975). Test methods for assessing the effects of chemicals on plants. Final report EPA 560/5-755-008 office of toxic substances, environmental protection agency, Washington, D.C.

- Environmental toxicology and ecotoxicology. Proc. of third international course held at Edinburg, U.K. 6-13 Sept. 1985, Published by WHO regional office for Europe Copenhagen, 1986.

- Fava, J.A., D. Lindsay, W.H. clement, G.M. Degraeve, J.D. Cooney, S. Jansen, W. Ruw, S. Moore P. Lannford (1989). Generalized methodology for conducting industrial toxicity reduction evaluations. EPA-600/2-88-070. Risk reduction engineering lab., Off., Research and Development, U.S. Environmental Protection Agency, Cincinnati, Ohio.

- Finney, D.J. (1971). Probit analysis, 3 ed. Cambridge Univ., Press, London & New York.

- Ghose S.K., Doctor P.B. and P.B. Kulkarni(1996). Toxicity of zinc in three metabolic systems. Env. Toxicol. *Water Qual.* **9**: 13-19.

- Goodfellow W.C., Kr W.C. McCulloch, J.A. Botts, A.G. McDearmon & D.F. Bishop (1989). Long-term multispecies toxicity and effluent fractionation study at a municipal wastewater treatment plant. In G.W. Suter II & M.A. Lewis, eds. Aquatic toxicology and Environmental Fate: Eleventh Volume. ASTM STP 1007, American Soc. Testing & Materials, Philadelphia, Pa, p. 139.

- Gopal K. (1975). Studies on the semipolluted chilwa (Gorakhpur) in relation to insect fauna. *Ind. J. Zool.* **16**: (3) 227-230.

- Hamilton, M.A., R. Russo & R.V. Thurston (1977). Trimmed separman-karber method for estimating median lethal concentrations in toxicity bioassays. *Environ. Sci. Technol.* **11**: 714.

- Hollstein M & J Mc Cann (1979). Short-term test for carcinogens and mutagens mutation Reg. **65**: 133.

- Kallquist T (1984). The application of an algal assay to assess toxicity and eutraphication in polluted streams in fresh water. biological Monitoring Pascoe R. and Edwards DW (eds.) pp. 121-129.

- Kopperdhal, F.R. (1976). Guidelines for performing static acute toxicity fish bioassays in municipal and industrial waste waters. Rep. To California State Water Resources Control Board, Sacramento.

- Litchfield J.T. and Wilcoxan F (1949). A simplified method for evaluating dose effect experiments. *J. Pharmac. Exp. Ther.* **96**: 99-113.

- Lowry O.H., Rosenbrough N.J., Farr A.L. and Randell R.J.(1951). Protein measurement with folin phenol reagent. *J.Biol. Chem.* **193**: 265-275.

- Mc Kim J.M. (1985). Early life stage toxicity tests pp. 58-95. In: Fundamentals of Aquatic Toxicology. G.M. Rand and S.R. Petrocelli (eds.) Hemisphere Publ. Corp. Washington.

- Mehrle P.M. and F.L. Mayer (1985). Biochemistry/Physiology pp. 262-282 In: Fundamentals of Aquatic Toxicology G.M. Rand and S.R. Petrocelli (eds.) Hemisphere Publ. Corp., Washington.

- Mayers T.R. and J.D. Hendricks (1985). Histopathology pp. 282-232. In: Fundamentals of Aquatic Toxicology. G.M. Rand and S.R. Petrocelli (eds.) Hemisphere Publ. Corp., Washington.

- Mount, D.I. & L. Aderson-carnahan (1988). Methods for aquatic toxicity identification evaluations: Phase I Toxicity characterization procedures. EPA-600/3-88-034. U.S. Environmental Protection Agency, Duluth, Minn.

- Mount, D.I. & L. Aderson-carnahan (1989).Methods for aquatic toxicity identification evaluations: Phase II Toxicity Identification procedures. EPA-600/3-88-035. Environmental Research Lab., Off., Research and Development, U.S. Environmental Protection Agency, Duluth, Minn.

- Mount, D.I. & L. Aderson-carnahan (1989). Methods for aquatic toxicity identification evaluations: Phase III Toxicity Confirmation procedures. EPA-600/3-88-036. Environmental Research Lab., Off., Research and Development, U.S. Environmental protection agency, Duluth, Minn.

- OECD (1981). The organization for economic co-operation and development guidelines for testing of chemicals effects on biotic systems (8000 TS-97-81-05-1) ISBN 92-62-12221-4.

- Parkhurst, B.R., C.W., Gehrs & I.B. Rubin (1979). Value of chemical fractionation for identifying the toxic components of complex aqueous effluents. In. L.L. Marking & R.A. Kimerle, eds. Aquatic Toxicology, ASTM STP 667, American Soc.Testing & Materials, Philadelphia, Pa, p. 122.

- Peltier, W.H. and C.I. Weber. Eds. (1985). Methods for measuring the acute toxicity of effluents to freshwater and marine organisms. EPA-600/4-85-013. Environmental monitoring and support lab., U.S. Environmental Protection Agency, Cincinnati, Ohio.

- Rand G.M., P.G. Wells and L.S. Mc. Carty (1995). Introduction to aquatic toxicology, In: Fundamentals of aquatic toxicology 2 ed. (Ed.)

- Robinson, J. Lazorchak, L. Wymer & R. Fryberg (1989). Short-term methods for estimating the chronic toxicity of effluents and receiving water to freshwater organisms. 2 ed. EPA-600/4-89-001 and supplement EPA-600/4-89-001A, Cincinnnati, Ohio.

- Samolloff M.R. et al., (1983). Combined bioassay-chemical fractionation scheme for the determination of toxic chemicals in sediments. Environ. Sci. Technol. 17: 329.

- Snedecor, G.W. and W.G. Cochran (1980). Statistical methods, 7 ed. Iowa State Univ., Press, Ames.

- Surber, E.W., J.N. English & G.N. McDermott, (1962). Tainting of fish by outboard motor exhaust wastes as related to gas and oil consumption. PHS Publ. No. 999-WP-25. Environmental Health Ser.: 170, U.S. Public Health Serv., Washington, D.C.

- U.S. Dept. of Health and Human Services (1984). Food and drug administration. Seed germination: environmental assessment. Technical guide No. 11.06 (draft) Centre for food safety and Applied Nutrition Centre for Veterinary Medicine, Washington D.C.

- Van Leenwen, C.J.P.S. Griftioen, W.H. A. Vergouw and J.L. mass Diepeveen (1985) Differences in susceptibility of early life stages of rainbow trout (Salmo gairdneri).

- Van Leenwen, ClJ.M. Rijkeboer and G.Niebeek (1986) Population dynamics of Daphnia magna as modified by chromic bromide stress. Hydrobiologia 133:277-285.

- Van Leeuwen, C.J.G. Niebeek and M. Rijkeboer (1987). Effects of chemical stress on the population dynamics of Daphnia magna: a comparison of two test procedures. Ecotoxicol. Environ. Saf. 14: 1-11.

- Walsh G.E. & R.L. Garnas (1983). Determination of bioactivity of chemical fractionations of liquid wastes using freshwater and saltwater algae and crustaceans. Environ. Sci. Technol., 17:180.

- Warren C.E. & P. Doudoroff (1971). Biology and water pollution control. W.B. Saunders co., Philadelphia, Pa.

- Weber, C.I., W.B. Horning, D.J. Klemm, T.W. Neiheisel, P.A. Lewis, E.L. Robinson, J. Menkedick & F. Kessler, eds. (1988). Short-term methods for estimating the chronic toxicity of effluents and receiving waters to marine and estuarine organisms. EPA-600/4-87-028. Environmental monitoring and support lab., U.S. Environmental Protection agency, Cincinnati, Ohio.

# 24

# Chemical Constraints of Water and their Management for Sustainable Health and Environment

*D.D. Ozha*

## Distribution

Earth is a water rich planet. The total available water on the basis of current estimate is 1370 million Km³. Ocean water accounts for 97.3 per cent and remaining 2.7 per cent is fresh water consisting of polar ice-caps and glaciers, ground water, soil moisture, lakes, swamps and streams etc. It is the surface waters in rivers, streams and lakes amounting to less than 0.5 per cent of available fresh water, that constitutes the basic water supply.

The population of the world was 2.8 billion in the year 1955, 5.3 billion in 1990 and over 6 billion in 1999 while that projected in the year 2025 is between 7.9 and 9.1 billion. The renewable fresh water falling on the continents and island each year is only about 41,000 cu. Km. which is hardly 0.03 per cent of the total water on the earth (Table 24.1). In our country the fresh water available in surface

### Table 24.1 : Status of World Water

| Sr. No. | Place/Source | Quantity of water in million KM³ |
|---|---|---|
| 1. | Earth Total | 1370 |
| 2. | All Oceans (97.3%) (Saline water, useful for fishing, water transport, disposal of waste/water and annual hydrological recycling of water) | 1331.64 |
| 3. | Remaining (Sweet) water (2.7%) | 38.36 |
| 4. | 80% of item 3 above is in surface sources in air as vapour and as soil-moisture near surface. | 30.14 |
| 5. | In underground sources item (4-3) | 8.22 |
| 6. | 75% of item 4 is in the polar ice caps and glaciers | 22.605 |
| 7. | Lakes and reservoirs on earth | 0.137 |
| 8. | Flowing Rivers | 0.00137 |
| 9. | Usable sweet water on the earth and underground (excluding that as water vapour in atmosphere and soil moisture) 0.36% of item (3) | 0.03 |

sources is estimated at 1680 Km³ and that easily extractable from underground sources is 420 Km³ (Table 24.2). All this quantity is again very much unevenly distributed. Thus Rajasthan with a population

### Table 24.2 : Status of Water in India

| Sr. No. | Place/source | Quantity of water in Cu. KM3 |
|---|---|---|
| 1. | Surface source (Rivers, lakes, impounded reservoirs etc. | 1680 |
| 2. | Water available for utilisation of item 1–41.7% | 700 |
| 3. | Total underground sources | 600 |
| 4. | Water available for utilisation of item 3–70% | 420 |
| 5. | In the Narrow Catchment Area of River Brahmaputra | 570 |

(very small part of the above can be usable)

of about 8 per cent of the country has got only 1 per cent of its water resources while the state of Bihar with 10 per cent population is having only 5 per cent of it. The country as a whole at present has about 2200 Cu.M of water available per capita per year, while Rajasthan gets only 500 which is less than

24 per cent of the country's average. When the availability of water at a place is more than 1700 mtr/ Cu. per capita per year, there is not much difficulty felt by the people in satisfying their different requirements. However, when it is less than that depending upon the actual availability, water stress of different orders is felt. The report of the United Nations in this respect states that about 1/3 of the world's population today is living in countries facing moderate to high water stress. The basinwise availability of surface water in our country alongwith the percapita availability in the year 1996 is depicted in Table 24.3.

**Table 24.3 : Basinwise Water Resources Availability (Surface)**

| Sr. No. | River Basin | Average Annual Annual Availability | | |
| --- | --- | --- | --- | --- |
| | | water Resources Potential (BCM) | per Capital (Cubic metre) | Per Ha of Cult Area (Cubic metre) |
| 1. | Indus | 73.31 | 1749 | 7600 |
| 2. | Ganga–Brahmaputra–Meghna | 1110.62 | 18061 | 52907 |
| 2 (a) | Ganga | 525.02 | 1471 | 8727 |
| 2 (b) | Brahmaputra and Barak | 585.60 | 16589 | 44180 |
| 3 | Godavari | 110.54 | 2048 | 5837 |
| 4 | Krishna | 78.12 | 1285 | 3847 |
| 5 | Cauvery | 21.36 | 728 | 3692 |
| 6 | Subernarekha | 12.37 | 1307 | 6533 |
| 7 | Brahmani–Baitarani | 28.48 | 2915 | 8903 |
| 8 | Mahanadi | 66.88 | 2513 | 8369 |
| 9 | Pennar | 6.32 | 651 | 1774 |
| 10 | Kahi | 11.02 | 1052 | 4977 |
| 11 | Sabarmati | 3.81 | 360 | 2455 |
| 12 | Narmada | 45.64 | 3109 | 7727 |
| 13 | Tapi | 14.88 | 1007 | 3285 |
| 14 | West flowing rivers from Tapi to Tadri | 87.41 | 3383 | 27900 |
| 15 | West flowing rivers from Tadri to Kanyakumari | 113.53 | 3480 | 36078 |
| 16 | East flowing rivers between Mahanadi and Godavari | 22.52 | 953 | 5199 |
| 17 | East flowing rivers between Pennar and Kanyakumari | 16.46 | 366 | 2400 |
| 18 | West flowing rivers of Kutch and Saurashtra incl. Luni | 15.10 | 683 | 644 |
| 19 | Area of Inland Drainage in Rajasthan | Negl. | – | – |
| 20 | Minor rivers draining into Bangladesh and Myanmar | 31.00 | 14623 | – |

A perusal of Table 24.3 reveals that 6 of our river basins are under water stres and 40 or 70 per cent of the basins have less than the average per capita availability of water. Alongwith the increase in population (Table 24.4) the demand for water for irrigation, energy, industries, domestic and other needs also goes on increasing (Table 24.5). The increasing standard of living and higher aspirations of the common man for increasing the per capita demand for water, thereby increasing the total demand on the water resources in all and especially in the developing countries of the world. According to

**Table 24.4 : United Nations' projections of India's population (million)**

| Year | 1990 | 1995 | 2000 | 2010 | 2020 | 2030 | 2040 | 2050 |
| --- | --- | --- | --- | --- | --- | --- | --- | --- |
| Total Population | 851 | 936 | 1022 | 1189 | 1327 | 1455 | 1564 | 1640 |
| % Urban Population | 26.7 | 28.6 | 30.6 | 33.8 | 37.2 | 41.2 | 45.3 | 50.0 |
| Urban Population | 227.2 | 267.7 | 315.8 | 401.9 | 493.6 | 599.4 | 708.5 | 820 |

a report jointly released by World Resource Institute (Washington DC), the United Nations Environmental programme and the World Bank (Washington DC) / Water Consumption in the World as a whole has risen 6 fold between the year 1990 and 1995.

**Table 24.5 : Present and future water demand in different sectors**

| Sector | Water Demand (BCM³) in the year | | |
|---|---|---|---|
| | 1990 | 2000 | 2025 |
| Irrigation | 460 | 630 | 770 |
| Drinking (including Lovestock) | 25 | 33 | 52 |
| Industrial | 15 | 30 | 120 |
| Energy | 19 | 27 | 71 |
| Others | 33 | 30 | 37 |
| Total | 552 | 750 | 1050 |

## Introduction

Provision of safe and adequate water supply and hygienic disposal of wastes is a basic necessity for healthy living of a community. In our country, having more than 8 per cent of its population living in rural areas, scores of villages yet do not have proper access to reliable water supply and people have to walk long distances in search of water.

It was not until 1885 that people realised the significance of invisible microbial life in the water. It is still a ccommon belief that apparently clean water is safe for consumption. Common man is not aware about the hidden enemies of life in water world. Very often when thirsty a common man does not bother about the quality of water, particularly in the hot days, when he/she is out of house, he drinks whatever water is available. This is why the percentage of illnesses are rather high during the summer months.

If everything that exists has life then everything that exists needs water. Water is the most ubiquitous material in the nature and is the most vital and fascinating of all God's creation. It is the most important raw material for mankind and is called "Liquid Gold".

65-70 per cent human body is composed of water. Similarly 88 per cent of milk, 87 per cent of apple, 80 per cent of fish, 77 per cent of beef, 75 per cent of potatoes and 66 per cent of eggs are water. It is only naturally occurring liquid compound on the surface of earth and is called "Universal solvent".

Recently, there has been considerable impact on hydro environmental conditions due to change in agricultural pattern, industrial development and urban expansions. All these factors have affected the ground and surface waters in some way or other. Therefore, it is exigence to educate the people about the adverse health effects of contaminated water as well as the role of water quality in sustainable development.

## Quality Concept of Water

The quality of water is much more important than quantity because water quality and health of organisms are interlinked. Water quality is judged by physico-chemical, bacteriological parameters, and sometimes, more detailed characteristics pertaining to biological growth forms, viruses and individual chemical compounds. Certain quality requirements are specified for routine potable use of water. These water characteristics specifications are called quality standards and specify two limits, the permissible and excessive limit.

The physical characteristics include colour, temperature, pH and electrical conductivity, taste and odour. The chemical parameters are the most important indices which charaterise the quality of water and enable to classify the water by chemical composition, evaluate the need to provide water bodies with nourishing additives for the development of aquatic organisms. The chemical parameter of water includes hardness, concentration of various cations viz. sodium, sotassium, calcium, magnesium, and arsenic, born and anions like carbonate, bicarbonate, chloride, sulphate, nitrate and fluoride.

## Factors Affecting Water Quality

It has been experienced that during traverse, water solubilises both organic and inorganic substances, however the extent of solubility of organic substamces are less as compared to inorganic. Paractically all waters contain dissolved salts and gases taken from air. Water acts as a transport medium as well as a chemical reagent in the conversion of rock to dissolved matter. Dissolution reactions take place because many constituents of earth crust are therm odynamically unstable in the presence of water. The presence of organic substances in natural waters either in finely dispersed or dissolved form is a result of continuous decay processes of remains of vegetative and animal origin. Presence of man made organics in natural water originates from either waste discharge or surface run off also inhibits the water quality. Amongst the other factors influencing water quality, the hydrogeological conditions prevails an important role. Achutta Rao[1] has described hydrogeological factor in typical desert areas of Western Rajasthan and has explained that how such factors govern the general salinisation in the ground waters'.

## Demand of Water

Water plays an important role in the manufacture of essential commodities, generation of power, transportation, recreation, domestic, commercial, agricultural and industrial activities. The demand of water is increasing day by day due to the rapidly growing population and industiral developments. The demand of water in various sector is described as under:

**(a) Domestic Purposes:** As per Bureau of Indian Standards, the average water demand for domestic purposes is 135 litres per capita per day *i.e.* a town of population 10,000 requires 1350,000 litres i.e. 1350 m$^3$/day to satisfy its domestic demand. The break up is as follows:

| Purpose | Amount of water (ltrs) | Purpose | Amount of water (ltrs) |
|---|---|---|---|
| Drinking | 5 | Cleaning Utensils | 10 |
| Cooking | 5 | Floor washing | 10 |
| Bathing | 55 | Flushing of water closets | 30 |
| Washing of clothes | 20 | | |

### The demand of water for domestic animals are as follows:

| Animal | Water Demand (Litre) | Animal | Water Demand (Litre) |
|---|---|---|---|
| Cow or buffalo | 50 | Dog | 10 |
| Horse | 50 | Sheep | 5 |
| Mule | 30 | Chicken | 0.1 |
| Hog | 20 | | |

Desert animals like gerbil, (rodent) tortoise, antelope etc. seldom drink water. They dig up plants and eat their moisture rich bulbs. An adult human produces about 300 ml. of water every day during metabolic process.

**(b) Commercial Purposes:** The water demand for commercial purpose may be taken as 10-20 per cent domestic demand. The various commercial activities include dairies, hotels and restaurants, laundries, motor garages, auditoria, theatres, educational institutions, offices, public gathering places and swimming pools etc. Following are the demands for some commercial units.

**(c) Municipal/Civil Purpose:** These include road washing, (about 5 LPcd) sanitation purposes *i.e.* cleaning public lavatories, large markets, sewers etc. and for carrying wastes from different places of the town (2-3 LPcd), ornamental purposes *i.e.*, aesthetics in town by beautifying it with gardens, lawns, fountains, artificial ponds, lakes and water falls. Water demand may be taken as 2 litre/m$^2$/day for public parks and 30 litres/Km/day for roadside trees.

| Units | Demand |
|-------|--------|
| Hospital with<100 beds | 340 1/bed |
| Hospital with > 100 beds | 450 1/bed |
| Hostel | 135 Lpcd |
| Office | 45 Lpcd |
| Hotel | 180 1/bed |
| Cinema hall/auditorium | 15 1/ seat |

(d) Fire Demand: Sufficient quantity of water should be available throughout the year for fire fighting purpose. It should be stored in the storage reservoirs and can be taken from water hydrants located at every 100-150 m. distance on the water mains. As per Bureau of Indian Standards[2], fire demand may be taken as 1800 1pm for every 50,000 population, if population is less than 3 lakhs, 6x1800/pm + 1800 / pm for every one lakh population in excess of 2 lakhs and the fire reserves should be provided for at least four hours.

## Water and Health

As stated earlier that water is indispensable part of hygiene and public health. The chemical constituents prevails great role in spreading disease. The drinking water standards laid by B.I.S. are shown in Table 24.6.

### Table 24.6 : Drinking Water Standards (B.I.S)

| Parameter | Desirable limit | Permissible limit in want of alternate source |
|-----------|-----------------|-----------------------------------------------|
| Colour (Hazen Units) | 5 | 25 |
| Odour | Unobjectionable | Unobjectionable |
| Taste | Agreeable | – |
| Turibidity (NT Units) | 5 | 10 |
| pH | 6.5–8.5 | 6.5–8.5 |
| Total Hardness | 200 | 600 |
| Anionic detergents | 0.02 | 1.0 |
| Phenoline compounds | 0.001 | 0.002 |
| Total dissolved solids | 500 | 1500 |
| Chloride | 200 | 1000 |
| Free residual chlorine | 0.2 | – |
| Calcium | 75 | - |
| Magnesium | 30 | 150 |
| Manganese | 0.05 | 0.5 |
| Iron | 0.3 | 0.1 |
| Copper | 0.05 | 0.5 |
| Zinc | 5 | 15 |
| Arsenic | 0.05 | 1.5 |
| Cadmium | 0.01 | 0.01 |
| Lead | 0.05 | 0.05 |
| Mercury | 0.001 | 0.001 |
| Selenium | 0.01 | 0.01 |
| Nitrate | 45 | 100 |
| Fluoride | 1.0 | 1.5 |
| Cyanide | 0.05 | 0.05 |
| Chromium | 0.05 | 0.05 |
| E.Coli /100ml | 0 | 0 |
| Coli from MPN/100ml | <10 | 10 |
| Gross alpha activity | 3 pci/1 | 2pci/1 |
| Gross beta activity | 30pci/1 | 30pci/1 |

The bacterial, viral and parasital diseases caused by water are shown in Table 24.7.

**Table 24.7 : Bacterial, Viral and Parasital Diseases caused by Water**

| Bacterial disease | Viral disease | Parasital disease |
|---|---|---|
| Cholera | Polio and Meningitis | Amoebiasis |
| Bacillary dysentry 1 | Herpingina | Giardiasis |
| Typhoid | | |
| Para typhoid | Hepatitis | Nutritional Deficiency |
| Gastro enterities | Infantile diarrhoea | |
| Infantile diarrhoea | Pneumonia | |
| Ceptospira | | |

## Toxicity of Nitrate

Nitrate is one of the several inorganic pollutants contributed by nitrogenous fertilizers, organic manures, human and animal wastes and industrial effluents through the bio chemical activities of microorganisms. The toxicity on health due to high nitrates in water and food uptake of animals and human beings are equally important. Nitrate itself is not toxic to health. Nitrate becomes a problem only when it is converted to nitrite in the human body and causes methemoglobinemia, alternatively called as Blue Baby Syndrome, gastric cancer and some other health disorders. Nitrate produced from nitrate in drinking water enters the blood stream mainly through the upper gastrointestianl tract[3]. Almost all the nitrate is taken up but the efficiency of the process depends on the food matrix. In our country ground waters of Haryana, Karnataka, Maharashtra, Bihar, Orissa and Rajasthan are severely affected with high nitrate problems.

When nitrate is absorbed in blood stream, it oxidizes haemoglobin, a Fe (lll) compound with reduced oxygen transport capacity, as this compound contains iron in its highest oxidation state which is in capable of binding oxygen. This way nitrate reduces the total oxygen carrying capacity of blood. As different parts of the body get deprived of oxygen, clinical symptoms of oxygen starvation start to appear, the main being cyanosis meaning dark blue lip. In severe condition the skin starts to take a blue colouration wherefrom the disease dervies its name, the Blue baby disease.

## Sickness in Livestocks

The investigation of deaths in a herd of cattle reveals that poisoning occurs when the cattle is fed on cornstalks having an unusually high conentration of potassium nitrate. The fatal of animals particularly amongst cattles and sheeps were observed during summer while drinking the high nitrate water and grazing low land having high nitrogen content[4].

It has also been seen that when pregnant cattle graze on land where the plants have high nitrogen content, they may abort without showing any of the acute symptoms of poisoning.

## Nitrate and Gastric Cancer

Nitrate, once produced, from different derivatives, can react with a variety of organic compounds in the human body to form nitrosamines and nitrosamides through nitrosation reactions in the stomach. Nitrosamines and nitrosamides are carcinogenic as they can be metabolized to potent electrophilic alkylating agents[5]. It is thought that carcinogenic nitroso compounds are involved in the aetiology of some types of cancers in human beings. Human oral cancer caused by tobacco chewing and snuff dipping and cancers related to smoking are thought to be the results of nitrosamines in tobacco products[6,7]. Nitrate derivative like $N_2O_3$, NOCl, NSCN are primarily responsible for the formation of nitrosamines and nitrosamides. Epidemiological studies in China found[8] an increased incidence of oesophageal cancer associated with several dietary factors including drinking water. Excess nitrate causes irritation of the mucous lining of gastro intenstinal tract and the bladder with symptoms of diarrhoea and diuresis.

## Environmental Hazards

Apart from health problems the high nitrates in water have adverse environmental effects[9-12]. They contribute eutrophication in the surrounding areas. The eutrophication of water bodies is known to imbalance the ecosystem. In some areas, large amount of soluble nitrate can lead to the depletion of subsurface organic carbon which in turn, may lead to a loss of denitrification capacity and high permeability for heavy metals. Similarly, lakes, ponds, rivers and in other water bodies due to high nitrate huge algal growth takes place which creates unaesthetic conditions. Some of the blue green algal species are toxic and due to anaerobic conditions fatal to of fishes are also possible.

## Remedial Measures

Prevention is always better than cure, which suggests that apart from judicious application of water and fertilizers in cultivated fields, water containing dangerous levels of nitrate should not be used as drinking water. This is possible only when the levels of nitrate in water are known, which can be done by regular monitoring of drinking water. Blending of water having very low nitrate content for drinking purposes may be one of the tool to combat the problem. Use of high doses of nitrgenous fertilizers in areas already enriched with high nitrate must be minimised. Nitrate can be removed effectively by deionisation, desalination, reverse osmosis, biological denitrifiation and electrodialysis[13] etc.

## Fluoride and its Crippling Effects

Fluoride is one of the most widely distributed potability hazard of water whose excessive concentrations in water and food have spread the disease fluorisis and thus have crippled millions of men, women, children and even the livestocks have not been spared. It affects young and old, poor and rich, rural and urban populations. Incidence of fluorosis has been reported from several countries including China, U.S.A., Italy, India, Mexico, West Indies, Spain and several other North Africans and South American countries.

In our country, Schroot[14] was the first Scientist who observed first time this disease in human being during 1937 in Andhra Pradesh. At present 15 States of our country have been declared as endemic for fluorosis. It has been observed that the onset of fluorosis and severity of the symptoms are governed by various factors *viz.* nutritional deficiencies, high ambient temperature, high alkalinity and low calcium and magnesium content. High values of sodium percentage were also observed in some high fluoride water.

In Rajasthan, particularly the arid region is severely affected with fluorosis. It is obvious that preventive measures should be taken immediately to protect people from the intake a large amount of fluoride through drinking water *i.e.* ground water. Therefore, it is necessary to know the fluoride status of well water. Ground Water Department has done detailed and systematic hydrogeo-chemical studies of fluoride enriched areas[15].

## Toxicity of Fluoride in Human & Livestocks Health

Ingestion and adsorption of excessive amount of fluoride produce toxic effects in both human beings and in livestocks. Acute poisoning occurs when large amounts are absorbed over short periods of time and chronic effects results from the cumulatve action of ingestion if smaller quantities for long periods. When the concentration of fluoride exceeds 1.5 mg/1, it induces a developmental disease of teeth in the calcification stage of children. The pathological condition becomes evident from the yellow to brown colouration of teeth and sometimes cracks develop in them and the conditions are known as mottling.

Excessive intake of fluoride is responsible for skeletal fluorosis. In this case deformities are found in persons particularly in the limbs, flexion deformity of knee and hip being the commonest. Fluoride toxicity can damage lungs, foetus and kidneys. In rural areas the affected persons can not bend their neck easily and are unable to see the moon. Results of epidemiological survey carried out in Nagaur district revealed that out of 1, 65,800 human population distributed in 181 villages of the Nagaer district, 1375 people have been suffering from skeletal fluorosis and 16,411 people are affected by dental fluorsis. In Didwana block of the district, highest number of patients were observed and also in Rani block of the Pali district. It is formidable that in the village Chotti-Chhapari itself there are more than 40 per cent cases of skeletal fluorosis. It was also observed that 1 mg. of fluoride in drinking water can dissolve 220 mg. of aluminium when it boiled in utensils made of aluminium. Excess intake of aluminium is also very dangerous for human beings. Generally in rural areas, aluminium utensils are often used for cooking and other domestic purposes.

Fluorosis in livestocks observed to be quite common in rock phosphate areas with increased intake of fluoride for prolonged period. Reserves of raw material for phosphatic fertiliser industeries have boomed the state. Excretion of calcium in feces increases and urine it decreases. The prominent symptoms of fluorosis in livestock are mottling and abrasion of teeth, Osteoporosis and intermittent lamensess. Bones lose their normal colour and lustre, become thickened and softened, leading to decreased breaking strength and formation of exostoses. Teeth also lose glistening white colour and become chalky, mottled and brittle. In certain spcies, teeth become abnormally elongated while in cattle, teeth becomes soft and wornout. In some cases pulp cavities are exposed particularly in young animals when permanent teeth are going to erupt. About 95 per cent of the total fluoride in animal body is found in bone, enamel, cementum and dentine. The teeth constitute a very reliable indicator of fluorine toxicosis.

During skeletal fluorosis, mineralization of tendons at the point of attachment of the long bones may also occurs so that joints become thickened and thus animals become stiff and lame.

## Prevention and Control

Although the disease fluorosis in incurable but it is preventable. Following measures must be adopted to combat this socio-economic problem.

1.  Blending of high fluoride and low fluoride water in endemic areas.
2.  Construction of wells/tubewells in low fluoride area.
3.  Prohibition on use of fluoride rich edibles, cosmetics and luxury items.
4.  Adequate use of vitamin C in diet.
5.  Appreciable use of high calcium rich diets and dietary products.
6.  Defluridation of water at domestic or community level.
7.  Public awareness and health educations.

## Toxicity of Arsenic

Arsenic contamination in ground water was detected in West Bengal in early eighties. A considerable number of people residing in the localised pocket of Murshidabad, Malda, Nadia, North 24 Parganas, and Bardhaman districts are affected by arsenic contamination. Studies so far revealed that such arsenic contaminations in ground water are caused due to natural geo-morphological changes. The symptom of chronic arsenic poisoning include various types of dermatological lesions, mascular weakness, liver disorder, paralysis of lower limbs etc. Arsenic is a potential carcinogen and skin cancer can occur after prolonged exposure.

There appears to be some confusion prevailing among the professionals and scientists as to the extent and magnitude of the problem of arsenic contamination and the number of people affected by the same.

While it has been established that parts of the districts mentioned above, are affected and substantial number of tubewells in these districts are contaminated with arsenic in varying degrees, it would be erroneous to presume that all the tubewells are polluted or the total population of these districts are at risk. Exact number of polluted tubewells could be ascertained only after a thorough water-equally survey is conducted, regarding which, it is understood that the State Government is taking nevessary actions. Meanwhile, however, under the sponsorship of the Rajiv Gandhi National Drinking Water Mission, a sample survey was conducted by the AIIH&PH in 1993 to assess the drinking water quality in the rural areas of West Bengal. Ground water spot sources were selected through statistically significant random sampling technique[16]. The analysis of the data reveals that while in Naida district, 50 per cent of the sampled tubewells are arsenic contaminated, the some in Bardhaman is only 1%,. In Murshidabad, Malda, South 24 Parganas, North 24 Parganas such tubewells are 10 per cent, 13 per cent and 16 per cent respectively (Table 24.8)

**Table 24.8 : Arsenic affected blocks in different districts of West Bengal (Upto 1995)**

| District | No. of Blocks affected | District | No. of Blocks affected |
|---|---|---|---|
| Malda | 5 | Burdwan | 2 |
| Murshidabad | 15 | Howrah | 2 |
| Nadia | 13 | Hooghly | 1 |
| North 24 Parganas | 14 | Total | 61 |
| South 24 Parganas | 9 | | |

Water quality analysis carried out by different agencies upto 1995 indicated that 61 Blocks in different districts as mentioned below are affected with arsenic contamination in ground water.

The people are not equally affected. A study conducted by All India Institute of Hygiene and Public. Health (AIIH& PH) and STM in 1985 in six arsenic affected villages indicated that of 127 families in the affected villages 48( 37.8%) were affected by arsenical dermatosis and 197 of 784 (25.1%) individuals were affected. A comprehensive epidemological study, with adequate sample size, covering all the districts, is required to be conducted, before it could correctly be estimated the actual number of people suffering from Arsenical dermatosis or other symptoms of chronic Arsenic poisoning.

## Remedial Measures

AIIH & PH is also working on the removal of arsenic from water. Various studies have been carried out both at laboratory and field. Different models have been developed for removal of arsenic. Such models include domestic filter, hand-pump attached ARP, deep tubewell attached ARP for pipe water supply schemes etc.

In arsenic prone areas, piped water supply scheme may be taken up to supply either treated water from surface water sources or from arsenic free under ground aquifer. During construction of tubewells appropriate sealing must be done so that arsenic from higher aquifer does not enter to the lower acquifer. Rain water harvesting and use of large village ponds (Dighis) with appropriate treatment (Horizonatal Roughfing Filter model developed by the AIIH&PH)., may also be tried in the affected village, whereever feasible.

In the existing hand pumps where arsenic is available beyond permissible limit, HP attached type Arsenic Removal Plant (ARP) may be constructed. However, before such construction, beneficiaries need to be motivated. The O&M responsibility must be taken by the people in the villages.

Manufacturing of domestic filters need to be encouraged. Such filters should be available at cheap price to the villagers.

Indiscriminate drawals of ground water in the arsenic affected areas are causing vertical movement of arsenic in the undreground soil strata. This may have aggravated in recent days due to overdrawal of water for BORO/cultivation. It is considered that a rational ground water management system need to be developed immediately in arsenic affected districts of West Bengal so that occurrences of arsenic contamination in ground water could be checked to a certain extent.

## SUMMARY

Interlinking of health of living organisams with water have enlightened the importance of qulality of water. Generally the planners have thoughts of quantity of water, however, quality of water of all natural sources is also equally important. No living entity can survive, grow and develop without water. Therefore, water is called 'Jeevan'. Water sustains all biological life, eco-systems and human activities. Owing to various adverse effects of unsuitable water in different field viz. drinking, irrigation and industries, quality of water has given utmost consideration in source development. Out of various constituents present in water, the chemical parameters have special significance due to their pivotal role in spreading diseases. As a result of alarmingly increasing population, unlimited expanded urbanisation and an intense industrialization the water and hygiene related problems are increasing. Studies carried out in our country reveals that toxicities of chemical constituents viz. nitrate, fluoride, arsenic and heavy metals are increasing which inturn is adversely affecting the health of human beings, livestocks and aquatic organisms.

Therefore, for sustainable health and enviornment water resources must be judiciously used, water quality awareness campaign must be encouraged and proper management practices must be adopted to combat the problems related to chemical constraints of water for sustainable health and environment.

Wastes also find their way by leaching into ground water or by direct discharge into the estuaries or the sea. Industrial and agricultural operations such as smelting or crop spraying introduce materials into the aquatic environment either directly or indirectly or via atmosphere. The control of water pollution is therefore essential for protecting if water resources are to be properly managed and damage to the wildlife, recreation, crops and human populations.

## REFERENCES

- Achutta Rao, A., (1975). Hydrogeological conditions in desert areas of Western Rajasthan. An evironmental analysis of Thar Desert. 1974.
- Bureau Indian Standards, Drinking Water Standards, (1983). Govt. of India, New Delhi.
- Solloman, T.A., (1957). Manual of Pharmacology, 8th ed. W.B. Saunders, Philadelphia.
- Ozha, D.D. (1998). Threat of high nitrate in ground water Trans. ISDT 25, 86-100.
- Bartholomew, B and Hill, M.J. (1984). Ground water pollution microbiology, wiley Interscience publication, John Wiley & Sons. N.Y. 156.
- Hecht, S.S. & Hoffman D, (1989). Chemistry, Agriculture & Environment, edited by M.L. Richardson, Royal Society of Chemistry, Cambridge, 377-388.
- Moncada S., Palmer, R.M.J., and Higgs, E.A., (1988). ibid.
- Yang, C.S. (1980). *Cancer Res.* **40**, 2653.
- Deshmuk, S.B., (1993) *J.I.A.E.M.*, **19**,48.
- Massey, A., and Robinson, J., (1971) *Water Sew. Works.*, **352**, 18-111.
- Schindler, D.W., (1971), *J. Physio* **7**, 321.
- Keeney, D.R. (1972), *Wat Res. Centre Univ.Lit Rev*.3
- Bernhardt, H.& Eberle., S.H., (1986). *Aqua*, **5**, 273.
- Schrott, H.E., Mc Robbert, G.R. Bernard, T.W. and Mannadinyer, (1937). *As Indian J, Med. Res.* 25,553
- Ozha, D.D. and Dutta, A.K. (1994) *J.I. W.W.A.*, **26**, 39.
- Nath, K.J. and Majumdar, A. 1997, *J.IWW* **29**, 342

# 25

# Heavy Metals and Nutritive Calories in Muscles of Select Fish and Prawn Harvested from Dahanu Creek, West Coast of India

*T. K. Ghosh*

Seven and six varieties of fish and prawn respectively were collected by bag nets from Dahanu creek, west coast of India, and the muscle tissues were processed for heavy metal and calorific value analyses in laboratory. Estimation of heavy metals by AAS (flame) revealed that barring iron all the metals were accumulated at negligible concentrations. The order of metal accumulation in fish and prawn tissues appeared to be as Fe>Zn>Mn>Cr>Cu>Pb>Ni>Cd. The accumulation of Fe and Cd in fish and prawn muscles varied between 0.1 & 0.68 and traces & 0.04 mg g$^{-1}$ dry wt. respectively. While considering total heavy metal burden, the sequence of fish species from highest to lowest was as A. Sona, H. nehereus, M. hamiltoni, B. dussumieri, T. savala, P. indicus and R. kanagurta. The same for prawn came as P. sculptilis, P. indicus, S. crassicornis, M. brevicornis, P. penicillatus and E. styliferus.

The average nutritive calories values (1000 times less of heat calories) of fishes indicated marginal increase (0.64 percent) over prawn tissues. The nutritive calories of fish and prawn muscles varied between 3.79 & 4.85 and 4.07 & 5.06 cal gm$^{-1}$ dry wt. respectively. Based on nutritive values, the fishes can be graded as P. indicus > B. dussumieri > A. sona > R. kanagurta > H. nehereus > M. hamiltoni > T. savala. In general, heavy metal and calorie contents of fish and prawn from Dahanu creek were within the desired range.

## Introduction

The universal concern caused by the diffusion of toxic metals into environment by industrial emissions and leaching from hazardous wastes has motivated the initiation of a number of sample surveys, pilot studies and biological monitoring programmes. The presence of mercury, lead, chromium and manganese in quantities above permissible limits has been reported in some estuaries, locations very close to alkali or rayon plants in the Trombay basin, coastal waters adjacent to Mumbai and Kochi, in the working area of some welding shops, electroplating and thermal processing units and the effluents of chrome tanneries (Krishnamurti, 1991). Maharashtra is the second leading state for marine fisheries in India with two-thirds of fish catch being at Greater Mumbai where sea fishes are very much in demand.

Monitoring of heavy metals in fish tissues is a measure to provide an early indication of levels that are considered unsafe for people. In view of installation of a 500 MW coal based thermal power station on the bank of Dahanu creek (northern Maharashtra) and Dahanu being a major marine fish landing station, there was a need to evaluate baseline status of heavy metal contamination and food value of the economically important fin and shell fish muscles of the creek.

## Materials and Method

Three specimens each of 7 (*Rastrelliger kanagurta, Arius sona, Harpodon nehereus, Mugil hamiltoni, Boleophthalmus dussumieri, Polynemus indicus* and *Trichiurus savala*) and 6 (*Penaeus indicus, Penaeus penicillatus, Exopalaemon styliferus, Solenocera crassicornis, Metapenaeus brevicornis* and *Parapenaeus sculptilis*) varieties of fish and prawn respectively were collected by bag net from Dahanu creek. The creek, which is about 10 km long, is on the west coast of India and is located at a distance of 111 km from Mumbai towards Ahmedabad. The depth of creek water varies from 1 to 5 m during low tide.

The fin and shell fishes were washed free of extraneous matter and were defreezed until dissection of muscle tissues in laboratory. The muscles were homogenized and digested with concentrated nitric acid – perchloric acid mixture. The resultant solutions were then diluted to known volume of deionized water and transferred to acid-washed test tubes with Teflon screw caps. Selective heavy metals (Cd, Cr, Cu, Pb, Fe, Zn, Mn and Ni) were analyzed by Perkin Elmer flame- AAS. The flame used for aspiration was air-acetylene. For estimating nutritive values of fish muscles, dry tissues, at $70^0C$ upto constant weight, were homogenized and subjected to combustion in bomb calorimeter. It may be mentioned that nutritive calorie values are 1000 times less of heat calories.

## Results and Discussion

The concentrations of different metals (Table 25.1) in muscle tissues of fin and shell fishes indicate that the levels of iron followed by zinc and manganese were comparatively more from those of other metals. The order of metal accumulation in fish and prawn tissues were as $Fe>Zn>Mn>Cr>Cu>Pb>Ni>Cd$. In an earlier study on fishes of Mumbai offshore, copper was not found in detectable amount in sizable number of samples (Ghosh and Kshirsagar, 1993). It is generally believed that fish actively regulates Cu and Zn concentrations in their muscles (Denton and Burdon-Jones, 1986). Further, average levels of all the metals studied were higher in prawn from those of fishes. Among the prawn, *Parapenaeus sculptilis* exhibited highest levels of all (except Mn) metals monitored. Similar conclusion could not be drawn for any specific fish.

**Table 25.1 : Heavy Metal Concentrations in Fish and Prawn Muscles Harvested from Dahanu Creek Region**

| SN | Fish /Prawn | Cadmium | Chromium | Copper | Lead | Iron | Zinc | Manganese | Nickel |
|---|---|---|---|---|---|---|---|---|---|
| | **FISH** | | | | | | | | |
| 1 | *Rastrelliger kanagurta* | 0.001 | BDL | 0.008 | 0.005 | 0.100 | 0.036 | 0.010 | 0.003 |
| 2 | *Arius sona* | 0.002 | 0.002 | 0.012 | 0.010 | 0.390 | 0.045 | 0.026 | 0.008 |
| 3 | *Harpodon nehereus* | 0.002 | 0.002 | 0.005 | BDL | 0.300 | 0.069 | 0.022 | BDL |
| 4 | *Mugil hamiltoni* | 0.002 | 0.004 | 0.008 | 0.008 | 0.266 | 0.074 | 0.032 | 0.006 |
| 5 | *Boleophthalmus dussumieri* | 0.004 | 0.002 | 0.004 | 0.026 | 0.260 | 0.049 | 0.035 | BDL |
| 6 | *Polynemus indicus* | 0.002 | 0.002 | 0.006 | 0.021 | 0.151 | 0.027 | 0.013 | 0.009 |
| 7 | *Trichiurus savala* | 0.007 | 0.007 | 0.010 | 0.010 | 0.148 | 0.058 | 0.031 | 0.010 |
| | **Mean** | **0.003** | **0.003** | **0.008** | **0.011** | **0.231** | **0.051** | **0.024** | **0.005** |
| | **PRAWN** | | | | | | | | |
| 8 | *Penaeus indicus* | BDL | 0.004 | 0.040 | 0.022 | 0.540 | 0.029 | 0.054 | BDL |
| 9 | *Penaeus penicillatus* | 0.002 | 0.002 | 0.040 | 0.017 | 0.400 | 0.019 | 0.029 | 0.004 |
| 10 | *Exopalaemon styliferus* | 0.003 | 0.003 | 0.024 | 0.008 | 0.168 | 0.062 | 0.024 | 0.013 |
| 11 | *Solenocera crassicornis* | 0.022 | 0.007 | 0.030 | 0.035 | 0.291 | 0.097 | 0.126 | 0.007 |
| 12 | *Metapenaeus brevicornis* | 0.006 | 0.003 | 0.078 | 0.022 | 0.297 | 0.075 | 0.072 | 0.028 |
| 13 | *Parapenaeus sculptilis* | 0.042 | 0.028 | 0.141 | 0.056 | 0.676 | 0.211 | 0.098 | 0.056 |
| | **Mean** | **0.013** | **0.008** | **0.059** | **0.027** | **0.395** | **0.082** | **0.067** | **0.018** |

Values are expressed as mg/gm dry weight; BDL: below detectable limit

Since the fishes under study are mostly animal feeders, the possibility of biomagnification of the metals cannot be ignored. Plankton, one of the basic food resources in marine system, are known to concentrate heavy metals in large quantities (Martin & Knauer 1973). They play an active role in removal of metals from the ambient sea water (Morris 1971) and also act as an indicator for pollution. Plankton are also known to concentrate metal from the ambient medium and pass them on to higher trophic levels. While evaluating the extent of distribution of select heavy metals (Cu, Zn, Cd & Pb) in water, sediment and plankton over a period of two years from Pondichery harbour, a distinct seasonal variation in the distribution of metals was observed (Senthilnathan & Balasubramanian 1999). The metals were high during monsoon and low during summer. The order of metal abundance in water, sediment and plankton was Zn > Cu > Pb > Cd. Plankton showed greater adsorption and absorption capacity for most of the heavy metals as revealed by the concentration factors.

Average concentrations of heavy metals in marine zooplankton is higher in the Arabian Sea than in the Bay of Bengal (Bhattacharya, 1986; George & Kureishy, 1979). While comparing metal levels in various marine animals of different regions of seas, Table 25.2 indicates that metal concentrations in fish of Dahanu creek area were comparable to majority of reported values. In general, metal burden in fishes from coastal waters of Pakistan and Oman were less (Jaffar & Ashraf, 1988 and Burn *et al.*, 1982). Accumulation of Cu in prawns and squilla of Gulf of Nicoya, Costa Rica & NE Pacific coast is comparable to those of Dahanu creek and the average value is about 8 times higher than that of fish of the same area. Similar fold of Cu enrichment in shrimps as compared to fish of NE Pacific coast was reported earlier by Harding and Goyette (1989). Even amongst mollusks, Gundacker (2000) concluded that gastropods accumulated 20 fold higher concentrations of Cd, Cu and Zn than the bivalves. Table 25.2 further indicates enhanced levels of metal accumulations in different varieties of invertebrates as compared to fish. The extent of occurrence or accumulation of trace metals by organisms in different tissues is dependent on the route of entry, that is, either from surrounding medium or in the form of food or chemical form of material available in the media. Based on laboratory studies with the crab *Scylla serrata*, Prasad and Neelakantan (1987) opined that the main route of entry of Cu, Hg and Ca seems to be through food, whereas in case of other metals (Zn, Mn, Co, Ni and Fe), it is water through which metal accumulation might have had occurred.

**Table 25.2 : Concentrations of Certain Heavy Metals in Tissues of Marine Organisms Collected from Different Regions**

| Organism | Tissues | Region | Heavy metals (mg kg$^{-1}$) | | | | | | Source |
|---|---|---|---|---|---|---|---|---|---|
| | | | Pb | Zn | Cr | Cu | Ni | Mn | |
| Zooplankton (dry wt.) | Total mass | Arabian sea | NR | 22494.00 | NR | 232.00 | 17.00 | NR | Bhattacharya (1986) |
| Zooplankton (dry wt.) | Total mass | Bay of Bengal | NR | 1701.00 | NR | 228.00 | 81.00 | NR | George and Kureishy (1979) |
| Clam *Anadara granosa* (dry wt.) | M | Mumbai harbour | 4.00 | 70.00 | 3.50 | 8.50 | 4.50 | 62.50 | Patel *et al.* (1985) |
| Mudskipper *Boleophthalmus boddaerti* (dry wt.) | M | Mumbai harbour | 6.50 | 75.00 | 0.60 | 5.00 | 1.50 | 34.00 | Patel *et al.* (1985) |
| Fish Saloman sole (wet wt.) | M | Coastal water of Pakistan | 0.03 | 1.10 | 0.12 | 0.16 | 0.03 | 0.06 | Jaffar and Ashraf (1988) |
| | L | (Arabian Sea) | 0.04 | 8.93 | 0.32 | 0.82 | 0.06 | 0.67 | |
| Fish *Sardinella longiceps* (wet wt.) | M | Coastal water of Pakistan | 0.09 | 2.11 | 0.09 | 0.21 | 0.03 | 0.06 | Jaffar and Ashraf (1988) |
| | L | (Arabian Sea) | 0.24 | 19.90 | 0.58 | 0.75 | 0.14 | 0.40 | |
| Fish *Scomberoides comersonianus* (wet wt.) | M | Coastal water of Pakistan | 0.03 | 3.71 | 0.12 | 0.31 | 0.03 | 0.05 | Jaffar and Ashraf (1988) |
| | L | (Arabian Sea) | 0.16 | 30.12 | 0.847 | 1.54 | 0.06 | 0.49 | |
| Oyster *Crassostrea madrasensis* (dry wt.) | M | SE Coast of India | NR | 211–370 | NR | 123–187 | NR | 25–87 | Rajendran *et al.* (1988) |
| Fifty varieties of fishes (dry wt.) | M | Great Barrier Reef, Australia | NR | 4.3–41.8 | NR | 0.47–2.4 | Rare | NR | Denton and Burdon–Jones (1986) |
| | L | | 38.90 | ND–2335 | NR | ND–334 | Rare | NR | |
| Two varieties of fishes (dry wt.) | M | Coastal water of Oman | 0.21–0.25 | 9.9–13.6 | 3.3 | 0.41–0.65 | 0.08–1.90 | 0.18–0.27 | Burns *et al.* (1982) |
| Arthropod *Squilla parva* (dry wt.) | Total mass | Gulf of Nicoya, Costa Rica | 1.4–2.6 | 75.212 | 0.07–0.9 | 134–65 | NR | NR | Dean *et al.* (1986) |
| Prawn *Penaeus brevirostris* (dry wt.) | Total mass | Gulf of Nicoya, Costa Rica | 0.06 | 214.60 | NR | 18.50 | NR | NR | Dean *et al.* (1986) |
| Shrimp *Pandalus platyceros* (dry wt.) | M | NE Pacific Coast | 0.7–1.25 | 49–53 | 0.5–0.6 | 14–20, | NR | NR | Harding and Goyette 1989) |
| English sole *Parophrys vetulus* (dry wt.) | M | NE Pacific Coast | 1.86 | 21.70 | 1.30 | 2.10 | NR | NR | Harding and Goyette (1989) |

*Contd....*

| Organism | Tissues | Region | Heavy metals (mg kg⁻¹) | | | | | | Source |
|---|---|---|---|---|---|---|---|---|---|
| | | | Pb | Zn | Cr | Cu | Ni | Mn | |
| Fish *Mullus barbatus* (dry wt.) | M | Eastern Mediterranean, Israel | NR | 22.00 | 0.50 | 3.70 | NR | NR | Hornung and Ramelow (1987) |
| Clam *Marcia recens* (dry wt.) | M | East Coast of India | 4.57–5.16 | 37.3–40.07 | NR | 7.87–10.05 | 1.61–1.62 | NR | Muralidharan and (1997) |
| Fish *Sardinella longiceps* (dry wt.) | M | SW Coast of India | NR | 20.52 | NR | 1.54 | BR | ND | Nair *et al.* (1997) |
| Fish *Mugil Cephalus* (dry wt.) | M | SW Coast of India | NR | 26.68 | NR | 1.51 | NR | ND | Nair *et al.* (1997) |
| Sea Turtle | Egg Shell | Orissa coast | 11.0 | 13.0 | 10.0 | 7.6 | 13.0 | 3.6 | Sahoo and |
| *Lepidocehelys olivacea* (dry wt.) | Hatchlings | Orissa coast | 20.0 | 17.3 | 10.3 | 9.3 | 25.0 | 23.6 | Sahoo (1996) |
| Seven varieties of fishes (wet wt.) | M | Arabian sea (off Mumbai) | 0.10–0.50 | 1.1–4.05 | 0.12–1.74 | ND–0.92 | ND–0.34 | 3.52–12.48 | Ghosh and Kshirsagar |
| | L | | 0.12–1.25 | ND–3.01 | 0.25–1.80 | ND–2.24 | ND–1.78 | 3.75–8.22 | (1993) |
| Fishes and prawns under present study (dry wt.) | M | Dahanu creek (near Mumbai) | BDL–0.06 | 0.02–0.21 | BDL–0.03 | 0.004–0.141 | BDL–0.06 | 0.01–0.13 | Present survey |

M: muscle; L: liver; NR: not reported

The mechanism (s) of metal uptake by the cells has not yet been fully elucidated; the evidence indicates that metals cross the cell membranes essentially by a passive transport process although endocytosis may also occur (George and Viarengo, 1984). When metals cross the cell membranes they react with the cytosolic component, and are usually complexed in different ways (by sulphydrylic binding, chelation, salt formation) to cytosolic compounds such as specific ligands (metallothioneins), substrates, products of enzymatic activity, or enzyme themselves.

The muscles of fish and shell-fish are valued principally by calories contributed by protein and small quantities of fat and carbohydrate. Fig 25.1 depicts calorie values varying between 3.79 and 5.06 cal gm⁻¹ dry wt. for fish and prawn of Dahanu creek. The average calorie value was marginally higher (0.64 percent) in fish over prawn. The estimated energy values were within the range (3.2 to 6.9 cal gm⁻¹ dry wt.) of various freshwater fishes from Gouri tank, Chambal (M.P.) and river Ganga (Saxena, 1990, Bilgrami and Dutta Munshi, 1979). While *Polynemus indicus* and *Solenocera crassicornis* exhibited highest calorie values amongst fish and prawn respectively, *Trichiurus savala* and *E. styliferus* encountered lowest values in respective groups.

Present study indicates that the levels of eight metals in different fish and prawn species of Dahanu creek are not alarming. The muscles of the fin and shell fishes which appeared to be harmless for human consumption are also good source of nutritive calories. In view of growing human activities and industrialization in this area, regular monitoring is necessary, in case there are any long term impact on biota.

## ACKNOWLEDGEMENTS

The author wishes to express his thanks to Director (Tech.), BSES Ltd., Mumbai and Director, NEERI, Nagpur for providing all sorts of facilities and co-operation during the course of investigation.

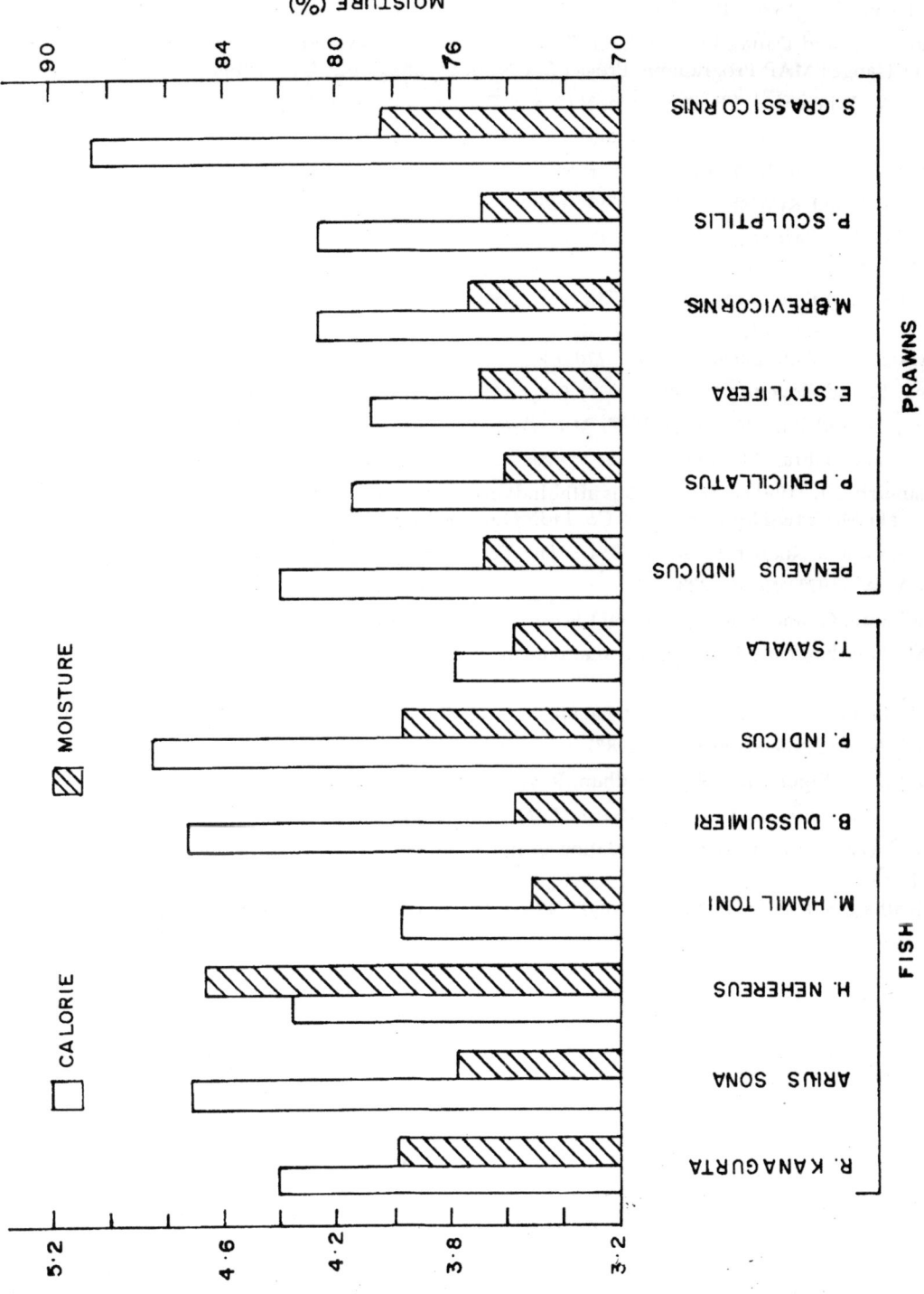

Fig. 25.1 : Calorie values and moisture contents of selective fishes and Prawns of Dahanu Creek

# REFERENCE

- Bhattacharya, S.S. (1986). Proc. Symp. Coastal Ecosystem. Acad. *Environ. Biol.,* India, p.21
- Bilgrami, K. S. and Datta Munshi, J.S. (1979).Limnological survey and impact on human activities on the river Ganges MAP Programme, Project 5, UNESCO, Bhagalpur Univ., Bihar
- Burns, K.A., Villeneuve, J.P., Anderlin, V.C. and Fowler, S.W. (1982). *Mar. Pollut. Bull.* 13: 240.
- Dean, H.K., Maurer, D., Vargas, J.A. and Tinsman, C.H. (1986). *Mar. Pollut. Bull.* 17: 128.
- Denton, G.R.W. and Burdon-Jones, C. (1986). *Mar. Pollut. Bull.* 17: 201
- George, M.D. and Kureishy, T.W. (1979). *Indian J. Mar. Sci.* 8: 190
- George, S.G. and Viarengo, A. (1984). Sixth Symposium on Pollution and Physiology of Marine Organisms. 1-3 Nov. 1983, Mystic, Connecticut, USA
- Ghosh, T.K. and Kshirsagar, D.G. (1993). of Proc. of National Academy of Sciences, India, 63 (B) III : 305
- Gundacker, C. (2000). *Environ. Pollut.* 110: 61
- Harding, L. and Goyette, D. (1989). *Mar. Pollut. Bull.* **20:** 187
- Hornung, H. and Ramelow, G.J. (1987) *Mar. Pollut. Bull.* **18:** 45
- Jaffar, M. and Ashraf, M. (1988). *Indian J. Mar. Sci.* **17:** 231
- Krishnamurti, C.R. (1991).*in* Toxic Metals in the Indian Environment. Krishnamurti, C.R. and Viswanathan, P. eds. **Tata** McGraw-Hill Publishing Co. Ltd., New Delhi, p. 1
- Martin, J. H. and Knauer, G. A. (1973) *Geochim Cosmochim Acta* **37:** 1639
- Morris A. W. (1971) *Nature:* **233:** 427
- Muralidharan, G. and Raja, P. V. (1997) *Indian J. Mar. Sci.* **26:** 383
- Nair, M., Balachandran, K. K., Sankaranarayanan, V. N. and Joseph, T. (1997). *Indian J. Mar. Sci.* **26:** 98
- Patel, B., Bangera, V.S., Patel, S. and Balani, M.C. (1985). *Mar. Pollut. Bull.* **16:** 22
- Prasad, P.N. and Neelakantan, B. (1987). *Sci. Cult.* **53:** 340
- Rajendran, N., Tagore, J. and Kasinathan, R. (1988). *Indian J. Mar. Sci.* **17:** 174
- Sahoo, G. and Sahoo, R. K. (1996). *Indian J. Mar. Sci.* **25:** 371
- Saxena, S. (1990).*in* Ecosystem Degradation in India, Sinha, B.N. ed. Ashish Publishing House, New Delhi, p. 72
- Senthilnathan, S. and Balasubramanian T. (1999). *Indian J. Mar. Sc.* **28:** 380

# 26

# Environmental Sustainability in Brackishwater Shrimp Aquafarming

*A. S. Ninawe*

Aquaculture is one of the fastest growing food production system in the world with an annual growth rate of 10 per cent annum since 1984 compared with 3 per cent for live stock meat and 1.6 per cent for capture fisheries production. Being more remunerative than agriculture and other livestock husbandry, a quafarming is developing as a prime farming activity tapping the enormous bio-energy to meet the challenges of starvation, malnutrition and nutritious food for the fast growing population. As a prioritised resort to improve the shortcomings in fishery production, aquaculture has been promoted for its potential to compensate for the low growth rate of capture fisheries and dwindling resources. As a result, aquaculture in general and shrimp farming in particular have become more popular among third world countries including India. An average productivity of fresh water fish ponds in Israel and China has been between 15 and 25 t/ha/year. In India 17 t/ha/year of carps and 6 t/ha/crop of shrimp are recorded. Thailand becoming number one shrimp producer in the world, producing 6-10t/ha/crop through intensive (85%) system (Menasveta, 1997). Across the globe there are records of capital intensive production system that may pose problems to the sustainability in the long run. Thus, intensive farming is more towards unsustainable development and hence needs to be changed globally for more sustainable extensive or semi- intensive farming with an integrated system approaches. The characteristics of shrimp farming at three levels of intensity *i.e.* traditional, semi-intensive and intensive are given in Table-26.1.

**Table 26.1 : Characteristics of shrimp culture at three levels of intensity**

| Characteristics | Level of intensity | | |
| --- | --- | --- | --- |
| | Traditional | Semi-intensive | Intensive |
| Land elevation (m MSL) | 0 to 1.0 | >1.0 to 2.0 | >2.0 |
| Pond area (ha) | >5 | 1.0 to 2.0 | <1.0 |
| Water depth (m) | 0.5 to 1.2 | 0.8 to 1.5 | 0.8 to 1.5 |
| Stocking density (PL/m2/crop) | <5 | > 5 to 15 | > 15 to 30 |
| Water exchange (% per day) | To compensate for the loss due to evaporation and seepage through tidal exchange tidal pumps | upto 15% | upto 30% |
| Aeration | Not required | In emergencies | Continuous |
| Feed | Natural | Natural+ Formulated | Formulated |
| Feeding frequency | —— | 1 to 4 times daily | 3 to 6 times daily |
| Level of water quality management | Low | Moderate | High |
| Need for dependable electric supply and generator back up | Not required | Partial backup necessary | Full back-up necessary |
| Size of shrimps at harvest (g) | 20 to 60 | 20 to 50 | 20 to 40 |
| FCR | —— | 1:1 to 1:15 | 1:1.5 to 1:1.7 |
| Survival (%) | 50 to 90 | 70 to 80 | 70 to 80 |
| Production level (kg/ha/crop) | 100 to1000 (kg/ha/year) | 1000 to 4000 kg/ha/4 to 5 months) | >6000 (kg/ha/6 months) |

(*Source*: Proc. of Workshop on Environmental Impact Assessment of Aquaculture Enterprises, 1997).

## Brackishwater Resources and Fish Production

India is endowed with rich natural resources in the coastal zone in the form of brackishwater/estuaries for taking up shrimp farming. In physical terms, the country has a long coastline of 8, 129 km, including the mainland, Andaman and Nicobar Islands and Lakshadweep. Fourteen large river systems and innumerable small seasonal coastal rivers drain into the seas. These forms extensive estuaries, backwaters, lagoons, coastal lakes, tidal creeks and mangrove swamps. The adjoining lands, due to salt incursion becomes not suitable for agricultural crops but would be suitable for brackishwater aquaculture. The brackishwater aquaculture activity has expanded significantly in recent years, particularly in the East Coast of Andhra Pradesh, Tamil Nadu and Orissa. Aquaculture contributes significantly to the overall shrimp production from the inland sector. The fish production in the country has increased from 2.8 million tonnes in 1984-85 to about 5.35 million tonnes, with a contribution of 2.97 million tonnes from marine and 2.38 million tonnes from inland sector during 1997-98. More than 70 per cent of inland production is through aquaculture. Carp culture in inland and shrimp culture in brackishwater sector are the two prominent culture operations in India. Coastal aquaculture has been recognised as a thrust area among the fisheries development programmes of country.

## Indian Scenario of Shrimp Farming

Across the globe shrimp farming technology paved the way to increase shrimp production by adopting extensive and semi- intensive systems of shrimp farming in the environmentally suited areas. India has about 1.19 million ha brackishwater area of which only around 1,00,000 ha are now under shrimp farming mostly by adopting the traditional practice (50,000 ha) and partly by extensive method of culture ( Paul Raj, 1995). Presently around 10 per cent of the available brackishwater areas has been developed for shrimp farming along with a number of supporting units like hatcheries, feed mills, processing and packaging industries etc. Thus the brackishwater area is still under-exploited. The major share of production comes from West Bengal, followed by Kerala, Andhra Pradesh and Orissa. The best species for culture in India are the tiger shrimp (*Penaeus monodon*), white shrimp (*P. indicus*), banana shrimp (*P. merguiensis*) and flower shrimp (*P. semisulcatus*) (Table 26.2).

**Table 26.2 : Production from coastal aquaculture-areas**

| Period | Area (ha) | Production rate (t/ha) | Production (t) |
|--------|-----------|------------------------|----------------|
| 1990–91 | 65,100 | 0.545 | 35,000 |
| 1991–92 | 68,227 | 0.581 | 40,000 |
| 1992–93 | 70,700 | 0.665 | 47,000 |
| 1993–94 | 82,500 | 0.752 | 62,000 |
| 1994–95 | 100,700 | 0.824 | 83,000 |
| 1995–96 | 100,700 | 0.695 | 70,000 |
| 1996–97 | 100,000 | 0.800 | 80,000 |

*Source*: MPEDA, Kochi

## Sustainable Eco-friendly Farming

Aquaculture has been practised for many centuries by small farmers and fisher-folk in Asia to improve their living conditions. However, there is a vast difference between the traditional methods and the new commercialised system. The traditional aquaculture, including shrimp, is usually small scale, using low inputs and relies on natural tidal action for water exchange. In some countries, such as India, Bangladesh and Thailand, there is a tradition of rice/shrimp rotating, with rice grown part of the year and shrimp and other fish species cultured rest of the year. In the traditional culture operations these naturally occurring post-larvae and juveniles are trapped in tidal impoundments and allowed to grow for short periods before they are caught. These ponds are constructed in suitable coastal brackishwater areas where there is a good tidal range and an abundant supply of prawn seed. This type of prawn culture is practised in the brackishwater *bheris* of West Bengal and in the paddy fields adjoining the Vembanad lake in Kerala. In Vypeen island about 1200 ha of paddy fields are utilised for traditional operation. Many of the fields are operated in extensive units upto 40 ha often ending in low prawn yields. The prawn catch from such fields varies from 500-1200 kg per hectare for the 6 months period. The case study on prawn production potentials of traditional paddy fields at Vypeen island in scientific manner can increase its life carrying capacity with definite positive impact on prawn yield. The division of bigger size prawn fields into 3-5 hectare size with common feeder canal, proper and well balanced flow systems and provision for potential prawn seeds and feed could be aimed at better production in two to three crops. The use of chemicals, antibiotics and processed feeds are not used in the traditional method. In this low yield, natural method, the harvest is small but sustainable over long periods and has no adverse effect on the environment and ecology.

## Employment Generation and Production Increase

During Eighth Plan high priority was given to aquaculture development due to its potential contribution to food security and foreign exchange earnings through export of high value products like shrimp. Its potential in employment generation is also quite high. Several socio-economic benefits have been reported arising from aquaculture development. (Pullin,1989; UNDP/Norvey/FAO,1987; Schmidt,1982). As an important coastal activity, it can provide livelihood not only for fisher-folk and their families but also for others in the fishing industry like people involved in the maintenance of fishing fleet (Raje and Singh,1995). The sector can create large number of employment opportunities in the farming sector and supported to produce thousand of tonnes of high quality nutritious food and earn valuable foreign exchange. It provides full time job to an average of 1 to 3 persons/ha through semi-intensive and intensive culture practices and upto 7 persons/ha through extensive farming. World-wide, shrimp farms covered approximately 9,62,600 ha in 1993, and employed over 1 million full time workers (FAO/NACA, 1994). It has also created indirect employment opportunities through allied services and industries like hatcheries, freezing, processing and packaging plants and manufacturing of feeds, chemicals, chemo-therapeutics and equipment and appliances. In the present shrimp production, 50 per cent is under traditional/extensive farming and the remaining is under modified extensive and semi-intensive farming, contributing to the employment and income of the local rural people. Currently there are 1,00,000 ha of shrimp farms providing employment at the rate of 5 persons/ha besides creating additional employment opportunities in several ancillary units (Sakthivel, 1999). Saline lands unfit for agriculture are being used for hatcheries and shrimp aquaculture resulting not only in increasing fish production, but also to engage number of displaced farm workers. The average labour requirement per ha of paddy cultivation is about 180 labour days per crop, whereas in shrimp farming it is about 600 labour days/crop. Moreover, regarding paddy, only one unrealistic crop may be raised in a year as against the possibility of two shrimp crops. Also the establishment of aquafarms has created subsidiary occupations like catering, transportation and handling of construction materials etc. Agricultural labourers, on an average, earn an annual income of Rs. 7500/- whereas the shrimp farm labourers earn Rs.12,000/- (Ninawe,1999).

## Intensification Problems

The demand for food increased due to population pressure. This lead to intensification of food production systems on land and water. Thus sustainability of shrimp aquaculture has been a focus these days due to the adoption of larger scale and intensive or semi-intensive farming practices. In such farming practices selected species are bred using a dense stocking rate to maintain crowded shrimp stocking density. The use of artificial feed, chemical additives and antibiotics are used to maintain crowded stocking density. This lead to the degradation, depletion and pollution of soil, water and other natural resources and disruption of social set up. The collapse of shrimp industry in Taiwan province of China, mainland provinces of China and subsequently in other countries in Asia including India reported disease and crop failures resulting in heavy economic losses (Dilip Kumar, 1999). In Asia and Latin America there are growing evidences that environmental impacts related to shrimp culture play an important role in outbreaks of disease, affecting shrimp ponds. The causes of disease and production losses are in many cases difficult to ascertain, but several studies link outbreaks of disease to environmental factors (Chen, 1990; Lin, 1989). It is yet to properly understood that intensive shrimp culture with high inputs such as feed and fertiliser caused stress on the water bodies, attracting disease incidence in many places.

## Effective Management Plan

In some South-east Asian countries, unregulated aquaculture practices, intensive and super-intensive culture operations have resulted in environmental and social problems like pollution due to discharge of waste water from the shrimp ponds. A similar situation was reported from some parts of India where intensive shrimp culture was carried out.

## Effluent Treatment in Aquaculture Ponds

The shrimp farm wastewater quality is dependent on the system of culture practice. The potential nutrient and organic loads from intensive culture tend to be higher than semi-intensive culture because of the increased inputs used. The impacts from external environmental change on shrimp culture represent a significant threat to the sustainability of shrimp culture in Asia (FAO/NACA,1994). The adverse effect of shrimp pond effluent on environment is considerably less than that of domestic or industrial waste water. The effluent quality during normal operation is similar to the quality of the water in pond, which if managed effectively will tend to be well mixed with water quality within acceptable ranges for shrimp (Satapornvanit, 1993). It is relatively difficult to assess the effects of external impact against those generated by shrimp farms themselves to identify the cause of the many water quality problems that crop up in shrimp culture ( Phillips, 1994). The sensitivity of shrimp, particularly in young stage to water contamination, in areas of intense agricultural, urban, industrial development always be considered as a high risky venture. Thus various environmental impacts need to be considered and understood in shrimp culture system.

In intensive farming, water quality is maintained by pumping as stocking rates are very high and proportionally high amounts of feed and chemicals etc. are used which lead to high amounts of waste materials loading in ponds and in water bodies discharged from the ponds. Feed conversion ratio (FCR) is an indirect indicator for the amount of nutrients lost in the pond ecosystem. Analysis of nutrient budgets in intensive shrimp farming has indicated that 63-78 per cent of nitrogen and 76-86 per cent of phosphorus inputs through feeds are lost as wastes (Phillips et al, 1993) (Table 26.3 & 26.4).

### Table 26.3 : Nitrogen and Phosphorous Budgets for an Intensive *Penaeus monodon* Farm

| | (Kg/t of shrimp produced) | | | |
|---|---|---|---|---|
| | Feed Conversion Ratio | | | |
| Parameters | 1.2:1 | | 2.0:1 | |
| | N | P | N | P |
| Free input | 91.2 | 17.0 | 152.0 | 28.4 |
| Shrimp harvest | 33.9 | 4.0 | 33.9 | 4.0 |
| Waste load | 57.3 | 13.0 | 118.1 | 24.4 |

(Source : Phillips *et al.*, 1993)

**Table 26.4 : Nutrient budgets estimated for 1 HA shrimp pond (Phillips, 1994)**

| | Semi–intensive | | | Intensive | |
|---|---|---|---|---|---|
| Potential harvest | | | | | |
| (mt/ha/crop) | 1.0 | | | 9.6 | |
| (mt/ha/yr) | 3.0 | | | 27.0 | |
| FCR | 1.4:1 | | | 1.0:1 | |
| | Nitrogen | Phosphorus | | Nitrogen | Phosphorus |
| Input with feed (mt/yr) | 2.98 | 0.45 | | 30.3 | 5.83 |
| Output with shrimp (mt/yr) | 2.65 | 0.18 | | 23.99 | 1.59 |
| Total waste loading (mt/yr) | 0.29 | 0.27 | | 14.34 | 4.24 |
| (kg/ha/yr) | 29 | 27 | | 1434 | 424 |
| kg/mt shrimp harvested | 9.7 | 9.0 | | 53.1 | 15.7 |

The intensification plays the most important role in shrimp culture operations and also on its sustainability. The quantity of waste produced is dependent on the FCR. There may be several other factors also determining the waste output. The efficiency of feed and fertiliser usage is considered to be less in intensive systems than in semi-intensive systems.

The pollution potential of shrimp farm effluents is considerably less than that of domestic or industrial wastewater (Macintosh and Phillips, 1992). However, in areas with significant concentrations of shrimp farms with poor flushing capacities, self pollution can occur. Nutrient and organic matter concentrations are highest during harvesting and subsequent cleaning of ponds. The farm water discharge and effluent could be monitored for salinity, temperature, pH, total phosphorus, total nitrogen, total ammonia, dissolved oxygen, chlorophyll and other suspended matter (Phillips et al 1990; Phillips,1994). The details of shrimp pond effluents and other types of effluents are given in Table 26.5.

**Table 26.5 : Shrimp Pond effluents and other types of effluents**

| Parameters | Shrimp pond effluent | Domestic waste water | | | Fish processing plant effluent |
|---|---|---|---|---|---|
| | | Untreated | Primary treatment | Biological treatment | |
| BOD (mg/l) | 4.0–10.2 | 300 | 200 | 30 | 10000–18000 |
| Total N (mg/l) | 0.03–5.06 | 75 | 60 | 40 | 700–4530 |
| Total P (mg/l) | 0.05–2.02 | 20 | 15 | 12 | 120–298 |
| Solids (mg/a) | 119–225 | 500 | – | 15 | 1880–7475 |

(Source : Office of Environmental Policy and Planning, 1994.)

Treatment of shrimp pond wastewater offers considerable potential for reducing impacts on the water quality in the estuarine environment. The studies on the treatment of shrimp pond waste are very few. These treatments could be physical, chemical and biological. The physical methods include filtration and sedimentation. Sedimentation of the suspended solids in settlement tanks is the cheapest method available. However, the main constraints in sedimentation are the high volume of effluent involved and the low concentration of solids. The effectiveness of sedimentation ponds also depends on the design, the surface area available for settling, the rate of flow and the retention time of the effluent. Recent studies have shown that upto 90 per cent of suspended solids, 60 per cent of BOD and 50 per cent of total phosphorus load can be removed by settlement treatment (Pillay, 1992). Some studies on water treatment systems for shrimp farms suggest that an integrated farming involving recycling of wastes from the primary systems can be a solution for pollution problems due to shrimp farming (Enandar and Hasselstrom, 1994).

Biological methods of waste treatment are still in experimental stage only. Culture of seaweed in the settlement tanks to remove the dissolved nutrients and culture of molluscs to remove the suspended particles are being suggested. The viability of the method and its cost-effectiveness should be worked out so that the same may be incorporated in the project. Hence intensive culture of shrimps is not advised in Indian conditions. Semi-intensive culture and improved extensive culture systems are generally practised.

Finally, there is a need to determine the environmental limits for sustainability of aquaculture development. Though, calculation of "Carrying Capacity" of coastal areas has been reported for cage culture (Makinen, 1991; Barg, 1992), yet its usefulness in case of shrimp culture is not known. Moreover, it will not be advisable to predict upper limits to aquaculture production based on national averages such as per capita productions per year; production per unit area / production per unit length of coastline etc. as reported by Csavas (1994a, b). Thus a more holistic approach can be taken into account by considering all possible factors interacting and influencing aquaculture, if essentially required to maintain the sustainability.

## Possible Impact on Environment

Many affecting impacts of shrimp farming are related to the intensity of farms in a given coastal area or the ability of the area to assimilate water materials. Major problems have surfaced in area where the level of farming has exceeded the carrying capacity of the local environment. Thus studying and understanding the environment in the context of aquaculture development are becoming imperative. Commercial shrimp culture has gained global attention not only due to its role in strengthening the economy of a country but also due to sudden collapse of industries in some parts of the globe. The impact of aquaculture on environment mainly depends on the location and type of farm and the production technology involved. Aquaculture had many positive impacts, if it can be practised as extensive or improved semi-intensive farming practices (Lee and Wickins, 1992; Macintosh and Phillips, 1992).

Though it is stated that the shrimp aquafarming effluent is less toxic than domestic and industrial waste water, crowding of shrimp farms and limited water flushing capacity, may create severe impact on the quality of receiving waters. A major shrimp mortality was reported in one of the waste coast of Sri Lanka due to discharge of pond effluent water to the main supply canal, "Dutch Canal" which serves as a water supply for several hundred shrimp farms (Sri Lanka report in FAO/NACA, 1994). In India, most of the ground water resources in the salt affected coastal areas are saline. Fresh water is available only at depths of above 100 m in most of the areas. Such freshwater resources are available even within the shrimp farm area which are not salinised by the sea-water stored in the farms. By seeing the present scenario of brackish- water aquaculture in India, it is utmost desirable to adopt scientific methods for its development. Models are available for predicting the capacity of coastal areas for Salmon cage culture (Makinen, 1991). Such models are yet to be developed for shrimp farming. A programme on Environment Monitoring undertaken by the Central Institute of Brackishwater Aquaculture (CIBA) for the World Bank assisted shrimp culture projects in West Bengal and Orissa are aiming towards the development of suitable models for shrimp farming. Several studies undertaken by them have clearly shown that the pollutional impacts of sea based farms in Nellore, Andhra Pradesh are negligible (Joseph et.al., 1997). In some parts of India, overcrowding of shrimp farms has happened earlier, since these farms were established without any logistics and inadequate infrastructure facilities available in those areas. This has resulted in mixing up the water intake and outlet systems in some of the farms. To maintain the sustainabilty in shrimp aquaculture ideal water quality parameters are proposed in Table 26.6.

**Table 26.6 : Ideal values of various water quality parameters for aquaculture in three types of water bodies**

| Sl. No. | Parameters | Freshwater | Brackishwater | Seawater |
|---|---|---|---|---|
| 1. | Colour (colour units) | clear water with greenish hue <100 colour units | clear water with greenish hue <100 colour units | clear water with greenish hue <100 colour units |
| 2. | Transparency (cm) | 20–35 | 26–35 | 26–35 |
| 3. | Clay Turbidity (mg⁻¹). | <30 | <30 | <30 |
| 4. | Solids (mgl⁻¹). | | | |
| | a. Total | <500 | >500 | >500 |
| | b. Suspended | 30–200 | 25–200 | 25–200 |
| 5. | Temperature (°C) | | | |
| | a. Tropical climate | 25–32 | 25–32 | 25–32 |
| | b. Temperate climate | 10–12 | 10–12 | 10–12 |
| 6. | pH | 6.7–9.5 | 7.0–8.7 | 7.0–8.5 |
| 7. | Hardness(mgl⁻¹) | 30–180 | >50 | >50 |
| 8. | Alkalinity(mgl⁻¹) | 50–300 | >50 | >50 |
| 9. | Chlorides (mgl⁻¹) | 31–50 | >500 | >500 |
| 10. | Salinity (ppt) | <0.5 | 10–25 | >30 |
| 11. | Dissolved oxygen (mg l⁻¹) | 5–10 | 5–10 | 5–10 |
| 12. | Total dissolved free carbondioxide (mg l⁻¹) | <3 | <3 | <3 |
| 13. | Ammonia nitrogen ($NH_3$-N) (mgl⁻¹) | | | |
| | a. Unionized ($NH_3$) | 0–0.1 | 0–0.1 | 0–0.1 |
| | b. Ionized ($NH_4^+$) | 0–1.0 | 0–1.0 | 0–1.0 |
| 14. | Nitrite nitrogen ($NO_2$-N, (mgl⁻¹) | 0–0.5 | 0–0.5 | 0–0.5 |
| 15. | Nitrate nitrogen (NO3-N, (mgl⁻¹) | 0.1–3 | 0.1–3 | 0.1–3 |
| 16. | Total nitrogen (mgl⁻¹) | 0.5–4.5 | 0.5–4.5 | 0.5–4.5 |
| 17. | Total phosphorus (mgl⁻¹) | 0.05–0.4 | 0.05–0.5 | 0.05–0.5 |
| 18. | Potassium (mgl⁻¹) | 0.5–10 | >0.5 | >0.5 |
| 19. | Calcium (mgl⁻¹) | 75–150 | >75 | >75 |
| 20. | Magnesium (mgl⁻¹) | 20–200 | 200–1350 | >1350 |
| 21. | Sulphate (mgl⁻¹) | 20–200 | 200–885 | >885 |
| 22. | Silica (mgl⁻¹) | 4–16 | >5 | >5 |
| 23. | Iron (mgl⁻¹) | 0.01–0.3 | 0.01–0.3 | 0.01–0.3 |
| 24. | Biochemical oxygen demand (B.O.D.) (mgl⁻¹) | <10 | <15 | <15 |
| 25. | Chemical oxygen demand (C.O.D.) (mgl⁻¹) | <50 | <70 | <70 |
| 26. | Hydrogen sulphide (mgl⁻¹) | <0.002 | <0.003 | <0.003 |
| 27. | Residual chlorine (mg l⁻¹) | <0.003 | <0.003 | <0.003 |
| 28. | Primary productivity (mgC/m³/day) | 1000–3000 | 1000–2500 | 1000–2500 |
| 29. | Chlorophyll-a (µgl⁻¹) | 20–275 | 20–250 | 20–250 |

(*Source* : Proc. of Workshop on Environmental Impact Assessment of Aquaculture Enterprises, 1997).

## Mangrove Productivity as Breeding Grounds

Mangroves are the most productive ecosystems after corals with high biodiversity. These are the nursery grounds for many species of finfish, shrimp and other crustaceans, molluscs, birds and mammals. It plays important role in nutrient cycling, as a source of nutrients for adjacent coastal ecosystems for many commercially important finfish, crustaceans and molluscs (Phillips *et al.*, 1993). The other impacts of intensive farming reported from Thailand, Taiwan, Philippines, Indonesia and China are destruction of coastal mangroves and degradation of land resources. The impact of shrimp farming on mangrove destruction has received considerable attention in countries like Philippines (Primavera, 1989), Ecuador (Aitken, 1990), Bangladesh (Sahid and Pramanik, 1986) and Indonesia (Chamberlain, 1991). In India the level of mangrove destruction is not quantified, The removal of mangroves can have a significant impact on the ecological, economic and social impact in relation to shrimp culture. This can also be a problem to both natural fisheries and shrimp culture through indiscriminate removal of mangroves.

## Effect of Salinisation

In inland areas shrimp farms located in elevated places might lead to salinisation of adjacent land through horizontal movement of saline water. Salinisation of soils surrounding shrimp farms have been reported from Sri Lanka resulting into economic losses (Jayasinge and DeSilva, 1990). In Taiwan, use of ground water for shrimp culture reported to lead to salinisation of freshwater supplies and land subsidence (Chiang and Lee, 1986). In India, most of the ground water resources in the salt affected coastal areas are saline. The available freshwater resources within the shrimp farm area are not salinised by seawater stored in the farms. In some parts of India, ground water is utilised for diluting the high saline water source to compensate the non availability of creek water. Such drawing of water, if done at large scale may lead to salinisation of ground water aquifers. In India definite proofs are not available on soil salinisation, since adequate information on the soil and water quality are not available prior to the establishment of shrimp farms. Studies conducted in Nellore (Andhra Pradesh) by Central Institute of Brackishwater Aquaculture (CIBA) have indicated that the salinisation of the soil depends on the quality of the soil. In sandy areas, upto 100 m from the farm, there was marginal increase in the salinity of the topsoil reported by Gupta *et.al.*1998.

## Remedial Measures

All the major shrimp farming countries of the world like Taiwan, China, Ecuador etc. have faced environmental problems which are mainly due to intensification. Improper and unplanned development by aquaculture community could lead to these problems. Commercial shrimp culture in India practices almost entirely in land-based ponds. The traditional tide-fed culture systems are generally located in low-lying inter-tidal coastal wetlands. But with the advent of pump fed semi- intensive and improved extensive type of culture systems, supra- tidal, elevated land is being used for shrimp farming. In India, shrimp farms have been constructed on a variety of coastal lands, unused agricultural land, salt-pans, waste land and wet lands such as mangroves and marshes.

In view of this, there is need to sustain the industry in the long run by proper environmental management operating both at farm level as well as the coastal management level. At farm level, more emphasis is to be given for proper site selection, designing and operation of farms to increase the farming efficiency and reducing the waste discharge. On the other hand, at the coastal management level, integration of farming in the coastal zone is to be taken in such a way that its impact on other activities and *vice versa*, can be avoided. In order to make the promising enterprise sustainable, it is essential that proper environmental monitoring plans and waste water treatment systems are developed. In India, maritime states are preparing their respective Coastal Zone Management Plan, indicating the areas and zones suitable for various users. Such comprehensive plan once prepared, could solve the problem and the major natural resources like mangroves can be protected.

The Ministry of Agriculture, Government of India realised the urgent need to develop guidelines to shrimp farmers, State Fisheries Departments, Pollution Control Boards and all other agencies involved in the process of promoting the enterprise. Proper farm management will reduce the nutrient load in the wastewater. Further, the guidelines prescribed by the Ministry of Agriculture, Government of India, if followed scrupulously, will prevent most of the adverse effects expected of shrimp farming.

While assessing the impacts on environment due to aquafarming the following points need to be taken into consideration.

1.  Monitoring and maintenance of significant soil, water and effluent quality is essential for maximising shrimp production as well as to reduce environmental problems. The water quality management is vital at all the three stages *viz.*, inlet water, pond water and discharge water. Good water quality management assures less disease occurrence.

2.  Aquaculture entrepreneurs should be made aware of these interactive impacts and impact on

environment. The net result of these interacting processes is reflected in good production, productivity and quality of the environment.

3.  The feed waste plays an important role in the total waste loadings in the environment. Quality feed with limited metabolite output and excellent FCR (Food Conversion Ration) may not affect the system much. Hence the use of wet diets such as fresh fish and invertebrates has to be reduced and preferably avoided in shrimp aquaculture systems and good quality pellet diets should be used. Guidelines on stocking density, feed management, waste water disposal should be strictly followed for a sustained growth in shrimp farming.

4.  As far as possible only organic manure/fertilisers and other plant products should be used and use of chemical pesticides in culture systems should be avoided. Also the use of anti-biotics/drugs in culture system should be avoided.

5.  Proper irrigation and drainage facility is must for sustainable farming. Moreover, reservoir facilities and effluent treatment facility will go a long way in successful shrimp farming. An environmental impact assessment (EIA) should be made even at the planning stage by all the aquaculture units above 40 ha size. R&D efforts in achieving remarkable breakthroughs in biological treatment of effluents by selected microbes, even genetically altered microbes, use of plant and animals such as sea-weeds, mussels and clams could pave the way for sustainable aquaculture to come.

6.  There is evidence that removal of mangroves leads to a decline in finifish and shellfish recruitment to the open waters through reduced availability of post-larvae. Construction activity within the natural mangrove areas or ecologically sensitive wetlands, swamps etc. should be prohibited. Agricultural land not fit for cultivation can be utilised for aquafarming.

7.  The introduction of imported shrimp seed may bring with it a number of problems including diseases, disease producing pathogens etc. Thus, introduction of exotic seed in the culture systems should be prohibited.

8.  Intensive culture which leads to over-capitalisation and more stress on the ambient environment should not be adopted. Suitable farming technology should be selected, depending on the infrastructure facilities available at the project implementation sites.

## SUMMARY

Commercial aquaculture has gained global attention in strengthening the economy of the country. As a result considerable investments have taken place in the coastal areas during the last few years and number of shrimp farms have increased significantly. Such expansion in most of the Asian countries at large scale could lead to several environmental and socio-economic problems. Thus environmental sustainability in brackishwater shrimp aquaculture has become relevant to the environmental issues. Proper environmental management plan based on the carrying capacity of culture system would help in monitoring the coastal aquaculture activity to run the industry for a longer period. Adoption of effluent treatment plants in aquaculture operations would also sustain the activity. Further government efforts would be needed on planning and legislation enforcement on various issues to bring the sustainability in coastal aquafarming.

## REFERENCES

● Aitken, D.,1990. Shrimp farming in Ecuador. An aquaculture success story. *World Aquaculture*, **21** (1): 7-16

● Anon, 1997. Environmental impact assessment of aquaculture enterprises. Proceedings of the workshop held at Rajiv Gandhi Centre for Aquaculture, Chennai during December 10-12, 1997, 188 p.

- Anon, 1999. Guidelines-Adopting improved technology for increasing production and productivity in traditional and improved traditional systems of shrimp farming. Publication by Aquaculture Authority, Govt. of India, New Delhi, 14 p.

- Barg, U.C., 1992. Guidelines for the promotion of environment of coastal aquaculture. FAO Fish. Tech. paper: 328. FAO, Rome, Italy.

- Chamberlain, G. W., 1991. Shrimp farming in Indonesia: 1-Growout techniques. *World Aquaculture*, 22: p.12-27.

- Chen, S. N., 1990. Collapse and remedy for the shrimp culture industry in Taiwan, Department of Zoology, National Taiwan University, Taiwan.

- Chiang, H.C. and J. C. Lee., 1986. Study of treatment and reuse of aquaculture waste water in Taiwan. *Aquaculture Engineering*, 5: p.301-312.

- Csavas, I. 1994a. Recommendations for sustainable aquaculture. Paper presented in SEAFDEC-AQD Seminar-Workshop on Aquaculture. Development in South-East Asia, p.26-28, Iililo City, Philippines.

- Csavas, I., 1994b. Important factors in the success of shrimp farming. *World Aquaculture*. 25(1): p.34-56.

- Dilip Kumar, 1999. Improving extension services system for sustainable development of shrimp aquaculture. Paper presented during the workshop on development of sustainable Management practices in shrimp farming during July 30-31, 1999 at Bhubaneswar

- Enander, M. and M. Hasselstrom, 1994. An experimental waste water treatment system for a shrimp farm. Infofish International. 4/94: p.56-61.

- FAO/NACA, 1994. Regional Study and Workshop on the Environment and Management of Aquaculture. FAO/UN and Network of Aquaculture Centres in Asia-Pacific, Bangkok.

- Gupta, B. P., K.O. Joseph, M. Muralidhar, K. K. Krishnani and P. Ravichandran. 1998. Studies on soil salinity in shrimp culture areas of Andhra Pradesh and Tamil Nadu. Abstract. In: Natl. Symp. on Combating pollutants accumulation in Eco-system for sustainable agriculture, October, 1998, Allahabad Agricultural Institute, Allahabad.

- Jayasinge, J.M. P. K. and J. A. De Silva., 1990. Impact of prawn culture development on the present land use pattern in the coastal areas of Sri Lanka. In: Symposium on Ecology and Landscape management of Sri Lanka held at Colombo in June 1990.

- Joseph, K.O., B.P. Gupta and M. Krishnan, 1997. A critical analysis of physico-chemical parameters for environmental evaluation in aquaculture, p. 110-121. In: Proc. of the workshop on Environmental Impact assessment of Aquaculture Enterprises held at Chennai during December 10-12, 1997, 168 p.

- Lee, D'OC and J.F. Wickins, 1992. Crustacean Farming. Blackwell Scientific Publication, Oxford, 392 p.

- Lin, C. K. 1989. Prawn culture in Taiwan: What went wrong? *World Aquaculture*, 20: p.19-20

- Macintosh, D.J. and M. J. Phillips., 1992. Environmental issues in shrimp farming. In: Saram, H. de and T. Singh (Eds) 1992. Shrimp'92 Hong Kong, Proc. 3 Global Conf. Shrimp Industry p.14-16, Sept. 1992.

- Makinen, T., 1991. Marine Aquaculture and Environment. Nordic Council of Ministers, Copenhagen, 1991.

- Menasveta, P.,1997. Intensive and efficient culture system- the Thai way can save mangroves., Aquaculture Asia Vol.II(1), Jan-March, 1997.

- Ninawe A.S.,1999. Coastal aquaculture versus environment: pros and cons. Infofish International 2/99: p.43-47

- Office of Environmental Policy and Planning, 1994. The environmental management of coastal aquaculture. An assessment of shrimp culture in Southern Thailand. OEPP, Network of Aquaculture centres in Asia Pacific (NACA), Bangkok, Thailand.

- Paul Raj R.,1995. Employment Opportunities in Aquaculture Paper presented at the Conference on Sustainable Aquaculture held at Anna University, Madras during, April 5-6, 1995.

- Phillips, M.J, Lin, C.K and Beveridge, M.C.M., 1990. Shrimp culture and the environment-Lessons from the world's most rapidly expanded warm water aquaculture sector. Paper presented at the Bellagion conference on Environment and aquaculture in developing countries, Sep. 1990, Bellagio, Italy.

- Phillips, M. J., 1994. Aquaculture and the Environment - Striking a balance In: Aquaculture Towards the 21st Century. Proc. of Infofish- Aquatech 94 held in Colombo, Sri Lanka during 29-31 August, p 26-56

- Phillips, M. J., C. K. Lin and M.C.M Beveridge., 1993. Shrimp culture and the Environment: Lessons from the world's rapidly expanding warm water aquaculture sector. In: R.S.V. Pullin, H. Rosenthal and J.L. Maclean. (Eds) Environment and aquaculture in developing countries. ICLARM Conf. Proc. 31: p.171-197

- Pillay, T.V.R. 1992. Aquaculture and the environment. Oxford, Fishing News Books, Blackwell, 189 p.

- Primavera, J. H., 1989. The social, ecological and economic implications of intensive prawn farming. *Asian Aquaculture*, **11** (1): p.1-6.

- Pullin, R.S.V., 1989 Third World aquaculture and the environment. NAGA ICLAM Quarterly, 12 (1): p.10-13

- Raje S. G. and V. V. Singh, 1995. Fishing fleet maintenance of Versova-An example of emancipation through cooperation "Fishing Chimes" 14 (11) p. 42-44

- Sahid, M. A. and M. A. H. Pramanik., 1986. The application of remote sensing to study the relationship between the shrimp/fish farms and the mangrove ecosystem of the Bangladesh coastal region. Proc. Regional Seminar on the Application of Remote sensing techniques to Coastal Zone Management and /environmental monitoring. Bangladesh Space Research and Remote Sensing Organisation, Dhaka, Bangladesh.

- Sakthivel M., 1999. Potential of Coastal Aquaculture-Constraints, options and Development Strategies. Newsletter *Ind. Soc. of Fish Professionals*. Vol.1(2): p.4-6.

- Satapornvanit, K. 1993. Master thesis of Asian Institute of Technology, Bangkok, Thailand.

- UNDP/Norway/FAO, 1987. Thematic evaluation of Aquaculture. FAO, Rome, 85p. Plus annexes.

# 27

# From Forest to Fish – A Catchment Modification Approach for the Environmental Management in Wetland Ecosystem

*T. K. Ghosh*

Forest is an ecosystem in itself, comprising all the living and non-living components. The main living components of a forest ecosystem are plants dominated by trees, forming the consumer element and decomposers of the microorganisms. Soil, water, air and sunshine form the non-living components of the ecosystem. These components interact with each other and evolve the ecological energy cycle which consists of two other cyclic processes, namely water cycle and matter (organic and inorganic) cycle. These processes maintain the dynamic equilibrium between the living components and non-living components within the ecosystem. Forests make the climate milder and help to ensure a continuous flow of clean water. In the Himalayas, most of the streams, which feed big rivers originate from dense forests. In the south, all rivers originate from forests and when forests from catchment areas disappear, rivers get flooded during monsoon and become completely dry during the rest of the year. Besides conserving water and maintaining humidity, forests also filter surface water. Forests are also regarded as soil manufacturer. The top soil is a forest product which has been formed over centuries below forest canopy by the accumulation of organic materials from leaves, branches and stems after they decay under the influence of bacteria, fungi etc. Most tree species produce leaf fertilizer. When a forest is cut down and burned, much of the nutrient and organic content of the ecosystem is lost as gases, wind-blown ash and leached out of the soils by the heavy rains. The soil beneath may be quickly exhausted and susceptible to rapid erosion. India is losing about 6,000 million tonnes of topsoil per annum through erosion. In terms of major nutrients (NPK), the annual loss was estimated to the order of Rs. 700 crores (Bahuguna 1986).

The catchment area or drainage basin from which, *via* its feeder streams, the river gets its water has important role on river water quality. By and large, the chemical composition of water is dependent on the geology, geography and cultural development of the catchment. The atmosphere has also a role to play and the composition of water, entering a river may be changed by industrial air pollutants, drafting in from kilometers away and dissolving in rainwater falling on the catchment. While evaluating nutrients in riverine, estuarine and adjoining coastal waters of Godavari, Bay of Bengal, Padmavathi and Satyanarayana (1999) reported that $NO_3$- N, $NH_4$–N, $PO_4$–P and $SiO_4$ – Si exhibited a decreasing trend from riverine to estuarine and coastal region indicating their dominant occurrence with river water.

According to Forest Survey of India (1997), present day forest cover of India is around 76.50 M ha (23.4% of total land mass). The distribution of the various categories of forest cover as per the 1997 assessment is given in Table 27.1. During 1951-52 to 1975-76 the country has lost about 4.2 M ha of forest area. If no remidial measures are taken, according to Khoshoo (1986) the forestry stock would decrease from 13.79 $m^3$ head$^{-1}$ in 1981 to 2.66 $m^3$ head$^{-1}$ in 2001.

The result of forest destruction is alteration in the microclimate, increasing intensity and frequency of floods, drought, soil erosion, siltation in receiving water bodies and finally adverse changes in the aquatic ecosystem. Present paper deals with impact of forest on river/ reservoir ecosystem and management of forest catchment areas for better environment.

### Table 27.1 : Forest Cover in India as per 1997 Assessment

| SN | Class | Area (Km²) |
|---|---|---|
| 1 | Dense forests (Crown density 40% and above) | 367,260 |
| 2 | Open forests (Crown density 10 to <40%) | 261,310 |
| 3 | Mangrove forests | 4,827 |
| 4 | Scrub area (tree lands with <10% crown density) | 57, 211 |
| 5 | Non–forest | 2596,655 |
| | Total | 3,287,263 |

*Source*: Bahuguna 2000

## Industrialization and Forests

In view of population pressure at an alarming rate, destruction of forests is going on at an estimated rate of 11 million ha a year. These forests are in poor countries and for them timber trade is a means to earn foreign exchange. The main customers are the three industrialized zones, *viz.* Japan (53%), Europe (32%) and USA (15%) (Bahuguna 1986). The pressure of industrial raw material on India's forest is very high. As a result, India is losing about 1.5 million ha of forests annually (Sodhi 1997). The alarming increase in human population, will demand at least four times more energy than today by the year 2040. The rich bamboo forests of South India have been consumed by the paper mills. Products of paper and paper board, newsprint and plywood have been 11,50,000, 50,000 and 1,16,800 tonnes per annum respectively in last decade.

Construction of big reservoirs on various rivers during last few decades have been responsible for destruction of forest lands. Vast forest areas were submerged under these reservoirs (*Plates 27.1 & 27.2*) resulting in deposition of organic matter and release of toxic gases.

Many industrial enterprises can be located according to environmental needs, but mines and mine-product dressing plants are existed where the minerals are found. This location is often in mountainous forests where the streams are small with a low and varying water flows. Therefore, mine is often the first source of pollution along a river (Sinha *et al.* 1990, Landner 1978). Apart from coal mine drainage, coal washery effluents are also potential pollutants to the receiving aquatic ecosystem.

In general, the potential pollution problems from the effluents of mineral industry may be summarized as follows:

- Pollution of receiving waters with slime and precipitates that sterilizes the bottom-reducing or eliminating the bottom fauna
- Toxic impacts of added organic or inorganic substances – their synergistic reaction products – that disrupt the normal biological cycles and ultimately production
- Overfertilization of receiving water by excessive discharge of nutrients causing high eutrophication followed by slow premature death of water bodies
- Water rendered unfit for recreational, communal or industrial use due to presence of slime, discoloration, objectionable taste and odours, *i.e.* loss of aesthetic value.

Forests in industrialized countries, especially in Europe, are dying due to acid rains. In Federal Republic of Germany, 34 per cent of forest is damaged. The worst affected areas are the Crunewald forests near West Berlin and Baverian Allagean Alps forests, where 100 and 80 per cent trees respectively are sick. In Switzerland, Australia and East Germany the percentages of damaged trees are 8, 11 and 12 per cent respectively (Bahuguna 1986). Acid rains caused due to air pollutants like $SO_2$ and nitrogen oxide are emitted by factories and automobiles. The acidic water finally drains into receiving reservoir/ river/estuary/sea causing hazard to aquatic life including fish. The sutley river indicating high providity has been shown in plate 2.

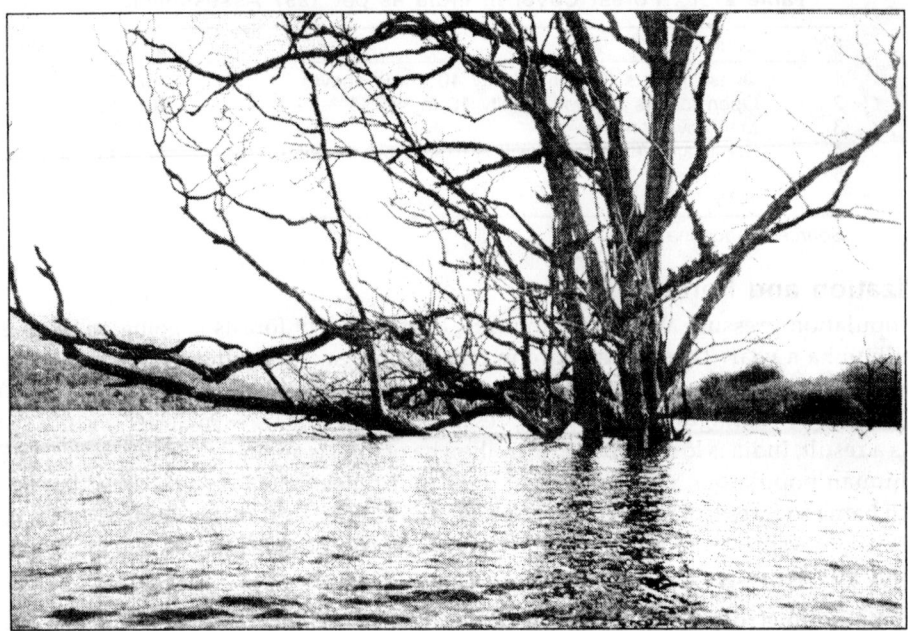

**Plate 27.1** : Submerged trees in Kadra reservoir due to construction of dam on Kali river at kadra in Utttar Kanada District of Karnataka (Photograph in July 2000)

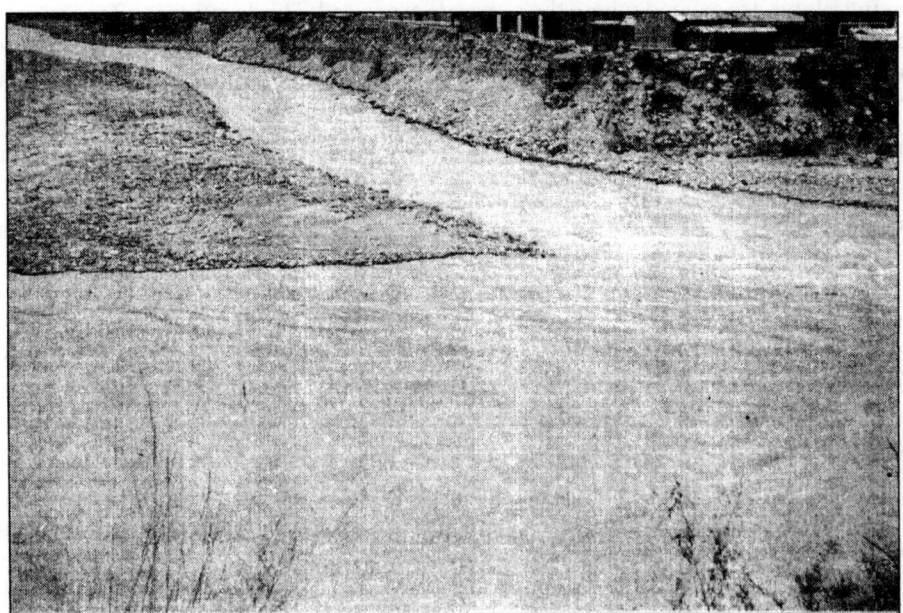

**Plate 27.2** : The Sutlej river showing high turbidity at Karcham in Kinnaur District of Himachal Pradesh receives Baspa river having comparatively clean water (Photograph in July 2000)

## Catchment Areas of Rivers in India

River basins of India can be broadly divided into three groups based on catchment areas. Besides these, there are a few desert rivers which flow for some distance and are then lost in the deserts. The flow of these rivers is uncertain. There are also completely arid areas where evaporation and rainfall are equal and there is no surface flow. River basins of 20,000 sq. km catchment area and above constitute the first group and are fourteen in number. There are three river systems to the north of Tropic of Cancer (23.5$^0$ latitude) which passes just north of Bhopal, seven systems between Tropic of Cancer and 20$^0$ latitude passing through Bhubaneshwar and four in Peninsular India. River basins with catchment area between 20,000 sq. km and 2,000 sq. km are classified as medium river basins. In this category there are forty-four rivers. Rivers with catchment area below 2,000 sq. km are called the minor rivers. These are in the coastal areas (i) on the east coast and in Kerala where the width of the land between mountains and sea is about 100 km and (ii) rest of the west coast where the rivers are much shorter as the width of the land between the sea and the mountains is less than 10 to 40 km. The reported catchment area in India is 3.05 million sq. km against the total geographical area of 3.28 million sq. km. The difference is due to areas for which statistics are not available such as remote mountains and inaccessible areas. Table 27.2 shows the details of catchment area for the four groups of river systems (Rao 1975).

**Table 27.2 : Details of catchment area for the four groups of river systems in India**

| River Basins | Catchment (million km$^2$) | Total area (%) | Run off (100 million M$^3$) | Run off (%) | Percentage of population in the basin |
|---|---|---|---|---|---|
| Group I. Major river basins | North 1.44 | 83 | 1,406 | 85 | 80 |
| | Central 0.42 | | | | |
| | South 0.72 | | | | |
| | Total : 2.58 | | | | |
| Group II Medium | 0.24 | 8 | 112 | 7 | 20 |
| Group III Minor | 0.20 | 6 | 127 | 8 | |
| Group IV Desert rivers | 0.10 | 3 | | | |
| Total | 3.12 | 100 | 1,645 | 100 | 100 |

*Source*: Rao 1975

The major river basins form 83 per cent of the total drainage area and together with the medium river basins cover practically 91 per cent of the total drainage area.

**Riverine Environment:** The characteristics of the surface runoff waters of a stream play the most important role on fisheries, since ecology determines the habitability and abundance of the flora and fauna in its different sections. Streams high in the catchment, flow turbulently and prevent much silt deposition, but benthic organisms including some caddis fly and diptera larvae filter fine organic particles from the water and some of the dissolved substances are used for growth of aquatic mosses, bryophytes or photosynthetic algae attached to the rocks. These are termed epilithic algae and they are grazed by other benthic invertebrates, *e.g.* mayfly (*Ephemeroptera*) and stonefly (*Plecoptera*) nymphs, snails etc. Carnivorous invertebrates (leeches, flatworms) and some insect larvae prey on the herbivores and detrivores, while fish is dependent on invertebrates and plant material as feed.

Organisms adapted to living suspended in water do not have time to develop significant populations in fast currents but as the moving water acquires greater volume and areas of reduced currents, there is time for build-up of distinctive plankton populations. The phytoplankton may be much denser than water and kept in suspension. The zooplankton include mostly small crustacea and rotifera. These feed on phytoplankton, either by filtration of the smaller ones or by grasping and chewing the larger ones, or, if carnivorous, on each other. Fish may feed on phytoplankton and zooplankton and in turn fish-eating fish, reptiles, birds and mammals may join the ecosystem.

## Forest Cover and Water Quality

There is a direct relationship between forest cover and water quality. From the surface which has a forest coverage, the amount of run-off will be less than that from open areas having no forest coverage. The flow of water (in terms of velocity and amount) influences the amount of soil erosion. In barren catchment areas, little rainwater soaks into the ground causing the level of groundwater depressed and poor seepage into streams (Fig. 27.1). Rivers run dry when the rain stops. Some of the impacts of catchment areas on water quality of river are summarised below: -

**Soil Erosion:** Soil erosion is a serious problem that leads to loss of fertile topsoil, siltation of reservoirs and even disaster like landslips. The primary cause for soil erosion is water moving over the surface of the ground. Severity of erosion, in turn, is determined by how much water is moving, how fast it travels and how readily the soil can be picked up and carried. Control, on the other hand, depends on how fast the surface water will soak into the soil, how effectively its speed can be slowed by obstructions, and how well the soil particles can be protected by vegetation.

Rivers in the world carry as much as three billion tons of material in solution and ten billion tons of sediment every year. Sediment content in water gives an indication of the nature of the catchment of the river. Figures based on the observations (Rao 1975) of a few years at different sites of select rivers are presented hereunder:

| | River/Site | m³ Sediment/km² of catchment/year | | River/Site | m³ Sediment/km² of catchment/year |
|---|---|---|---|---|---|
| 1. | Sutlej at Bhakra | 600 | 7. | Brahmaputra at Pandu | 508 |
| 2. | Chenab at Kanthan | 600 | 8. | Narmada at Garudeshwar | 502 |
| 3. | Chambal at Gandhi Sagar | 365 | 9. | Tapi at Ukai | 1,094 |
| 4. | Ganga at Farakka | 560 | 10. | Godavari at Polavaram | 192 |
| 5. | Kosi at Barahakshetra | 2,000 | 11. | Manjira at Nizam Sagar | 560 |
| 6. | Teesta at Anderson Bridge | 5,148 | 12. | Damodar at Panchet | 1,075 |

The sediment content in river varies from month to month. While it is negligible in the winter and summer months, it attains the maximum value in the monsoon season. The sediment load carried by some rivers is indeed very heavy. While the rivers in the Indian peninsula like the Krishna and the Godavari carry about 100 mg/l, the silt carried by the Ganga often exceeds 2,000 mg/l. In the Kosi, silt content is much larger, being 3,310 mg/l. Difference of colour in Plate 27.2 shows high silt content in Sutlej river water as compared to that of Baspa at their confluence in Karcham area, Kinnaur District in Himachal Pradesh. Some of the rivers in other countries also have high levels of silt (Table 27.3). The Mississippi (US), the Nile (several countries) and the Yellow (China) rivers carry 1,750, 1,500 and 240,000 mg/l silt respectively. Silting of reservoirs reduces their total life and carrying capacity of fisheries potential. The deposition of silt in Nizamsagar, in the course of the last 40 years, has reduced the live capacity of the reservoir from 725 million m³ to practically half. Similarly, in the Bhakra reservoir, the calculated annual sediment deposition is about 33 million tonnes a year or 600 m³ per km² of catchment. In general, soil loss in well managed forest land is low as compared to degraded forests, agricultural land and poorly managed sloping terraces (Table 27.4).

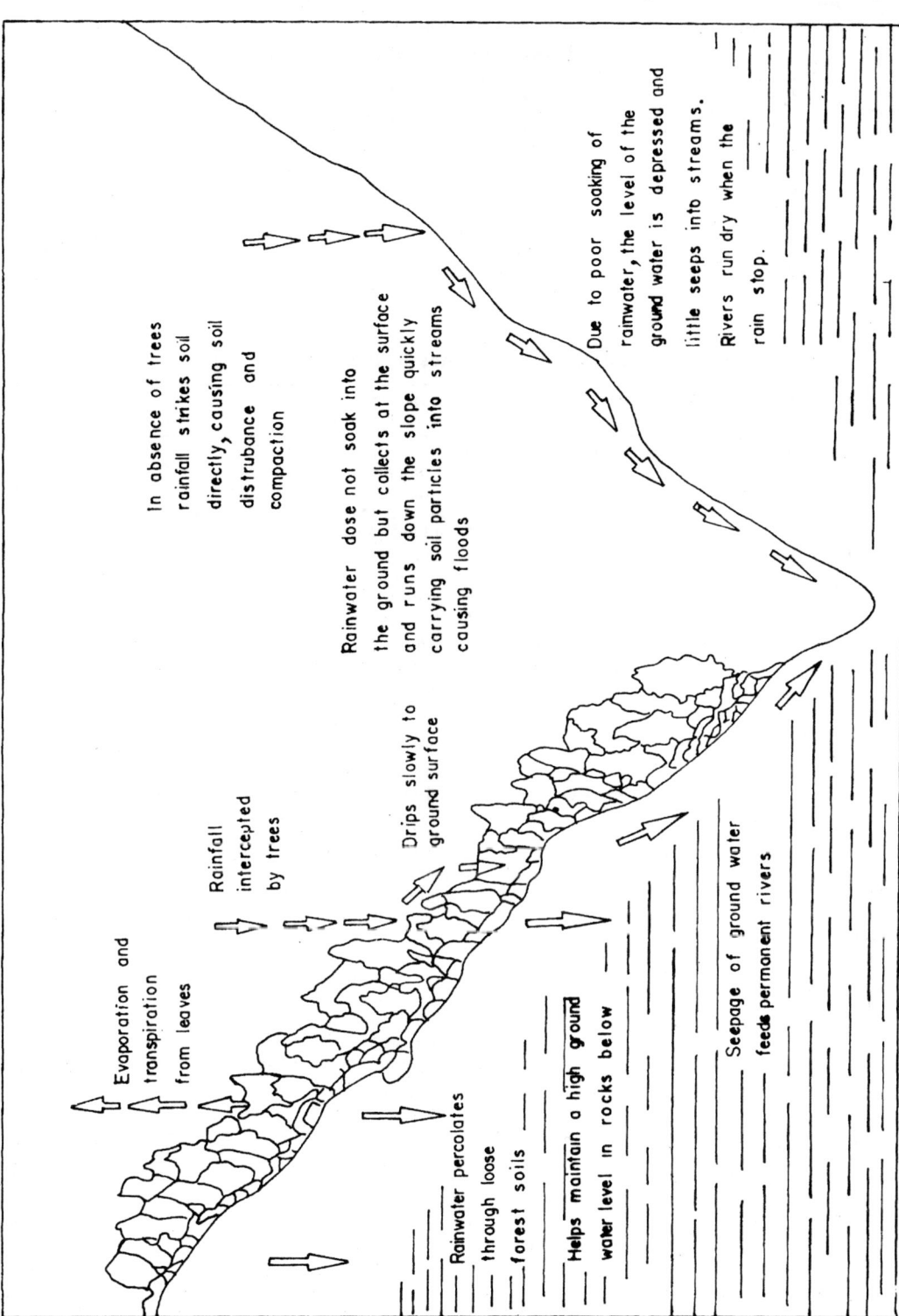

**Fig. 27.1** : Deforested slopes drain more water and more sediment quicker than forested slopes to stream / rivers

**Table 27.3 : Sediment load of selected major rivers**
**(after Brown and Wolf 1984)**

| River | Countries | Annual sediment load (million metric tones) |
|---|---|---|
| Yellow | China | 1,600 |
| Ganges | India | 1,455 |
| Amazon | Several | 363 |
| Mississippi | United States | 300 |
| Irrawaddy | Burma | 299 |
| Kosi | India | 172 |
| Mekong | Several | 170 |
| Nile | Several | 111 |

**Table 27.4 : Surface erosion rates in the Himalaya**

| Source | Estimated/ measured | Area | Type of land | Soil loss (tonnes/ha/yr) |
|---|---|---|---|---|
| Laban 1978 | Estimates | Middle mountains of Nepal | Well managed forest land | 5-10 |
| | | | Well managed rice terraces (bunded) | 5-10 |
| | | | Well managed maize terraces | 5-15 |
| | | | Poorly managed sloping terraces | 20-100 |
| | | | Degraded rangeland | 40-200 |
| Carson 1985 | Estimates | Nepal | Irrigated rice land | 0 |
| | | | Level terraces | 5 |
| | | | Sloping terraces | 20 |
| | | | Shifting cultivation | 100 |
| Carson 1985 | Estimates | Watershed in Dailekh district, Middle mountain of Nepal | Undisturbed forest | 5 |
| | | | Scrub forest, surface protected | 5 |
| | | | Degraded scrub forest | 15 |
| | | | Irrigated bench terraces, good condition | 2 |
| | | | Non-irrigated bench terraces, good condition | 7 |
| | | | Abandoned terraces (Open to grazing) | 20 |
| Mathur, et al., 1976 | Measured | Dehradun | Small forest watershed with secondary shrub growth (control) (average of 5 years) | 0.8 |
| | | | Small forest watershed | |
| | | | ♦ before deforestation (average of 2 years) | 0.4 |
| | | | ♦ year of clearfelling | 0.54 |
| | | | ♦ average of two years after plantation | 0.25 |
| Sastry and Narayana 1984 | Measured | Doon Valley | Agricultural watershed | |
| | | | – before treatment (average of 8 years) | 2.4 |
| | | | – after treatment (average of 9 years) | 0.2 |
| | | | Forest watershed covered with sal trees but open to grazing | |
| | | | – before treatment (average of 4 years) | 4.7 |
| | | | – after treatment (construction of brushwood check dams) (average of 5 years) | 2.8 |
| Das et al., 1981 | Measured (sediment production rate of catchment result of both surface erosion and mass wasting) (Figures given in cum/ha/yr and converted using soil density of 1.4 t/cum) | Western Himalaya | Sutlej (Bhakra) | 14.47 |
| | | | – before soil conservation programme (1962) | |
| | | | – after soil conservation programme | |
| | | | (1966) | 9.13 |
| | | | (1968) | 8.85 |
| | | | (1972) | 8.51 |
| | | | (1976) | 8.39 |

*Contd....*

| Source | Estimated/ measured | Area | Type of land | Soil loss (tonnes/ha/yr) | |
|---|---|---|---|---|---|
| | | Eastern Himalaya | Tessta | 137.48 | |
| | | | Gumti (Tripura) (1973) | 4.98 | |
| | | | Pagladiya (at Nalbari) | 43.96 | |
| Singh et al. 1983 | Measured | Southwestern part of central Himalaya | Forested sites | | |
| | | | Mixed oak-pine forest | 0.032 | |
| | | | Pine forest | 0.025 | |
| | | | Oak forest (average of six sites) | 0.023 | |
| | | | Non forested sites | 0.056 | |
| | | | Damaged by landslides 6-40 years ago (average of four sites) | | |
| | | | corresponds to Cropland (maize) | 0.064 | |
| Narayana and Ram Babu 1983 | Estimates | Entire Himalaya | North Himalaya forest region | Nil – 2.87 | |
| | | | Northeastern Himalaya, Alpine grass and meadow region | Nil – 0.50 2.87 | |
| | | | Northeastern forest region (including Meghalaya, Nagaland etc.) | Nil – 40.95 | |
| | | | | Average 1974–76 | Average 1986–87 |
| CSWCRTI 1986, 1987 | Measured | Microwatersheds (0.8 ha to 4.5 ha) near Chandigarh, protection provided in 1978 | Annually burnt watershed changes to mixed forest | 28 | 0.004 |
| | | | Watershed with afforestation and contour trenches changes to mixed forest | 1 | 0.0035 |
| | | | Watershed with cutting of trees and shrubs and overgrazing changes to mixed forest | 97 | 0.0035 |
| | | | Overgrazed watershed changes to one with a bhabhar grass cover | 35 | 0.025 |
| | | | Control watershed | 2 | 0.016 |

**Enrichment of Chemical:** Rain and any other form of precipitation is not pure water. It contains significant quantities of dissolved gases ($O_2$, $N_2$, $CO_2$), cations ($H^+$, $Na^+$, $K^+$, $Ca^+$, $Mg^{2+}$ etc.), anions ($SO_4^{2-}$, $Cl^-$, $NO_3^-$, $PO_4^{3-}$ etc.), cation trace elements ($Cu^{2+}$, $Mn^{2+}$, $Fe^{3+}$ etc), organic compounds and both organic and inorganic particles. The rain picks up some of these from tiny droplets of sea spray carried upward into the atmosphere by wind, some from dust blown from the land and others from atmospheric gases in it by lightning.

The concentrations of commonly analysed substances are generally low in rainwater, but as the water percolates through or runs off a catchment, it changes chemically through leaching of substances from soil and rocks. The harder the rock, the less the chemical modification, but on softer rocks with deep soils and consequent cultivation there are greater changes (Table 27.5). Significant increase of ions in stream water over rainfall water due to disturbance of forest area has been demonstrated in Table 27.6.

The spoils excavated during coal mining contain appreciable quantities of iron pyrites which, under the influence of abundant water and physical and chemical weathering, release large quantities of both iron and aluminium. Release of heavy metals through different mining ctivities and their contamination in riverine system through leaching can not be ignored.

**Table 27.5 : Rates of removal of substance in mg m⁻² yr⁻¹ from different sorts of catchment area**

|  | Phosphorus | Nitrogen |
|---|---|---|
| Forest (USA) | 8.3 | 440 |
| Mostly agricultural (USA) | 22.7 | 630 |
| Entirely agricultural (USA) | 30.8 | 982 |
| Tundra, Surden | 4.1 | 97 |
| Tropical forest | 10.0 | 470 |
| Lowland agriculture, Norfolk, UK | 13.0 | * |
| Forest on igneous rock | 4.7 | * |
| Forest on sedimentary rock | 11.4 | * |
| Forest plus pasture on igneous rock | 10.2 | * |
| Forest plus pasture on sedimentary rock | 23.2 | * |

*: Values not reported
*Source*: Likens *et al.*, 1977, Omernik 1976

**Table 27.6 : The effect of catchment area on some aspects of drainage water chemistry (Values are in mg/l except pH)**

| Ions | Undistrubed forest on igneous rock, New Hamshire, USA (Likens et al. 1977) | | Lowland chalk and glacial drift, agricultural Norfolk, U.K. (Moss 1980) | |
|---|---|---|---|---|
|  | Rainfall | Stream | Rainfall | Stream |
| Na⁺ | 0.12 | 0.87 | 1.2 | 32.5 |
| K⁺ | 0.07 | 0.23 | 0.74 | 3.1 |
| Mg²⁺ | 0.04 | 0.38 | 0.21 | 6.9 |
| Ca²⁺ | 0.16 | 1.65 | 3.7 | 100.0 |
| Cl⁻ | 0.47 | 0.55 | < 1.0 | 47.0 |
| HCO₃⁻ | 0.006 | 0.92 | 0.0 | 288.0 |
| pH | 4.14 | 4.92 | 3.5 | 7.7 |

Particles are added to the water as it drains through the catchment. There may be inorganic clay, silt or sand particles or they may be organic. These will include fine remains of the decomposition of organic matter in soil and also large and small pieces of barely degraded plant litter washed into the stream.

**Migration of Nutrients:** Phosphorus is, on an average, the scarcest element in the earth's crust of those required absolutely for algal and higher plant growth. It is also relatively insoluble, being readily precipitated as complexes of iron, aluminium, calcium and other relatively abundant metals in rocks and soils. Table 27.7 shows the ratios of amounts of various other necessary elements to the amounts of phosphorus required for algal and plant growth. It also shows the ratio in the soils and rocks which make up the lithospheric supply of these elements. The third column gives the ratio of the first two column (lithosphere: plants) and indicates the relative supply to the relative need. Ratios greater than 1 in third column indicate that the need is more likely to be met by the supply than it is in the case of phosphorus, and all of the elements supplied from the lithosphere that plants require are in this category. Certain elements like sulphate, chloride, borate, nitrogen and carbon which are needed by plants and have vast supply in the environment have not been included in the table.

The loading of a substance carried in water from the land draining into a water body depends on two things, viz. the size of the catchment in relation to the area of the waterbody, and the rate of removal of the substance per unit area of catchment. Sedimentary rocks have greater removal rates than igneous rocks, and agricultural areas have greater rates than undisturbed ecosystems. Surveys in the USA show that perhaps only 40 per cent of the total phosphorus carried by streams is in unavailable form, the rest rapidly becoming locked into the sediments of the rivers and lakes. The loading rate

**Table 27.7 : The relative supply and demand of elements required by plants and algae and derived from soils and rocks (lithosphere) of the catchment area (modified from Hutchinson 1973)**

| Elements | Ratio of amount of element to that of phosphorus in the lithosphere (1) | Ratio of amount required of element to amount required of phosphorus in plants and algae (2) | Ratio of (1) to (2 |
|---|---|---|---|
| Na | 32.5 | 0.52 | 43.0 |
| Mg | 22.2 | 1.39 | 16.0 |
| Si | 268.1 | 0.65 | 410.0 |
| P | 1.0 | 1.0 | 1.0 |
| K | 19.9 | 6.1 | 3.3 |
| Ca | 39.5 | 7.8 | 5.1 |
| Mn | 0.90 | 0.27 | 5.3 |
| Fe | 53.6 | 0.06 | 880.0 |
| Co | 0.02 | 0.0002 | 110.0 |
| Cu | 0.05 | 0.006 | 8.5 |
| Zn | 0.07 | 0.04 | 1.5 |
| Mo | 0.0014 | 0.0004 | 3.6 |

of phosphorus and nitrogen on a waterbody may be independent of the catchment area as such under certain conditions. These are due to discharge of excreta, directly or indirectly, to a watercourse by groups of men and domestic or wild animals.

**Pollutants from Plants:** Continuous losses of branches, flowers and pollens from catchment areas are common in many streams. Substances transported to water bodies and producing allelopathic effects on aquatic lives are commonly liberated by three following general routes:

*Weathering:* Leaves and plant parts falling to the ground may be decomposed by weathering and soil micro-organisms. Certain micro-organisms may change non-toxic compounds to toxic ones, as in the case of amygdalin in peach residues or phlorizin in apple residues (Datta and Chatterjee 1979).

*Leaching:* Water soluble inhibitors leach out of plant residues after death when the various membranes usually lose their differential permeability, thereby adding soil pollutants. Leachates of bark of *Aesculus hippocastanum* and *Malus* sp., top residues of *Avena fatua*, wheat straw etc. are rich in phytotoxins.

*Exudation:* Toxins, exuded from roots of crop and non-crop plants pollute the soil medium. The crop plants include corn, cowpea, oat, wheat etc. The non-crop plants include *Calluna vulgaris*, *Digitaria sanguinalis*, *Pinus elliottii* etc.

## Impact of Catchment on Aquatic Lives: Select Case Studies

At low and high levels, major ions may determine the nature of the biota in an aquatic ecosystem. Directly or indirectly, aquatic organisms are affected by incoming pollutants of catchment areas in different ways as summarized below:

- increase in osmotic pressure
- mechanical injury or blocking of gills from silt or other suspended materials
- alteration of pH
- toxic ingredients
- destruction of biota - fish is indirectly affected when its habitual food organisms are destroyed
- destruction of spawning ground.

Most wetland ecosystem are in varying stages of degradation. In general, water bodies are at the receiving end of the fallout of upland deforestation. In the absence of active root systems in the river catchments, rainwater — instead of percolating downwards, washes fertile topsoil away and deposits it as silt into dams and riverbeds reduced water carrying capacity of the wetlands. Select site specific impacts are summarized hereunder.

**Laktak catchment:** Situated 38 km south of Imphal in Manipur, Laktak is the largest freshwater lake in the North-East. The lake covers an area of 286 km² at an elevation of 768.5 m. A number of streams and rivers drain into the lake. Of the total catchment of 980 km², 430 km² is under paddy cultivation, 150 km² under habitation and 400 km² under unclassed forests to the west and NW of the lake.

The lake is threatened by excessive silting and inflow of nutrients from various anthropogenic sources which has been reflected through higher levels of BOD (Singsit and Karnatak 1999). Deforestation and shifting cultivation, uncontrolled use of fertilizers on agricultural lands and discharge of domestic waste combinely contribute silt, nutrients and biogenic salts to the lake. This turns collectively into a recipe for eutrophication of the lake which may lead eventually to massive mortality among fish from oxygen deficiency owing to excessive growth of floating weeds and algae.

**Kashmir Wetlands:** Situated in the northern part of India within the western Himalayan region, Kashmir has a number of freshwater wetlands. These wetlands exhibit a great diversity primarily owing to variations in their origin, latitudinal situation and the nature of the biota they contain. Basically, all are high altitude lakes (1,500-4,000m above sea level) compared to those situated in the plains of India.

The total forest cover in the State is 20,182 sq. km., which is about 9.98 per cent of its geographic area. A comprehensive assessment made between 1987 and 1989 indicates a decrease of 2.1 per cent in the forest cover (450 sq. km.). Extensive deforestation, overgrazing, unsustainable agricultural practices, especially on sloping lands and the overexploitation of biomass for fuel, fodder and timber purposes, have, over the years stripped the land of its natural vegetation cover resulting in soil erosion. It has been estimated that about 36,200 cu. m. of silt is annually deposited in the Dal lake. The data on the silt load between 1970 and 1980 indicates that on an average, 3,331 acre feet of silt is deposited annually in the Wular Lake. These values, however, appear to be on the lowest side as data from all the tributaries has not been taken into consideration. The open water surface area of the Wular lake has reduced from an original 202 sq. km. to the present 24 sq. km. (Trisal 1998). The present open area of about 12 sq km. of the Dal lake is but a vestige of what it was even in the 18th century. The Anchar lake, another urban lake in Srinagar, is on the verge of extinction due to the combined effects of siltation and urbanization.

**Catchment of the Rio Negro:** The Rio Negro is a large acidic black-water river which drains predominantly undisturbed lowland tropical forest in the North Western portion of the Amazon river basin. Its characteristic black colour and acidity are due to low concentrations of suspended solids and high concentrations of dissolved organic acids derived from extensive areas of podzol soils in the upstream portion of the basin (Forsberg et al. 1988, Klinge 1967). A small placer gold-mining operation developed in the upper Rio Negro near Santa Isabel do Rio Negro in the beginning of 1993.

The exceptionally high levels of mercury contamination encountered in the upper Rio Negro reflect a high input of mercury to this river system and/ or high rates of bioaccumulation through its aquatic food chain. Chemical weathering in the river's drainage basin is the most likely source of mercury inputs. The tertiary ferralitic soils which cover most of the lowland Amazon (Lucas et al. 1996) are exceptionally rich in mercury. Roulet et al. (1996) encountered mercury concentrations up to 200 ng g$^{-1}$ in isolated ferralitic soils of the Tapojos basin, a value several times higher than those commonly found in temperate soils. Mercury concentrations as high as 4.2 ppm have been reported in common food fish collected from the river (Malm et al. 1995).

**Galloway, SW Scotland:** A detailed investigation towards relationships between high flow water chemistry and conifer forest cover in 94 streams over an area of about 2000 km² in Galloway, south west Scotland, was carried out by Puhr et al. (2000). Of the 94 stream sites, 29 were classified as granitic catchments, 51 ordovician catchments and 14 silurian catchments. The results indicated that over the entire region pH levels were lower with increasing catchment afforestation whilst aluminum concentrations were higher. Concentrations of sulphate were also higher with increasing afforestation, which suggested that conifers play a primary role in increasing the acidity levels of streams by exacerbating aerial acid deposition in the entire region. Areal acid deposition in Galloway is relatively high, particularly when wealth systems travel from a south-easterly direction and have thereby crossed the heavily industrialized areas of the United Kingdom and other parts of Europe (Fowler *et al.* 1982). Most scientists now agree that conifer plantations enhance levels of dry and occult acid deposition (Harriman *et al.* 1987, Hughes *et al.* 1994, Rees and Ribbens 1995) causing low pH of water of the streams nearby.

**Murray Darling Basin, Australia:** The Australian National Eutrophication Management Programme (NEMP) has published a statement representing the agreed scientific consensus on sources and the transport of phosphorus to inland surface waters. The aim was to provide managers with generally accepted guidelines for identifying the action priorities. This statement was the conclusion of a joint workshop convened by NEMP and Environment Australia - The scientists at the workshop concluded that although phosphorus is a natural element in water and is essential for animals and plant life, levels currently reaching many rivers are too high. Overall, diffused sources of phosphorus are the dominant component in most Australian catchments.

Most phosphorus in Australian catchment derives from soil erosion, in particular caused by water. Transport of phosphorus from diffuse landscape sources can occur in both dissolved and particulate forms. Storms are the cause of most of the transport of phosphorus from land to rivers, when land is eroded from hill slopes, from the beds and blanks of gullies and streams. Heavily grazed lands, irrigated areas, intensive livestock farms and the horticultural areas are particularly at risk. An example of eutrophication in Australia refers to the Murray Darling Basin. In the Murray Darling Basin the gullies are widespread. The P associated with soil particles in these gullies is generally from natural sources and not from fertilizer use. Although much of the soil erosion which caused the gully formation occurred several decades ago, active gullies continue to input phosphorus to rivers. In the river systems such as the Murray Darling Basin, most of the diffuse-source phosphorus input comes from gully erosion and stream bank collapse of readily dispersible soils. It is very likely that most of the phosphorus is "native" phosphorus coming from subsoils as a result of weathering of naturally occurring phosphorus containing rocks (Anonymous 1999).

## Catchment Management to Protect Wetland

In order to check massive environment degradation in terms of floods, soil loss, landslides, lives, property etc. call for following steps towards rational management of forest ecosystem is urgently needed. Natural environment is composed of climatic conditions, soil and water status, vegetational conditions, land characteristics etc. All these singularly or collectively affect the nature, growth, prosperity etc. related to forest ecosystem.

**Management of Soil Environment:** The principal soil management is to check the heavy loss of soil and its transportation. Control of rapid soil runoff can be exercised through the following measures:

(a) **Identification of Critical Area:** It is true that all parts of the catchment do not erode equally. Hence to plan a soil conservation management, the foremost task is to identify the critical areas of the catchment, which are prone to soil erosion.

(b) **Terracing:** The practice of terracing of land requires some knowledge of surface gradient, nature of parent rock and intensity of rainfall. The regions of steep slope with high intensity of rainfall require inward terracing instead of outward or flat terracing.

(c) **Gully Checking:** Since increasing gully action leads to tremendous increase of soil erosion, it is advisable to plant fast growing native herbs and shrubs to check expansion of gullies.

(d) **Check Dams:** Soil erosion can be reduced considerably by constructing check dams at suitable sites and elevations. The number and size of check dams depend on water catchment area. Dams are to be constructed in a series of successive height intervals rather than in isolation.

(e) **Soil Moisture and Water Management:** Water loss through evaporation is reduced considerably due to canopy of tree leaves, grasses, seedlings, herbs alongwith dense litter of leaves and twigs. In general, natural forest posses high leaf litters. The estimated annual leaf litters in Nilgiris were 1650, 1240, 1791 and 3055 kgha$^{-1}$ in bluegum, black wattle, bluegum and black wattle mixture and shoal (natural forest) respectively (Chinnamani 1987). In catchments, vegetation plays the duel role in tropical condition, such as:

● Reduction of surface runoff
● Increase of infiltration

Infiltration rates of select forests are referred in Table 27.8. It is evidenced that through afforestation

**Table 27.8 : Infiltration rate (cm hr$^{-1}$) under different plant covers in hills**

| Plant covers | Study 1 | Study 2 |
|---|---|---|
| Shola (natural forest) | 16.8 | 12.5 |
| Bluegum Plantation (*Eucalyptus globulus*) | 20.7 | 11.3 |
| Grazed natural grassland | 5.1 | 6.3 |
| Broom – Shrub | 11.3 | – |

*Source:* Chinnamani 1987

programme, soil moisture of a given area can be maintained or even be enhanced. Besides increasing the capacity of the soil as water reservoir, humus also imporves drainage and contributes balanced nutrients for plants, leading to overall increase in biological productivity of cropland.

## Management of Slope Failures

In many cases the failure of slope is due to destruction of vegetation. Management of slope failure is necessary because of 2 reasons. Firstly, the places where slope failures occur, vegetations are lost. Secondly, downward movement of loosened materials damage downslope vegetations. Such failures can be checked by controlling haphazard construction of road networks and by planting vegetation in affected areas. The construction should be avoided on steep slopes.

## Control of Wild Fire and Grazing

Fires burn off the protective vegetation and destroy the water-holding capacity of the humus mantle. Increased erosion and runoff generally follow. Heavy grazing reduces plant density. Palatable grasses and shrub lose their vigor by continual close cropping. As a result productivity drops, tops and roots die back and valuable litter dwindles. Proper care should be taken on overgrazing and wild fire.

## Woodland and Revegetation

For a consistent use of a waterbody for human, animal, crops and fishes, it is necessary that its catchment area is ideally vegetated by species that are native of that catchment. River and stream bank plantings act as strong vegetative barriers against bank erosion.

In order to meet the shortages of wood one can have 2 major objectives of forestry:

● Affording long-term ecological security, and
● Supply of goods and services to the people and industry through well plan of production.

To achieve these objectives 3 broad types of forestry, namely conservation, production and social ,orestry need to be practiced.

Conservation forestry will cover natural vegetation in watersheds and fragile ecological areas and biosphere reserves, national parks etc. where no commercial exploitation is allowed. Production forestry aims at meeting the raw material demands of all forest-based industry. The third type of forestry is social forestry or agroforestry. By and large, social forestry appears to have good prospects in the catchment areas where villagers occupy. Villagers should be encouraged to plant more trees in village surrounds, on roadsides, river banks, school and office compounds etc. Some areas should be grown with firewood species and some small timber and bamboos. Infact, depending upon the situation one can mix 3 basic elements, *e.g.* agriculture, forestry and animal husbandry. Some of the important agroforestry system that can be profitably adopted are as follows:

- Silviculture, *e.g.* energy plantation of casuarina, subabul etc.
- Agri-silvicultural, *e.g.* growing of crops with trees on boundary or intermixed, *e.g.* khejri with bajra, subabul, casuarina, tad palm on boundary with agricultural crop in the centre
- Silvipastural: growing trees with grasses, livestock or both, *e.g.* khejri+grass, subabul + grass, babul + grass etc.
- Silvi horticultural: here fruit yielding trees are combined with fuel as wood yielding trees, *e.g.* casuarina + sapota, jackfruit + teak, subabul + ber etc.
- Agri-silvi-pastured: here tree, crops, grasses are grown together as intermixture, e.g. tree + grass + crop
- Agri-Silvi-horticultural: this is a combination of wood as fuel or timber yielding trees + fruit yielding tree + crop
- Multistorey: here several tiers of crops are grown under one piece of land, *e.g.* coconut + ragi + pepper + cocoa in humid tropics

## Publicity, Community Participation and Involvement of Panchayats

The catchment treatment work as a whole and afforestation programme in particular should be given adequate publicity through various media, so that public awareness is aroused in favour of protection of forests and plantations and sound land management in the catchment. The panchayats could play an important role not only in protecting the forestry assets, but also in planning, planting and distribution of forest produce.

## REFERENCES

- Anonymas (1999). Scope Newsletter, No. 33, CEEP
- Bahuguna, S. (1986). Deforestation and its impact, p. 167-173 *in* B. P. Radhakrishna and K. K. Ramachandran *ed.* India's environment: Problems and perspectives. Proc. of the Seminar at Trivandrum, Nov. 26-28, 1984, Geological Soc. India, Bangalore
- Bahuguna, V. K. (2000). Forests in the economy of the rural poor: an estimation of the dependency level. *Ambio.* **29** (3): 126-129
- Brown, L. R. and Wolf, E. C. (1984). Soil erosion: Quiet crisis in the world economy. Worldwatch paper 60
- Carson Brian (1985). Erosion and sedimentation processes in the Nepalese Himalaya, ICIMOD Occasional Paper No. 1, ICIMOD, Kathmandu
- Chinnamani, S. (1987). Improper landuse in western and eastern ghats and its impact on environment, Proc. Nat. Conf. Env. Impact on Biosystem. Loyala College, Madras

- CSWCRTI (1986), Soil Conservation: Annual Report 1986, Central Soil and Water Conservation Research and Training Institute, Dehra dun

- CSWCRTI (1987), Soil and Water Conservation: Annual Report 1987, Central Soil and Water Conservation Research and Training Institute, Dehra dun

- Das, D. C., Bali, Y. P. and Kaul, P. C. (1981). Soil conservation multipurpose river valley catchments: Problems, programme approach and effectiveness, *Indian Journal of Soil Conservation*, Vol. 9, No. 1

- Datta, S. C. and Chatterjee, A. K. (1979). Pollution by plant. P. 195-214 *in* S.P. Raychaudhuri and D. S. Gupta ed. Environ. Pollut. and Toxicol. Today and Tomorrow's Printers and Publishers, New Delhi

- Forest Survey of India (1997) State of forest report, FSI, Govt. of India, Dehradun, pp. 1-72

- Forsberg, B. R., Devol, A. H., Richey, J. E., Martinelli, L. A. and dos Sanos, H. (1988) Factors controlling nutrient concentration in Amazon floodplain lakes. *Limnol. Oceanogr.* 33: 41-56

- Fowler, D., Cape, J. N., Leith, I. D., Paterson, I. S., Kinnaird, J. W. and Nicholson, I. A. (1982). Rainfall acidity in northern Britain. *Nature* 297: 383 - 386

- Harriman, R., Morrison, B. R. S., Caines, L. A., Collen, P. and Watt, A.W. (1987). Long-term changes in fish population of acid stream and locks in galloway south west Scotland. *Water, Air and Soil Pollut.*, 32: 89 - 112

- Hughes, S., Norris, D.A., Steveres, P. A. , Reynolds, B. and Williams, T. G. (1994) Effects of forest age on surface drainage water and soil solution aluminum chemistry in Stagnopodzols in Wales. *Water, Air and Soil Pollut.* 77: 115 - 139

- Hutchinson, G. E. (1973). Eutrophication. *Amer. Sci.* 61; 269-279

- Khoshoo, T. N. (1986). Environmental priorities in India and sustainable development. Presidential address, Indian Sci. Cong. Assoc. New Delhi

- Klinge, H. (1967). Podzol soils: A source of blackwater in Amazonia. Atal do Simposio sobre a Bota Amazonica 3 (Limnologia), 117-125

- Laban P. (1978,). Field measurements on erosion and sedimentation in Nepal, department of soil conservation and watershed management, FAO/UNDP. IWM/SP/05

- Landner, L. (1978). Wastes from extraction and refining ores, p. 192-204. FAO/SIDA workshop on aquatic pollution in relation to protection of living resources. Manila, Philippines, Jan. 17-Feb. 27, 1977

- Likens, G. E., Bormann, F. H., Pierce, R. S., Eaton, J. S. and Johnson, N. M. (1977). Biogeochemistry of a forested ecosystem. Springer-Verlag, New York

- Lucas, R., Nahon, D., Cornu, S. and Eyrolle, F. (1996). Genese et fonctionnement des sols en milien equatorial. *Compt. Rend. Acad. Sci., Paris* 322 (11a) 1-16

- Malm, O., Castro, M.B., Branches, F. J. P., Zuffo, C. E., Padovani, C., Viana, J. P., Akagi, H., Bastos, W. R., Silviera, E. G., Guimaraes, J. R. D. and Pfeiffer, W. C. (1995). Fish and human hair as bio-indicators of Hg contamination on Tapajos, Madeira and Negro river basins, Amazon, Brazil, pp. 25-32 In: Proc. Int. Workshop Environ. Mercury Pollut. Health Effects Amazon River Basin. Kato, H. and Pfeiffer, W. C. (eds) National Institute for Minamata Disease, Minamata, Japan,

- Mathur, H. N., Ram Babu, Joshie, P. and Singh, Bakshish (1976). Effect of clearfelling and reforestation on runoff and peak rates in small watershed, Indian Forester, Dehra dun

- Moss, B. (1980). Ecology of freshwaters, Blackwell Scientific Publications, London

- Narayana, V. V. Dhruva and Ram Babu (1983). Estimation of soil erosion in India, Journal of Irrigation and Drainage Engineering, Vol. 109, No. 4,

- Omernik, J. (1976). The influence of land use on stream nutrient levels - U. S. Environ. Protec. Agency Report EPA - 600/3 -76- 014; 1-105

- Padmavathi, D and Satyanarayana D. (1999). Distribution of nutrients and major elements in riverine, estuarine and adjoining coastal waters of Godavari, Bay of Bengal. *Indian J. Mar. Sc.* **28** (4): 345-354

- Puhr, C. B., Donoghur, D. N. M., Stephen, A. B., Tervet, D. J. and Suiclair, C. (2000). Regional patterns of stream water acidity and catchment afforestation in Galloway, SW Scotland. *Water, Air and Soil Pollut.* **120** (1-2): 47-70

- Rao, K. L. (1975). India's water wealth: its assessment, uses and projections, Orient Longman, N. Delhi

- Rees, R. M. and Ribbem, J. C. H. (1995). Relationships between afforestation, water chemistry and fish stocks in an upland catchment in South- west Scotland. *Water, Air and Soil Pollut.* **85**: 303 - 308

- Roulet, M., Lucotte, M., Rheault, I., Tran, S., Farella, N., Canuel, R., Mergler, D. and Amorim, M. (1996). Mercury in Amazonian soils: Accumulation and release. In: Proc. 4th Int. symp. Geochem. Earth's surface, Bottrell, S. H. (ed) Ilkely, England pp 453-457

- Sastry, G. and Narayana ,V. V. Dhruva (1984). Watershed responses to conservation measures, Journal of Irrigation and Drainage Engineering, Vol. 110, No. 1, March Singsit, S. and Karnatak, D. C. (1999) Laktak lake and the syndrome of ecological disaster. Himalayan Paryavaran Vol. 6: 6-9

- Singh, J. S., Pandey, A. N. and Pathak, P. C. (1983). A hypothesis to account for the major pathway of soil loss from Himalaya, Environment Conservation, Switzerland, Vol. 10, No. 4

- Sinha, M. P., M. K. Singh, S.N. Singh and M. M. P. Singh (1990). Some problems of pisciculture in particular reference to coal industry effluents, p. 121-142 *in* R. K. Trivedi and M. P. Sinha (ed) Impact of mining on environment, Ashish Publishing House, N. Delhi.

- Sodhi, S. S. (1997). Significance of forests in ecosystem: adopt a tree. *Employment News* **22** (11): 1-3

- Trisal, C.L. (1998). Kashmir: fast disappearing p: 95-99, The Hindu Survey of the Environment, India

# 28

# Role of Vermitechnology in Pollution Abatement

*G. Tripathi, S. S. Suthar and B. M. Sharma*

The living planet earth is rich in earthworm resources. These important and interesting biological resources inhabit different ecological conditions on the globe and remain active day and night in upper layer of soil. Earthworm aerate and mix soil and enrich the exhausted soil with their mucus and excreta. They modify physics, chemistry and biology of soil and provide a suitable environment for growth and development of useful organisms in soil to combat pests and Pethogens. Thus the presence of earthworm in soil reduce the requirement of fertilizers and pesticides. Earthworms decontaminate soil from effects of pollutants and toxicants. They are the food source for various animals and have also got medicinal importance in old and new literature. These unparalleled properties of earthworms define them as valuable biological resources for benefits of human being in the present millennium. Potential application of earthworms have led the development of vermitechnology or vermicultural biotechnology (VBT) in different parts of the world for management of agricultural, industrial waste and sewage wastes. Application of earthworms in detoxification and their biomass production for protein source are the attractive aspects of vermitech. Some eathworms bioindustries has come up in developed countries for socio-economic upliftment. Further research in the area of vermicology will potentiate the regional economy all over the world. Popularization of ecologically sound, economically viable and socially acceptable vermitechnology will be very useful for developing countries.

## Introduction

Every creature of nature from microscopic bacteria and viruses to giant metazoan plays an important role in sustainable development of our natural resources and ecosystem. Earthworm is one of these which have a major role in ground soil ecosystem. They are the friend of farmers and have been known since the time of Aristotle (384-322 B.C) and Darwin (1881). Darwin in his famous book 'The Formation of Vegetable Mould through the Action of Worms, with Observation of their Habits'; decribed the litter consuming efficiency of earthworms and referred them as nature's ploughman. Aristotle called earthworm 'the intestine of earth'. As name 'earthworm' indicates, it dwells below the surface of eath in tunnels and galleries. It has a great importance in delaing with physics, chemistry and biology of soil. It makes soil porous and nutrient rich by adding excreta which contains calcium, magnesium, nitrogenous compunds, phosphorous, mucus etc. The importance of earthworm is being globally recognised in the areas of vermicomposting, detoxification, pollution monitoring, animal food production. and land reclamation.

Vermicomposting of solid waste deals with the management of industrual and agricultural waste, cattle yard produce , municipal garbage, municipal sewage and kitchen waste and its utilization as a bilogical tool for mankind is invariably known as vermitechnology, vermitech or vermiculture biotechnology (VBT). Detoxication is concerned with the accumulation of certain heavy metals, toxic substances and residues of pesticides in the body of earthworms. Due to having high concentration of protein and certain essential amino acids like lysine, vitamins etc. earthworm may act as an important food source for poultry, rats and pigs. Earthworms sub terrestrial habitat Effects the soil particle breakdown, soil aggregation, turnover, moisture, porosity, aeration, microbiology and energy budget. Thus they help in improvement and reclamation of land. Medicinal importance of eathworms has also been reported because they have certain pharmacologically active materials like antipyretic (Hori *et al.*, 1974). In Unani system of medicine earthworms may be applied in dry form to cure hernia, creomic boils, piles, wounds, respiratory aliment, jaundice and rheumatic pains etc. (Jairapuri, 1993). The use of earthworms as bioindicator can be helpful for evaluating the effects of agriculture practices, acidic rain, pollution etc. They may act as a bioindicator for tree growth (Ghilarov., 1978; Bouche, 1981; Paoletti *et al.*, 1991). Earthworm biomass is a outable indicator for detecting trends in soil pH, soil humidity and humus quality. It is possible to couple earthworm distribution as site indicators for wood production and forest development practices (Muys and Granval, 1997).

The unsafe and rapid use of our natural resources for fulfilment of everexpanding demand of human population has caused cartain unmendable losses. It has questioned the existence of biodiversity on this living planet. Unsolved problem of waste production and pollution is gradually imbalancing our biosphere. Almost all existing technologies for waste treatment and disposal are costly. Earthworms have tremendous power to regulate various types of organic wastes. Therefore, at this crucial juncture, the popularization of vermiculture biotechnology (VBT) or vermitech becomes important for abatement of pollution.

## Vermitechnology

Vermicomposting refers to the production of energy and nutrient rich excreta of worms. Manipulation of bilogical potential of earthworms in waste management and biofertilizer production is the vermitechnology. It opens a new dimension in the area of biotechnology for sustainable development of low cost technologies and referred to as vermiculture biotechnology (VBT). The role of earthworm in decomposition processes has been demonstrated by several workers (Edward and Lofty, 1977; Senapati and Dash 1984; Lee, 1985; Reinecke *et al.*, 1992; Vincellas-Akpa and Loquet, 1997; Singh, 1997; Tripathi and Singh, 2000). Earthworm increases the nutrient concentration of soil and soil fertility when introduced to a new soil by adding their castes and excreta. Some organic and inorganic compounds can not be directly used by plants. Earthworm break down these compounds for easy availability to plants. They may consume all kinds of organic wastes equal to their body mass per day in soil (Fig.28.1).

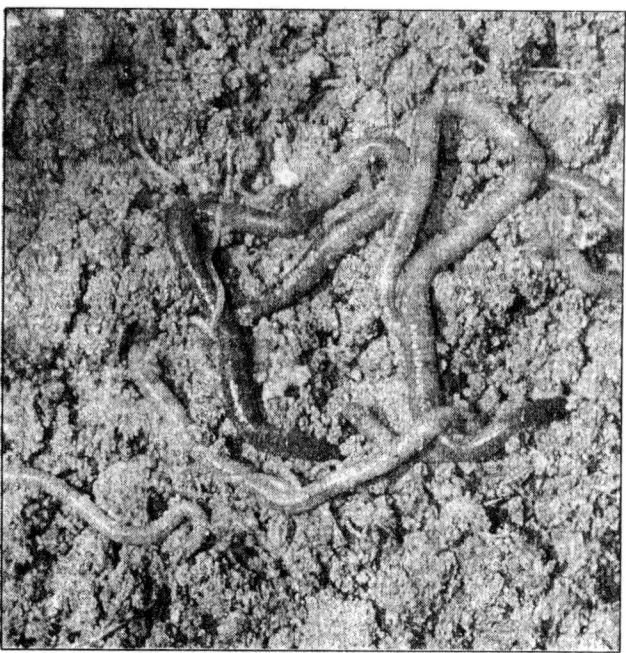

**Fig. 28.1 :** Earthworms, consuming organic Wastes in soil (Photo : by Suthar)

The process of decomposition of organic matter by earthworms promotes growth of bacteria and actinomycetes. Vermitechnology plays a significant role in the treatment of feedlot cattle manure (Mitchell, 1997). *Eisenia fetida anderi* (Bouche) is often utilized for vermicomposting (Bouche, 1972; Satchell, 1983; *Albanell et al.,* 1988, Harvas *et al.,* 1989). It is very easy to breed litter dwelling earthworms such as *Eisenia Fetida,* (Loehrel *et al.,* 1985.) On the other hand breeding and culture of large and deep burrowing earthworm such as *Lumbricus terrestris* is more difficult. Aside form the traditional fish bait market, waste processing and biomass production, the application of vermitechnology may be useful for the production, of large number of selected species of earthworm for the purpose of restoration (Butt *et.at.,* 1992). Vermitechnology can be combined with traditional existing green waste composting operations in order to maxmize the potential of both processes (Frederickson *et al.,* 1997). Many types of organic material are suitable for vermitechnology. Vermitech mainly deals with the following steps:

i)   Use of solid wastes in the form of bedding material
ii)  Addition of organic material for earthworm feeding
iii) Seperation of nutrient rich excreta as vermicompost product.
iv)  Production and sepration of wormbiomass for further use.

## Vermitechnology Species

Many species of eathworms are suitable for vermitechnology but intensive work has been done on the biological potential of only few species specially *Eisenia Eudrulus and Eudirlus eugeniae;* in U.S.A., Africa, Japan, Germany and Latin America. *Eisenia fetida* is suitable for production of vermicompost by using animal dung, household refuses and sewage sludges (Graff, 1974; Hartenstein *et al.,* 1979., Vincelas-Akpa and Loquet, 1997; Mitchell, 1997). *Eudrilus eugeniae* the African night crawler originated from Africa have cosmopolitan distribution and now widely cultured in the United States of America. In Philippines *Perionyx excavatus* has been sucessfully used as a source of protein for animal food. *Dendrobaena veneta* shows good results when used for managing the paper pulp sludges and yeast extract (Fayolle *et al.* 1997). There are about 4,200 species of Oligochaetes in the world. Among these 280 are microdrili and remaining about 3200 belongs to megadrili (earthworm) (Julka, 1993). On the basis of their characteristic features they can be classified into three major categories. epigeic ; (litter dweller), endogeic; (top soil layer dwellers) and aneceic: (deep burrowing species). The main differences among these three catagories have been shown in Table. 28.1. The names of some commonly found vermicomposting species of earthworms are mentioned in Table 28.2.

**Table 28.1 : Differnece among epigeic, endogeic and aneceic earthworms**

| S.No. | Character | Epigeic | Endogeic | Aneceic |
|---|---|---|---|---|
| 1. | Habitat | Litter dweller | Live in upper most organic rich layer of soil | Deep burrowing |
| 2. | Size | About 10 to 30 mm | 100 to 120 mm | 200 to 1100 mm |
| 3. | Body colour | Uniformly coloured | Weakly pigmented | Anterior and posterior parts dark brown in colour |
| 4. | Cocoon production rate | Highet | Moderate to high | Low |
| 5. | Life cycle | Short | Intermediate | Long |

In fact all known species of earthworms are nc suitable for vermiculture. The earthworm species used for vermiculture technology should have following features:

(1) High efficiency to consume all types of organic wastes.
(2) Tolerance for extreme changes in environment.
(3) short life cycle
(4) High rate of cocoon production.

**Table 28.2 : Some common earthworm speices (Julka, 1993)**

| | Peregrine species | | | Endemic species | |
|---|---|---|---|---|---|
| S.No. | Family | Species | S.No. | Family | Species |
| 1. | Lumbricidae | Bimastos parvus Dendrobaena rubida Eisenia fetida Eisenia nortensis | 1. | Megascolecidae | Comarodrilus lennoscolex Nelloscolex, Perionyx, Tonoscotex |
| 2. | Eudrilidae | Eudrilus eugeniae | 2. | Moniligastridae | Moniligaster |
| 3. | Megascolecidal | Amynthas diffrengens Lampito mauritii Metaphire anomala | 3. | Ocherodrilidae | Deccania malabaria, thabonia |
| | | Metaphire biramanica Perionyx excavatus Perionyx sansibaricus | 4. | Octochacitidae | Rehila, Barogaster, Calebiella, Dashiella Cennogaster, Octocraetoides Octochaetona, Octonocracta, Periodoscolex, Scolioscolides |
| 4. | Octochaetidae | Dichogater bolaui Dichogaster saliens Ramiella bishambari Hoplochaetella khandalaensis Haplochaetella suctoria | | | |
| 5 | Ocherodrillidae | Ocherodrilus accidentalis | | | |
| 6 | Moniligastridea | Drawida willsi Moniiigaster perrieri | | | |

The waste consuming efficiency of *Eisenia fetida* and *Lumbricus rubellus* is so high that these two species have provided foundation for vermicomposting industries. *Lampito mauritti* is a litter dwelling species, commonly feeds on the plant litter or deep roots and other plant debrises. *Perionyx excavatus* which is endogeic species consumes large quantity of soil rich in humus. The *E.fetida and Lubricus rubellum* are better for composting in temperate climate. Whereas *Eudrilus eugeniae and Perionyx excavatus* are good for tropical climate. The other useful species for India climate are *lampito mauritti, dichogaster bolaui, drawida willsi and perionyx excavatus* (Dash and Senapati, 1985; Singh, 1997). The scientists at Sambalpur University has suggested vermicomposting by mixed culture of Dichogaster bolaui, Drawida willsi, Lampito mauritti and Perionyx excavantus rather than a monoculture. *pheretima elongata* and *eisenia fetida* are used at Pune in Maharashtra.

## Earthworm Culture

Our living planet earth is rich in earthworm resources Vermicullture program can be launched in different parts of globe in order to convert organic wastes into assets and to save the earth from pollution. Earthworm culture involves the following steps:

**(a) Selection of Culture Containers:** Containers for earthworm culture should be made up of cement, wood, plastic, stone etc. Containers of 2m x 2m x 0.6m size can contain about 4000 worms and each worm needs about 1.8 cm area for better development. These containers can have about 4 kg. worms and these worms can consume about 20 kg. waste per day (Prakash, 1996). The wall of container should have holes of about 0.5 to 0.1 cm for aeration and excess water flow. The inner surface of container should be lined with cover of Jute to stop the coming out the worms through holes.

**(b) Placement of Containers:** The Containers should be placed in humid and proper shadow place for better development of worms. Containers should be protected from predators like ants, rats, frogs and birds etc.

**(c) Preparation of Culture Media:** Soild wastes like dry leaves, old newspapers, crop residues, animal yard wastes, stubbles, dung, kitchen wastes should be mixed with soil in certain ratios and filled in containers upto one third part with required quantity of water. The ratio of earthworm and waste should be 2:1 In other words if there is 1 gm. waste the earthworm should be 2 gm: about 10 kg adult worms can convert 3 tone waste per month.

**(d) Worm Cast and Mass Production and Collection:** After 4 and to 6 weeks the solid wastes are changed into nutrient rich, blackish brown vermicompost which is the excreta of worms. The worm cast and worm mass produced during vermicomposting are replaced from time to time. The container should be empty on clear surface and divide the compost in to small heaps. Then earthworms and cocoon should be separated. The cocoons should be introduced to hatch. These cocoons can also be utilized for next vermicomposting. The nutrient level of vermin compost has been given in Table 28.3.

**Table 28.3 : The nutrient level of vermicompost (Prakash, 1996)**

| Nutrient | Range | Nutrient | Range |
|----------|-------|----------|-------|
| Organic Carbon | 9.15–18.0% | Ca&mg (MEC/100 gms) | 22.6–46.7% |
| N | 0.5-0–1.5% | Cu | 2.0to 9.5 (ppm) |
| P | 0.1–0.3% | Fe | 2.0 to 9.3 (ppm) |
| K | 0.15–0.6% | Zn | 5.7 to 11.5 (ppm) |
| Na | 0.06–0.3% | S | 128 to 548 (ppm) |

The worms starts multiplying in specific season specially from March to July. Worm is hermephrodite but cross fertilization takes place and cocoon is produced. After a fortnight of regular managing of vermibed the breeding worms began to produce cocoon. In *Eisenia fetida* two cocoons are produced after mating. They are yellowish brown or red coloured having lemon shape. Each cocoon is 3 to 4 mm in size and contains about 20 ova of these a maximum of a 8 ova usually develop completely. During this 2 hatching take place. (Hand, 1989). The life cycle of *Eisenia fetida* is shown in Fig 28.2.

## Limiting Factors for Vermiculture

Vermiculture process is influenced by certain external factors. They may act as limiting factors for population growth in a culture medium. Some of the important factors are as follows:

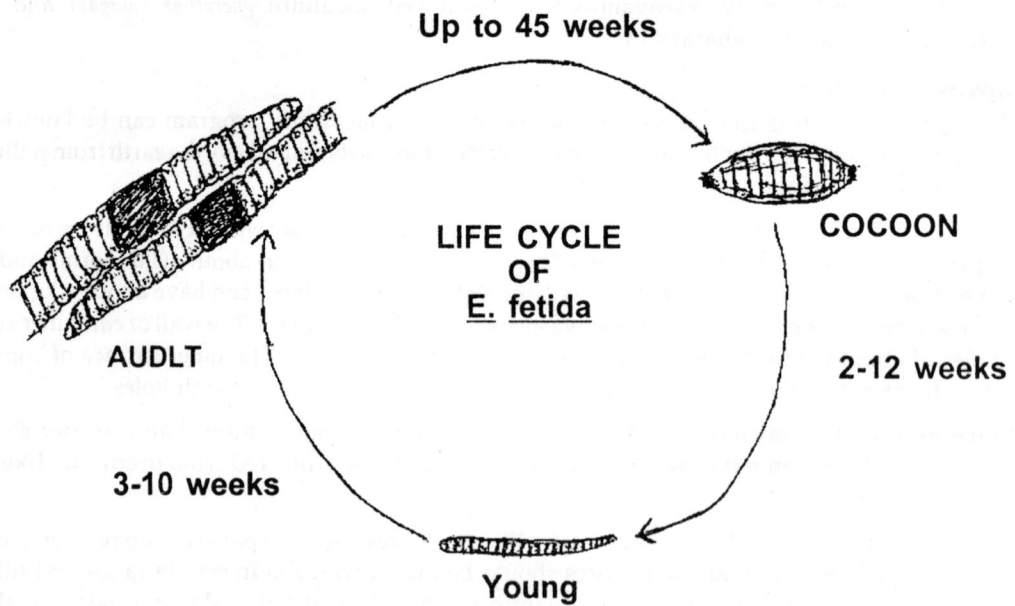

**Up to 45 weeks**

**LIFE CYCLE OF E. fetida**

**COCOON**

**2-12 weeks**

**AUDLT**

**3-10 weeks**

**Young**

**(i) pH:** The worm shows maximum activity and growth at normal pH. The lower pH (acidic) in the medium reduces the activity of worms and it leads to weight loss and population decline. The *Amynthas hawayanus* worm dies quickly in a moist substrate with a pH value less than 5 and greater than 8. (Kaplan *et al,* 1980). Some times it has been seen that water logging leads to anaerobes and change in the pH of the medium takes place.

**(ii) Temperature:** Earthworms have maximum activity at $25^0$ C. Worms can tolerate $10^0$ to $30^0$C temperature but more than $40^0$C and less than $10^0$C is lethal to them (Fayolle *et al.,* 1997). In *Derdrobaena veneta* cocoon production on paper sludge begins between 42-90 days at $25^0$ C and 62-83 days at $20^0$C. The cocoon production is influenced by temperature and significantly higher in paper sludge compared with horse manure. The *Amynthus* species grow optimally on horse manure at $29^0$C and on activated sludge in horse manure at $20^0$C to $28^0$C (Kaplan *et al.,* 1980). The hatching of cocoon remains faster in the range of $20^0$C to $25^0$C with mean incubation time of 36 days in brown peal and 90 days at $10^0$C (Fayolle *et al.,* 1997).

**(iii) Moisture:** Successful survival of worms in the culture medium effectively depends upon the moisture contents of the medium which should be optimum. It should be between 60 to 65 per cent. There is a direct relationship between moisture content and the growth rate of earthworm *Eisenia andrei* in pig manure grow and mature between 65 to 90 per cent moisture content and the optimim being 85 per cent (Dominguez and Edward, 1997). According to Reincke and Ventor (1987), *Eisenia fetida* shows better growth and reproduction at moisture contend of more than 70 per cent in cow manure.

**(iv). Ventilation:** The air is a vital factor in vermiculture process. The culture medium should be turned and mixed after an appropriate time to make medium aerobic for better results. The growth of microbial communities in culture medium is badly affected by oxygen. These microorganisms plays a significant role in earthworm digestion. However, conditons must remain aerobic. So feedstock materials should permit the flow of air.

## Vermitechnology and Pollution Reduction

Pollution has now become a globally recognized serious problem. Due to lack of certain ecofriendly technologies for waste management, rapid industrialization and deforestation have made the environment warm and imbalance. The result can be seen in the form of soil erosion, low soil fertility, soil toxicity, diseases and pretime deaths. The ever growing population, increased industrialization and intensive agriculture generate a lot of wastes and impose the problem of waste disposal. The heavy use of pesticides, fertilizers and other agrochemicals has not only contaminated soil, degraded soil productvity, destroy soil fauna but also their residues cause toxicological effects on animal system. Industrial effluents contain heavy metals, dyes and other disease causing agents. The household and agriculture wastes, dairy and livestock wastes accumulate in quantity of several million of tons. They are the main agents for ground and surface water pollution.

In our country about 2000 million animal and human solid and liquid excreta and about 200 million tonnes of crops straws are produced. One million worms can convert about 120 tonnes organic wastes into vermifertilizer in about one moth (Jairajpuri, 1993). So the role of vermitechnology in pollution abatement can not be ignored.

Earthwarm has efficiency to consume all the types of organic rich solid waste material and can accumulates certain toxic substances, heavy metals and dyes. Earthworm is very useful in breakdown of vegetable, industrial and organic wastes (Edward, 1988). By using vermitehnology or vermiculture biotechnology (VBT) we not only manage waste materials but can also recycle organic wastes. India produces about 3000 million tones of organic wastes annually, which may be utilized to produce vermifertilizer. This huge quantity of wastes has potentiality to produce about 400 million tons of plant nutrients besides biogas and alcohol (Das and Senapati, 1986). Therefore, vermitechnology may be effectively employed for management of various types of wastes as described below:

**(a) Agricultral Wastes:** Million of tons of agriculture wastes are produced per annum in our country. It comprises of livestock excreta including chicken, duck, pig, cattle, sheep, goat and horse yard manure, dairy wastes, mushroom culture waste, food processing wastes and plant residues etc It generates bad odour and pollutes soil and the water bodies by mixing through rain water flow. It also gives shelter to several disease causing agents, vectors and pathogenic insect larvae in rural areas and farm houses. It creates major problem due to lack of adequate place for safe disposal. The agricultural wastes contain high concentration of cellulose compounds, organic nutrients, protein, phosphorus, nitrogen and fats, organic acids and other plant nutrients. These types of wastes are good food in the form of bedding materials for development of vermiculture biotechnology (Harwood, 1976).

Worm plays a valuable role in recycling of agriculture wastes for best reutilization of nutrients in the form of worm cast or excreta or vermicompost. Vermicomposting can play a significant role in the treatment of feed cattle manure. The earthworm's activity can recover a portion of the more labile nutrients and also promote favourble physio-chemical conditions of soil (Mitchell, 1997). The poultry waste is the suitable feed for earthworm in terms of productivity. Alternative to this is the mixed feed prepared from poultry manure and cow dung (1:1). This has been suggested as an appropriate diet in the mass cultivation and production of earthworms for their proteins (Kale and Bano, 1986). Such experiments has been done with *Eisenia fetida* using potato wastes. One estimation shows that 2.1 million tons of potato wastes give a turnover of 10,500 tons of earthworm biomass (Edward, 1983). *Eisenia fetida* when allowed to feed on cellulose (plant residues rich in cellulose) mixed with sludge, a considerable amount of energy is derived and selectively remove a larger proportion of ambient cellulose matrix from the medium (Hartenstein, 1981).

Animal effluents from housed livestock is very useful for earthworm culture Meadows *et al.* (1990) and Mitchell (1997) calculated an interesting mathematics for feedlot cattle manure and through it total protein yielding. According to them feedlot cattle manure typically produces an average of 1300 kg (dry weight) manure per head per year and increase live weight from 300 to 450 kg in a feeding period of 90 days giving annual beef protein -N production 6.6 kg. While earthworm protein-N produced from 1300 kg manure was 6.2 at the maximum rate of trial. Cow manure is known to be one of the best natural feeds for the earthworm, *Eisenia fetida*. Its population increases in numbers and biomass when allowed to feed on sludge cake derived from dairy waste supplemented with cellulose material such as rice straw (Hatanaka *et al*, 1983). Kale (1986) demonstrated the biomass production of *Perionyx excavatus and Eudrilus eugeniac* by using cow dung with different agricultural and wastes like gram barn, rice barn, wheat barn and poultry dropping in different ratios. She found maximum biomass of earthworms when cultured in wheat, rice barn and poultry dropping with dung.

Earthworm shows high cocoon production rate when feed on animal organic matter containing more nitrogen *i.e.,* biogas slurry. Biogas slurry contain 50 per cent organic nitrogen and 50 per cent ammonical nitrogen. In preservation of cow dung in a heap, there are loss of nitrogen (clearly 50% as ammonia) and water soluble salts (90% as water soluble potassium) through volatilization and leaching when exposed to sun and rain (Poonuraj *et al*, 1998). Therefore, the vermicoposting of dung is better than composting of dung. According to Sabine (1978) cattle dung is very good food for vermitech which contains about 3.5 per cent nitrogen (74% in organic from and 26% in as similable ammonical form). Breeding potential of some important species of earthworm have been tested on different culture media in laboratory (Table: 28.4)

**Table 28.4 : Breeding potentials of some earthworm species in different culture media**

| S. No. | Culture medium | Earthworm speices applied | Breeding decomposition efficiency | References |
|---|---|---|---|---|
| 1. | Cattle manure+soil | Amynthas morroso | Moderate breeding and decomposition | Singh, (1997) |
| 2. | Straw+Soil | Amynthas moorrisi | Shows fast breeding and moderate decomposition | Singh, (1997) |
| 3. | Leaf litter+soil | Dichogaster bolaui | Shows low breeding and moderate decomposition | Singh, (1997) |
| 4. | Cattle manure | Dichogaster bolaui | Shows moderate breeding and decomposition | Singh, (1997) |
| 5. | Straw litter | Dichogaster bolaui | Very fast breeding and decomposition | Singh, (1997) |
| 6. | Hay+soil | Perionyx sansibaricus | Fast breeding and moderate decomposition | Singh, (1997) |
| 7. | Feet lot cattle manure | Eisenia Fetida | Very fast breeding and decomposition | Mitchell, (1997) |
| 8. | Potato wate | Eisenia Fetida | Very fast breeding and decomposition | Edward, (1980) |
| 9. | Horse manure | Dendrobaena veneta | Low breeding and moderate decomposition | Fayolle, et al. (1997) |
| 10. | Poultry manure | Eudrilus eugeniae | Very faset breeding and decomposition | Kale & Bano (1986) |
| 11. | Green waste | Eisenia andrei | Low breeding and high decompostition | Frederickson et al. (1997) |
| 12. | Pig manure | Eisenia andrei | Fast breeding and moderate decomposition | Domingueza & Edward (1997) |

*Eudrilus eugeniac* shows highest population when allowed to feed on biomass sludge and popultry manure and cow dung (in a ratio of 1:1). It also shows maximum biomass when feed on poultry manure and cow dung (1:1) as compared to biogas sludge (Kale and Bano; 1986). According to Singh (1997) straw litter is very good bedding material for *Dichogster bolaui*. This species shows fast breeding, quick decompostion when allowed to feed on straw litter. Thus, the vermitechnology plays a valuable and significant role in minimization of disposal of agriculture wastes as well as worm mass and cast production.

**(b) Industrial Wastes:** Industrial wastes are produced in a qunatity of several million tons per annum. They conatin inorganic and organic chemical substances. Industrial wastes include sugar mill wastes, distillery wastes, cotton mill wastes, dairy industry wastes, wood industry wastes, agriculture based industrial wastes and chemical industry wastes. The wastes from these industries contain high level of organic compounds, heavy metals, toxins, cellulose, lignin, sugar and its derivatives. These wastes flow through streams and at last fall into rivers and other large water bodies. It is the reason why most industries have been established near or aside the bank of rivers or large water bodies to drain the water according to the need of industry. These industrial wastes create bad odour and cause lethal biochemical toxicity and pathogenic problems in aquatic flora and fauna. These harmful chemical compounds enter in human body through food chain. These industrial effluents when applied directly to soil shows adverse effects on soil quality, soil fauna as well as productivity of soil. Recently it has been found that the BOD (Biological Oxygen Demand) has increased seriously from 2 tons/million gallon water to more than 230/tons in some popular rivers of country due to mixing of different industriual effluents. Industries of Mumbai account for only 13 per cent of the total waste dumped into water bodies and in Calcutta 11 per cent waste is of industrial origin (Dash and Mishra, 1998). In Mumbai about 600 million litre industrial effluent is produced per day. Tripathi and Singh, (2000) have discussed the importance of earthworm resources in industrial waste management through application of vermiculture biotechnology (VBT).

The solid paper and pulp mill sludge are produced from paper mill industries. Paper and pulp waste consists of adequate amount of organic wastes like lignea and cellulose. It have a high COD rate. One estimation shows that one tons paper production generates 225 to 320 m$^3$ waste materials.

The vermicomposting plays a significant role in paper pulp and waste sludge treatment. The vermicomposting is suitable and low cost technology to manage paper pulp mill wastes as demonstrated by several workers (Hartenstein, 1978; Edward, 1988; Hand and Hayes, 1983; Butt, 1993; Elvira *et al.,* 1997). The paper and pulp mill waste comprises of low nitrogen content and large amount of polysaccharides. This low nitrogen content leads to limited biooxidation process, therefore, it can be mixed with nitrogen rich materials like sewage sludge, pig manure poultry slurry etc. It facilitates better conditions and provides good population of microbial communities for better biological oxidation of wastes. However, solid paper pulp mill sludge is not able to support earthworm growth by itself. The mixture procedure could be a suitable technique for its utilization as food source in vermicomposting (Elvira et al., 1997). Chemical characteristics of SPPMS (solid paper pulp mill sludge) has been shown in Table 28.5.

**Table 28.5 : Chemical characteristics of solid paper pulp mill sludge (Elvira *et al.,* (1997)**

| Characteristic | Values in percentage except pH and C/N ratio |
|---|---|
| pH | 9.2 |
| total solids | 18.9 |
| Ash | 87.5 |
| total organic carbon | 47.6 |
| Total Kjeldani nitrogen | 0.24 |
| C/N ratio | 188.3 |
| Crude fibre | 67.9 |

The flyash which is produced from thermal industries have major disposal problems. It has been estimated that about 60 million tons of flyash are produced per annum from thermal power plants situated in different parts of India (Saxena *et al.,* 1998). Its chemical composition is similar to soil except organic components, humus and it contains several toxins, heavy metals and therefore, it cannot be used directly in the soil agroecosystem. The disposal of thermal power wastes on soil may result in hyper accumulation of heavy metals in soils. The vermicomposting of flyash mixing with different organic rich components results into valuable vermicompost. Flyash contains several utilizable elements and it could be decomposed by the activity of microbial community (Rippon and Wood, 1976). The microbial activity during vermicomposting of flyash produces soluble nutrients for easy availability to plants and other soil organisms (Saxena *et al.,* 1998). Saxena and others (1998) have successfully evaluated this flyash in vermicomposting. According to them organcic waste like grass cutting mixed with flyash provide a potentially valuable material for Eisenia fetida. The NPK content is found in a comparatively higher amount in vermicompost than the commercially available organic manure. Scientists working at Bangalore University are successfully employing African night crawler (*Eudrillus eugenae)* for management of effluents of distillery industries around Bangalore. Scientists working at NEERI (National Environmental Engineering Research Institute) also recommended some potential earthworm species for break down of industrial wastes. Japan imports several tons of earthworms from U.S.A. every year for managing its paper pulp mill wastes. Different organizations like E.E.C. (European Economic Community), O.E.C.D. (Organization for Economics of United Nations) and Pesticide Registrations Authorities and Environmental Pollution Communities are recommending earthworms for ecotoxicological testing of industrial pollutants (Singh and Rai, 1998).

(c) **Sewage Sludge:** In the urban and rural areas several tons of sewage wastes is produced per year. In England about 1.2 million dry tons of sewage sludge is produced per year and in the USA this figure reaches upto 7 million tons dry sludge per annum. This municipal sewage sludge contains high organic matter, toxins, detergents, fecal material. Kitchen refuses, polybag, plastic articles, paper bags, packing wastes etc. These sewage wastes reach water bodies and rivers which not only produce bad odour but also cause bad effects on water quality. Sewage sludge when fall into river, cause pollution and makes the water undrinkable. It imbalances the fresh water ecosystem. Due to presence of organic rich substances it gives shelter to many pathogenic organisms like bacteria, viruses, protozoans and nematodes, helminthes and many insect larval forms. Sewage sludge causes lethal effects on animals physio-chemical systems due to presence of toxic substances. Yamuna receives 200 million litre of untreated human wastes and 20 million litre of industrial waste water per day (Dash and Mishra, 1998). The recent report of Central Pollution Control Board shows alarming datas, according to it the BOD of Yamuna (Delhi) unit has increased 117.3 ton/day to 211.0 ton per day between the period of year 1982 to1998. Sewage sludge contains a large amount of organic materials which can be degraded or recycled by manupulating biological potential of an organism. The organic material present in such a waste can be determined by using certain devices like by measiring the chemical oxygen demand (COD) and biological oxygen demand (BOD). It is thus an indication of amount of dissolved oxygen (DO) that will be depleted from water during the natural biological assimilation of organic pollutants. Polluted water bodies, sewage, industrial wastes have high BOD rates.

The treatment of waste water include physical, chemical and biological processing. A single device cannot be a success therefore we have to introduce these physical, chemical as well as biological methods of sewage treatment. The biological or secondary treatment includes application of natural decomposers and detritus feeders which break down organic matter into simple organic and inorganic substances. The sewage sludge treated through anaerobic respiration (Bacteria of different groups) or by composting through worms ( i.e., vermicomposting) shows better results without any extra economical burden at a low tech level. The manipulation of earthworms efficiency for sewage treatment have been described by several workers (Edward and Lofty, 1977; Satchell, 1967; Neushuser at al., 1980; Mitchell 1977; Mitchell et at., 1980, Hartenstein, 1979). The treatment of sewage sludge includes primary, secondary and tertiary treatment. Primary treatment involves separation of indigestible or non recycling substances like slit, grit, polythene bags, stones, plastic articles, sand etc. from sewage sludge. It does settling and screening of solid material. Secondary treatment or biological treatment deals with the purification of sewage. It also includes conversion of sewage waste into vermifertilizer and products of micronutients. Tertiary treatment includes micro strainers, sand filters and chemical treatment. Appelhof (1990) has demonstrated that the vermicomposting of municipal waste water has low costs as compared to other treatment methods of water management. In United States of America earthworms has been successfully employed in breakdown of activated sludges very effectively (Hartenstein et al., 1979). Neuhauser et al. (1988) pointed out that vermicomposting of sewage sludge could accelerate organic matter stabilization as compared to sludge without earthworms. Thus vermitechnology is a part of biological treatment of waste water sludge. The anaerobic activities of other microorganism (Bacteria, Protozoans etc.) not only accelerate the vermicomposting process but also make the waste treatment easy when employed simultaneously with vermicomposting. The entire process of utilization of earthworms in waste water/sludge treatment has been shown in Fig .28.3.

**(d) Green Waste:** Green wastes from garden pruning and trimming of plants and shrubs, weeds, leaves, grasses etc. cause a problem of disposal. These waste contains large quntity of cellulose, lignin, suberin, protein, lipids and other inorganic plant nutrients. The best use of these wastes is traditional composting. Composting is a biological process which involves microorganisms. These microorganisms viz., bacteria, fungi, actinomycetes, algae, protozoan break down the green waste and produce an organic nutrient rich compost and dead or living microorganisms. The composting process may be of aerobic and anaerobic type. The breakdown of these organic substances through microoganisms is a thermobiochemical process and produces heat and sometimes during this process temperature reaches upto $60^0$C. The micrbial composting may be improved by the combined action of earthworm and microflora living in their intestine and the surrounding. Worms may help to accelerate the transformation of organic matters by aeration, by excreta and qualitative or quantitative influence of the microflora (Vincellas-Akpa and Loquet, 1997).

The Lignin is abundant in green wastes. The lignolytic activity can be imporved by combining green waste composting with vermicomposting. The vermitechnology and composting of green waste may be combined in order to maximize the potential of both processes and stabilization (Frederickson et· al.,1997). The thermophilic reaction of composting process kills the harmful pathogens larvae, cysts, eggs of different pests, parasites and spores of fungus. When composting is combined with vermicomposting we acquire useful vermicompost and production of earthworm biomass.

Six weeks vermicomposting of partially composted organic matter of about two weeks by *Eisenia andrei* reduces volatile solid contents significantly more than those of the composting of fresh waste for 8 weeks (Frederickson *et al.*, 1997). According to Vincellas-Akpa and Loquet, (1997) the total loss

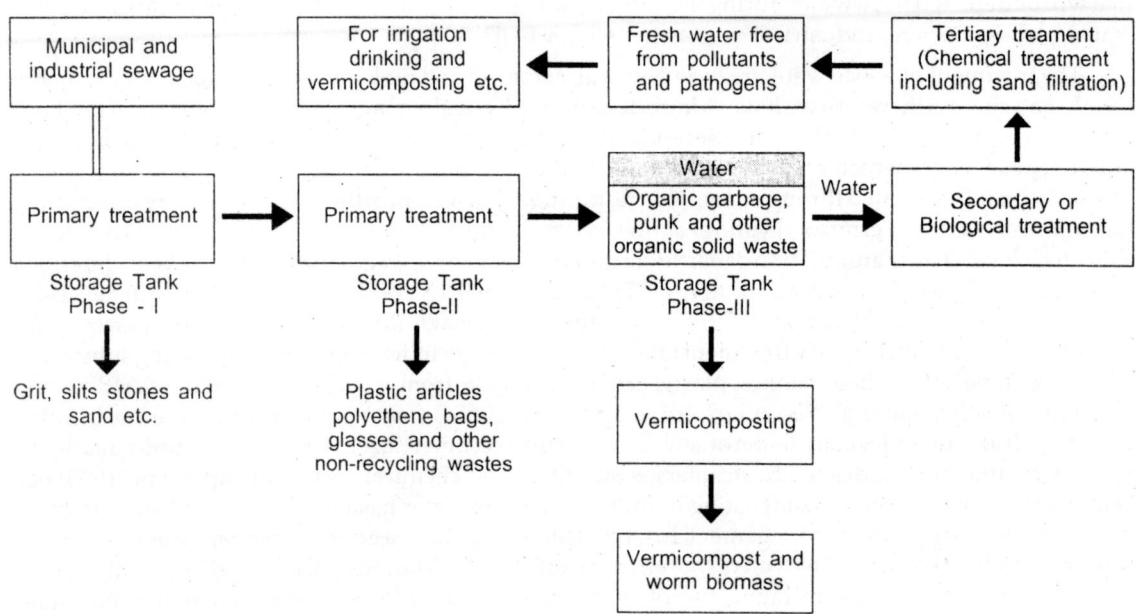

**Fig 28.3** : A model for utilization of vermitech in sewage treatment.

of organic matter and carbon in vermicomposting remains faster than the composting. The loss remain continuous in composting whereas it increased in vermicomposting after a certain period. The growth of earthworm becomes slow when allowed to feed on precomposted wastes because there is a correlation in microorganisms and earthworm digestion which results in the organic waste transformation (Edward and Fletcher, 1988; Thorpe *et al.*, 1993). Hence precomposted matter contains less quality of microorganisms and progressively it is reduced, so earthworm shows less growth and biomass in the composted matter as compared to the fresh green wastes.

The combination of composting with vermicomposting has two advantages:

1. It maximizes the recycling of organic wastes by using biopotential of microorganisms and worms.
2. Precomposting phase play a good role in pathogen control. The green waste sometime contains larvae, eggs, spores and cysts of different pathogens and pests. The thermophilic stages of composting process kills these pathogens and pest larvae.

(e) **Detoxification:** Earthworms have a wonderful property of detoxification. For the heavy metal and toxic substances the worm can act as bioconcentrators. It has been reported by several workers that earthworm is very much useful in assesment of heavy metals, pesticides and their residues, radio active residues and other toxic substances (Edward and Thompson, 1973; Satchell, 1955). They can accumulate various heavy metal ions such as zinc, lead, cadmium, chromium, nickel, zinc, copper, mercury etc. in their body (Harteinstein et al, 1980; Beyer, 1981). In this way they play an important role in environment monitoring. Many chemical toxins are present in sewage sludge, industrial effluents of agrochemicals and chemical industries. If these industrial effluents are applied directly in non-treated form in agricultural field they may cause hazards to plant community and enter into food chain and reach the human beings. These toxic substances specially Mn, Pb, arsenic act as slow poison and causes lethal effects on body systems. In this way earthworms play a major role in minimization of soil pollution.

There are several reports dealing with the aspect of toxicants on earthworm biomass and population in field. Some experminets show the effects of heavy metals on reproduction in earthworms (Neuhauser et al.; 1984, Reinecke and Reinecke; 1997). Accumulation of heavy metals and pesticidses may some times cause biohazard to animals which feed on earthworms specially birds. These pesticide residues when appear in birds biosystem through food chain cause physiological disorder especially on vitellogenin and egg formation. The use of untreated sewage sludge and paper mill wastes which contains heavy metals, chemicals and toxins may be hazard to crops and soil fauna. Vermicomposting of these wastes not only help in assessment of toxicants but also produce valuable vermicompost for better crop production.

(f) **Protein Source:** The earthworms have been universally accepted as a protein source for fish meal and poultry industries (Guerreo, 1983, Kale and Bano, 1988). The earthworm dry matter contains about 60-70 per cent protein with a high concentration of essential amino acids specially lysine (6.9 - 0.9%), fat (14-21%), carbohydrates (0.3 - 0.54%), calcium and about 0.7% - 0.9% phosphorous. In this way earthworm dry mass have a great nutritional value. In addition to these it also contains niacin and vitamins i.e. Vitamin $B_{12}$ at a suitable concentration (McInory, 1971; Schulz and Graff, 1977; Hartenstein, 1981; Edward, 1985).

The presence of essential amino acids (Table 28.6) in earthworm tissues adequately fulfil the recommendation of FAO/WHO particularly in terms of tyrosine all of which are important components

Table 28.6 : **Different Amino acids in worm protein in gm (Taboga, 1980)**

| Amino acid | Amount in gm/100gm | Amino acid | Amount in gm/100gm |
|---|---|---|---|
| Ala | 5.4 | Met | 2.0 |
| Arg | 7.3 | Phe | 5.1 |
| Asp | 10.5 | Pro | 5.3 |
| Cys | 1.8 | Ser | 5.8 |
| Glu | 13.2 | Tyr | 4.6 |
| His | 3.8 | Val | 4.4 |
| Ile | 5.;3 | Thr | 4.6 |
| Leu | 6.2 | Try | 2.1 |
| Lys | 7.3 | Gly | 4.3 |

of animal foods (Singh and Rai, 1998). Due to this high food value they can be utilized in poultry and piggery, diet of rats and as a bait for fishery. Thus vermitechnology have been proved to be advantageous to solve food problems for man and domestic animals as well as poultry industries (McInory, 1971; Yashida and Hoshii, 1978). During 1980 at least 500 million Canadian night crawlers (Lumbricus terrestis) were exported from Ontario to the U.S.A. as the diet worms at an average whole sale price of $35 per thousand worms. The total value of export was $175 million (Tomlin, 1983). Amino acid spectrum of earthworms show that they can be considered as a better food source for protein as compared to other animal derived protein sources. Production of *Perionyx excavatus* as a protein source has been demonstrated in Philippines (Guerrero, 1983). The earthworm bait market has continued to expand rapidly over the past few years because of the shortage of traditional bait such as shrimps and coarse fish (Tomlin, 1983). In North America specially the African night crawler (*Eudrilus eugeniae*) and tiger worm (*Eisenia fetida*) are commonly used for the purpose of bait industries. In *Eudrilus eugeniae* the nutrient levels of worm meal are found on dry matter basis as 65 per cent protein, 11 per cent carbohydrate and 6.5 per cent to fat. Replacement of 50 per cent fish meal by earth worm meal in the diets of poultry shows encouraging results (Kale and Bano, 1986).

## Work in Progress

Vermiculture biotechnology has been universally accepted as an ecofriendly technology for sustainable development and abatement of pollution caused by municipal garbage, sewage sludge, agricultural and industrial wastes. Earthworms as a protein rich food source for animal as well as their utilization in land reclaimation has no less importance. Therefore, much efforts have been made to study the earthworm biodiversity in different parts of world (Edward and Lofty 1977; Satchell 1983; Lee, 1985; Daube *et al.*, 1994; Fayolle *et al.*, 1997). In the northern region of Europe, Asia and North America the Lumbricidae is the important group of earthworm of forest, grassland, sownpasture, cropland and gardens. The Worm Depot Inc. in California and South Resources Management Group Inc. in Washington are doing well with low and high tech vermicomposting. Biosystem Research group in U.K. has combined vermiculture with traditional green waste composting system. Scientists in France, Belgium, Spain, Japan and Australia have initiated investigations on earthworm ecology and waste transformation efficiencies (Fayolle *et al.*, 1997, Vincellas - Akpa and Loquet; 1997; Muys and Granval, 1997; Mitchell, 1997; Elvira *et al.* 1997). Several studies has been done on *Eudrilus eugeinae, Perionyx excavatus and Prsenia foetida* for vermicomposting in South Africa (Reinecke *et al.*, 1992). Cuba in 1980 started vermiculture programme with only 2 small boxes and have established 172 centres up to 1992 with annual production of 93,000 tones of worms humus (Rosset and Benjamin, 1993). United States of America is encouraging vermicomposting bioindustries under private and government sectors. In our country the diversity, distribution, seasonal dynamics, abundance and ecology of earthworm in different soil strata have been studied by various workers (Dash and Patra, 1977; Julka and Senapati, 1987, Kale and Krishanamurti, 1981; Ismail 1986; Tripathi *et al.*,1995). Scientists working at Sambalpur University, Orissa have suggested vermicomposting by mixed culture. Some species of earthworms are being successfully developed for culture under laboratory conditions at Agriculture University, Bangalore.

Pune based centre has suggested two earthworm species viz., *Pheretima elongata* and *Eisenia fetida* for vermicomposing. At Parrys tea garden of Coimbatore through financial support from European Economic Community (EEC) has attracted attention of tea grower for vermicomposting in India. The work at Banaras Hindu University, Varansi, supported by United States India fund project has identified *Amynthas morrisi, Dichogaster bolaui* and Perionyx sansibricus as potential decomposers (Singh and Rai, 1988). The scientists working at National Environmental Engineering Research Institute (NEERI), Nagpur recommended a suitable earthworm species for the break down of negligible waste. Madras based workers have identified few suitable species for vermiculture (Ismail, 1997). Scientists working at International Crops Research Institute for the Semi Arid Tropics (ICRISAT) have identified a potential and abundant earthworm species. Some reports on vermitechnology are also available from other states including Gujrat, M.P. and Rajasthan. The work on earthworm biodiversity and vermiculture technology is in progress at J.N.V. University, Jodhpur for benefits of desert region of Rajashtan (Table 28.7). Infact efforts should be made to identify suitable species of earthworms inhabiting the globe for pollution abatement and welfare of animal and mankind undoable the work on earthworm resources will facilitate the development of vermitech bioindustries all over the world.

## Table 28.7 : The scope of vermiculture biotechnology

| | | |
|---|---|---|
| 1. House hold waste (Waste papers, garbage, garden pruning waste etc.)<br><br>2. Kitchen waste (Old vegetables, pealoff vegetables and fruits, packing papers and kitchen refuges etc.)<br><br>3. Agriculture waste (Crop stubbles, Crop resifdues, leaves and other agro-industrial wastes etc.)<br><br>4. Municipal waste and sewage sludges (City refuge, municipal garbage and sewage etc.)<br><br>5. Farm Yard manure (Manure and dung of domestic animals like Cow, Horse, Sheep, Pig etc.)<br><br>6. PESTICIDES AND RESIDUES OF OTHER TOXIC SUBSTANCES. (Residues of pesticides, fungicides, nematicides, other agrochemicals, heavy metals and fertilizers etc.)<br><br>7. INDUSTRIAL EFFLUENTS (Effluents from chemical industries, distilleries, paper mills, food processing and fertilizer industries and solid waste from other industries.) | → VERMI-TECHNOLOGY → | • Nutrient rich vermicompost<br>• Worm mass production for vermicomposting<br>• Solid waste management<br>• Worm tissue as a protein rich food for rat, poultry and piggary industries.<br>• Production of worm as a bait for fish market<br>• Improvement of soil fertility by the physio-chemical activity of worm<br>• Detoxification and accumulation of certain heavy metals and toxins<br>• Role in pollution minimization<br>• Improvement of soil microbiology<br>• Soil reclaimation and amelioration<br>• Medicinal product from worm biomass<br>• Bioindicator for development of silvipasture and agrisilviculture practices in barren land<br>• Agriculture based sustainsable development.<br>• Upliftment of rural economy. |

## Conclusion

The man and its surrounding environment influence each other. The interference of human being in nature has caused certain drastic problems. Pollution which is an anthrogenic problem. Unsafe utilization of our natural resources to fulfill the demand of ever expanding population, rapid industrialization, reduced fossil energy based inputs, intensive agriculture, heavy use of agrochemicals to achieve the goal of high crop production have not only damaged to out environment but also changed the physio-chemical as well as productivity of soil systems. Rapid urbanization, disposal of domestic and municipal sewage, industrial effeuents, agricultural waste and other organic solid wastes have caused certain eco-biological imbalances. In the present millennium much effort will be made to trap the potentials of organisms for abatement of solid waste pollution. At this juncture the role of earthworm biopotential in pollution abatement can not be neglected. Solid waste input based vermitechnology gives output in the form of valuble nutrient rich worm cast and protein rich worm biomass which can be used in vermicomposting and sustainable agricultural land development to reduce pollution and solve the food crises for human beings and animals. Hence there is a vast scope of vermitechnology in coming decades in India and abroad.

## ACKNOWLEDGEMENT

Authors gratefully acknowledge the financial support received from DBT, New Delhi for work on earthworm biodiversity and vermiculture.

# REFERENCES

- Albanell, E., Plaixants, J. and Cabrero, T. (1988). Chemical changes during vermicomposting (*Eisenia fetida*) of sheep manure mixed with cotton industrial wastes. *Biology and Fertility of Soils,* **6**, 266-269.

- Appelhof, M. (1980). House hold scale vermicomposting In: *Research Needs Workshops on the Role of Earthworm in the Stablization of Organic Residues.* April 9-12, Hickert Cornes, Michigan, U.S.A.

- Beyer, W.N. (1981). Metals and Terrestrial Earthworms (Annelida Oligocheata). In: *Workshop on the Role of Earthworms in the Stabilisation of Organic Residues.* (M.Appelhof, Compiler), Vol. I, Proc. Beech Leaf Press, Kalamazoo, MI, pp. 137-150.

- Bouche, M.B. (1972). Lombriciens de France : Ecologie et Systematique. INRA, Annales de Zoologie ecologiqe - animals speical number 72 (2).

- Bouche, M.B. (1981). Development of lombriciens:bio stimulations des sols et bio-indication. In:compte rendu des journees science ecologique et development, pp. 281-295, 19-20 Sept. 1979. AFIE, Grenoble.

- Butt, K.R. (1993). Utilization of solid paper-mills sludge and spent brewery yeast as a feed for soil dwelling earthworms. *Bioresources Technology,* **44**, 105-107.

- Butt, K.R.; Frederickson, J. and Morris, R.M. (1992). The Intensive production of *Lumbricus terrestris* for soil amelioration. *Soil Bilogy and Biochemistry,* **24**, 1321-1325.

- Darwin, (1881). The formation of vegetable mould through the action of worms with observation of their habits, Murrary London, 298p.

- Dash, M.C. and Mishra, P.C. (1998). Role of cynobateria in water pollution abatement. *Indian J. Env. Ecoplan,*:1-11(1998).

- Dash, M.C,. and Patra. V.C. (1977). Density biomass and energy budget of a tropical earthworm population from a grass land site in Orissa. *Indian Rev. Ecol. Biol. Sol.,* 4:461-471.

- Dash, M.C. and Senapati, B.K. (1985). Vermitechnology potentially of Indian earthworms, for vermicomposting and vermifeed. In Soil Biology M.M Mishra and K.K. Kapoor, Eds) pp. 61-69. Haryana Agriculture University Press, Hissar.

- Dash, M.C and Senapati, B.K. (1986). Vermitechnology an option for Organic Waste Management in India. In: *Proc. Nat. Sem. Org. Waste Utiliz. Vermicom.* Part B. *Vermes and Vermicomposting* 157-172 (M.C. Dash, B.K.. Senapati and P.C. Mishraeds. Sri Artatrana Routfor Five Star Printing Press, Burla, Orissa.

- Domingues, J. and Edward, C.A. (1997). Effects of stocking rate and moisture content on the growth and maturation of *Eisenia andrei* (Oligochaeta) in pig manure. *Soil Biol. Biochem.,* 29:743-746.

- Doube, B.M., Stephens, P.M., Davoren, C.W. and Ryder, M.H. (1994) Interactions between earthworms, beneficial soil micro organisms and root pathogens. *Appl. Soil Ecol.,* 1:3-10.

- Edwards, C.A. (1983). *Earthworms Organic waste and food-span.* Shell Chem. Co. 26(3): 106-108.

- Edwards, C.A. (1985). Production of feed protein from animal waste by earthworms. *Phil. Trans. R. Soc. Lond* B 310: 299-307.

- Edwards, C.A (1988). Breakdown of animal, vegetable and indistrial organic wates by earthworms. In: *Earthworms in Waste and Environmental management.* (C.A. Edwards and E.F Neuhausereds). pp. 21-34, SPB Academic Publishing, The Netherlands.

- Edward, C.A. and Lofty, J.R. (1977). Biology of earthworms. Chapman and Hall, New York, 333 p.

- Edwards, C.A. and Thompson, A.R. (1973). Pesticides and soil fauna. *Residue Rev.,* **45**:1-79.

- Elvira, C., Sampedro, I. Dominguez, J.and Mato, S.(1997). Vermicomposting of waste water sludge from Paper-Pulp Industry with Nitrogen Rich Material. *Soil Biol Biochem. Vol.* 29, No. 3/4, pp. 759-762.

- Fayolle, L., Michaud, H., Clauzeau, D. and Starviecki, J. (1997). Influence of temperature and food source on the life cycle of the earthworm *Dendrobaena veneta* (Oligochaeta). *Soil Biol. Biochem.* **20**: 747-750.

- Frederickson, J., Butt, K.R., Morris, R.M. and Dahiel, C (1997). Combining vermiculture with traditional green waste composting systems. Soil Biol. Biochem. Vol. 29, No.3/4 pp. 725-730.

- Ghilarov, M.S. (1978). Bodenwirbellose als India Katoren des Bodenhaushaltes and von bodenbildenden Prozessen. *Padobiologia, 18,* 300-309.

- Graff, O. (1974). Crrewinnung von Biomasse aub Ablalstoffen durch kultur des kompostre genwarms *Eisenia fetida* (savigny), 1826 Londan bforsch. volk. 24, 134-142.

- Guerrero, R.D. (1983). The culture and use of *Perionyx excavatus* as a protein resource in the philippines In: Earthworm *Ecology from Darwin to vermiculture* (Eds. J.E. Satchell.) Chapman & Hall, New York.

- Hand, P. (1989). Earthworm Biotechnology (Vermicomposting In: *Resources and Appication of Biotechnology* (Eds. R. Green Shields), Macmillan Press Ltd., London.

- Hand, P. and Hayes, W.A. (1983). The composting of slurries by earthworms In: *International conference on composting of solid waste and slurries,* pp. 246-260. Department of Civil Engineering, Leeds University.

- Hartenstein, R. (1978). Proc. Utilization of soil organisms in sludge management syracase, NY. 171 pp.

- Hartenstein, R (1981) Production of earthworm as a potentially economical source of protein. *Bioeng. Biotech.,* **23,** 1797-1811.

- Hartenstein, R.; Neuhauser, E.F. and Kaplan, D.L. (1979). A progress report on the potential use of earthworms in sludge management *In: Proc. 8th Nat. sludge conf. silver springs,* Md; pp. 238-241.

- Hartenstein, R.; Neuhauser, E.F. and Collier, J. (1980). Accumulation of heavy metals in the earthworm *Eisenia fetida J. Environ. Qual.,* **9,**23-26.

- Harvas, L.; Mazuelos, C.S.; Senesi, N. and Saiz-Jimenez, C. (1989). Chemical and physio-chemical characterization of vermicomposts and their humic acid fractions, *The science of the total Environment* 81/82,543-550.

- Harwood, M. (1976). Recovery of Protein from poultry waste by earthworms. *Proc. Ist Austr. Poult. Stockfeed conv. Melbourne,* pp. 138-143.

- Hatanaka; K; Ishioka, Y and Furuichi, E. (1983). Cultivation of *Eisenia fetida* using dairy waste sludge cake In: *Earthworm Ecology from Darwin to vermiculture* (Ed.Z.E. Satchell). Chapman and Hall, London.

- Hori, M.; Kondon, K.; Yoshida, T., Konishi, E and Minami, S(1974). Studies of antipyretic components in the Japanese earthworm. *Biochem Pharmaco.,* **23,** 1583-1590.

- Ismail., S.A. (1986). Earthworm Resources of Madras. In: *Proc. Natl. Sem. Org. Waste utiliz. vermicom.* Part B. *Verms and Vermicomposting* (M.C. Das, B.K. Sanapati and P.C. Mishra, eds), Five Star Printing Press, Burla, pp 8-15

- Ismail, S.A. (1997). *Vermicology: The Biology of Earthworms.* Orient Longman, Hyderabad, India.

- Jairajpuri, M.S. (1993). *Earthworm and Vermiculture: An Introduction, Earthworm Resources and Vermiculture:* 1-5, Zoological Survey of India, Calcutta.

- Julka, J.M (1993) Earthworm Resources of India and their utilization in vermiculture. *Earthworm Resources and Vermiculture:* 51-56. Zoological Survey of India, Calcutta.

- Julka, J.M. and Senapati, B.K. (1987). *Records of the Zoological Survey of India,* Miscellaneous Publication. Occasional paper no. 92, Grafic Printall, Calcutta.

- Kale, R.D. (1986) Earthworm feed for poultry and aquaculture In: *Proc. Nat. Semi. Org. Wate utiliz. vermicomp,* Part B. *Verms and Vermicomposting* 137-146 (M.C. Dash, B.K. Senapati and P.C. Mishra, eds), Sri Artatrana Rout for Five star printing press, Bula, Orissa.

- Kale, R.D. and Bano, K. (1986). Fields trails with vermicompost (Vee Comp. E. 83 UAS) an organic fertilizer: In *Proc. Nat. Sem. Org. waste utiliz. vercomp.* Part B *Verms and Vemicomposting* (M.C. Dash, B.K. Senapati and P.C Mishraeds) Five Star Printing Press, Bural, Orrisa.

- Kale, R.D. and Krishnamoorthy, (1981). What effects the abundance and diversity of earthworms in soils? *Proc. Indian Acad Sci.* (Annual Sci.) 90:117-211.

- Kaplan, D.L.; Hartenstein, R.; Neuhauser, E.F. and Maleckp, M.R. (1980). Physio-chemical requirements in the environment of the earthworms *Eisenia fetida. Soil Biol. Biochem,* **12**: 347-352.

- Lee, K.E. (1985). Earthworms: *Their Ecology and Relationships with the soils and Land use,* Academic Press, New York, 411P.

- Loehrol, R.C.; Neuhouser, E.F. and Malecki, K. (1985). Factors affecting the vermistablization process: Temperature, Moisture content and polyculture water research and technology 19, 1311-1317.

- McInroy, D.M. (1971). Evaluation of earthworm *Eisenia fetida* as a food for man and domestic animals feed stuffs fed, 20th, 37-46.

- Meadows, R; Andrews, B.; Johnston B. and Granam, J. (1990). The feedcot manual. NSW Department of Agriculture and fisheries, Sydney.

- Mitchell, A. (1997). Production of Eisenia fetida and vermicompost from feed lot cattle manure Soil Biol.Biochem. Vol. 29, No.3/4, pp. 763-766.

- Mitchell, M.J.; Mulligan, R.M. Hartenstein, R. and Neuhanser, E.F. (1977). Conversion of sludge into Topsoils by earthworms. *Compost Science* **18(4)**, 17-26.

- Mitchell, M.J.; Hornor, S.G. and Abrams, B.I. (1980). Decomposition of sewage sludge in drying beds and the potential role of the earthworm, *Eisenia fetida. J. Environ Qual.* **9**, 373-373.

- Muys, B. and Granval, P.H. (1997). Earthworms as bioindicator of forest site quality. *Soil Biol. Biochem.,* **29**: 763-766.

- Neuhauser, E.F.; Hartenstein R. and Kalpan, D.L. (1980). Growth of the earthworm *Eisenia fetida* in relation to population density and food rationing Oikos, 38, 93-98.

- Neuhanuser, E.F.; Malecki, M.R. and Leohr, R.C. (1984). Growth and reproduction of the earthworm *Eisenia fetida* after exposure to sublethal concentration of metal. *Pedobiologia* **27**, 89-97.

- Neuhauser, E.F.; Loehr, R.L. and Malecki, M.R. (1988). The potentioal of earthworms of managing sewage sludge In: *Earthworms in Waste and Environmental Management* (C.A. Edwards and E.F Neuhauser, Eds.), pp. 9-20, SPB Academic Publishing, The Hauge.

- Paolett; M.G.; Favretto, M.R.; Stinner, B.R.; Purrington, F.F. and Bater, J.E., (1991). Invertebrates as bioindicatrs of soil use. *Agriculture Ecosystems and Encvironment,* **34**, 341-362.

- Poonuraj, M.; Murugesan, A.G. and Sukumarna, N. (1998). Effect of different organic wastes on fecurity of two earthworms. *Lempito mauritii* (King berg ) and *Perionyxs excavatus,* (E. Ferrier) *J. Environ. Biol.* **19(1)**, 57-61.

- Prakash, J. (1996). The Appropriate Application at Farmers Lavel In: *Biovillage* (Apreport), 1996.

- Reincke, A.J. and Venter, J.M. (1987). Moisture preferences growth and reproduction of the compost worm *Eisenia fetida* (Oligochaeta). *Biology and Fertility of Soils.* 135-141.

- Reincke, A.J.; Viljoen, S.A. and Soayman, R.J. (1992). The suitability of *Endrilus eugeneae, Perionyse excavatus* and *Eisenia fetida* (Oligochaeta) for vermicomposting in S. Africa in terms of their temperature requirements. *Soil Biol. Biochem.* **12**: 1295-1307.

- Reincke, A.S. and Reincke, A.J. (1997). The influence of lead and maganese on spermatozoa of *Eisenia fetida* (Oligochaeta). *Soil Biol. Biochem* Vol. 29, No. 3/4. pp. 732.742.

- Rippon, J.E. and Wood, M.J. (1976). Microbiological aspects of pulverized fuel ash. p. 331-349. In: *The Ecology or Resource Degradation and Renewal.* M.J. Chadwick and G.J. Gooman eds John Wiley and Sons., New York.

- Rosseat, P. and Benjamin, M. (1993). Soil conservation, a key to the new model. In: *Two Stops Back one Step Forward: Cubas National wide Experiment with Organic Agriculture,* Global Exchange, California, pp. 38-50.

- Sabine, J.R. (1978). The nutritive value of earthworm mean. In *Utilization of Soil Organisms is Sludge Management* (ed. R. Hartenstein). State Univ. New York, Syracuse, pp. 122-130.

- Satchell, J.E. (1955). Some aspects of earthworm ecology. In *Soil Zoology* (D.K., McE Kevar, Ed.) pp. 356-364. Butter worths, London.

- Satchell, J.E,. (1967). Lumbricidae. In *Soil Biology* A Burges and F. Raw eds) Academic Press, London, 259-322.

- Satchell. J.E. (1983). *Earthworm Ecology from Darwin to Vermiculture.* (Ed, J.E Satchell) Chapman and Hall, London.

- Saxena, M.; Chauhan, A. and Asokan, P. (1998) Flyash Vermicompost from Non-ecofriendly organic wastes. *Poll.Res.* **17**(1): 5-11.

- Schulz. E. and Graff, O. (1977). Zur Bewertung von Regenwurmmene ous *Eisenia fetida* (Savigny 1826). als Eiweiss futtermittel *Land b Fersch volkenrode,* **27**, 216-218.

- Senapati, B.K. and Dash, M.C. (1984). Fundamental role of earthworms decompose sub-system. *Trop. Eco.* **25**:54-73.

- Singh, J. (1997). Habit at preferences of selected Indian earthworm species and their efficiency in reduction of organic materials. *Soil Biol. Biochem.* **29**: 585-588.

- Singh, J. and Rai. S.N. (1998). Potential of earthworms in sustainable agriculture. *Yojna,* (Nov.) pp. 10-12.

- Taboga, L. (1980). The nutritional value of earthworm for chickens. *Br. Poull. Sci.* **21**, 405-410.

- Therpe, I.S.; Killham, K; Prosser, J.I. and Glover, L.A. (1993) Novel method for the study of the population dynamics of a genetically modified micro organism in the gut of the earthworm *Lumbricus terrestris. Biol Fertil. Soils.* **15**:55-59.

- Tomlin, A.P. (1983). The earthworm bait market in North America. In: *Earthworm Ecology from Darwin to Vermiculture.* (Ed. J.E. Satchell). Chapman and Hall, London.

- Tripathi, G.; Rai, S.N. and Singh, J. (1995). Ecology and vermitechnology of some Indian Earthworms In: *Proc. Conf. sustain Agril. Environ.* pp. 92, Hissar, India.

- Tripathi, G. and Singh, J. (2000). Earthworm biodiversity and vermitechnology in industrial waste management. In: *Industry Evnironment and Pollution* (Eds. A. Kumar and P.K. Goel), *PP. 60-74, Technoscience,* India.

- Vincellas- Akpa; M. and Loquet, M. (1997). Organic matter transformation in Lignocelluosic waste products composted or vermicomposted (*Eisenia fetida anderi*): Chemical analysis and C13 CPMAS NMR Spectoscopy. *Soil Biol; Biochem.* **29**:751-758.

- Yosida, M. Hoshu, H. (1978). Nutritional value of earthworms for poultry feed. *Jpn. Sci.,* **15**, 308-311.